W0036817

OXFORD HANDBOOK OF

Infectious Diseases and Microbiology

Published and forthcoming Oxford Handbooks

OXFORD HANDBOOK OF
Infectious Diseases and Microbiology

THIRD EDITION

EDITED BY

Fiona Cooke

Consultant Medical Microbiologist, Addenbrookes
Hospital, Cambridge, UK

Ed Moran

Consultant in Infectious Disease, Southmead Hospital,
Bristol, UK

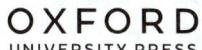
OXFORD
UNIVERSITY PRESS

OXFORD
UNIVERSITY PRESS

Great Clarendon Street, Oxford, OX2 6DP,
United Kingdom

Oxford University Press is a department of the University of Oxford.
It furthers the University's objective of excellence in research, scholarship,
and education by publishing worldwide. Oxford is a registered trade mark of
Oxford University Press in the UK and in certain other countries

© Oxford University Press 2025

The moral rights of the authors have been asserted

First Edition published in 2009
Second Edition published in 2017
Third Edition published in 2025

All rights reserved. No part of this publication may be reproduced, stored in
a retrieval system, or transmitted, in any form or by any means, without the
prior permission in writing of Oxford University Press, or as expressly permitted
by law, by licence or under terms agreed with the appropriate reprographics
rights organization. Enquiries concerning reproduction outside the scope of the
above should be sent to the Rights Department, Oxford University Press, at the
address above

You must not circulate this work in any other form
and you must impose this same condition on any acquirer

Published in the United States of America by Oxford University Press
198 Madison Avenue, New York, NY 10016, United States of America

British Library Cataloguing in Publication Data
Data available

Library of Congress Control Number: 2023946135

ISBN 978–0–19–289683–4

DOI: 10.1093/med/9780192896834.001.0001

Printed in Italy by
L.E.G.O. S.p.A. Lavis (TN)

Oxford University Press makes no representation, express or implied, that the
drug dosages in this book are correct. Readers must therefore always check
the product information and clinical procedures with the most up-to-date
published product information and data sheets provided by the manufacturers
and the most recent codes of conduct and safety regulations. The authors and
the publishers do not accept responsibility or legal liability for any errors in the
text or for the misuse or misapplication of material in this work. Except where
otherwise stated, drug dosages and recommendations are for the non-pregnant
adult who is not breast-feeding

Links to third party websites are provided by Oxford in good faith and
for information only. Oxford disclaims any responsibility for the materials
contained in any third party website referenced in this work.

MIX
Paper | Supporting
responsible forestry
FSC
www.fsc.org   FSC® C023419

Foreword

I like to ask medical students the following question: which part of the body is *not* susceptible to infection? After a moment's hesitation, I quickly add that it is a trick question as the answer, of course, is there is none. There are obvious corollaries: practitioners in almost every area of medicine can expect to encounter and manage infections; and there is a lot to know about them. This third edition of the *Oxford Handbook of Infectious Diseases and Microbiology* is an invaluable tool. It authoritatively and concisely addresses first, a core understanding of infectious agents and their treatments; and then, how to recognise, diagnose and manage a panoply of infectious syndromes and problems. A wealth of real-life experience and expertise has been skilfully curated and presented by the editors to meet the needs of busy students and practitioners. It amounts to a very informative and practical guide. To return to the beginning, doctors in almost every specialty, nurses, pharmacists, biomedical scientists and students in these professions will have much to gain from this *Handbook*—it will help them develop core knowledge and skills and deliver the best possible care to patients with infection.

Dr Sir Michael Jacobs
Keble College, University of Oxford
November 2024

Preface to the third edition

Hippocrates (it is alleged) asked us to 'Declare the past, diagnose the present, foretell the future', and rarely in medicine has the future many foretold become the diagnosable present so rapidly. In the years since the publication of the first edition of this book, the treatment of viral hepatitis has transformed to the extent that drugs have been introduced and withdrawn as obsolete, novel classes of antivirals and antibiotics are now mainstream, new infections have emerged and traversed the globe, and the coronavirus pandemic has revolutionized the speed at which research findings lead to licensed treatments.

Health systems have had to adapt to changing needs, increasing demand, and limited resources—and infection training has consequently evolved alongside. In the UK, the distinction between classic 'Infectious Diseases' and 'Microbiology' is ever harder to spot and the increasing number of dual-accredited consultants are developing their jobs to fit their training and expectations. This handbook has always supported the belief that infection training should reflect a bedside-to-bench-to-bedside philosophy, with practitioners able to deliver compassionate care holistically from initial presentation to laboratory diagnostics, and ultimately supervising and supporting patients with their treatment.

For this edition, we invited busy hospital clinicians working at the 'coalface' to come alongside us to update the text and add new topics. We are incredibly grateful for their invaluable contributions. While, as ever, no single book—or at least no single portable book—can tell you everything you need to know, we hope that this third edition of the *Oxford Handbook of Infectious Diseases and Microbiology* will continue to prompt, guide, and educate those caring for people with infections.

Ed Moran, Fiona Cooke

Contents

Contributors

Alison Burgess
Specialist Registrar in Infectious
Diseases and Microbiology, North
Bristol NHS Trust, Bristol, UK
*Chapter 14: Respiratory, head, and
neck infections;*
Chapter 15: Cardiovascular infections

Frances Edwards
Specialist Registrar in Infectious
Diseases and Medical Microbiology,
North Bristol NHS Trust, Bristol, UK
Chapter 1: Basics of antimicrobials;
Chapter 22: Bone and joint infections;
Chapter 23: Pregnancy and childhood;
*Chapter 24: Immunodeficiency and
HIV;*
Chapter 25: Health protection

Donall Forde
Consultant Virologist & Infectious
Disease Physician, Public Health
Wales, Cardiff, UK
Chapter 4: Antivirals;
Chapter 8: Viruses

Jasmin Islam
Infectious diseases & Microbiology
Consultant, Kings College Hospital,
London and UK Health Security
Agency, London, UK
Chapter 2: Antibiotics;
Chapter 3: Antifungals;
Chapter 9: Fungi

Megan Jenkins
Consultant in Infectious Disease,
North Bristol NHS Trust,
Bristol, UK
Chapter 13: Fever;
*Chapter 14: Respiratory, head, and
neck infections;*
Chapter 16: Gastrointestinal infections

Matthew Powell
Specialist registrar in Infectious
Diseases and Microbiology, Public
Health Wales, Cardiff, UK
Chapter 5: Antiparasitic therapy;
Chapter 7: Bacteria;
Chapter 10: Protozoa;
Chapter 11: Helminths;
Chapter 12: Ectoparasites

James R Price
Senior Lecturer and Honorary
Consultant in Infection, Brighton
and Sussex Medical School,
University of Sussex, Brighton, UK
Chapter 6: Infection control;
Chapter 7: Bacteria

Ameeka Thompson
Specialist Registrar in Infectious
Diseases and Microbiology, North
Bristol NHS Trust, Bristol, UK
Chapter 17: Urinary tract infections;
*Chapter 18: Sexually transmitted
infections;*
Chapter 19: Neurological infections;
*Chapter 20: Ophthalmological
infections;*
*Chapter 21: Skin and soft tissue
infections*

George Trafford
Consultant in Infectious Diseases
and Microbiology, Royal Devon
University Hospitals, Exeter, UK
Chapter 7: Bacteria

Shannon Bernard Healey
Academic Clinical Fellow
(Neurology), University College
London, London, UK
Chapter 25: Health protection

Abbreviations

23-PPV	23-valent pneumococcal polysaccharide vaccine	ATS	American Thoracic Society
3TC	lamivudine	ATU	area of technical uncertainty
A1AT	α1-antitrypsin deficiency	ATV	atazanavir
ABC	abacavir	AUC	area under the curve
ABG	arterial blood gas	AV	atrioventricular
ABPA	allergic bronchopulmonary aspergillosis	AWaRe	Access, Watch, Reserve
ABPI	ankle–brachial pressure index	BA	blood agar; bacillary angiomatosis
ACA	acrodermatitis chronica atrophicans	BAL	bronchoalveolar lavage
		B-ALL	B-cell acute lymphoblastic leukaemia
ACDP	Advisory Committee on Dangerous Pathogens	BASHH	British Association for Sexual Health and HIV
ADA	adenosine deaminase	BBV	blood-borne virus
ADEM	acute disseminated encephalomyelitis	BC	blood culture
ADH	antidiuretic hormone	BCG	bacille Calmette–Guérin
ADP	adenosine diphosphate	BCRP	breast cancer resistance protein
AFB	acid-fast bacilli	BCYE	buffered charcoal yeast extract (agar)
AFLP	amplified fragment length polymorphism	bd	twice daily
AHA	American Heart Association	BHIVA	British HIV Association
AHP	allied health professional	BIA	British Infection Association
AKI	acute kidney injury	BIC	bictegravir
ALP	alkaline phosphatase	BLNAR	β-lactamase-negative, ampicillin-resistant
ALT	alanine aminotransferase		
AMP	adenosine monophosphate	BMA	British Medical Association
AMR	antimicrobial resistance	BMI	body mass index
AMS	antimicrobial stewardship	BMT	bone marrow transplant/ation
ANA	antinuclear antibody	BNF	British National Formulary
ANCA	antineutrophil cytoplasmic antibody	bp	base pair
		BP	blood pressure; bacterial peliosis
ANTT	aseptic non-touch technique		
aP	acellular pertussis	bpm	beats per minute
APACHE	acute physiology and chronic health evaluation (score)	BSA	body surface area
		BSAC	British Society for Antimicrobial Chemotherapy
API®	Analytical Profile Index		
ARDS	acute respiratory distress syndrome	BSE	bovine spongiform encephalopathy
ARK	Antibiotic Review Kit (study)	BSI	bloodstream infection
ART	antiretroviral therapy	BTS	British Thoracic Society
ASOT	anti-streptococcal O titre	BV	bacterial vaginosis
AST	antimicrobial susceptibility testing; aspartate aminotransferase	CagA	cytotoxin-associated gene A
		cAMP	cyclic adenosine monophosphate
ATP	adenosine triphosphate		

CA-MRSA	community-acquired MRSA
CAN	colistin–nalidixic acid
CAP	community-acquired pneumonia
CAPD	continuous ambulatory peritoneal dialysis
cART	combination antiretroviral therapy
CAR-T	chimeric antigen receptor T-cell
CAUTI	catheter-associated urinary tract infection
CBD	common bile duct
cccDNA	covalently closed circular DNA
CCDA	charcoal–cefoperazone–deoxycholate agar
CCDC	Consultant in Communicable Disease Control
CCEY	cefoxitin cycloserine egg yolk
CCF	congestive cardiac failure
CCFA	cefoxitin cycloserine fructose agar
CCHF	Crimean–Congo haemorrhagic fever
CCP	cyclic citrullinated peptide
ccr	cassette chromosome recombinase
CCU	clean-catch urine
CDAD	Clostridioides difficile-associated disease/diarrhoea
CDC	Centers for Disease Control and Prevention
CDDEP	Center for Disease Dynamics, Economics & Policy
CDI	Clostridioides difficile infection
cDNA	complementary DNA
CF	cystic fibrosis
CFT	complement fixation test
CFTR	cystic fibrosis transmembrane conductance regulator
cfu	colony-forming unit
CGD	chronic granulomatous disease
CIN	Cefsulodin–Irgasan–Novobiocin (agar)
CJD	Creutzfeldt–Jakob disease
CK	creatine kinase

CKD	chronic kidney disease
Cl	chloride
CL	containment level
CLABSI	central line-associated bloodstream infection
CLED	cystine, lactose, electrolyte-deficient (agar)
CLSI	Clinical and Laboratory Standards Institute
cmH_2O	centimetre of water
CMI	cell-mediated immunity
CMO	Chief Medical Officer
CMV	cytomegalovirus
CNS	central nervous system
CO_2	carbon dioxide
COBI	cobicistat
CoNS	coagulase-negative staphylococci
CONSORT	Consolidated Standards of Reporting Trials
COPD	chronic obstructive pulmonary disease
COSHH	Control of Substances Hazardous to Health
CoV	coronavirus
Covid-19	coronavirus disease 2019
CPA	Clinical Pathology Accreditation
CPE	carbapenemase-producing Enterobacterales
CQC	Care Quality Commission
CRBSI	catheter-related bloodstream infection
CrCl	creatinine clearance
CRF	circulating recombinant form
CRP	C-reactive protein
CRTD	cardiac resynchronization therapy device
CSF	cerebrospinal fluid
CSU	catheter specimen of urine
CT	computed tomography
CVC	central venous catheter
CVID	common variable immunodeficiency
CXR	chest X-ray

CYP450	cytochrome P450	eGFR	estimated glomerular filtration rate
DAA	directly acting antiviral		
DAIR	debridement and implant retention	EIA	enzyme-linked immunoassay
		EIEC	enteroinvasive Escherichia coli
DAT	direct agglutination test	ELAM-1	endothelial leucocyte adhesion molecule 1
DCA	deoxycholate citrate		
DEC	diethylcarbamazine	EM	electron microscopy; erythema chronicum migrans
DEET	diethyltoluamide		
DFA	direct fluorescent antibody; direct immunofluorescence assay	EMG	electromyography
		ENT	ear, nose, and throat
		EO	ethylene oxide
DHF	dengue haemorrhagic fever	EPIC	European Prevalence of Infection in Intensive Care
DHFR	dihydrofolate reductase		
DHP-1	dehydropeptidase-1	EPP	exposure-prone procedure
DHPS	dihydropteroate synthase	EQA	external quality assessment
DHSC	Department of Health and Social Care	ERCP	endoscopic retrograde cholangiopancreatography
DIC	disseminated intravascular coagulopathy	erm	erythromycin ribosomal methylase
		ESBL	extended-spectrum β-lactamase
DIPC	Director of Infection Prevention and Control		
		ESC	European Society of Cardiology
DKA	diabetic ketoacidosis		
DMSA	dimercaptosuccinic acid	ESCKAPPM	Enterobacter spp., Serratia spp., Citrobacter freundii, Klebsiella aerogenes, Acinetobacter spp., Proteus vulgaris, Providencia spp., Morganella morganii
DNA	deoxyribonucleic acid		
DNAse	deoxyribonuclease		
DOR	doravirine		
DPD	dihydropyrimidine dehydrogenase		
		ESR	erythrocyte sedimentation rate
DRV	darunavir	ET	exfoliative toxin; (o) edema factor
ds	double-stranded (DNA)		
dsDNA	double-stranded DNA	ETEC	enterotoxigenic Escherichia coli
DTG	dolutegravir		
DTP	differential time to positivity; diphtheria, tetanus, polio (vaccine)	ETT	endotracheal tube
		ETV	etravirine
		EUCAST	European Committee on Antimicrobial Susceptibility Testing
DVT	deep vein thrombosis		
DWI	diffusion-weighted imaging	EVAR	endovascular aneurysm repair
E	ethambutol	EVD	external ventricular drain
EASL	European Association for the Study of the Liver	EVG	elvitegravir
		FAT	fluorescent antibody test
EBNA	Epstein–Barr nuclear antigen	FBC	full blood count
EBV	Epstein–Barr virus	FDA	Food and Drug Administration
ECDC	European Centre for Disease Prevention and Control	FDG	fluorodeoxyglucose
		FEV1	forced expiratory volume in 1s
ECG	electrocardiography	FHA	filamentous haemagglutinin
ECOFF	epidemiologic cut-off value		
eDNA	extracellular DNA	FLAIR	fluid-attenuated inversion recovery
EDTA	ethylenediaminetetraacetic acid		
		FMT	faecal microbiota transplant
EEG	electroencephalography		
EFV	efavirenz		

FTA-ABS	fluorescent treponemal antibody absorption		HBeAg	hepatitis B e antigen
FTC	emtricitabine		HBIG	hepatitis B immunoglobulin
g	gram		HBsAg	hepatitis B surface antigen
G6PD	glucose-6-phosphate dehydrogenase		HBV	hepatitis B virus
GAS	group A Streptococcus		HBZ	HTLV basic zipping factor
GBS	group B Streptococcus; Guillain–Barré syndrome		HCAI	healthcare-associated infection
			HCC	hepatocellular carcinoma
gCJD	genetic Creutzfeldt–Jakob disease		HCO3–	bicarbonate ion
			HcoV	human coronavirus
G-CSF	granulocyte colony-stimulating factor		HCV	hepatitis C virus
			HCW	healthcare worker
GDH	glutamate dehydrogenase		HDAg	hepatitis D antigen
GDP	guanosine diphosphate		HDV	hepatitis D (delta) virus
GFR	glomerular filtration rate		H&E	haematoxylin and eosin
GGT	gamma glutamyltransferase		HE	Hektoen enteric (agar)
GI	gastrointestinal		EPA	high-efficiency particulate air
GISA	glycopeptide-intermediate Staphylococcus aureus		HEV	hepatitis E virus
			HFM	hand, foot, and mouth
GMC	General Medical Council		Hfr	high-frequency recombination
GMP	good manufacturing practice		HFRS	haemorrhagic fever with renal syndrome
GNR	Gram-negative rod			
GORD	gastro-oesophageal reflux disease		HHV	human herpesvirus
			HHV-6	human herpesvirus 6
GP	general practice; general practitioner		HHV-7	human herpesvirus 7
			Hib	Haemophilus influenzae type b
GPA	granulomatosis with polyangiitis		HIDA	hepatobiliary iminodiacetic acid
GPC	Gram-positive cocci		HIV	human immunodeficiency virus
GPR	Gram-positive rod		HLA	human leucocyte antigen
GSS	Gerstmann–Sträussler–Scheinker		HLH	haemophagocytic lymphohistiocytosis
GU	genitourinary		HMPV	human metapneumovirus
GUM	genitourinary medicine		HNIG	human normal immunoglobulin
GVHD	graft-versus-host disease		H2O2	hydrogen peroxide
h	hour		HPA	Health Protection Agency
H	isoniazid		HPLC	high-pressure liquid chromatography
HA	haemagglutinin			
HACEK	Haemophilus, Aggregatibacter, Cardiobacterium, Eikenella, Kingella		HPS	hantavirus pulmonary syndrome
			HPU	health protection unit
HadV	human adenovirus		HPV	human papillomavirus; hydrogen peroxide vapour
HAI	hospital-acquired (associated) infection			
			HpyV	human polyomavirus
HA-MRSA	healthcare-acquired MRSA		HRP II	histidine-rich protein II
HAP	hospital-acquired pneumonia		H2S	hydrogen sulfide
HAV	hepatitis A virus		HSCT	haematopoietic stem cell transplantation
HbA1c	glycated haemoglobin			
HBcAg	hepatitis B core antigen		HSV	herpes simplex virus
HBcrAg	hepatitis B core-related antigen		HT	haemorrhagic toxin

HTLV-1	human T-cell lymphotropic virus 1	IPCN	infection prevention and control nurse
HTM	Health Technical Memorandum	IPCT	infection prevention and control team
HUS	haemolytic uraemic syndrome	IPV	inactivated polio vaccine
HVS	high vaginal swab	IQA	internal quality assurance
IAV	influenza A virus	IQC	internal quality control
IBD	inflammatory bowel disease	IRIS	immune reconstitution inflammatory syndrome
IBMS	Institute of Biomedical Science	IS	insertion sequence
IBV	influenza B virus	ISAGA	immunosorbent agglutination assay
ICAM-1	intercellular adhesion molecule 1	IU	international unit
ICC	infection control committee	IUCD	intrauterine contraceptive device
ICD	implantable cardiac defibrillator; intercostal drain/age	IUGR	intrauterine growth restriction
ICP	intracranial pressure	IV	intravenous/intravenously
ICED	implantable cardiac electronic device	IVC	inferior vena cava; intravascular catheter
iCJD	iatrogenic Creutzfeldt–Jakob disease	IVIG	intravenous immunoglobulin
ICTV	International Committee on Taxonomy of Viruses	K+	potassium
		K13	Kelch 13
ICU	intensive care unit	kb	kilobase
ID	infectious diseases; implanted device	kbp	kilobase pair
		KOH	potassium hydroxide
IDSA	Infectious Diseases Society of America	KPC	Klebsiella pneumoniae carbapenemase
IE	infective endocarditis	KS	Kaposi's sarcoma
IFAT	immunofluorescence antibody test	L	litre
		LAD	leucocyte adhesion deficiency
IFD	invasive fungal disease	LAMP	loop-mediated isothermal amplification
IFN	interferon		
IgA	immunoglobulin A	LCM	lymphocytic choriomeningitis
iGAS	invasive group A Streptococcus	LCMV	lymphocytic choriomeningitis virus
IgE	immunoglobulin E	LDH	lactate dehydrogenase
IgG	immunoglobulin G	LES	Liverpool epidemic strain
IgM	immunoglobulin M	LF	lethal factor
IGRA	interferon-γ release assay	LFT	liver function test
IL	interleukin	LGV	lymphogranuloma venereum
IM	intramuscular; infectious mononucleosis	LIPS	luciferase immunoprecipation system
INH	inhaled	LMIC	low- and middle-income country
INI	integrase inhibitor	LOS	lipo-oligosaccharide
INR	international normalized ratio	LP	lumbar puncture
INSTI	integrase strand transfer inhibitor	LPS	lipopolysaccharide
		LPV	lopinavir
IPC	infection prevention and control	LRTI	lower respiratory tract infection
		LT	lethal toxin

LTR	long terminal repeat
LVF	left ventricular failure
m	metre
MAC	Mycobacterium avium complex
MAI	Mycobacterium avium intracellulare
MALDI	matrix-assisted laser desorption/ionization
MALDI-TOF	matrix-assisted laser desorption/ionization time-of-flight mass spectroscopy
MALT	mucosa-associated lymphoid tissue
MASCC	Multinational Association for Supportive Care in Cancer
MAT	micro-agglutination test
MATS	Meningococcal Antigen Typing System
MBC	minimum bactericidal concentration
MBL	metallo-β-lactamase
MC&S	microscopy, culture, and sensitivity
MDR	multidrug-resistant
MDRD	Modification of Diet in Renal Disease
MDT	multidrug therapy; multidisciplinary team
MEC	minimum effective concentration
MERS	Middle East respiratory syndrome
MESS	MRSA Enhanced Surveillance
MeV	measles virus
Mf	microfilariae
Mg2+	magnesium
MGE	mobile genetic element
MGIT	Mycobacteria Growth Indicator Tube
MHC	major histocompatibility complex
MHRA	Medicines and Healthcare products Regulatory Agency
MIC	minimum inhibitory concentration
MIF	micro-immunofluorescent antibody
MIRU-VNTR	mycobacterial interspersed repetitive unit variable-number tandem repeats

MISC-C	multisystem inflammatory syndrome in children associated with Covid
mL	millilitre
MLSB	macrolides, lincosamides, and streptogramin type B
MLST	multiple locus sequence typing
MLVA	multiple locus variable-number tandem repeat analysis
Mm	millimetre
MMR	measles, mumps, and rubella (vaccine)
MOTT	mycobacteria other than tuberculosis
MR	magnetic resonance
MRCP	magnetic resonance cholangiopancreatography
MRI	magnetic resonance imaging
mRNA	messenger RNA
MRSA	meticillin-resistant Staphylococcus aureus
MRV	minority resistance variant
MSA	mannitol salt agar
MSCRAMM	microbial surface components recognizing adhesive matrix molecules
MSM	men who have sex with men
MSSA	meticillin-sensitive Staphylococcus aureus
MSU	midstream urine
MTB	Mycobacterium tuberculosis
MuV	mumps virus
MVC	maraviroc
NA	neuraminidase
NAAT	nucleic acid amplification test
NaCl	sodium chloride
NAD	nicotinamide adenine dinucleotide
NAD(P)	nicotinamide adenine dinucleotide (phosphate)
NADPH	nicotinamide adenine dinucleotide phosphate
NASH	non-alcoholic steatohepatitis
NCCR	non-coding control region
NEC	necrotizing enterocolitis
NEQAS	National External Quality Assessment Service for Microbiology
NEWS	National Early Warning Score
NG	nasogastric
NGS	next-generation sequencing

NGU	non-gonococcal urethritis		PABA	para-aminobenzoic acid
NH4+	ammonium ions		PAE	post-antibiotic effect
NHS	National Health Service		PAIR	puncture, aspiration, injection, and re-aspiration
NHSBT	NHS Blood and Transplant		PAN	polyarteritis nodosa
NICE	National Institute for Health and Care Excellence		PaO2	partial pressure of arterial oxygen
NICU	neonatal intensive care unit		PAS	para-aminosalicylic acid; periodic acid–Schiff
NINSS	Nosocomial Infection National Surveillance Scheme		PBMC	peripheral blood mononuclear cell
NK	natural killer		PBP	penicillin-binding protein
nm	nanometre		PCD	primary ciliary dyskinesia
NNRTI	non-nucleoside reverse transcriptase inhibitor		PCP	Pneumocystis pneumonia
NPA	nasopharyngeal aspirate		PCR	polymerase chain reaction
NPV	negative predictive value		PCV	pneumococcal conjugate vaccine
NRTI	nucleoside reverse transcriptase inhibitor		PD	pharmacodynamics; peritoneal dialysis
NS	non-structural protein		PE	pulmonary embolism
NSAID	non-steroidal anti-inflammatory drug		PEA	phenyl ethanol agar
NTCP	sodium taurocholate cotransporting polypeptide		Peg	polyethylene glycol
			PEG-IFN	pegylated interferon
NTD	neglected tropical disease		PEL	primary effusion lymphoma
NTM	non-tuberculous mycobacteria		PEP	post-exposure prophylaxis
NTS	non-typhoidal Salmonella species		PET	positron emission tomography; post-exposure treatment
NVE	native valve endocarditis			
NVP	nevirapine		PeV	parechovirus
NVS	nutritionally variant streptococci		PfEMP1	Plasmodium falciparum-infected erythrocyte membrane protein 1
NYC	New York City (agar)			
O2–	superoxide		PFGE	pulsed-field gel electrophoresis
OATP	organic anion transporting polypeptide		PFOR	pyruvate ferredoxin oxidoreductase
OCP	oral contraceptive pill, ova cysts parasites		P-gp	P-glycoprotein
			PHMB	polyhexamethylene biguanide
OCV	oral cholera vaccine		PI	protease inhibitor
od	once daily		PIA	polysaccharide intercellular adhesin
OHS	oral hydration salt			
OI	opportunistic infection		PICC	peripherally inserted central cannula
OMP	outer membrane protein			
ONPG	o-nitrophenyl-β-D-galactopyranoside		PICU	paediatric intensive care unit
			PID	pelvic inflammatory disease
OPAT	outpatient parenteral antimicrobial therapy		PIE	pulmonary infiltrates with eosinophilia
OPV	oral poliovirus vaccine			
ORION	Outbreak Reports and Intervention Studies of Nosocomial Infection		PIMS	paediatric inflammatory multisystem syndrome
			PIV	parainfluenza virus
ORS	oral rehydration salt		PJI	prosthetic joint infection
PA	protective antigen		PK	pharmacokinetics

PKDL	post-kala-azar dermal leishmaniasis
pLDH	plasmodial lactate dehydrogenase
PLWH	people living with HIV
PML	progressive multifocal leukoencephalopathy
PNP	purine nucleoside phosphorylase
PO	oral/orally
PPD	purified protein derivative
PPE	personal protective equipment
PPI	proton pump inhibitor
ppm	part per million
PPM	permanent pacemaker
PPROM	preterm premature rupture of the membranes
PPV	positive predictive value
PR	per rectum
PRCA	pure red cell aplasia
PrEP	pre-exposure prophylaxis
PROM	premature rupture of membranes
PrPC	cellular prion protein
PrPSc	scrapie prion protein
PSA	prostate-specific antigen
Psa	pneumococcal surface adhesin
PT	prothrombin time; pertussis toxin
PTC	percutaneous transhepatic cholangiography
PTLD	post-transplant lymphoproliferative disorder
PUO	pyrexia of unknown origin
PV	per vagina; poliovirus
PVC	peripheral venous catheter
PVE	prosthetic valve endocarditis
PVL	Panton–Valentine leucocidin
PVL-SA	Panton–Valentine leucocidin-associated Staphylococcus aureus
PWID	people who inject drugs
QAC	quaternary ammonium compound
qds	four times daily
qPCR	quantitative PCR
R	rifampicin
R0	basic reproduction number R nought
RAL	raltegravir
RAPD	random amplification of polymorphic DNA
RAS	resistance-associated substitution
RBC	red blood cell
RBD	receptor binding domain
rcDNA	relaxed circular DNA
RCT	randomized controlled trial
RDT	rapid diagnostic test
REA	restriction endonuclease analysis
rep-PCR	repetitive element polymerase chain reaction
RF	rheumatoid factor
RFLP	restriction fragment length polymorphism
RIDDOR	Reporting of Injuries, Diseases and Dangerous Occurrences Regulations
RIG	rabies immunoglobulin
RIPL	Rare and Imported Pathogens Laboratory
RMAT	rapid micro-agglutination test
RMSF	Rocky Mountain spotted fever
RNA	ribonucleic acid
RNP	ribonucleoprotein
ROM	rupture of membranes
RPR	rapid plasma reagin
RPV	rilpivirine
RR	rifampicin-resistant
rRNA	ribosomal RNA
RSV	respiratory syncytial virus
RT	reverse transcriptase
RTV	ritonavir
RUQ	right upper quadrant
RuV	rubella virus
RVF	Rift Valley fever
s	second
SaBTO	Advisory Committee on the Safety of Blood, Tissues, and Organs
SaO2	arterial oxygen saturation
SARS	severe acute respiratory syndrome
SARS-CoV-2	severe acute respiratory syndrome coronavirus 2
SBP	spontaneous bacterial peritonitis
s/c	subcutaneous
SCC	staphylococcal cassette chromosome

SCID	severe combined immunodeficiency disease		Stx	Shiga toxin
sCJD	sporadic Creutzfeldt–Jakob disease		SVR	sustained virological response
			SVT	supraventricular tachycardia
SDD	selective decontamination of the digestive tract		T3SS	type III secretion system
			TAC	transient aplastic crisis
SE	staphylococcal enterotoxin		TAF	tenofovir alafenamide
SENIC	Study on the Efficacy of Nosocomial Infection Control		TB	tuberculosis
			TBE	tick-borne encephalitis
SHOT	Serious Hazards of Transfusion		TBM	tuberculous meningitis
			TBW	total body weight
SIADH	syndrome of inappropriate antidiuretic hormone		TCBS	thiosulfate–citrate–bile salts–sucrose
SICP	standard infection control precautions		TCT	tracheal cytotoxin
			TDF	tenofovir disoproxil
siRNA	small interfering RNA		tds	three times daily
SIRS	systemic inflammatory respiratory syndrome		TFT	thyroid function test
			TK	thymidine kinase
SIV	simian immunodeficiency virus		TMA	transcription-mediated amplification
SLE	systemic lupus erythematosus			
slpAST	surface layer protein A gene sequence typing		TNF	tumour necrosis factor
			TOC	test of cure
SLST	single locus sequence typing		TOE	transoesophageal echocardiography
S-MAC	Sorbitol MacConkey			
SMIs	Standards for Microbiology Investigations		TOP	topical
			TORCH	Toxoplasma, other, rubella, cytomegalovirus, herpes simplex virus
SNP	single-nucleotide polymorphism			
SOFA	Sequential Organ Failure Assessment		TP	tube precipitin
			TPHA	Treponema pallidum haemagglutination assay
SOP	standard operating procedure			
SOT	solid organ transplant		TPN	total parenteral nutrition
SPA	suprapubic aspirate		TPPA	Treponema pallidum particle assay
SPE	streptococcal pyogenic exotoxin			
			TQM	total quality management
SPECT	single-photon emission computed tomography		tRNA	transfer RNA
			TSE	transmissible spongiform encephalopathy
SPI-1	Salmonella pathogenicity island 1			
			TSP	tropical spastic paraparesis
spp.	species		TSS	toxic shock syndrome
SPS	sodium polyanetholesulfonate		TSST	toxic shock syndrome toxin
SRSV	small round structured virus		TST	tuberculin skin test
ss	single-stranded		TTE	transthoracic echocardiography
SSA	streptococcal superantigen			
SSI	surgical site infection		TTP	thrombotic thrombocytopenic purpura
SSPE	subacute sclerosing panencephalitis			
			U	unit
SSRI	selective serotonin reuptake inhibitor		UBT	urea breath test
			UCV	ultraclean ventilation
SSSS	staphylococcal scalded skin syndrome		UKAP	UK Advisory Panel
STI	sexually transmitted infection			

UKAS	United Kingdom Accreditation Service
UKHSA	UK Health Security Agency
ULN	upper limit of normal
URTI	upper respiratory tract infection
USS	ultrasound scan
UTI	urinary tract infection
U&Es	urea and electrolytes
UV	ultraviolet
VA	ventriculo-atrial
VAP	ventilator-associated pneumonia
VAPP	vaccine-associated paralytic poliomyelitis
VATS	video-assisted thoracoscopic surgery
VCA	viral capsid antigen
VCAM-1	vascular cell adhesion molecule 1
vCJD	variant Creutzfeldt–Jakob disease
VDRL	Venereal Disease Research Laboratory
VHF	viral haemorrhagic fever
VIP	Visual Infusion Phlebitis
VISA	vancomycin-intermediate Staphylococcus aureus
VL	viral load
VNTR	variable-number tandem repeat
VOC	variant of concern
VOI	variant of interest
VP	ventriculoperitoneal
VRE	vancomycin-resistant Enterococcus
VRSA	vancomycin-resistant Staphylococcus aureus
VTEC	verocytotoxigenic
VUR	vesico-ureteric reflux
v/v	volume by volume
VVC	vulvovaginal candidiasis
VZIG	varicella-zoster immunoglobulin
VZV	varicella-zoster virus
WCC	white cell count
WGS	whole genome sequencing
WHO	World Health Organization
XDR	extensively drug-resistant
XLD	xylose–lysine–deoxycholate
Z	pyrazinamide
ZN	Ziehl–Neelsen

Part 1

Antimicrobials

Basics of antimicrobials

A history of antibiotics

Definitions

An 'antimicrobial' is an umbrella term for drugs with activity against microorganisms (e.g. antibacterials, antivirals, antifungals, antiparasitics—including both antiprotozoal and antihelminth agents). An 'antibiotic' is, strictly speaking, a chemical compound made by a microorganism that inhibits or kills other microorganisms at low concentrations. This does not include synthetic agents, although, in practice, the term is often used for any antibacterial.

A history

Substances with some form of anti-infective action have been used since ancient times; the Chinese used 'mouldy' soybean curd to treat boils and carbuncles, and the South American Indians chewed cinchona tree bark (which contains quinine) for malaria.

In Europe, one of the earliest recorded examples was the use of mercury to treat syphilis in the 1400s.

- In 1877, Louis Pasteur showed that injections of extracts of soil bacteria cured anthrax in animals.
- In 1908–10, Paul Erlich, Nobel Prize winner and father of chemotherapy, synthesized arsenic compounds effective against syphilis.
- In 1924, the compound actinomycetin, so named because it is produced by *Actinomycetes*, was discovered.
- In 1932, Domagk discovered the dye prontosil that cured streptococcal infections in animals. The active group turned out to be the sulfonamide attached to the dye, and by 1945, over 5000 sulfonamide derivatives had been developed. Adverse effects and drug resistance have limited clinical use of these compounds.
- In 1944–5, Waksman isolated streptomycin from the soil microbe *Streptomyces griseus*. It was active against *Mycobacterium tuberculosis* some Gram-negative organisms, Waksman was awarded the Nobel Prize.

History of penicillin

Alexander Fleming returned to St Mary's Hospital after a weekend away in 1928 to discover that the mould *Penicillium notatum* had contaminated his culture plates. He observed that the colonies of *Staphylococcus aureus* nearest to the mould had lysed, while those further away had not, and hypothesized that the *Penicillium* mould had released a product that caused bacterial cell lysis. He called this product penicillin. Although Fleming discovered penicillin, he was unable to purify sufficient quantities for clinical trials. In 1939, Howard Florey, Ernst Chain, and Norman Heatley, working in Oxford, obtained the *Penicillium* fungus from Fleming. They overcame the technical difficulties and conducted clinical trials to demonstrate the efficacy of penicillin. Mass production soon began in the United Kingdom (UK) and the United States. Initially, penicillin was used almost exclusively for soldiers injured during the Second World War. It became widely available by 1946. As soon as he discovered penicillin, Fleming warned of the development of penicillin resistance, and indeed resistance was seen almost immediately (See Table 1.1.).

Table 1.1 A non-exhaustive antibiotic timeline

Year	Antibiotic	Class of antibiotic
1928	Penicillin discovered	β-lactam
1932	Prontosil discovered	Sulfonamide
1942	Penicillin introduced	β-lactam
1943	Streptomycin discovered	Aminoglycoside
1947	Chloramphenicol discovered	Protein synthesis inhibitor
1947	Chlortetracycline discovered	Tetracycline
1952	Erythromycin discovered	Macrolide
1960	Flucloxacillin introduced	β-lactam
1961	Ampicillin introduced	β-lactam
1963	Gentamicin discovered	Aminoglycoside
1964	Cephalosporins introduced	β-lactam
1964	Vancomycin introduced	Glycopeptide
1971	Rifampicin introduced	Rifamycin
1974	Co-trimoxazole introduced	Sulfonamide and trimethoprim
1979	Ampicillin/clavulanate introduced	β-lactam/β-lactamase inhibitor
1987	Ciprofloxacin introduced	Quinolone
1995	Meropenem introduced	Carbapenem
2000	Linezolid introduced	Oxazolidinone
2003	Daptomycin introduced	Lipopeptide
2005	Tigecycline introduced	Glycylcycline
2010	Ceftaroline introduced	Anti-MRSA β-lactam
2012	Fidaxomicin introduced	Macrocyclic
2014/15	Ceftolozane/tazobactam and ceftazidime/avibactam introduced	β-lactam/β-lactamase inhibitor
2017	Dalbavancin introduced	Glycopeptide
2019	Delafloxacin introduced	Quinolone
2021	Imipenem/cilastatin/relebactam introduced	β-lactam/β-lactamase inhibitor/non-β-lactamase inhibitor

MRSA, meticillin-resistant *Staphylococcus aureus*.

Over the last century, natural penicillins have been chemically modified to produce semi-synthetic penicillins. Flucloxacillin has an isoxazoyl side chain, enabling it to resist penicillinase produced by *S. aureus* and to retain activity. Amoxicillin, also developed in the 1960s, has a positively charged amino group that enables uptake through the cell membrane of Gram-negative bacteria, expanding its spectrum of activity. In the late 1970s, piperacillin was developed, with the addition of a polar side chain, allowing even better penetration of Gram-negatives, including *Pseudomonas*. The rise in prevalence and increased distribution of the β-lactamase enzyme produced by bacteria have resulted in a greater importance of β-lactamase inhibitors such as clavulanic acid and tazobactam. More recently, non-β-lactam β-lactamase inhibitors, such as avibactam and vaborbactam, have become available to overcome extended-spectrum β-lactamases and carbapenemases.

The global picture

In 2015, the World Health Organization (WHO) declared that antimicrobial resistance (AMR) is a global health and development threat, citing AMR as one of the top 10 global public health threats facing humanity. The rise in antimicrobial-resistant pathogens not only threatens safe and effective healthcare, but also results in wider societal threats such as on food security. Strategies to target AMR have grown in prominence over the last decade, and antimicrobial stewardship (AMS) is high on both the health and political agenda. In the UK, the Department of Health and Social Care (DHSC) has published its 5-year action plan for AMR (2019–24) to support the UK 20-year vision for AMR in 2040. However, resistant pathogens are not limited by borders and success in the fight against AMR will only be achieved by a concerted global effort, encompassing human, animal, and environmental domains. Fortunately, the scale of the AMR threat, and the need to contain and control it, is widely acknowledged by governments, international agencies, researchers, and private companies alike. A selection of resources regarding AMR and the global response can be seen in Table 1.2, and AMS is discussed further in ➔ Chapter 6, p. 34.

Methods to tackle antimicrobial resistance

Resistance to antimicrobials develops when selective pressure is exerted on the microorganism from use of antibiotics and other agents (see ➔ Mechanisms of resistance, pp. 11–12). Antimicrobials are required to treat infection and can save lives. However, they are often taken when they have no benefit such as in viral infections or if there is no infection at all. In these instances, they will drive resistance while giving no benefit to the user. Reducing inappropriate antibiotic use is a key factor in tackling AMR and will be discussed in more detail below. However, many other factors, such as improved sanitation, good infection control measures, vaccination, widespread availability of diagnostic tests and diagnostic stewardship, appropriate use of antibiotics in agriculture and the environment, and reducing poverty, will all have an impact. The UK strategy focuses on three key ways of tackling AMR:

- reducing the need for, and unintentional exposure to, antimicrobials;
- optimizing the use of antimicrobials; and
- investing in innovation, supply, and access.

Table 1.2 Sources of information on antimicrobial resistance

Information	Web address
Department of Health and Social Care: UK 5-year action plan for antimicrobial resistance 2019 to 2024	℘ https://www.gov.uk/government/publications/uk-5-year-action-plan-for-antimicrobial-resistance-2019-to-2024
Public Health England: Antimicrobial Resistance: resource handbook	℘ https://www.gov.uk/government/publications/antimicrobial-resistance-resource-handbook
British Society for Antimicrobial Chemotherapy	℘ https://bsac.org.uk
Eurosurveillance (European data)	℘ https://www.eurosurveillance.org
National Antimicrobial Resistance Monitoring System for Enteric Bacteria (USA)	℘ https://www.cdc.gov/narms/
World Health Organization: Antimicrobial resistance	℘ https://www.who.int/health-topics/antimicrobial-resistance
Center for Disease Dynamics, Economics & Policy (CDDEP)	℘ https://resistancemap.cddep.org/AntibioticUse.php ℘ https://cddep.org/wp-content/uploads/2021/02/The-State-of-the-Worlds-Antibiotics-in-2021.pdf
ReAct: Action on Antibiotic resistance	℘ https://www.reactgroup.org/
Start smart then focus: antimicrobial stewardship toolkit for hospitals in England (updated March 2015)	℘ https://www.gov.uk/government/publications/antimicrobial-stewardship-start-smart-then-focus
TARGET antibiotics toolkit hub	℘ https://www.rcgp.org.uk/clinical-and-research/resources/toolkits/amr/target-antibiotics-toolkit.aspx

United Kingdom

The National Action Plan (NAP) outlines an overall target to reduce total UK antimicrobial use in humans by 15% by 2024, from the 2014 baseline. The majority of antibiotics prescribed in 2020 were within the general practice (GP) setting (73%), followed by hospital inpatients (13%), hospital outpatients (6%), dental practice (5%), and other community settings. However, prescribing in the GP setting has seen continuous year-on-year decreases, including in 2020 (reduction of 10% between 2016 and 2019 and a further 9% reduction between 2019 and 2020). In contrast, in hospital settings, antibiotic use, measured by using hospital admissions as the denominator, showed a 2% increase in prescribing between 2016 and 2019 and there was a 5% increase in total antibiotic prescribing between 2019 and 2020. This reflects the changes in hospital populations since the start of the coronavirus disease 2019 (Covid-19) pandemic; more acutely ill patients were admitted, whereas elective procedures were cancelled. National stewardship programmes, such as 'Start smart then focus' for secondary care and the TARGET toolkit (Treat Antibiotics Responsibly, Guidance, Education and Tools) for primary care, aim to reduce unnecessary prescribing.

Although total antibiotic consumption has reduced over time nationally, there remains unexplained variation in prescribing across the country. Higher prescribing tends to occur in more deprived communities and areas. Research which accounted for patient demographics (age, gender), chronic conditions, comorbidities, and smoking status found that disparate consumption rates prevail, with more deprived areas having the higher prescribing rates. Patient healthcare-seeking behaviours may, in part, explain these differences. However, there is a need to better understand why such variation persists. Infection with a resistant organism not only causes increased mortality and morbidity, but also results in longer hospital stays and increased healthcare costs.

Low- and middle-income countries

In low- and middle-income countries (LMICs), there was a 76% increase in antibiotic consumption rates between 2000 and 2018, with the highest rates in North Africa/the Middle East (111% increase) and South Asia (116%). Globally, there are large variations in the rates of total antibiotic consumption across countries and in the proportion of antibiotic classes in different geographical contexts. Reasons are multifactorial and include availability of antibiotics without prescriptions, difficulty accessing medical care, higher rates of 'fake' drugs, lack of clean water/sanitation, and inadequate infection prevention and control. Studies analysing antibiotic consumption on a global scale and evaluating time trends still remain scarce, reflecting the lack of surveillance data in LMICs.

Antimicrobial consumption in animals is nearly triple that of humans and is related to the global rise in demand for animal protein. Since 2000, meat production has reached a plateau in high-income countries but has grown by 64%, 53%, and 66% in Asia, Africa, and South America, respectively. The enormous increase in demand has rapidly increased the use of antimicrobials in the animal health sector where these drugs are used not only to treat and prevent infection, but also to promote rapid growth. The animals then excrete both the antibiotics and resistant organisms into the environment, so affecting the ecosystem around them. Other examples of non-human use include:

• tetracycline sprayed on apple plantations to treat fireblight;
• oxytetracycline added to water in commercial fish farms to treat infections;
• antibiotics used to eliminate bacterial growth inside oil pipelines.

Mechanisms of action

Antibiotics show 'selective toxicity' (i.e. they target parts of the bacterial cell that differ from human cells). These are the cell wall, cell membrane, bacterial ribosome, and bacterial DNA and folate synthesis pathways. For mechanisms of antibiotic action, see Fig. 1.1.

For definitions and examples of bactericidal and bacteriostatic antibiotics, see Table 1.3.

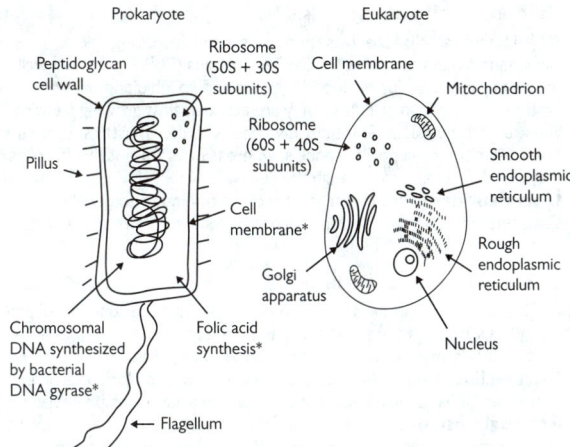

Fig. 1.1 Diagrams of prokaryotic and eukaryotic cells and their components that are targeted by antibiotics (indicated by an asterisk).

Table 1.3 Examples of bactericidal and bacteriostatic antibiotics

Bactericidal: killing all susceptible bacteria during the exponential phase of growth	Bacteriostatic: stopping bacteria from reproducing (i.e. keeping them in the stationary phase of growth, without necessarily killing them)
β-lactams	Macrolides/lincosamides
Aminoglycosides	Chloramphenicol
Glycopeptides	Linezolid
Quinolones	Trimethoprim
Trimethoprim–sulfonamide combination	Tetracyclines

Inhibition of cell wall synthesis

- All **β-lactam antibacterials** (penicillins, cephalosporins, and carbapenems) bind to penicillin-binding proteins (PBPs) in the cell wall, preventing cross-linking of peptidoglycans and so inhibiting cell wall synthesis, resulting in cell lysis. They are active against growing bacteria and are bactericidal. In Gram-negative bacteria, they must first cross the outer membrane via porin channels, whereas in Gram-positive bacteria, they can diffuse directly through the cell wall.
- **Glycopeptides** (vancomycin and teicoplanin) bind to the D-alanyl D-alanine side chain of the peptidoglycan precursor, again preventing cross-linking and so inhibiting cell wall synthesis.

Inhibition of protein synthesis

The 70S bacterial ribosome is made up of a 50S and a 30S subunit. All protein synthesis inhibitors are bacteriostatic, except aminoglycosides which have at least two mechanisms of action and are bactericidal.

- **Tetracyclines** bind to the 30S ribosomal subunit, and block attachment of transfer RNA (tRNA) and addition of amino acids to the protein chain.
- **Aminoglycosides** also bind to the 30S ribosomal subunit and prevent its attachment to messenger RNA (mRNA). They can also cause misreading of the mRNA, resulting in insertion of the wrong amino acid or interference in the ability of amino acids to connect with each other.
- **Macrolides** and **lincosamides** attach to the 50S ribosomal subunit, causing termination of the growing protein chain.
- **Chloramphenicol** also binds to the 50S ribosomal subunit and interferes with binding of amino acids to the growing chain.
- **Linezolid** (an oxazolidinone) binds to the 23S ribosomal RNA (rRNA) of the 50S subunit and prevents formation of a functional 70S initiation complex which is necessary for protein synthesis.

Inhibition of nucleic acid synthesis

- **Fluoroquinolones** interfere with DNA synthesis by blocking the enzyme DNA gyrase. This enzyme binds to DNA and introduces double-stranded breaks that allow the DNA complex to unwind. Fluoroquinolones bind to the DNA gyrase–DNA complex and allow broken DNA strands to be released into the cell, resulting in cell death.
- **Rifampicin** binds to DNA-dependent RNA polymerase, which blocks synthesis of RNA and results in cell death.

Inhibition of folate synthesis

For many organisms, para-aminobenzoic acid (PABA) is an essential metabolite which is involved in the synthesis of folic acid, an important precursor to the synthesis of nucleic acids.

- **Sulfonamides** are structural analogues of PABA and compete with PABA for the enzyme dihydropteroate synthetase.
- **Trimethoprim** acts on the folic acid synthesis pathway at a point after the sulfonamides, inhibiting the enzyme dihydrofolate reductase (see Fig. 1.2).
- **Co-trimoxazole**—both trimethoprim and sulfonamides are bacteriostatic. When they are used together (e.g. in **co-trimoxazole**), they produce a sequential blockade of the folic acid synthesis pathway. and have a synergistic effect.

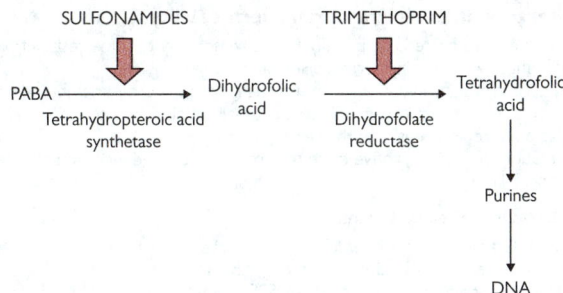

Fig. 1.2 Inhibition of folate synthesis.

Disruption of the cytoplasmic membrane

Polymyxin molecules bind to the lipopolysaccharides in the outer membrane of Gram-negative cells, causing reduced membrane integrity. The inner membrane also loses its stability due to the inclusion of hydrophilic molecules in fatty acid chains, resulting in leakage of cytoplasm and cell lysis.

Daptomycin conversely is only active against Gram-positive organisms. It binds directly to the cell membrane, causing ions to leak out of the cell. This results in cell depolarization, which rapidly leads to cell death.

Mechanisms of resistance

Bacteria can develop to avoid being killed by antibiotics; this is known as antibiotic resistance. It can be intrinsic (such as Gram-negative organisms resistant to vancomycin) or acquired. Examples of acquired resistance are discussed below.

Production of enzymes

B-lactamases are enzymes that hydrolyse β-lactam drugs. In Gram-negative bacteria, the β-lactam drug enters the cell through the porin channels and encounters β-lactamases in the periplasmic space. This results in hydrolysis of the β-lactam molecules, before they reach their PBP targets. In Gram-positive bacteria, β-lactamases are secreted extracellularly into the surrounding medium and destroy the β-lactam molecules before they enter the cell.

Aminoglycoside-modifying enzymes produced by Gram-negative bacteria may produce adenylating, phosphorylating, or acetylating enzymes that modify aminoglycosides, so that the latter are no longer active.

Chloramphenicol acetyltransferase, produced by Gram-negative bacteria, can modify chloramphenicol, so that the antibiotic is no longer active.

Alteration in outer membrane permeability

Gram-negative bacteria (especially *P. aeruginosa*) may become resistant to antibiotics by developing permeability barriers.

Mutations resulting in the loss of porin channels in the outer membrane no longer allow the entrance and passage of small antibiotic molecules, such as β-lactam or quinolones, into the cell.

Alterations in proton motive force may result in reduced inner membrane permeability.

Alteration of target sites

PBPs in Gram-positive and Gram-negative bacteria may be altered through mutations, so that β-lactams can no longer bind to them.

Even minor alteration of the 30S or 50S subunit can prevent binding and confer resistance. Methylation of rRNA confers resistance to macrolides, lincosamides, and streptogramins. Mutations in the chromosomal genes for DNA gyrase and topoisomerase IV confer quinolone resistance. The latter is a single base change, so resistance may develop rapidly (see below).

Efflux pumps

Transmembrane proteins form channels that actively export an antimicrobial agent out of the cell as fast as it enters. They are present in both Gram-positive and Gram-negative bacteria, and can be antibiotic-specific (e.g. to tetracyclines) or multidrug transporters (e.g. quinolones, macrolides, tetracyclines), so contributing to multidrug resistance.

Alteration of metabolic pathways

Some microorganisms develop an altered metabolic pathway that bypasses the reaction inhibited by the antimicrobial. Mutations that inactivate thymidylate synthetase block the conversion of deoxyuridylate to thymidylate. These mutants use exogenous thymine or thymidine for DNA synthesis and therefore are resistant to folate synthesis antagonists.

Molecular genetics of resistance

Bacteria replicate by binary fission, with one cell producing two identical daughter cells. This process is fast; for example, *Escherichia coli* has a doubling time of 20min, resulting in rapid expansions in bacterial populations. There is an associated error rate, and although some errors result in a survival disadvantage and the death of the mutant bacteria, some mutations result in a survival advantage. Additionally, to benefit microbial evolution, bacteria have evolved to transfer genetic material both within a population and across species.

Some definitions related to bacterial genetics are listed in Table 1.4.

Point mutations or single-nucleotide polymorphisms (SNPs)

Bacteria are constantly undergoing mutations, some of which will, by chance, result in a survival advantage (e.g. increased virulence or antibiotic resistance). In the presence of an antibiotic, resistant bacteria will be preferentially selected for. The mutation will be passed to future generations

Table 1.4 Definitions in bacterial genetics

Definition	Description	Example
Isolate	A population of bacteria in pure culture derived from a single clinical sample	*Escherichia coli* isolated from a specific patient's blood culture
Clone	A group of organisms that are so similar phenotypically and genotypically that the most likely explanation is that they arose from a common ancestor. Cannot be distinguished by multiple genetic tests	MRSA epidemic clones
Strain	Phenotypically and/or genotypically similar group of isolates (no agreement on minimal set of characteristics)	VRE strains
Type	Bacteria identified as having the same pattern or set of markers by using a defined system, allowing them to be classified	M-protein typing (emm) in group A *Streptococcus*
Species	A group below genus level whose members display a high degree of similarity (no accepted species definition for bacteria)	*Staphylococcus argenteus* is a novel staphylococcal species, also considered as a part of the *S. aureus* complex
Vertical gene transfer	Transfer of genetic material from a parent cell to its offspring	Point mutation in PBP Rearrangements in large sections of DNA
Horizontal gene transfer	Transfer of genetic material from one cell to another, that is not to its offspring	ESBL transfer via MGE
Heteroresistance	Growth of one bacterial subpopulation at a higher antibiotic concentration than predicted by the MIC for most cells. Difficult to diagnose and may result in poor response to treatment	*S. aureus* or *Enterococcus faecium* and vancomycin *Acinetobacter baumanii* and carbapenems and colistin *Streptococcus pneumoniae* and penicillin

ESBL, extended-spectrum β-lactamase; MGE, mobile genetic element; MIC, minimum inhibitory concentration; MRSA, meticillin-resistant *Staphylococcus aureus*; PBP, penicillin-binding protein; VRE, vancomycin-resistant *Enterococcus*.

(vertical transfer), and a resistant clone will emerge. This explains why new resistance patterns tend to emerge in areas of the hospital where antibiotic use is the highest (e.g. intensive care units). Examples of point mutations include β-lactamase and fluoroquinolone resistance.

Mobile genetic elements

These are pieces of DNA that can move between bacteria and result in the horizontal transfer of resistance genes. Bacterial genomes consist of core genes and accessory genes; it is the latter that are defined by acquisition and loss. There are several different MGEs described in the following list:

- **plasmids**—extrachromosomal circular DNA, which vary from 10kbp to over 400kbp (kilobase pairs) in size. Can carry resistance genes, virulence factors, and metabolic capabilities. They are autonomous self-replicating genetic elements that possess an origin for replication and genes that facilitate their maintenance in the host bacteria. Conjugative plasmids require additional genes to initiate self-transfer;
- **insertion sequences (IS)**—short DNA sequences, usually only 700–2500bp (base pairs) long. They encode an enzyme needed for transposition and a regulatory protein which either stimulates or inhibits the transposition activity. They are thus different from transposons, which also carry accessory genes such as antibiotic resistance genes. The coding region in an IS is usually flanked by inverted repeats;
- **transposons**—these are often called 'jumping genes' and may contain IS. They cannot replicate independently but can move between one replicating piece of DNA to another (e.g. from a chromosome to a plasmid). Conjugative transposons mediate their own transfer between bacteria, whereas non-conjugative transposons need prior integration into a plasmid to be transferred;
- **integrons**—these may be defined as a genetic element that possesses a site (*attI*) at which additional DNA in the form of gene cassettes can be integrated by site-specific mutation. They also encode nintegrase, which mediates these site-specific recombination events. Gene cassettes normally consist of an antibiotic resistance gene and a 59-base element that functions as a site-specific recombination site. The largest integrons (e.g. in *Vibrio cholerae*) can contain hundreds of gene cassettes;
- **bacteriophages**—a bacteriophage is a virus that infects bacteria and may become integrated into the bacterial chromosome (and is then called a prophage). They typically consist of an outer protein enclosing genetic material (which may be single- or double-stranded DNA or RNA). Bacteriophages may be considered MGEs but are rarely involved in the transfer of resistance genes. They have been used as an alternative to antibiotics (phage therapy) in Eastern Europe and the former USSR since the early twentieth century.

Transfer of mobile genetic elements
(See Table 1.5 and Fig. 1.3.)

Table 1.5 Transfer of mobile genetic elements

Conjugation	Plasmid transferred directly from one cell to the next via a conjugation pilus	R plasmid harbouring antibiotic resistance genes
Transduction	Transfer of DNA via a bacteriophage	*Corynebacterium diphtheriae* toxin phage
Transformation	Uptake of naked DNA from the environment	*Streptococcus pneumoniae* from smooth (capsulated) to rough colonies
Transposition	Excising a segment of DNA from one position in the chromosome and inserting it elsewhere	Multiple examples of chromosomal rearrangement exist

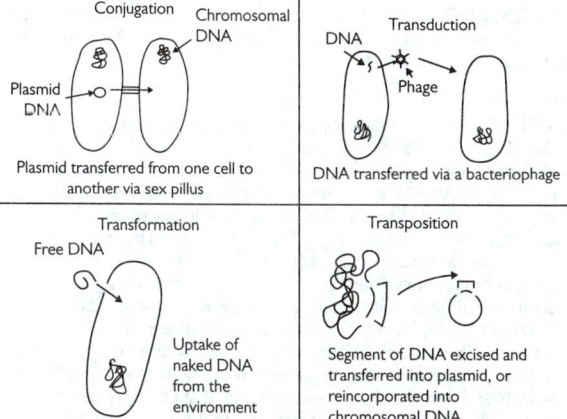

Fig. 1.3 Transfer of mobile genetic elements.

Susceptibility testing

It is important to standardize both the methods used in antimicrobial susceptibility testing (AST) and interpretive criteria, to allow for comparison
of results between different centres. Prior to 2016, the UK followed the
British Society for Antimicrobial Chemotherapy (BSAC) guidelines but now
follows the EUCAST (European Committee of Antimicrobial Susceptibility
Testing) protocols. Other reference bodies exist such as the Clinical and
Laboratory Standards Institute (CLSI) in the United States. Methods below
are described using the EUCAST protocols.

Minimum inhibitory concentration

The minimum inhibitory concentration (MIC) is the concentration of an
antimicrobial required to completely inhibit the growth of an organism
after a defined time period (usually overnight). Performing MIC testing on a
number of strains of a single species allows estimation of the concentration
that will inhibit 90% (MIC_{90}) or 50% (MIC_{50}) of that isolate *in vitro* and can
detect shifts in antibiotic susceptibility in bacterial populations.

Minimum bactericidal concentration

The minimum bactericidal concentration (MBC) is the concentration of an
antimicrobial required to kill a bacterium. It can be determined from broth
dilution tests by subculturing an overnight culture to agar containing no antibiotic. The MBC is considered the lowest concentration capable of reducing the original inoculum by a factor of 1000 (e.g. from 10^5 colony-forming
units (cfu)/mL to 10^2 or less).

Susceptibility testing techniques

See Table 1.6 for the advantages and disadvantages of each method.
- Disc diffusion—the bacterial colony is made into suspension of 0.5
  McFarland turbidity standard and inoculated evenly onto Mueller–
  Hinton agar. Antibiotic-impregnated discs are placed on the plate,
  which are incubated for 16–20h. The zone of inhibited growth around
  each disc is measured (see Fig. 1.4 and Box 1.1), and the zone size
  can be compared to clinical breakpoints for each organism/antibiotic
  combination. Note some organisms require alternative agars.
- Broth microdilution—a panel contains wells of antibiotic in broth.
  There is a 2-fold difference in antibiotic concentration in each well.
  A standardized volume of bacterial suspension is dropped into each
  well, and the panel is incubated. A cloudy appearance indicates bacterial
  growth, and thus the lowest concentration of antibiotic required to
  inhibit growth (the MIC) can be determined. An alternative method of
  agar microdilution is used for mecillinam and fosfomycin testing.
- Antimicrobial gradient method—a plastic strip containing a steadily
  decreasing concentration of a single antibiotic is placed on an agar plate
  inoculated with the test organism. Commercial versions include Etest.
  The MIC can be read from the strip at the point that bacterial growth is
  inhibited. This can be complicated—for example, whether to include or
  ignore microcolonies (see manufacturer's guidance).

Table 1.6 Advantages and disadvantages of different susceptibility testing techniques

	Advantages	Disadvantages
Disc diffusion	Simple to perform and interpret Cheap	Qualitative (resistant/intermediate/susceptible)
Dilutional method	Gold standard (good reproducibility) Quantitative (MIC)	Labour-intensive
Gradient	Quantitative (MIC) Easy to perform	MIC may not correlate with dilutional method Expensive if more than a few drugs are tested
Automated	Fast Standardized and reduce errors Can insert 'expert rules'	Machines can be very expensive to purchase and maintain
Mechanism-specific	Rapid and cheap—good for screening	
Genotypic	Rapid	Do not always correlate with phenotypic resistance Absence of genotypic resistance does not mean no other mechanism of resistance is present

MIC, minimum inhibitory concentration.

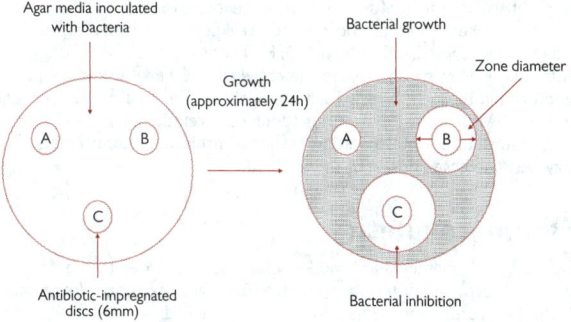

Fig. 1.4 Disc diffusion.

> ### Box 1.1 Key points about interpretation of zone size
>
> - It is important to measure the zone size for each 'bug drug' combination and check the cut-off with EUCAST guidelines.
> - Some antibiotics (e.g. vancomycin) can produce a small zone and be susceptible (vancomycin is a large molecule, so it diffuses a small distance).
> - Some antibiotics (e.g. ciprofloxacin) can produce large zones and be resistant.
> - Length of incubation, temperature, depth of agar, and concentration of the inoculum also affect the zone size.

- Automated systems—reagent cards containing differing quantities of antibiotics in a series of wells are inoculated with the test organism. Optical systems allow detection of subtle changes in bacterial growth. Some systems can run hundreds of tests simultaneously.
- Mechanism-specific tests—certain phenotypic tests may enable inference of the presence of a resistance mechanism (e.g. chromogenic systems for detection of meticillin-resistant *S. aureus* (MRSA) or cephalosporinase).
- Genotypic methods—using molecular methods such as polymerase chain reaction (PCR) or other techniques to detect resistance genes. Examples include *mecA* (MRSA) and *vanA* and *vanB* (vancomycin-resistant *Enterococcus* (VRE)).

Clinical breakpoints

Clinical breakpoints are set by a committee, such as EUCAST (⌛ https://www.eucast.org/clinical_breakpoints), to guide clinicians on therapy and predict treatment success. Comparing the measured MIC or disc diameter to the breakpoint will define whether an organism is classed as susceptible, intermediate, or resistant. The breakpoint will take into account *in vitro* potency, pharmacokinetics/dynamics, clinical experience, and infection site.

In cases where there are no defined breakpoints, clinicians can refer to the epidemiologic cut-off value (ECOFF). These are measures of drug MIC distribution, allowing one to see the range of MICs in a 'wild-type' population and in those with resistance mechanisms. The area of technical uncertainty (ATU) warns laboratories about interpretative difficulties for zone sizes. Reproducible interpretation cannot be achieved. Results in the ATU may need increased dosing of the antibiotic.

Pharmacokinetics

Expresses in a mathematical model 'what the body does to the drug'. It allows absorption, distribution, metabolism, and excretion (mnemonic ADME) of a drug over a time period to be quantified.

Absorption

To be effective, a drug must reach the site of the infection. In some cases, this is possible by topical (TOP) application (e.g. nystatin drops for oral candidiasis), but in most cases, drugs are absorbed in the gut and then transported around the body by the circulation.

Some drugs are poorly absorbed when given by mouth (e.g. aminoglycosides, glycopeptides) and are therefore given parenterally. The lack of absorption can be utilized, as the drug will then stay in the gut lumen, for example in the use of vancomycin or fidaxomicin for *Clostridioides difficile*.

If a drug is absorbed when given by mouth, the proportion that is absorbed into the systemic circulation is called the bioavailability. Drugs given intravenously (IV) have 100% bioavailability. The time profile of absorption versus elimination is usually more important than the total amount of drug absorbed (➔ see Pharmacodynamics (often referred to as PD), pp. 20–1).

Absorption may be affected by interactions with other drugs or food that may bind the drug (e.g. tetracyclines should not be given with milk). Altered physiology (e.g. diarrhoea) may reduce absorption. None of the commonly prescribed antibiotics are subject to significant first-pass metabolism in the liver.

Distribution

The volume of distribution is not a 'real volume'. It is a proportionality factor that relates the amount of drug in the body to the drug concentration in the blood. The larger the volume of distribution, the more likely that the drug is found in tissues of the body. The smaller the volume of distribution, the more likely that the drug is confined to the circulatory system.

Metabolism

The liver is the principal site of drug metabolism. Drug metabolism rates vary among patients. Some patients metabolize a drug so rapidly that therapeutically effective blood and tissue concentrations are not reached; in others, metabolism may be so slow that usual doses have toxic effects. Individual drug metabolism rates are influenced by genetic factors, coexisting disorders (particularly chronic liver disorders and advanced heart failure), and drug interactions (especially those involving induction or inhibition of metabolism). For many drugs, metabolism occurs in two phases. The most important enzyme system of phase I metabolism is cytochrome P450 (CYP450). CYP450 enzymes can be induced or inhibited by many antibiotics, resulting in drug interactions in which one drug enhances the toxicity or reduces the therapeutic effect of another drug. With ageing, the liver's capacity for metabolism through the CYP450 enzyme system is reduced by ≥30% because hepatic volume and blood flow are decreased. Thus, drugs that are metabolized through this system reach higher levels

---

Box 1.2 Antimicrobials metabolized by CYP3A4

- Inducers—rifampicin, some non-nucleoside reverse transcriptase inhibitors (NNRTIs)
- Inhibitors—macrolides, chloramphenicol, azole antifungals, protease inhibitors
- Substrates—macrolides, azole antifungals, ritonavir, saquinavir, indinavir, nelfinavir

and have prolonged half-lives in older people. Similarly, because neonates have partially developed hepatic microsomal enzyme systems, they also have difficulty metabolizing many drugs. Some antibiotics are metabolized in the liver by isoforms of CYP450, of which the CYP3A4 isoform is the most abundant (see Box 1.2). Rifampicin induces the activity of CYP3A4, leading to increased metabolism (and reduced efficacy) of drugs that share this pathway (e.g. human immunodeficiency virus (HIV) protease inhibitors). In contrast, azole antifungals and macrolides inhibit the activity of CYP3A4, which will reduce the metabolism (and may increase toxicity) of drugs also metabolized by this isoform. Always check for interactions before starting or stopping antibiotics, and seek expert advice if unsure.

Excretion

This can be divided into renal (water soluble substances, e.g. aminoglycosides, glycopeptides) and non-renal (biliary tree, e.g. ceftriaxone; gastrointestinal tract, e.g. azithromycin). Clearance determines the half-life of the drug (the time for the blood concentration to decrease by half). Steady state generally occurs when a patient has taken the drug for a period of time equal to 5–7 half-lives. Calculating the creatinine clearance (CrCl) (➔ see Antimicrobials in renal impairment, pp. 26–28) as a measure of renal function can be essential for safe dosing of some renally excreted drugs such as once-daily aminoglycosides (➔ see Aminoglycosides, pp. 52–4).

Pharmacodynamics

Is often described as 'what the drug does to the body' and describes the biochemical, molecular, and physiological effects of a drug on the body or microorganism. This involves receptor binding, post-receptor binding effects, and chemical interactions. PD explains the relationship between dose and response to a drug (i.e. the drug's effect). The pharmacological response depends on the drug binding to its target. The concentration of the drug at the receptor site influences the drug's effect.

Antibiotic dosing regimens have traditionally been determined by PK parameters only. However, PD plays an equal, if not more important, role. In this age of increasing AMR, PD becomes even more important because these parameters may be used to design dosing regimens which counteract or prevent resistance.

Effects on the body

These may be desirable (the therapeutic action of the agent) or undesirable (side effects, e.g. diarrhoea, neuropathy, ototoxicity). The balance between these effects is influenced by the therapeutic window—the difference between the dose that is effective (desired) and the dose that gives more adverse undesired effects than desired. Drugs with narrow windows may require therapeutic drug monitoring (e.g. gentamicin).

Synergism

This occurs when the activity of two drugs together is greater than the sum of their actions if each were given separately. An example is the use of ampicillin and gentamicin for enterococcal infections (➔ see Enterococci, pp. 275–7) where ampicillin acts on the cell wall to enable gentamicin to gain entry into the cell and act on the ribosome.

Antagonism

One drug diminishes the activity of another drug, so giving both antibiotics together may result in a worse clinical outcome than just giving one antibiotic. For example, co-administration of a bacteriostatic agent (e.g. tetracycline) with a β-lactam may inhibit cell growth and prevent the bactericidal activity of the β-lactam.

A pharmacokinetic/pharmacodynamic response to antibiotic therapy

The primary measure of antibiotic activity is the MIC. The MIC is the lowest concentration of an antibiotic that completely inhibits the growth of a microorganism *in vitro*. While the MIC is a good indicator of the potency of an antibiotic, it indicates nothing about the time course of antimicrobial activity.

PK parameters quantify the serum level time course of an antibiotic. The three PK parameters that are most important for evaluating antibiotic efficacy are the peak serum level (Cmax), the trough level (Cmin), and the area under the serum concentration time curve (AUC). However, while these parameters quantify the serum level time course, they do not describe the killing activity of an antibiotic.

Integrating the PK parameters with the MIC gives us three PK/PD parameters which quantify the activity of an antibiotic (see Table 1.7):
- peak/MIC ratio—Cmax divided by MIC;
- time above MIC (T > MIC)—percentage of dosage serum level > MIC;
- 24h AUC/MIC ratio.

There are three PD properties of antibiotics that best describe the killing activity. These are:
- time-dependent killing—the rate of killing is determined by the length of time above the MIC; important when adjusting doses of glycopeptides;
- concentration-dependent killing—the effect of increasing concentrations results in increased killing (e.g. once-daily dosing of aminoglycosides);
- post-antibiotic effect—persistent suppression of bacterial growth following antibiotic exposure.

Eagle effect

This is a paradoxical effect, first described by Eagle in 1948, whereby there is reduced killing activity at antibiotic concentrations above the MIC or MBC. It has been extensively reported in Gram-positive and Gram-negative bacteria, mycobacteria, and fungi, with a diverse range of antibiotics from

Table 1.7 Pattern of antibiotic activity and pharmacokinetics/pharmacodynamics

Pattern of activity	Antibiotics	Goal of therapy	PK/PD parameter
Type I Concentration-dependent killing and prolonged persistent effects	Aminoglycosides Daptomycin Fluoroquinolones Ketolides	To maximize concentrations	Peak/ MIC
Type II Time-dependent killing and minimal persistent effects	Carbapenems Cephalosporins Erythromycin Linezolid Penicillins	To maximize duration of exposure	T > MIC
Type III Time-dependent killing and moderate to prolonged persistent effects	Azithromycin Clindamycin Oxazolidinones Tetracyclines Vancomycin	To maximize amount of drug	24h AUC/ MIC

AUC, area under the curve; MIC, minimum inhibitory concentration; PD, pharmacodynamic; PK, pharmacokinetic; T, time.

different classes. The Eagle effect resembles some elements of bacterial persistence and tolerance, yet has a number of distinguishing attributes, most notably an increased number of surviving bacteria at supra-MIC antibiotic concentrations. This phenomenon demonstrates that microorganisms have multiple means to evade antimicrobials.

Preventing the development of resistance

Studies are focusing on defining the breakpoints that predict the emergence of resistance. An ideal antibiotic should have a low rate of resistance mutation, a high-fitness cost of resistance, and a low rate of fitness-restoring complementary mutation. Novel parameters that are being investigated include:
- mutant prevention concentration—the ability to restrict the selection of resistant mutants;
- mutant selection window—the concentration range between the minimal concentration required to block the growth of wild-type bacteria, up to the concentration needed to inhibit growth of the least susceptible single-step mutant. There are different concentration ranges for each organism/drug combination.

Routes of administration

(See Box 1.3.)

Oral administration

Most antibiotics used in human medicine are given orally (PO) in the community. If a drug is absorbed when given by mouth, the proportion that is absorbed into the systemic circulation is called the bioavailability (➔ see Pharmacokinetics (often referred to as PK), pp. 18–20). This depends on the formulation of the drug and how it is taken; for example, some tetracyclines should not be taken with milk or antacids, as these decrease antibiotic absorption. Antibiotics with high bioavailability include quinolones, metronidazole, and clindamycin. Antibiotics with low bioavailability include many β-lactams.

Intravenous administration

Indications for intravenous therapy

- Life-threatening infections (e.g. meningitis, bacteraemia, endocarditis). In these instances, high concentrations, reliable dosing, and penetration to the source of infection are reasons to give drugs IV.
- Inability to take/absorb PO medications (e.g. nil by mouth, severe vomiting or diarrhoea, oesophageal or intestinal obstruction, post-operative ileus).
- Poor oral bioavailability—some drugs are not absorbed if given PO (e.g. aminoglycosides, glycopeptides, colistimethate sodium).

Disadvantages

- Side effects, which may be local (e.g. phlebitis) or systemic (e.g. rapid infusion may result in anaphylactoid reactions such as the 'red man syndrome' with vancomycin).
- Line infections, which may be local (e.g. exit site, tunnel, or pocket infections) or systemic (e.g. bacteraemia, endocarditis).
- Inconvenience to the patient.
- Need to stay in hospital. This may be overcome by outpatient parenteral antimicrobial therapy (OPAT).
- Usually more expensive than PO formulation.

Box 1.3 Practical points

- Many people believe that IV antibiotics are somehow 'stronger' than PO antibiotics. This is **not** necessarily the case; for example, ciprofloxacin is as effective when given PO as when given IV and is much cheaper.
- The PO and IV doses of the same antibiotic may be different (e.g. metronidazole).
- The volume of fluid associated with IV medications can be significant.
- Continuous infusions are sometimes used in critically ill patients.
- With the introduction of intermediate susceptibility (EUCAST guidelines), more frequent or higher doses may be recommended (e.g. ciprofloxacin and piperacillin–tazobactam).

Intravenous to oral switch

Due to problems associated with IV therapy, 'IV to PO switch' protocols encourage clinicians to change to PO antibiotics as soon as it is safe. Some conditions are specifically excluded (e.g. endocarditis, meningitis). Consult with an infection specialist if unsure.

Criteria include:
- availability of a suitable PO agent;
- the patient can tolerate, swallow, and absorb PO antibiotics;
- no symptoms or signs of ongoing sepsis.

Intramuscular administration

This is an infrequent method of administration, largely because absorption is unpredictable and the injection may be painful. Local side effects include irritation and development of a sterile abscess. The advantages are that there is no question of compliance and the agent can be administered easily in the community. Intramuscular (IM) administration is commonly used in genitourinary (GU) clinics, and for tuberculosis (TB) treatment in the developing world.

Never give IM injections to patients with bleeding/clotting disorders (e.g. thrombocytopenia, haemophilia).

Examples of drugs given intramuscularly
- Benzylpenicillin for meningitis if IV access delayed (e.g. in the community).
- Procaine benzylpenicillin to treat syphilis.
- Ceftriaxone for gonococcal infection.

Topical administration

Many antimicrobials are available as TOP preparations. They are most commonly used in general practice and dermatology. However, they are not without risk and should be used with caution. Before prescribing a TOP antimicrobial, consider the following.
- Does the condition require treatment? Not all skin conditions that are oozing, crusted, or pustular are infected. Would improving hygiene resolve the situation? Even if an organism is cultured from a swab, it may represent colonization and not require treatment.
- Would systemic antibiotics be more appropriate? Some skin infections (e.g. erysipelas, cellulitis) require systemic antibiotics, as the infection is too deep for TOP antibiotics to penetrate adequately.
- Development of resistance—TOP antibacterials should be limited to those not used systemically, in order to prevent the development of resistance.
- Duration of treatment—TOP agents should only be used for short periods in defined infections.

Examples of drugs given topically

Fusidic acid may be used to treat impetigo, although PO therapy is often required. Mupirocin may also be used to treat impetigo (if MRSA-positive) or given as part of MRSA decolonization regimens. Chloramphenicol may be given as eye drops or ear drops for conjunctivitis or otitis externa, respectively. Aciclovir cream may be used for treatment of oral and genital herpes simplex infections. Nystatin drops can be used for oral candidiasis.

Clotrimazole cream is used for vulvovaginal candidiasis or athlete's foot. Permethrin and malathion are used for scabies. Malathion, pyrethroids, or dimeticone may be used for head lice.

Aerosolized administration

Aerosolized antibiotics are usually given for treatment or prophylaxis of respiratory infections. They are administered directly to the site of action and may have fewer systemic adverse effects. However, they are usually more difficult to give, and there may still be some systemic absorption. One of the main groups to benefit from aerosolized antibiotics are cystic fibrosis (CF) patients who may acquire multiresistant organisms (➔ see Cystic fibrosis, pp. 663–5).

Examples of antimicrobials given by inhalation

- Tobramycin (➔ see Aminoglycosides, pp. 52–4)—an aminoglycoside used in *Pseudomonas aeruginosa* infection in CF patients. Resistance can develop.
- Colistimethate sodium (➔ see Polymyxins, pp. 73–4)—a polymyxin antibiotic active against many Gram-negative organisms, including *P. aeruginosa* and *Acinetobacter* spp. Used as an adjunct to other treatment in CF patients.
- Pentamidine isetionate (➔ see Antiprotozoal drugs, pp. 128–33)—used as a second-line agent for the treatment or prophylaxis of pneumocystis pneumonia (PCP) (➔ see *Pneumocystis jirovecii*, pp. 522–4). Side effects include hypotension following administration, and severe, sometimes fatal, reactions due to hypotension, hypoglycaemia, pancreatitis, and arrhythmias.
- Ribavirin (➔ see Antivirals for respiratory syncytial virus, p. 100) is licensed for the treatment of severe respiratory syncytial virus (RSV) bronchiolitis in infants and children, especially if they have other serious diseases. There is no evidence of mortality benefit. Side effects include worsening respiration, bacterial pneumonia, and pneumothorax.

> CAUTION: ribavirin is teratogenic, and exposure should be avoided in pregnant and breastfeeding women.

Outpatient parenteral antimicrobial therapy

OPAT services are useful in allowing patients who require IV antibiotics (for the reasons listed in ➔ Routes of administration, pp. 23–5) but are otherwise well enough to remain at home. Benefits include reduced healthcare costs, shorter admissions, and lower rates of healthcare infections.

Various resources have been produced, including the Infectious Diseases Society of America (IDSA)-sponsored *Handbook of Outpatient Parenteral Antimicrobial Therapy (OPAT) for Infectious Diseases* (third edition available online) and the BSAC-supported OPAT strategy for the UK. Good practice recommendations for a successful OPAT service are outlined below.

OPAT team

The team should have a clear lead clinician and formal processes for referral and patient review. Studies show that having an infection specialist and/or an infection specialist pharmacist adds value in both adhering to monitoring and optimizing treatment, and importantly in considering the principles of antibiotic stewardship. Specialist nurses with experience in intravascular devices are also required.

Patient selection

Suitability criteria for inclusion should be well defined, and patients assessed before acceptance. It must include infection-related criteria (such as severity of infection), as well as other factors which may influence treatment success (e.g. comorbidities, lifestyle factors).

Antimicrobial management and drug delivery

The first dose of a new antibiotic should be given in a hospital or another supervised setting. Antibiotics can be given through a peripheral cannula, but often a longer-lasting line (e.g. peripherally inserted central cannula (PICC)) is used. Often antibiotics will be selected that can be given once a day to allow for ease of administration in the community. More recently, elastomeric devices which allow continuous infusions of drugs are being used for selected antibiotics. Some services require patients to visit a central hub each day, whereas some have staff visiting patients' homes.

Monitoring of the patient

Careful patient monitoring is important, as it has been shown that up to 25% of patients will develop complications while on OPAT. Regular clinical review, review of drug interactions and monitoring, and laboratory tests including full blood count and renal function are recommended.

Outcome monitoring

Prospective data should be collected for the purposes of audit and clinical governance. This should include demographics, agents used, and any complications (e.g. line infection, drug reaction, readmission).

Antimicrobials in renal impairment

The use of drugs in patients with renal impairment can cause several problems:
- reduced excretion of a drug or its metabolites may cause toxicity;
- nephrotoxic drugs may cause further kidney damage;
- increased sensitivity to some drugs;
- side effects may be poorly tolerated in patients with renal impairment;
- some drugs are not effective when renal function is impaired;
- administration of fluid or excess sodium (e.g. with use of piperacillin–tazobactam) must be considered.

Assessment of renal function

Renal function can be assessed in a number of ways.

- Serum creatinine concentration is the most commonly measured parameter. It is affected by muscle mass; lower muscle mass results in lower creatinine concentration. Renal impairment may therefore be underestimated in elderly patients or overestimated in certain races (e.g. black people). Serum creatinine concentration does not rise until 60% of total renal function is lost.
- Direct measure of the glomerular filtration rate (GFR) can be done by measuring plasma or urinary clearance of a substrate. This is difficult to do and rarely done in clinical practice.
- There are a number of formulae for calculating the estimated glomerular filtration rate (eGFR); the most commonly used is the CKD-EPI (Chronic Kidney Disease Epidemiology Collaboration). Variables include body surface area (BSA), serum creatinine concentration, age, sex, and race (see Box 1.4).
- An alternative is the MDRD (Modification of Diet in Renal Disease) formula, although this is less accurate when the eGFR is >60 and in elderly patients.
- CrCl is used in patients at extremes of muscle mass or in the elderly. It is calculated using the Cockcroft and Gault formula (see Box 1.5), which is based on age, weight, sex, and serum creatinine concentration. These are commonly available as online calculators.

Dose modification in renal impairment

- At what level of renal impairment a drug dose must be reduced depends on the proportion of drug eliminated by the kidneys and its toxicity. For drugs with minor or no dose related side effects, a simple scheme for dose reduction is sufficient. For more toxic drugs with a small safety margin, dose regimens based on the GFR are used.
- When both efficacy and toxicity are closely related to the plasma drug concentration, recommended regimens should be regarded only as a guide to initial treatment; subsequent doses must be adjusted according to clinical response and plasma drug concentration (e.g. vancomycin, gentamicin).

Box 1.4 CKD-EPI

$$eGFR = 142 \times \min(\text{standardized Scr/K}, 1)^a \times \max(\text{standardized Scr/K}, 1)^{-1.200}$$

$$\times 0.9938^{Age} \times 1.012 \text{ [if female]}$$

Abbreviations / Units
- eGFR (estimated glomerular filtration rate) = mL/min/1.73 m2
- Scr (serum creatinine) = mg/dL
- K = 0.7 (females) or 0.9 (males)
- $\alpha = -0.241$ (females) or -0.302 (males)
- min= indicates the minimum of Scr/K or 1
- max= indicates the maximum of Scr/K or 1

Box 1.5 Cockcroft and Gault formula

$$CrCl = \left[(140 - age) \times lean\ body\ weight\ \times N\right] / serum\ creatinine$$

Where:
- CrCl is creatinine clearance in mL/min;
- age is in years;
- body weight is in kilograms;
- $N = 1.23$ for men; 1.04 for women;
- serum creatinine concentration is in μmol/L.

- The total daily maintenance dose of a drug can be reduced either by reducing the size of the individual doses or by increasing the interval between doses.
- For some drugs, although the size of the maintenance dose is reduced, it is important to give a loading dose if an immediate effect is required. The loading dose should usually be of the same size as the initial dose for a patient with normal renal function.
- Seek specialist advice from your hospital pharmacist for patients on haemodialysis, haemofiltration, or chronic ambulatory peritoneal dialysis.

Drugs to be used with caution in renal impairment

- For up-to-date guidance, always consult your hospital pharmacist, the *British National Formulary (BNF)*, or the *Electronic Medicines Compendium* (available at: ✋ https://www.medicines.org.uk/emc/).
- Particular antibiotics to use with caution include:
  - aminoglycosides (high chance of toxicity);
  - tetracycline (can exacerbate renal failure);
  - nitrofurantoin (ineffective as not secreted into the collecting system and high chance of side effects);
  - co-trimoxazole (can elevate creatinine concentration without changing the eGFR);
  - β-lactams (dose adjustment frequently required).

Antimicrobials in liver disease

Metabolism by the liver is the main route of elimination for many drugs, but hepatic reserve is large and liver disease has to be severe before important changes in drug metabolism occur. Routine liver function testing is a poor guide to metabolic capacity, and it is not possible to predict the extent to which the metabolism of a particular drug may be impaired in an individual patient. Drug prescribing should be kept to a minimum in all patients with severe liver disease, especially if there is evidence of decompensation (jaundice, ascites, encephalopathy).

Effect of liver disease on response to drugs

Liver disease may alter the response to drugs in several ways:

- impaired drug metabolism may lead to increased toxicity (e.g. rifampicin and fusidic acid);
- hypoproteinaemia results in reduced protein binding and increased toxicity of highly protein-bound drugs (e.g. phenytoin);
- reduced synthesis of clotting factors increases the sensitivity to PO anticoagulants;
- hepatic encephalopathy may be precipitated by certain drugs (e.g. sedative drugs, opioids, diuretics, drugs that cause constipation);
- fluid overload (ascites, oedema) may be exacerbated by drugs that give rise to fluid retention (e.g. non-steroidals, corticosteroids);
- hepatotoxicity is either dose-related or unpredictable (idiosyncratic), and is more common in patients with liver disease.

Drugs to be used with caution

- For up-to-date guidance, always consult your hospital pharmacist or the *BNF*.
- Drugs to be used with particular caution and that may require dose adjustments include tetracyclines, fusidic acid, metronidazole, chloramphenicol, rifampicin, isoniazid, and pyrazinamide.

Antimicrobials in pregnancy

Many antibiotic agents have very limited data available on their use in pregnancy. The prescriber must balance the risk between undertreating an infection in the mother and the risk of damage to the fetus from the drug. Up-to-date advice should be sought from a current formulary (e.g. the *BNF*) or online resources such as BUMPS (Best Use of Medicines in Pregnancy). (See Table 1.8.)

Table 1.8 Specific agents

	First trimester	Second/third trimesters	Breastfeeding
Penicillins	++	++	++
Co-amoxiclav	++	/ Possible association with NEC in neonates	++
Cephalosporins	++	++	/ Manufacturers recommend avoiding ceftaroline and cefixime
Trimethoprim/ co-trimoxazole	! Folate antagonist, so risk of teratogenicity	++ Can cause neonatal haemolysis and methaemoglobinaemia	++ Small risk of kernicterus or haemolysis

(Continued)

Table 1.8 (*Contd.*)

	First trimester	Second/third trimesters	Breastfeeding
Nitrofurantoin	++	/ Can cause haemolysis. Avoid if delivery is imminent	++
Erythromycin	++ Considered to be safe		++
Other macrolides (eg azithromycin)	/ Less evidence with use—avoid unless no alternative	++	++
Clindamycin	++	++	++ Rarely causes infant diarrhoea or colitis
Quinolones	/ Use with particular caution	/ Risk of fetal/neonatal cartilage abnormalities in animal studies. Risk/benefit decision	
Tetracyclines	! Affect skeletal development and deposit in bones and teeth	/ Maternal hepatotoxicity; discoloration of teeth and possible effect on bone growth. Avoid prolonged/repeated courses	
Glycopeptides	/ Limited data	++	++ Not absorbed from GI tract
Gentamicin	/ Possibility of oto-/nephrotoxicity in neonates. Risk/benefit decision, with careful monitoring if used		++ Poorly excreted in breast milk
Metronidazole	++	++	++
Fluconazole	/ Avoid high doses or prolonged courses. Topical preferred if possible		++
Aciclovir	++	++	++

++ This drug is generally safe.

/ Avoid if safer alternative, but can be used if benefit outweighs risk.

! Avoid.

GI, gastrointestinal; NEC, necrotizing enterocolitis.

Antimicrobials in children

Many medications, including antibiotics, lack evidence for their efficacy in children, and so they do not have a licence from the Medicines and Healthcare products Regulatory Agency (MHRA). It is accepted that 'off-label' use is often required in children. Care must be taken with dosing, as the PD may be very different in children, particularly those in the neonatal period. Where possible, expert advice should be sought. Below are some specific cautions to be aware of:

- nitrofurantoin can cause haemolysis in infants aged <3 months and should be avoided;
- co-trimoxazole can cause kernicterus in neonates;
- chloramphenicol is linked with grey baby syndrome (abdominal distension, pallid cyanosis, and circulatory collapse) in neonates. It can also cause marrow suppression. Caution is advised;
- ceftriaxone is used with caution in neonates due to risks of hyperbilirubinaemia. It must not be given at the same time as calcium supplementation; Cefotaxime is more commonly used in this age group.
- tetracyclines are known to deposit in growing bones and teeth of children causing tooth staining. They should be avoided in children aged <12 years (unless the benefit outweighs the risk, e.g. in Rocky Mountain spotted fever);
- quinolones have been linked with arthropathy in animal studies, although there is no clear evidence of this in humans. Short courses may be considered if the benefit is deemed to outweigh the risk.

Other special populations

Extremes of weight

Both being significantly over- or underweight can affect the PD of antimicrobials, and thus impact their efficacy. Consequences of weight can be hard to predict; for example, being overweight can increase the GFR, thus increasing renal clearance. However, obese patients may also have comorbidities, such as kidney disease and hypertension, which may negate this effect.

Different weights used in dosing

- Total body weight (TBW) is the measured weight.
- Body mass index (BMI) takes into account the height and gives an idea of a patient's stature.
- Ideal body weight uses a formula based on height and gender, and is based on tables linked to life expectancy.
- Lean body weight estimates the fractional fat mass but is not commonly used in clinical practice.

Obese patients have more adipose tissue, and so when using lipophilic drugs (which will be distributed into adipose tissue), dosing based on TBW should be used to account for this. Conversely, hydrophilic drugs are expected to stay in the circulation, and so ideal body weight should be used to calculate dosing.

Overall, there is very little information on dosing at extremes of weight. Prescribers must be cautious in looking out for drug activity and toxicity. There may be a role for therapeutic drug monitoring in certain circumstances.

Elderly patients

When prescribing for the elderly, consider weight, concurrent liver and kidney disease, and other medications, which can be numerous. The risk of *C. difficile* infection is greatly increased with age, and particular care should be taken in avoiding unnecessary antibiotics.

Concurrent comorbidities

Antimicrobials can exacerbate certain medical conditions. Examples of specific conditions and some trigger antibiotics include:

- myasthenia gravis—aminoglycosides, quinolones, macrolides;
- porphyria—macrolides, tetracyclines, co-trimoxazole;
- glucose-6-phosphate dehydrogenase (G6PD) deficiency—sulfonamides, quinolones, nitrofurantoin.

Antimicrobial prophylaxis

Definitions

Prophylaxis is the administration of antibiotics to prevent an infection from developing. Primary prophylaxis aims to prevent initial infection or disease (e.g. to cover potential site contamination during a surgical procedure), whereas secondary prophylaxis aims to prevent recurrent disease (e.g. giving penicillin to a patient who has had rheumatic fever).

Surgical prophylaxis

All hospitals have a policy for antimicrobial prophylaxis for common procedures. The following factors should be considered.

Patient factors
- Any drug allergies?
- Recent antibiotics?
- Colonization with resistant organisms?

Drug
- Spectrum should cover the likely infecting organism(s).
- Penetrates the likely site of infection.
- Favourable safety profile.
- Bactericidal.

Dose?
- Aim to maintain the drug concentration above the target MIC.
- Repeat dosing might be needed, based on length of the procedure and likely blood loss.

Route
- Depends on the nature of the procedure and the PK of the drug.

Table 1.9 Examples of antibiotic prophylaxis (also check the UK Health Security Agency, *Green Book*, and *British National Formulary*)

Infection	Criteria	Notes	Recommendation
Invasive group A *Streptococcus* (iGAS)	1. Contact* with symptoms (sore throat, cellulitis, etc.) 2. Mother or neonate if other is infected	Other contacts advised of symptoms of iGAS	Phenoxymethyl-penicillin(10 days) or Azithromycin (5 days)
Neisseria meningitidis (invasive disease)	Contact* of confirmed or probable disease		Ciprofloxacin (one dose) or Rifampicin twice daily (2 days)
Haemophilus influenzae (invasive disease)	Contact* and children aged <10 years or vulnerable person in household		Rifampicin (4 days)
Diphtheria	Contact* or HCW with close respiratory or cutaneous contact	Contacts require testing	Erythromycin (7 days) or Benzylpenicillin IM (one dose)
Pertussis	All household contacts* where ≥1 contact is at risk (e.g. pregnant women, neonates, HCW)		Macrolide (7 days; 3 days if azithromycin) or Co-trimoxazole (7 days)
Tuberculosis	Risk assessment for household and close contacts	Perform Mantoux test and/or IGRA	Isoniazid (6 months) or Isoniazid + rifampicin (3 months)

* Definition of contact varies; check individual guidance.

HCW, healthcare worker; IGRA, interferon-γ release assay; IM, intramuscular.

Time of administration
- Ideally would be administered 0–2h prior to the procedure, in order to ensure adequate tissue levels.

Duration
- Usually not given for >24h.
- If there is suspicion of ongoing infection, the patient should be carefully reassessed, Consider changing the antibiotics in case of resistance.

Risks to consider
- Adverse effects of the drug (e.g. anaphylaxis, nephrotoxicity).
- Selection of antibiotic-resistant organisms.
- Alteration of patients' normal flora.

Prophylaxis after exposure to infectious diseases

Bacterial diseases which usually necessitate antibiotics to be prescribed for contacts of the index case include those listed in Table 1.9. For specific advice, contact your local Health Protection Unit.

Other examples of antimicrobial prophylaxis

- Prevention of pneumococcal infection in asplenia or sickle-cell disease.
- Prevention of gas gangrene in high-lower limb amputations or following major trauma.
- Use of antibiotic-impregnated materials (e.g. gentamicin in cement in prosthetic joint replacement or antibiotic-impregnated Dacron graft in vascular surgery).
- Some viral diseases, including hepatitis B, varicella, and measles have recommendations for prophylaxis (➔ see Chapter 8).

NB antibiotics to prevent endocarditis in high-risk patients (valvular or structural heart disease) undergoing surgery or dental procedures are NO LONGER recommended (see National Institute for Health and Care Excellence, Clinical guideline 64 (2008, updated 2016), available at: ℀ https://www.nice.org.uk/guidance/cg64).

Antimicrobial stewardship

AMS requires a multidisciplinary approach. There are numerous factors which contribute to an AMS programme. ➔ Antimicrobial stewardship/ antimicrobial resistance, 6–8m pp. 177, 273, 274. Also, see ➔ Intravenous to oral switch, p. 24; ➔ Optimal duration of therapy, p. 714; and ➔ Antimicrobial prophylaxis, pp. 32–4. Consider these initiatives every time you review a patient on antibiotics. AMS is discussed further in ➔ Chapter 6, p. 34.

Antibiotics

Penicillins

Penicillin was discovered by Alexander Fleming in 1928 but did not become widely available until the 1940s. Penicillins are closely related compounds comprising a β-lactam ring, a five-membered thiazolidine ring, and a side chain (see Fig. 2.1). The ring structures are essential for antibacterial activity, and the side chain determines the spectrum and pharmacological properties. Most penicillins in current use are semi-synthetic derivatives of 6-aminopenicillanic acid. They inhibit bacterial cell wall synthesis and are thus bactericidal.

Classification

- Group 1—benzylpenicillin and its long-acting parenteral forms.
- Group 2—PO absorbed penicillins (e.g. phenoxymethylpenicillin).
- Group 3—antistaphylococcal penicillin (e.g. flucloxacillin).
- Group 4—extended-spectrum penicillins (e.g. amoxicillin).
- Group 5—antipseudomonal penicillins (e.g. ticarcillin, piperacillin).
- Group 6—β-lactamase-resistant penicillins.

Mode of action

Penicillins inhibit cell wall synthesis by binding to penicillin-binding protein (PBPs) and inhibiting transpeptidation of peptidoglycans.

Resistance

Bacteria may become resistant to penicillins via a number of mechanisms:
- destruction of the antibiotic by β-lactamases (➲ see β-lactamases, pp. 40–1)—this is the commonest mechanism;
- failure to penetrate the outer membrane of Gram-negative bacteria;
- efflux across the outer membrane of Gram-negative bacteria;
- low-affinity binding of the antibiotic to target PBPs.

Some bacteria may display more than one resistance mechanism; for example, in meticillin-resistant *Staphylococcus aureus* (MRSA), the *mecA* gene encodes an additional PBP (i.e. an altered target site) and most also produce a β-lactamase.

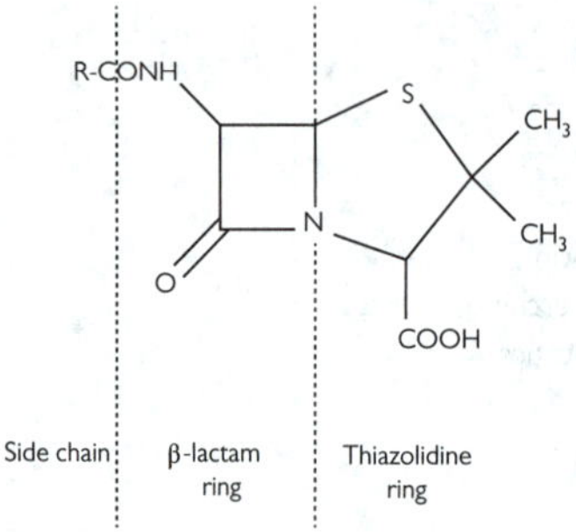

Fig. 2.1 Structure of penicillin.

Clinical use

- Benzylpenicillin is used in infections due to group A and group B streptococci, meningitis due to *Streptococcus pneumoniae* (if penicillin-susceptible) and *Neisseria meningitidis*, streptococcal and enterococcal endocarditis, and neurosyphilis.
- Aminopenicillins are used in respiratory tract infections, endocarditis, meningitis, and urinary tract infections (UTIs) caused by susceptible organisms, and treatment of *Helicobacter pylori*.
- Extended-spectrum and antipseudomonal penicillins are used in infections due to resistant Gram-negative bacteria, usually in combination with an aminoglycoside.
- Phenoxymethylpenicillin is used prophylactically to prevent recurrent rheumatic fever, secondary cases in outbreaks of group A *Streptococcus* (GAS) disease, and pneumococcal and *Haemophilus influenzae* infections in asplenic patients.
- Pivmecillinam is a narrow-spectrum antibiotic active against PBP-2 in cell walls of Gram-negative bacteria. It has limited susceptibility to most β-lactamases. Used to treat acute uncomplicated UTI.
- Temocillin is a beta-lactamase resistant penicillin. It is not active against Gram-positive bacteria, its primary use being against susceptible enterobacteriales producing ESBL or AmpC beta-lactamases.

Pharmacology

- Penicillins differ markedly in their PO absorption (phenoxymethylpenicillin 60%, amoxicillin 75%, antipseudomonal penicillins 0%).
- They vary in their degree of protein binding, and metabolism is minimal.
- They are rapidly excreted by renal tubular cells; excretion may be blocked by probenecid. Dose modification may be required in renal failure.

Toxicity and side effects

- Allergic reactions (rashes, serum sickness, delayed hypersensitivity)—occur in <10% of those exposed. Anaphylactic reactions are rare (0.004–0.4%).
- Gastrointestinal (GI)—diarrhoea, enterocolitis (2–5%, usually ampicillin).
- Haematological—haemolytic anaemia, neutropenia, thrombocytopenia (1–4%).
- Laboratory—elevated transaminase levels (usually with flucloxacillin), electrolyte abnormalities (hypernatraemia, hypo- or hyperkalaemia).
- Renal—interstitial nephritis, haemorrhagic cystitis.
- Central nervous system (CNS)—encephalopathy or seizures may rarely occur. The risk is higher with prolonged high dosing (e.g. certain endocarditis treatment regimens), and in those with renal impairment.

Cephalosporins

Giuseppe Brotzu first demonstrated the antimicrobial activity of culture filtrates of the mould *Cephalosporium acremonium* in 1945. However, the cephalosporin class of antibiotics did not become widely used for another 20 years. Cephalosporins consist of a β-lactam ring and a six-membered dihydrothiazine ring modified at certain positions to produce different compounds. Most available cephalosporins are semi-synthetic derivatives of cephalosporin C.

Classification

The classification into 'generations' is the most commonly used, with each successive generation acquiring better Gram-negative activity, usually at the expense of some Gram-positive activity, until more broad-spectrum activity appears in generations 4 and 5.

- First generation—primarily active against Gram-positive bacteria (e.g. cefazolin, cefalotin, cefradine, cefalexin).
- Second generation—enhanced activity against Gram-negative bacteria and varying activity against Gram-positive bacteria (e.g. cefuroxime, cefamandole, cefaclor). The cephamycin group (e.g. cefotetan, cefoxitin) have additional anaerobic activity against, for example, *Bacteroides fragilis*.
- Third generation—markedly increased activity against Gram-negative bacteria (e.g. cefotaxime, ceftriaxone, ceftazidime (NB poor activity against Gram-positives), cefdinir, cefixime, cefpodoxime).
- Fourth generation—broad spectrum of activity against Gram-positive cocci and Gram-negative bacteria, including *Pseudomonas* spp. (e.g. cefepime, cefpirome).
- Fifth generation—active against MRSA (e.g. ceftaroline—no pseudomonal or vancomycin-resistant *Enterococcus* (VRE) activity; ceftobiprole—active against *Pseudomonas* and enterococci).
- Novel cephalosporin compounds approved to address the problem of multidrug resistance:
  - Cefiderocol is an injectable, active against all Ambler classes of carbapenemases. It is licensed for aerobic Gram-negative infections, in patients with limited treatment options.
  - ceftazidime–avibactam is a third-generation cephalosporin combined with a β-lactamase inhibitor, and is active against serine-carbapenemases, but not against metallo-β-lactamases (MBLs);
  - ceftolozane–tazobactam is a novel fifth-generation cephalosporin combined with a different β-lactamase inhibitor, and is particularly useful against resistant *Pseudomonas*.

Mode of action

They inhibit cell wall synthesis by binding to PBPs and inhibiting transpeptidation of peptidoglycans. They are bactericidal and exhibit significant post-antibiotic effect (PAE) against Gram-positive (but not Gram-negative) bacteria.

Resistance

- Due to destruction of the antibiotic by β-lactamases (➲ see β-lactamases, pp. 40–1), reduced penetration through the outer membrane of Gram-negative bacteria, and enhanced efflux or alteration in the PBP target, resulting in reduced-affinity binding.

- *Listeria*, 'atypical' organisms (*Mycoplasma*, *Chlamydophila*), MRSA, and enterococci ('LAME') were considered intrinsically resistant to cephalosporins—however, some fifth-generation agents have activity against the latter two.

Clinical use

- First generation—staphylococcal and streptococcal skin and soft tissue infections, UTIs.
- Second generation—severe community-acquired pneumonia (CAP), otitis media, sinusitis, streptococcal pharyngitis, early Lyme disease.
- Cephamycins—intra-abdominal, pelvic, and gynaecological infections, infected decubitus ulcers, diabetic foot infections, mixed aerobic–anaerobic soft tissue infections.
- Third generation—penicillin-resistant pneumococci, meningitis, upper respiratory tract infections (URTIs) and lower respiratory tract infections (LRTIs), sinusitis, otitis media, nosocomial infections caused by Gram-negative bacilli, *Neisseria gonorrhoeae*, chancroid, Lyme disease, typhoid, severe *Shigella* spp. and non-typhoidal *Salmonella* infection, outpatient antibiotic therapy for endocarditis and osteomyelitis.
- Fourth generation—severe Gram-negative infections such as *Pseudomonas aeruginosa*, *Enterobacter* spp., *Citrobacter* spp., and *Serratia* spp.

Pharmacology

May be given PO, IV, or IM. Fourth-generation drugs are all parenteral. PO preparations have 80–95% bioavailability. Protein binding is variable (10–98%). Drugs are largely confined to the extracellular compartment. Poor CNS penetration, unless meningeal inflammation. Cross the placenta. Most drugs are not metabolized, except cefotaxime and cephalothin which are metabolized in the liver. Most drugs are excreted by the kidneys. Ceftriaxone and cefoperazone are excreted by the biliary system (see Box 2.1).

Toxicity and side effects

- Hypersensitivity—rash (1–3%), urticaria and serum sickness (<1%), anaphylaxis (0.01%).
- GI—diarrhoea (1–19%), nausea and vomiting (1–6%), transient hepatitis (1–7%), biliary sludging (ceftriaxone).
- Haematological—eosinophilia (1–10%), neutropenia, thrombocytopenia, clotting abnormalities, platelet dysfunction, haemolytic anaemia.

Box 2.1 CAUTION!

Second- and third-generation cephalosporins are susceptible to in-activation by inducible β-lactamases (➜ see β-lactamases, pp. 40–1). They should never be used to treat organisms that may have these enzymes (e.g. *Enterobacter* spp., *Serratia* spp., *Citrobacter freundii*, *Klebsiella aerogenes*, *Acinetobacter* spp., *Proteus vulgaris*, *Providencia* spp., *Morganella morganii* (ESCKAPPM).

- Renal—interstitial nephritis.
- CNS—seizures.
- False-positive laboratory tests—Coombs' test, glycosuria, serum creatinine.
- Other—drug fever, disulfiram-like reaction, phlebitis.

β-lactamases

β-lactamases are enzymes that bind covalently to the β-lactam ring, hydrolyse it, and make the antibiotic ineffective. Emergence of resistance to β-lactam antibiotics began even before penicillin was widely available, with the first β-lactamase (penicillinase) being described in *Escherichia coli* in 1940. This was followed by the emergence of resistance in *S. aureus*, due to plasmid-encoded penicillinase. Many genera of Gram-negative bacilli possess naturally occurring chromosomally mediated β-lactamases (AmpC); these enzymes are thought to have evolved from PBPs, to which they are very similar. The first plasmid-mediated β-lactamase in Gram-negative bacteria TEM-1 was described in 1960. Within a few years, it had spread worldwide and was found in many different species. Over the past 20 years, many antibiotics have been developed to be resistant to these β-lactamases. However, with each new class of drugs, new β-lactamases have emerged.

Classification

There are two classification systems for β-lactamases:
- molecular (Ambler)—four classes (A to D) based on the nucleotide/amino acid sequences of the enzymes:
  - classes A, C, and D are serine β-lactamases;
  - class B are zinc-dependent enzymes (MBLs) that hydrolyse the β-lactam ring by a different mechanism;
- functional (Bush–Jacoby–Medeiros)—three groups, each with subgroups:
  - group 1 β-lactamases are cephalosporinases that are not inhibited by clavulanic acid. They correspond to Ambler group C;
  - group 2 β-lactamases are penicillinases and/or cephalosporinases that are inhibited by clavulanic acid. This group corresponds to Ambler groups A and D, and includes the TEM and SHV enzymes;
  - group 3 β-lactamases are zinc-dependent (MBLs) and are not inhibited by clavulanic acid. They correspond to Ambler group B;
  - group 4 is no longer used—it included enzymes that would have been included in one of the other groups, if more information had been available.

AmpC β-lactamases

These are chromosomally mediated β-lactamases that are active against third-generation cephalosporins and are not inhibited by clavulanic acid. They fall into molecular group C/functional group 1. They are found in the ESCKAPPM group of organisms (e.g. **E**nterobacter spp., **S**erratia spp., **C**itrobacter freundii, **K**lebsiella aerogenes, **A**cinetobacter spp., **P**roteus vulgaris, **P**rovidencia spp., and **M**organella morganii). Use of third-generation cephalosporins to treat these infections results in the selection of stably derepressed mutants that hyperproduce AmpC, and has been associated with clinical failure. These infections are therefore usually treated with carbapenems.

Extended-spectrum β-lactamases

These are β-lactamases which are capable of conferring bacterial resistance to penicillins, first-, second-, and third-generation cephalosporins, and aztreonam (but not cephamycins or carbapenems) by hydrolysis of these antibiotics, and which are inhibited by β-lactamase inhibitors such as clavulanic acid. They fall into functional groups 2be and 2d. Extended-spectrum β-lactamases (ESBLs) are most commonly found in *E. coli* and *Klebsiella pneumoniae*, but have been described in many other Gram-negative bacilli. Most ESBLs are derivatives of the TEM and SHV enzymes (see below).

- TEM β-lactamases—TEM-1 is the commonest β-lactamase in Gram-negative bacteria and is able to hydrolyse penicillins and early-generation cephalosporins. TEM-2 has a similar spectrum. TEM-3 was the first ESBL reported in 1989. Since then, over 160 TEM enzymes have been described. Most of these are inhibited by clavulanic acid, but some inhibitor-resistant variants exist, particularly in Europe. TEM enzymes are commonest in *E. coli* and *K. pneumoniae*, but are increasingly found in other species of Gram-negative bacilli.
- SHV β-lactamases—SHV-1 β-lactamase is most commonly found in *K. pneumoniae* and accounts for ≤20% of ampicillin resistance in this species. Unlike TEM, there are relatively few SHV-1 derivatives.
- CTX-M β-lactamases—this family of plasmid-mediated β-lactamases preferentially hydrolyses cefotaxime. They have been found in *Salmonella enterica* serovar Typhimurium and *E. coli*, as well as in other enterobacteria. These enzymes are quite different from TEM and SHV enzymes, and show greater similarity to the chromosomal AmpC enzyme of *Kluyvera ascorbata*, suggesting CTX-M may have originated from this species. CTX-M β-lactamases have previously been associated with outbreaks in Europe, South America, and Japan, although they are now reported worldwide.
- OXA β-lactamases—these are characterized by their high hydrolytic activity against oxacillin and cloxacillin, and are poorly inhibited by clavulanic acid. They belong to molecular group D/functional group 2d. OXA-type ESBLs are mainly found in *P. aeruginosa* but have been detected in other Gram-negative bacteria. More recently, non-ESBL OXA derivatives have been described.
- Other ESBLs—a number of ESBLs that are unrelated to the established families of ESBLs have been described (e.g. PER-1, PER-2, VEB-1, GES, BES, TLA, SFO, and IBC).

ESBL detection methods

In general, ESBL detection methods use a β-lactamase inhibitor (clavulanate) in combination with an oximino-cephalosporin (e.g. ceftazidime or cefotaxime). Clavulanate inhibits ESBLs, thereby reducing the level of resistance to cephalosporin. A number of methods exist (e.g. Jarlier double disc method, Etest® for ESBLs).

β-lactamase inhibitors

β-lactamase inhibitors are clavulanic acid and penicillanic acid sulfone derivatives. They have weak antibacterial activity but are potent inhibitors of many β-lactamases (e.g. penicillinases produced by *S. aureus*, *H. influenzae*, *Moraxella catarrhalis*, and *Bacteroides* spp.) and of TEM and SHV β-lactamases produced by *Enterobacterales*. They can restore the antibacterial activity of certain antibiotics (e.g. amoxicillin, ampicillin, piperacillin, mezlocillin, cefoperazone). Four β-lactamase inhibitors are in clinical use: clavulanic acid, sulbactam, tazobactam and avibactam. All are only available in combination with a β-lactam antibiotic; the antibiotic spectrum is determined by the companion antibiotic. Although there are minor differences in potency, activity, and pharmacology among the four compounds, they can be considered therapeutically equivalent (except for some *Klebsiella* spp. where clavulanate inhibits isolates resistant to sulbactam and tazobactam).

Co-amoxiclav

- Clavulanate is a potent inhibitor of many plasmid-mediated β-lactamases and a weak inducer of some chromosomal β-lactamases.
- It is available as a combination with amoxicillin and used for the treatment of a wide range of infections where β-lactamase-producing organisms may be present. Examples include otitis media, sinusitis, pneumonia, skin and soft tissue infections, diabetic foot infections, and bite infections.
- It is available as PO or parenteral formulations. In the PO formulation, the ratio of amoxicillin to clavulanic acid is 2:1 (e.g. 250mg/125mg), whereas in the IV formulation, it is 5:1 (e.g. 1000mg/200mg).
- Side effects are similar to ampicillin. Cholestatic jaundice may occur during/after therapy and is six times commoner than with amoxicillin alone.

Ticarcillin/clavulanic acid

- This combination is useful against infections caused by *Pseudomonas* spp. and *Proteus* spp.
- It has been used for the treatment of pneumonia, intra-abdominal infections, gynaecological infections, skin and soft tissue infections, and osteomyelitis.
- It is only available in parenteral form and is given IV.
- Side effects are similar to those of other β-lactams. Cholestatic jaundice may also occur because of the clavulanic acid component.

Ampicillin–sulbactam

- Sulbactam is 6-desaminopenicillin sulfone. It has a broader spectrum of activity but is less potent than clavulanic acid. It is used for the treatment of skin and soft tissue infections, intraabdominal infections, and gynaecological infections.

Piperacillin–tazobactam

- Tazobactam is penicillanic acid sulfone β-lactamase inhibitor, with a similar structure to that of sulbactam. Its spectrum of activity is similar to that of sulbactam, but its potency is comparable to that of clavulanic acid.

- It is available as a combination with piperacillin (an antipseudomonal penicillin) and is given parenterally.
- It has a broad spectrum of activity and is used in the treatment of pneumonia (especially *P. aeruginosa*), skin and soft tissue infections, intra-abdominal infections, UTIs, polymicrobial infections, bacteraemia, and febrile neutropenia (in combination with an aminoglycoside).
- Side effects are similar to those of piperacillin.

Ceftazidime–avibactam

- avibactam is a β-lactamase inhibitor, and is active against serine carbapenemases, but not against metallo- β-lactamases (MBLs)
- it is available with ceftazidime and is given parenterally
- it has a broad spectrum of activity and is used for complicated intra-abdominal infections, complicated UTI including pyelonephritis, HAP including VAP and infections due to gram-negative bacteria with limited treatment options
- side effects are similar to those of ceftazidime and include thrombocytosis

Ceftolozane–tazobactam

- see above for details on tazobactam
- it is available with ceftolozane and is given parenterally
- it has a broad spectrum of activity and is used for complicated intra-abdominal infections, complicated UTI including pyelonephritis, HAP and VAP. It is particularly useful against resistant *Pseudomonas*
- side effects are similar to those of cepahslosporins

Carbapenems

Carbapenems are β-lactam antibiotics derived from thienamycin, a compound produced by *Streptomyces cattleya*. Three carbapenems are licensed for use in the UK: imipenem, meropenem, and ertapenem. Other drugs in the same class include panipenem, doripenem, biapenem and faropenem.

Mode of action

These agents show high affinity to most high-molecular-weight PBPs of Gram-positive and Gram-negative bacteria. Carbapenems, particularly imipenem, traverse the outer membrane of Gram-negative bacteria through different outer membrane proteins (OprD) than those that are used by penicillins and cephalosporins (OmpC and OmpF). They also have excellent stability to β-lactamases. Consequently, carbapenems have the broadest antibacterial spectrum of all the β-lactam antibiotics. Imipenem is slightly more active against Gram-positive bacteria, whereas meropenem and ertapenem are slightly more active against Gram-negative species. Meropenem is the most active against *P. aeruginosa*. Ertapenem has poor activity against *P. aeruginosa* and *Acinetobacter* spp.

Resistance

Resistance is due to one of four mechanisms: production of a low-affinity PBP target; reduced outer membrane permeability due to the absence of OprD in Gram-negative bacteria; efflux of the drug in Gram-negative bacteria; or production of β-lactamases ($\bigodot$ see β-lactamases, pp. 40–1) that hydrolyse carbapenems (carbapenemases). Carbapenem resistance in *Enterobacterales* may be due to a combination of porin loss PLUS an ESBL or AmpC enzyme (such strains rarely spread) OR an acquired carbapenemase (such a strain being more likely to spread, and often occurring in strains already resistant to many antibiotics). For a summary of carbapenemases, see Table 2.1.

Clinical use

- Carbapenems may be used to treat a wide variety of severe infections (e.g. bacteraemia, pneumonia, intra-abdominal infections, obstetric and gynaecological infections, complicated UTIs, soft tissue and bone infections).
- Imipenem and meropenem are most appropriate for treatment of infections caused by the cephalosporin-resistant AmpC-producing organisms, ESCKAPPM group (e.g. *Enterobacter* spp., **S**erratia spp., **C**itrobacter freundii, **K**lebsiella aerogenes, **A**cinetobacter spp., **P**roteus vulgaris, **P**rovidencia spp., and **M**organella morganii).
- Imipenem and meropenem are also used for the treatment of serious infections (e.g. patients with polymicrobial infections, febrile

Table 2.1 Summary of the main carbapenemases

Enzyme	Class	Characteristics
IMP-type	Metallo (class B)	Plasmid-mediated, at least 17 varieties, originated in Japan in 1990s in enterics. Now worldwide. Also found in *Pseudomonas* and *Acinetobacter*
VIM	Verona Integron-encoded metallo (class B)	Originally from Italy (1999), at least 10 types, now wide geographic distribution. Mainly found in *P. aeruginosa* and *Pseudomonas putida*, only rarely in *Enterobacterales*
OXA	Oxacillinase (class D)	Occurs mainly in *Acinetobacter*. Also OXA-48 *K. pneumoniae* in the Middle East and North Africa, and imported into the UK. Both plasmid and clonal spread
KPC	*K. pneumoniae* carbapenemase (class A)	Ten variants, KPC-2 to KPC-11 which differ by one or two amino acid substitutions. Also clonal spread, including global *K. pneumoniae* ST258 lineage
CMY	Class C	First class C carbapenemase, isolated from *Enterobacter aerogenes* in 2006 on plasmid pYMG-1
SME, IMI, NMC, CcrA	Class A	Little clinical significance at present
NDM-1	New Delhi metallo-β-lactamase	Described originally in New Delhi in 2009. Mainly plasmid spread in *E. coli* and *K. pneumoniae*

neutropenia, and nosocomial infections such as those caused by *P. aeruginosa* and *Acinetobacter* spp.).

- Meropenem is also licensed for the treatment of bacterial meningitis—imipenem should not be used because of its propensity to cause seizures.
- Ertapenem has similar uses to those of imipenem and meropenem, but cannot be used in infections caused by *P. aeruginosa* and *Acinetobacter* spp. Its long plasma half-life means that it can be administered once daily (od), making it useful for outpatient parenteral antimicrobial therapy (OPAT).

Pharmacology

- Imipenem, meropenem, and ertapenem have poor PO absorption and are given parenterally.
- Imipenem and meropenem are pharmacologically similar, with a plasma half-life of 1h, whereas ertapenem has a plasma half-life of 4h, which permits once-daily dosing.
- All carbapenems are widely distributed and penetrate inflamed meninges.
- All are renally excreted and require dose modification in renal failure.
- Imipenem is a substrate for renal dehydropeptidase-1 (DHP-1) enzyme and is therefore co-administered with cilastatin, a DHP-1 inhibitor.

Toxicity and side effects

- Carbapenems are generally well tolerated.
- β-lactam allergic reactions are the commonest side effects (e.g. rash, urticaria, immediate hypersensitivity, cross-reactivity with penicillin).
- Imipenem causes nausea (if infused too quickly) and can cause seizures.

Carbapenem with broad-spectrum beta-lactamase inhibitor

The addition of a broad-spectrum beta-lactamase inhibitor to a carbapenem can restore efficacy. Vaborbactam and relebactam inhibit class A carbapenemases (but not B or D).

- Meropenem-vaborbactam is used mostly in the treatment of KPC-producing Enterobacterales. It is not useful against carbapenem resistant *Pseudomonas aeruginosa nor against Acinetobacter* species. It is licensed for complicated UTIs and intra-abdominal infections, HAP and VAP, bacteraemia associated with these licensed indications and aerobic Gram–negative infections in patients with limited treatment options.
- Imipenem-cilastatin-relebactam is similarly used in the treatment of KPC-producing Enterobacterales and has activity against some imipenem resistant *P. aeruginosa*. It is not useful against *Acinetobacter* species. It is licensed for aerobic Gram–negative infections in patients with limited treatment options.

Carbapenemases

Carbapenem antibiotics (➲ see Carbapenems, pp. 43–6) are the cornerstone agents for treating ESBL infection. The emergence of carbapenem-hydrolysing β-lactamases has prompted great concern. (Table 2.1) Enzymes have been identified belonging to classes A and B (MBLs) and can be chromosomally or plasmid-mediated, the latter facilitating transmission between strains and species. *K. pneumoniae* carbapenemase (KPC) is the most clinically important of class A carbapenemases—they are plasmid-mediated and confer resistance to all β-lactams. NDM-1, a novel MBL, was first described in 2009 in a European patient hospitalized in India with a *K. pneumoniae* infection. It has been identified in other *Enterobacterales*, including *E. coli* and *Enterobacter*. In general, bacteria carrying NDM-1 are sensitive to colistimethate sodium or tigecycline.

Carbapenemase Detection Methods

Detecting carbapenemases is difficult, as resistance can be low level, which complicates detection and interpretation. In addition not all carbapenemase producers are resistant to carbapenems and carbapenem-resistance can be due to other mechanisms (such as a combination of ESBL / AmpC plus imperme-ability or increased efflux pump production). Gold standard for detecting the carbapenemase genes are genotypic methods: multiplex PCR assays are avail-able that detect common carbapenemases. However, phenotypic methods (such as biochemical tests, growth-based assays, immunochromatography, MALDI to detect carbapenem hydrolysis) are convenient and manageable. This is a fast-moving field, but the following may provide guidance:

- Ertapenem resistance may suggest possible CPE
- Temocillin resistance may indicate presence of an OXA-48
- Some organisms such as Stenotrophomonas maltophilia are inherently resistant to Carbapenems
- Ceftolozane-tazobactam resistance in pseudomonas may predict 'exotic' b-lactamases (suggest liaison with reference lab)

Monobactams

Monobactams are monocyclic β-lactam antibiotics produced by some bac-teria (e.g. *Chromobacterium violaceum*). They are only active against Gram-negative bacteria.

Aztreonam

- Aztreonam is the only commercially available compound.
- It is active against most *Enterobacterales*, *H. influenzae*, and *Neisseria* spp. *Stenotrophomonas maltophilia*, *Burkholderia cepacia*, and many *Acinetobacter* spp. are resistant. Some strains of *P. aeruginosa*, *Enterobacter cloacae*, and *C. freundii* are resistant.
- Aztreonam passes through the outer membrane and binds to PBP3 of Gram-negative bacteria. It is resistant to hydrolysis by most β-lactamases, apart from AmpC β-lactamases.
- Aztreonam is not absorbed PO and is given IV or IM. It is widely distributed and penetrates inflamed meninges. It is mainly renally excreted and requires dose modification in renal failure.
- It is used for the treatment of a variety of infections (e.g. UTIs, pneumonia, septicaemia, skin and soft tissue infections, intra-abdominal infections, gynaecological infections, and wound and burn infections).
- Aztreonam should never be used alone as empirical therapy, as it has no activity against Gram-positive organisms.
- Side effects are similar to those of other β-lactams, except for hypersensitivity which does not occur.

Other cell wall agents

Bacitracin

Bacitracin binds to isoprenyl phosphate and prevents dephosphorylation of the lipid carrier that transports the cell wall building block across the membrane. Without dephosphorylation, the native compound cannot be regenerated for another round of transfer. Similar reactions in eukaryotic cells may account for this agent's toxicity, and it is therefore used topically. It is also used to identify GAS (bacitracin-resistant) in the diagnostic laboratory.

Fosfomycin

Fosfomycin inhibits pyruvyl transferase, and therefore formation of *N*-acetylglucosamine from *N*-acetylmuramic acid. It is a naturally occurring antibiotic with a fairly broad spectrum, particularly against Gram-negative rods. It is mainly used to treat UTIs.

Cycloserine

This drug is often part of the second-line regimen for drug-resistant TB. It is a structural analogue of *D*-alanine, and acts on alanine racemase and synthetase to inhibit the synthesis of terminal *D*-alanyl-*D*-alanine. It thus prevents formation of the pentapeptide chain of muramic acid (➔ see Antituberculous agents, pp. 75–9).

Isoniazid and ethambutol

These are first-line drugs used in the treatment of TB. They interfere with mycolic acid synthesis in mycobacterial cell walls (➔ see Antituberculous agents, pp. 75–9).

Glycopeptides

The glycopeptide antibiotics vancomycin and teicoplanin are bactericidal against most Gram-positive bacteria. Vancomycin was first isolated from *Nocardia orientalis* and introduced into clinical practice in 1958. Teicoplanin was obtained from *Actinoplanes teichomyceticus* in 1978 and is available in Europe and Asia, but not in the USA.

Mode of action

Glycopeptides inhibit cell synthesis by binding to the *D*-alanyl-*D*-alanine tail of the muramyl pentapeptide. This complex cannot be processed by the enzyme glycosyltransferase, inhibiting the incorporation of murein monomers (*N*-acetylmuramic acid and *N*-acetylglucosamine) into the growing peptidoglycan chain.

Antimicrobial activity

Glycopeptides have broad activity against Gram-positive organisms (e.g. staphylococci, *Enterococcus faecalis*, *S. pneumoniae*, groups A, B, C, and G streptococci, *Streptococcus bovis*, *Streptococcus mutans*, viridans group streptococci, *Listeria monocytogenes*, *Bacillus* spp., *Corynebacterium* spp., *Peptostreptococcus* spp., *Actinomyces* spp., *Cutibacterium* (formerly known as *Propionibacterium*) spp., and most *Clostridioides* spp.). Glycopeptides show no activity against Gram-negative species (except non-gonococcal *Neisseria* spp.).

The minimum inhibitory concentration (MICs) of teicoplanin against coagulase-negative staphylococci (CoNS) is more variable than that of vancomycin.

Resistance

Vancomycin resistance may be intrinsic or acquired.

- Intrinsic vancomycin resistance occurs in *Leuconostoc*, *Pediococcus*, *Lactobacillus*, and *Erysipelothrix rhusiopathiae*. Intrinsic teicoplanin resistance is seen in *Staphylococcus haemolyticus*.
- Enterococci—six types of glycopeptide resistance have been described (VanA, VanB, VanC, VanD, VanE, and VanG), named on the basis of their ligase genes (*vanA*, *vanB*, etc.; see Table 2.2). These result in the formation of a peptidoglycan precursor with decreased affinity for glycopeptides. Resistance may be intrinsic (e.g. in *Enterococcus gallinarum*, *Enterococcus casseliflavus*) or acquired (e.g. in *Enterococcus faecium*, *E. faecalis*).
- *S. aureus*—the first clinical isolate of *S. aureus* with diminished susceptibility to vancomycin was reported in Japan in 1997. This is referred to as a vancomycin-intermediate *S. aureus* (VISA) or glycopeptide-intermediate *S. aureus* (GISA). VISA isolates have a thickened cell wall, which may prevent glycopeptides from reaching their target sites. In 2002, two isolates of truly vancomycin-resistant *S. aureus* (VRSA) were reported, both of which carried the *vanA* gene, suggesting horizontal transfer of this gene from enterococci.
- *S. pneumoniae*—vancomycin tolerance has been reported recently.

Clinical use

Glycopeptides are used to treat the following conditions:

- severe infections caused by MRSA;
- meningitis due to penicillin-resistant *S. pneumoniae*;
- *Clostridioides difficile*-associated diarrhoea (PO vancomycin);
- febrile neutropenia;
- continuous ambulatory peritoneal dialysis (CAPD) peritonitis;
- endophthalmitis;
- empirical treatment of intravascular catheter-related infections and cerebrospinal fluid (CSF) shunt infections.

Pharmacology

- Vancomycin is usually given IV, but may also be given PO, intraperitoneally, intrathecally, or intraocularly. It is widely distributed but has poor CSF penetration in the absence of meningeal inflammation. Vancomycin is excreted unchanged in the kidneys, and dose reduction is required in renal impairment. Vancomycin shows time-dependent killing—if the trough level is too high, it is better to reduce the dose rather than increase the dosing interval.
- Teicoplanin is usually administered IV and IM, but may also be given intraperitoneally. It has a long plasma half-life (83–168h), enabling daily dosing. Teicoplanin has better bone penetration than vancomcyin. It is excreted by the kidneys.

Toxicity and side effects

Toxicity is commoner with vancomycin than with teicoplanin.

Table 2.2 Vancomycin resistance in enterococci and staphylococci

	VanA	VanB	VanC	VanD	VanE	VanG
Vanc MIC	64–>500	4–>500	2–32	64–128	16	12–16
Teic MIC	16–>500	0.5–2	0.5–2	4–64	0.5	0.5
Expression	Inducible	Inducible	Constitutive, inducible	Constitutive	Inducible	
Location	P, C	P, C	C	C	C	C
Species	Enterococcus faecalis and faecium, Staphylococcus aureus	E. faecalis, E. faecium	Enterococcus gallinarum and casseiflavus, Enterococcus flavescens	E. faecium	E. faecalis	E. faecalis

C, chromosome; MIC, minimum inhibitory concentration (microgram/mL); P, plasmid; Teic, teicoplanin; Vanc, vancomycin.

- Ototoxicity is rare, unless there is renal impairment.
- Nephrotoxicity occurs with high doses and is often associated with concomitant aminoglycoside usage.
- Infusion-related reactions can occur (e.g. 'red man syndrome' with rapid infusion of vancomycin).
- Others (e.g. neutropenia, thrombocytopenia, rashes, drug fever).

Glycopeptide monitoring

Basic principles of glycopeptide monitoring are described in ➋ Glycopeptide monitoring, pp. 50–1. Please consult your hospital guidelines, antibiotic pharmacist, or infection specialist for specific advice.

- Recommended initial dose of vancomycin or teicoplanin depends on the type of infection, patient weight, and renal function. Loading doses (based on actual body weight) are commonly given if creatinine clearance (CrCl) is >20mL/min.
- Vancomycin trough (pre-dose) levels are usually monitored to reduce the risk of nephrotoxicity and guide future dosing. Always review any other nephrotoxic drugs your patient is taking (e.g. gentamicin) (see Table 2.3).
- Teicoplanin trough (pre-dose) levels are usually monitored in severe infections to ensure therapeutic levels. Monitoring is not needed for toxicity (see Table 2.4).
- Information: always state the time of last dose, time of sample, and current dosing regimen, to aid interpretation of result.
- Timing of levels: vancomycin is usually monitored before the third dose (unless CrCl is <10mL/min, then before the second dose). Teicoplanin is usually monitored after 7 days of treatment.

Table 2.3 Interpretation of vancomycin pre-dose (trough) levels

<10mg/L	Subtherapeutic	Check sample timing. If a true sample, increase the dose (usually by 500mg increments, either as once daily or in divided doses)
10–20mg/L	Optimum dose*	Continue on current dose; reassay 1–2 times a week if no change in renal function
20–25mg/L	Above recommended target level	Reassessment/extend dosing interval (e.g. from twice daily to once daily). Reassay after third dose
>25mg/L	Above recommended target level	Omit further dosing until level <20mg/L. Reassessment/extend dosing interval

* For severe infections (e.g. MRSA pneumonia, osteomyelitis, endocarditis, bacteraemias), many experts aim for a target concentration of 15–20mg/L.

Table 2.4 Interpretation of teicoplanin pre-dose (trough) levels

<20mg/L	Subtherapeutic level, especially if severe infections	Increase dose (usually by ~50%). Reassay after five doses
20–60mg/L	Optimum dose	Continue on current dose, and reassay in 1 month if no change in renal function
>60mg/L	Above recommended target level	Reassess dose according to renal function. Consider reducing daily dose or extending the dosage interval (e.g. to every 48h)

Lipoglycopeptides

Dalbavancin and oritavancin are semi-synthetic lipoglycopeptides licensed in the UK for acute bacterial skin and skin structure infections. They have been developed to treat infections with multiresistant Gram-positive pathogens. The heptapeptide core (common to all glycopeptides) results in inhibition of cell wall synthesis (transglycosylation and transpeptidation), and the lipophilic side chain prolongs the half-life, helping to anchor the drug to the cell membrane. Oritavancin also disrupts bacterial membrane integrity increases membrane permeability, inhibits RNA synthesis. Both agents are active *in vitro* against *S. aureus* (including MRSA), *Staphylococcus epidermidis*, *Streptococcus* spp., and VanB-VRE. Oritavancin is active against VISA, VRSA, and VanA-VRE, whereas dalbavancin is active against VISA, but not against VanA-VRE or VRSA. Dalbavancin is given once weekly, which may facilitate outpatient treatment.

Fidaxomicin

Fidaxomicin is the fermentation product of the actinomycete *Dactylosporangium aurantiacum* subspecies *hamdenesis*. It is the first in a new class of macrocyclic antibiotics, and is bactericidal, poorly absorbed systemically, and more selective for *C. difficile*, with minimal disruption to normal gut flora. Evidence from two double-blind randomized controlled trials (RCTs) indicates it is non-inferior to vancomycin in curing patients with mild to severe *C. difficile* infection (CDI). It reduces the recurrence rate of CDI, and its side effect profile is similar to that of PO vancomycin. The National Institute for Health and Care Excellence (NICE) guidance in 2021 recommended fidaxomicin. Second-line antibiotic for a first episode of mild, moderate or severe *C. difficile* infection if vancomycin is ineffective; first-line for a relapse and as an alternative to vancomycin for a recurrence.[1] Consult an infection expert, and weigh up the potential benefits alongside the medical need, risks of treatment, and relatively high cost of fidaxomicin (➔ see *Clostridioides difficile* diarrhoea, pp. 698–701).

References

1 National Institute for Health and Care Excellence (2012). *Clostridium difficile infection: fidaxomicin*. Available at: ℞ https://www.nice.org.uk/guidance/ng199/chapter/Recommendations.

Aminoglycosides

Streptomycin, produced by *Streptomyces griseus*, was the first aminoglycoside used in the initial treatment trials of TB in the 1940s. Today aminoglycosides remain an important part of the antibiotic arsenal. All aminoglycosides have an essential six-membered ring with amino group constituents (aminocyclitol). The term aminoglycoside results from the glycosidic bonds between aminocyclitol and two or more sugars. Aminoglycosides are active against many Gram-negative, and some Gram-positive, organisms. In the UK, currently available aminoglycosides are: streptomycin, neomycin, kanamycin, paromomycin, gentamicin, tobramycin, amikacin, netilmicin, and spectinomycin. Other drugs (e.g. sisomicin, dibekacin, isepamicin) are available in Japan and continental Europe.

Mode of action

Aminoglycosides bind to the A site of the 30S ribosomal subunit, resulting in a conformational change that interferes with messenger RNA (mRNA) translation and translocation, and hence inhibit protein synthesis. Avidity of binding varies across aminoglycosides. Transport of aminoglycosides into the cell by energy-dependent mechanisms (energy-dependent phase (EDP)-I and EDP-II) results in accumulation of high concentrations of the drug in the cell. The onset of cell death is coincident with the transition from EDP-I to EDP-II.

Resistance

Resistance to aminoglycosides may be intrinsic or acquired.

- Intrinsic resistance may be non-enzymatic or enzymatic:
  - anaerobes are unable to generate a sufficient electrical potential difference across the membrane and are intrinsically resistant;
  - mutations in the 16S ribosomal subunit can result in resistance to streptomycin in *Mycobacterium tuberculosis* (MTB);
  - methylating enzymes that modify 16S ribosomal RNA (rRNA) may cause intrinsic resistance; this has not yet been seen in clinical isolates.
- Acquired resistance may occur by a variety of mechanisms:
  - reduced drug uptake;
  - efflux pumps (e.g. activation of the Mex XY pump in *P. aeruginosa*);
  - enzymatic modification of the drug may occur as a result of aminoglycoside-modifying enzymes (AMEs) that phosphorylate, acetylate, or adenylate exposed amino or hydroxyl groups. The enzymatically modified drugs bind poorly to ribosomes, resulting in high levels of resistance.

Clinical use

- Empirical therapy—aminoglycosides may be given as empirical therapy for serious infections suspected to be due to Gram-negative bacteria. Depending on the clinical indication, they are usually combined with a β-lactam, vancomycin, or an anaerobic agent.

- Specific therapy—once culture results are available, aminoglycosides may be useful for specific treatment (e.g. infections due to *Pseudomonas* spp. or resistant Gram-negative species, endocarditis).
- Prophylaxis—aminoglycosides are sometimes used prophylactically (e.g. to prevent enterococcal endocarditis in 'at-risk' patients undergoing genitourinary (GU) or GI procedures).
- Gentamicin is the most commonly used aminoglycoside in the UK. Its main use is in empirical treatment of serious infections (e.g. septicaemia, febrile neutropenia, biliary sepsis, acute pyelonephritis, endocarditis). It is often incorporated into cement in orthopaedic procedures. Gentamicin drops are used in superficial eye infections and bacterial otitis externa.
- Amikacin is used in gentamicin-resistant infections, mycobacterial infections, and nocardiosis.
- Tobramycin is slightly better for *P. aeruginosa* than gentamicin, and may be used in cystic fibrosis (CF) patients.
- Neomycin is given PO for bowel sterilization pre-surgery or for selective decontamination of the digestive tract (➔ see Antimicrobial prophylaxis, pp. 32–4).
- Netilmicin is used in Gram-negative infections that are resistant to gentamicin.
- Streptomycin is used to treat TB, particularly in the developing world. It is sometimes used synergistically in enterococcal endocarditis (if there is gentamicin resistance).
- Spectinomycin is used to treat gonococcal infections.
- Paromomycin is used to treat cryptosporidiosis.

Pharmacology

- Aminoglycosides share a number of important characteristics (➔ see Pharmacodynamics (often referred to as PD), pp. 20–1):
  - concentration-dependent bactericidal activity;
  - significant PAE;
  - synergism, particularly with cell wall-active agents.
- Aminoglycosides have poor PO absorption and are usually administered IV or IM. They may also be administered PO (e.g. neomycin, paromomycin), TOP, intrapleurally, intraperitoneally, or intrathecally.
- Aminoglycosides are highly soluble with low protein binding, resulting in distribution in the vascular and interstitial compartments. CSF penetration is poor, apart from in neonates. Aminoglycosides are excreted unchanged in the urine (99%).
- Aminoglycosides may be given od or in multiple daily doses. Dosing od is simpler and as efficacious as multiple dosing and may lower the risk of drug-induced toxicity. The usual suggested dose of gentamicin is 5–7mg/kg/day. The dose is reduced in renal failure to 3mg/kg/day. Exceptions: children, pregnancy, burns, and endocarditis. If patients need to continue therapy beyond 48h, trough drug levels should be monitored, and the dosing interval adjusted according to the Hartford nomogram (see Fig. 2.2).

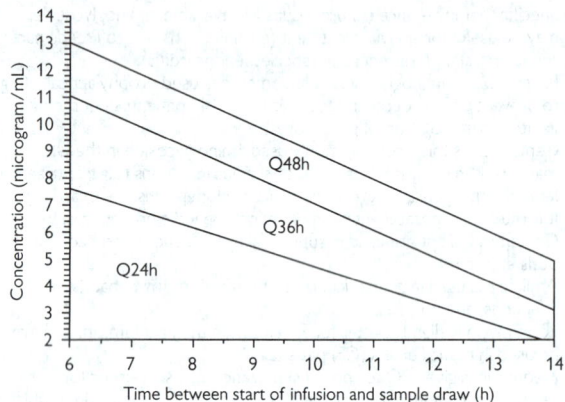

Fig. 2.2 Hartford nomogram for once-daily aminoglycosides.

Reproduced from Nicolau et al. (1995). 'Experience with a once-daily aminoglycoside program administered to 2,184 adult patients' Antimicrob Agents Chemother **39**:650–5 with permission from the American Society of Microbiology.

Toxicity and side effects

- Nephrotoxicity is the commonest adverse effect (5–25%).
- Ototoxicity (cochlear and vestibular) may be irreversible.
- Neuromuscular blockade is rare.
- Aminoglycosides are associated with increased risk of deafness in patients with mitochondrial mutations (MHRA, 2021).

Macrolides

Macrolides (erythromycin, clarithromycin, and azithromycin) and lincosamides (lincomycin and clindamycin), although chemically unrelated, have some similar properties such as antimicrobial activity, mechanisms of action, resistance, and pharmacology. Ketolides are a new class of antibiotics, derived from erythromycin, with activity against macrolide-resistant strains (see Box 2.2).

Box 2.2 MLS$_B$ resistance (also known as inducible resistance)

Macrolides, lincosamides, and streptogramin type B (MLS$_B$) antibiotics bind to closely related sites on the 50S ribosome of bacteria. One consequence is that some bacteria (e.g. staphylococci, streptococci, enterococci) with inducible resistance to erythromycin also become resistant to the other MLS$_B$ agents, in the presence of erythromycin. The methylase enzyme involved is not induced by lincosamides or streptogramins, which therefore remain active in the absence of macrolides. Over 20 erm genes encode the MLS$_B$ resistance, and it is becoming commoner in GAS and pneumococci.

Erythromycin

- Erythromycin was derived from *Saccharopolyspora erythraea* in 1952. Erythromycin A is the active component. It consists of a 14-membered macrocyclic lactone ring attached to two sugars.
- Mode of action—inhibits RNA-dependent protein synthesis at the step of chain elongation by interacting with the peptidyl transferase site. It also inhibits the formation of the 50S ribosomal subunit.
- Resistance—there are four resistance mechanisms:
  - decreased outer membrane permeability; for example, *Enterobacterales*, *Pseudomonas* spp., *Acinetobacter* spp. are intrinsically resistant;
  - efflux pumps (e.g. *msr(A)* gene of *S. aureus* and *mef(A)* gene of *S. pneumoniae* and GAS);
  - alterations of 23S rRNA by methylation of adenine. This confers resistance to MLS$_B$ and is referred to as the MLS$_B$ phenotype. It is encoded by *erm* (erythromycin ribosomal methylase) genes;
  - enzymatic inactivation by phosphotransferases, mediated by *mph* genes. Hydrolysis of the macrocyclic lactone is encoded by the esterase genes *ere(A)* and *ere(B)* on plasmids.
- Clinical use—CAP, atypical pneumonia (e.g. *Mycoplasma pneumoniae*, *Chlamydia pneumoniae*, *Legionella pneumophila*), *Bordetella pertussis*, *Campylobacter* gastroenteritis.
- Pharmacology—given PO (stimulates GI motility) or IV. Widely distributed in tissues. Excreted in the bile and urine; some is inactivated in the liver.
- Toxicity and side effects—GI symptoms (nausea, vomiting, abdominal cramps, diarrhoea) are common; skin rash, fever, eosinophilia, cholestatic jaundice, transient hearing loss, QT prolongation, torsades de pointes, candidiasis, pseudomembranous colitis, infantile pyloric stenosis.

Clarithromycin

- Structure—14-membered ring with a methoxy group at position 6.
- Mode of action—same as erythromycin. More active than erythromycin against *S. pneumoniae*, GAS, MRSA, *M. catarrhalis*, and *L. pneumophila*. Also active against *Mycobacterium leprae*, *Mycobacterium avium* complex (MAC), and *Toxoplasma gondii*.
- Resistance—similar to erythromycin.
- Clinical use—similar to erythromycin. Treatment of MAC and other non-tuberculous mycobacteria (NTM) infections, *H. pylori* eradication, Lyme disease.
- Pharmacology—given PO or IV. Metabolized in the liver to active metabolites.

Azithromycin

- Structure—15-membered lactone ring (azalide).
- Mode of action—same as erythromycin. Greater activity against Gram-negative species than with erythromycin and clarithromcyin. Also active against MAC and *T. gondii*.
- Resistance—similar to erythromycin.

- Clinical use—similar to erythromycin. Also used for treatment of trachoma, *Babesia microti*, *Borrelia burgdorferi*, cryptosporidiosis.
- Pharmacology—given PO, but should be taken 1h before or 2h after food. Widely distributed in tissues, with a half-life of 2–4 days. Mostly not metabolized and excreted in the bile.
- Toxicity and side effects—similar to erythromycin.

Spiramycin

- Used in treatment of cryptosporidia and prevention of congenital toxoplasmosis.

Lincosamides

This group of antibiotics includes lincomycin (not available in the UK) and clindamycin. Lincomycin was isolated from *Streptomyces lincolnensis* in 1962. Clindamycin, which was produced by the chemical modification of lincomycin, has better PO bioavailability and increased bacterial potency, compared to lincomycin. Although chemically unrelated to erythromycin, many of the biological properties of lincosamides are similar to those of macrolides.

Mode of action

Lincosamides inhibit protein synthesis by interacting with the peptidyl transferase site of the 50S ribosomal subunit. They also inhibit the formation of the 50S ribosomal subunit. Clindamycin is highly active against anaerobes (e.g. *B. fragilis*), pneumococci, GAS, meticillin-sensitive *S. aureus* (MSSA), *T. gondii*, and *Plasmodium falciparum*.

Resistance

There are several resistance mechanisms.
- Alteration of 50S ribosomal proteins of the receptor site confers resistance to macrolides and lincosamides.
- Alteration in the 23S subunit by methylation of adenine results in the MLS_B phenotype (see Box 2.2) and confers resistance to MLS_B. This MLS_B phenotype is encoded by *erm* genes.
- Inactivation by 3-lincomycin, 4-clindamycin *O*-nucleotidyltransferase. This is plasmid-mediated and encoded by *linA* and *linA'* genes.
- Decreased membrane permeability in Gram-negative species (e.g. *Enterobacterales*, *Pseudomonas* spp., *Acinetobacter* spp.).

Clinical use

- Alternative to β-lactams in penicillin-allergic patients with skin and soft tissue infections.
- Staphylococcal bone and joint infections.
- Severe GAS infections (e.g. necrotizing fasciitis, toxic shock syndrome (TSS)).
- Anaerobic infections (e.g. intra-abdominal sepsis, anaerobic bronchopulmonary infections).
- *P. jirovecii* pneumonia (in combination with primaquine).
- *P. falciparum* malaria (in combination with quinine).

Pharmacology

- Clindamycin is given PO or IV, or by deep IM injection.
- Well absorbed PO and widely distributed, with good tissue penetration, especially bone. CSF penetration is negligible.
- Most of the drug is metabolized to products with variable antibacterial activity.
- Excreted in the bile and urine—dose modification required in severe renal and liver disease.

Toxicity and side effects

- *C. difficile* colitis—discontinue clindamycin.
- Allergic reactions—rashes, fever, erythema multiforme, anaphylaxis.
- Laboratory abnormalities—transient hepatitis, neutropenia, thrombocytopenia.

Streptogramins

Streptogramins are a group of antibiotics derived from various *Streptomyces* spp. They consist of two macrocyclic lactone peptolide components referred to as streptogramin A and streptogramin B. Two key agents are in clinical use:

- pristinamycin (used for treatment of skin and soft tissue infections)
- quinupristin/dalfopristin (Synercid ®, a combination available only in IV formulation)

Mode of action

Streptogramins exert their action on the second stage of protein synthesis. The two components act synergistically:

- streptogramin A molecules bind to the 50S ribosomal subunit and prevent aminoacyl-transfer RNA (tRNA) from attaching to the catalytic site of the peptidyl transferase, thus inhibiting transfer of the growing peptide chain;
- streptogramin B molecules prevent the peptide bond from forming, resulting in the premature release of incomplete polypeptides.

Resistance

- Modification of the ribosomal target site results in resistance to MLS_B (the MLS_B phenotype), which is encoded by various *erm* genes (➔ see Lincosamides, pp. 56–7; see Box 2.2).
- Enzymatic inactivation by acetyltransferases, encoded by *vat(A)*, *vat(B)*, and *vat(C)* in staphylococci, and by *vat(D)* in *E. faecium*; active transport out of cells by efflux pumps, encoded by *vga(A)* and *vga(B)* in staphylococci.

Clinical use

- Vancomycin-resistant *E. faecium* (not active against *E. faecalis*).
- Serious Gram-positive infections where there is no alternative antibiotic available.

Pharmacology

- Wide volume of distribution, but poor CSF penetration.

Toxicity and side effects

- Commonest side effect is injection site reactions that occur in >30%, so the drug should be given via a central vein.
- Inhibition of hepatic CYP3A4.

Lipopeptides

Daptomycin, a fermentation product of *Streptomyces roseosporus*, was discovered in the 1980s. It is a 13-membered cyclic amino acid lipopeptide antibiotic with a lipophilic tail. It was approved in the UK in 2003 for the treatment of complicated skin and soft tissue infections.

Mode of action

The exact mechanism of action is unknown, although it appears to bind to the cell membrane of Gram-positive bacteria in a calcium-dependent manner, disrupting the cell membrane potential. Daptomycin is active against Gram-positive organisms (e.g. staphylococci and streptococci), including those that are glycopeptide-resistant.

Resistance

Resistance to daptomycin is rare, but strains with reduced susceptibility have been obtained after serial passage *in vitro*.

Clinical use

Daptomycin is used for complicated skin and soft tissue infections caused by Gram-positive bacteria. It is also licensed for right-sided endocarditis caused by *S. aureus*, administered on expert advice.

Pharmacology

Daptomycin is given by IV infusion. The area under the curve (AUC)/MIC profile and prolonged PAE enable od dosing. Daptomycin is highly protein-bound and is eliminated largely unchanged by the kidneys.

Toxicity and side effects

- Common side effects—nausea, vomiting, diarrhoea, headache, rash, injection site reactions.
- Muscle toxicity—myalgia, muscle weakness, and myositis are uncommon; rhabdomyolysis is rare. Serum creatine kinase (CK) should be checked before starting treatment, and weekly during treatment. Stop treatment if symptoms develop.
- Interference with prothrombin time (PT)/international normalized ratio (INR) assay—clotting sample should be taken just prior to administration of daptomycin.

Oxazolidinones

Oxazolidinones are a purely synthetic class of antimicrobials with activity against staphylococcal and streptococcal species. Linezolid was introduced in 2001. It is active against Gram-positive bacteria and is used for infections that are resistant to other antibiotics (e.g. MRSA, VRE). Always involve an infection specialist when initiating therapy.

Mode of action

Oxazolidinones are protein synthesis inhibitors that are bacteriostatic against Gram-positive organisms. They bind to the 50S ribosomal subunit at its interface with the 30S ribosomal subunit, preventing formation of the 70S initiation complex.

Resistance

Despite its recent introduction, resistance to linezolid among strains of MRSA and VRE has already been reported. The mechanism appears to be mutation in the 23S RNA domain V region. It is usually associated with long durations of therapy or prior exposure to linezolid.

Clinical use

* Linezolid is approved for use in Gram-positive pneumonia and complicated skin/soft tissue infections, and serious infections due to resistant Gram-positive bacteria (e.g. MRSA, VRE, penicillin-resistant pneumococci).
* Tedizolid is a related agent currently approved for acute Gram-positive skin and skin structure infections only.

Pharmacology

Linezolid may be given PO (100% bioavailability) or IV. Linezolid is widely distributed, with good tissue and CSF penetration. It is metabolized by oxidation in the liver and excreted in the urine (85%) or faeces. No dose adjustment is required for renal or hepatic disease. It is given bd; tedizolid is given daily.

Toxicity and side effects

Linezolid is generally well tolerated.

* GI symptoms (e.g. nausea, vomiting, diarrhoea) are common.
* Myelosuppression—thrombocytopenia, neutropenia, and pancytopenia have been reported. Commoner with prolonged therapy (>10 days) and usually reversible. Full blood count (FBC) should be monitored weekly in patients taking linezolid.
* Monoamine oxidase inhibition—linezolid is a monoamine oxidase inhibitor. Patients should be told to avoid tyramine-rich foods. Linezolid has been associated with serotonin syndrome in patients taking concomitant selective serotonin reuptake inhibitors (SSRIs).
* Optic neuropathy has been reported in patients taking >28 days' treatment. Patients should be told to report visual symptoms and referred to an ophthalmologist, if necessary.
* Lactic acidosis has been associated with prolonged treatment.

Chloramphenicol

Chloramphenicol, initially called Chloromycetin®, was first isolated from *Streptomyces venezuelae* in 1947. It has a broad spectrum of activity against a wide range of bacteria, spirochaetes, rickettsiae, chlamydiae, and mycoplasmas. Soon after its introduction in 1949, reports of aplastic anaemia emerged, limiting its use. Furthermore, widespread use in the developing world has resulted in resistance, particularly in *Salmonella* typhi. Despite this, chloramphenicol remains useful for the treatment of serious infections that are resistant to other antibiotics.

Mode of action

Chloramphenicol inhibits protein synthesis by binding to the 50S subunit of the 70S ribosome at a site that prevents the attachment of tRNA—this prevents association of the amino acid with peptidyl transferase and peptide band formation. This is a bacteriostatic effect in most organisms but is bactericidal in some meningeal pathogens (e.g. *H. influenzae*, *S. pneumoniae*, *N. meningitidis*).

Resistance

There are several resistance mechanisms:
- reduced permeability or uptake;
- ribosomal mutation;
- production of acetyltransferase, an enzyme that acetylates the antibiotic into an inactive form. This mechanism also confers resistance to tetracyclines (⊙ see Tetracyclines, pp. 61–3) and is responsible for widespread epidemics of chloramphenicol resistance to *S. typhi* and *Shigella dysenteriae* seen in the developing world.

Clinical use

In the developed world, chloramphenicol is rarely used (because of toxicity), but it remains a commonly used antibiotic in the developing world.
- Enteric fever due to *S. typhi* and *S. paratyphi*—high rates of drug resistance have been reported in India, Vietnam, and Central and South America.
- Severe infections, such as meningitis, septicaemia, and epiglottitis, due to *H. influenzae*.
- Sometimes used in infective exacerbations of chronic obstructive pulmonary disease (COPD).
- An alternative agent for infections in pregnancy, young children, or patients with immediate penicillin hypersensitivity.
- Eye drops/ointment are widely used for superficial eye infections.
- Ear drops are used for bacterial otitis externa.

Pharmacology

Chloramphenicol may be administered PO, IV, IM, or TOP. It has high lipid solubility and low protein binding, resulting in a wide volume of distribution in body fluids and tissues. CSF and ocular penetration is good. Chloramphenicol is metabolized in the liver by glucuronidation and excreted in the bile. Only 5–10% is excreted in the urine.

Toxicity and side effects

- Bone marrow suppression is common, dose-related, and reversible. It is a direct pharmacological effect of the antibiotic, resulting from inhibition of mitochondrial protein synthesis. Manifestations include anaemia, reticulocytosis, leucopenia, and thrombocytopenia. Monitor FBC twice weekly during treatment.

- Aplastic anaemia is a rare, idiosyncratic, and often fatal complication, which may occur during or after completion of therapy. It occurs in 1 in 25 000–40 000 patients. The pathogenesis of this condition is incompletely understood. Monitor FBC twice weekly during treatment, and discontinue the drug if the white cell count (WCC) falls below $2.5 \times 10^9/L$.
- There are also reports of haemolytic anaemia in patients with glucose-6-phosphate dehydrogenase (G6PD) deficiency and childhood leukaemia after chloramphenicol therapy.
- Grey baby syndrome—high doses in neonates may result in grey baby syndrome (abdominal distension, vomiting, cyanosis, circulatory collapse) due to inability to metabolize and excrete the drug. If the drug is required in neonates, the dose should be reduced and drug levels monitored.
- Other side effects—rash, fever, Jarisch–Herxheimer reactions, GI symptoms, glossitis, stomatitis, optic neuritis, bleeding disorders, acute intermittent porphyria, interference with development of immunity after immunization.

Tetracyclines

Tetracyclines are a group of broad-spectrum bacteriostatic antibiotics active against Gram-positive, Gram-negative, and intracellular organisms (e.g. *Chlamydophila*, mycoplasmas, rickettsiae, and protozoan parasites). The first tetracycline chlortetracycline was isolated from *Streptomyces aureofaciens*, a soil organism. Since then, a number of other tetracyclines have been developed. Tetracyclines differ in their pharmacological properties, rather than in their spectrum of cover, although minocycline has a slightly broader spectrum.

Classification

- First generation—tetracycline, chlortetracycline, oxytetracycline, demeclocycline, lymecycline, and metacycline.
- Second generation—doxycycline and minocycline.
- Third generation (glycylcyclines)—tigecycline.

Mode of action

- Tetracyclines inhibit bacterial protein synthesis by reversibly binding to the 30S ribosomal subunit. This blocks binding of aminoacyl-tRNA to the ribosomal 'A' site, preventing the addition of new amino acids. As their binding is reversible, these agents are mainly bacteriostatic.
- Tetracyclines also inhibit mitochondrial protein synthesis by binding to 70S ribosomal subunits in mitochondria in eukaryotic parasites. The mechanism of their antiprotozoal activity is unknown.

Resistance

The widespread use of tetracyclines has been accompanied by increasing drug resistance. This is mediated by acquisition of genes on mobile genetic elements (MGEs) (see Molecular genetics of resistance, pp. 12–15). Many tetracycline resistance genes have been identified; most belong to the *tet* family, and some belong to the *otr* family. These genes confer resistance by the following mechanisms:

- efflux pumps—these membrane-associated proteins pump tetracyclines out of the cell. They confer resistance to first-generation tetracyclines;
- ribosomal protection proteins are cytoplasmic proteins that release tetracyclines from their binding site by guanosine diphosphate (GDP)-dependent mechanisms. They protect the ribosome from first- and second-generation tetracyclines;
- enzymatic inactivation—this mechanism is seen in *B. fragilis* where the *tet(X)* gene codes for a protein that modifies tetracyclines in the presence of nicotinamide adenine dinucleotide phosphate (NADPH) oxidase and oxygen.

Clinical use

- Chlamydial infections—trachoma, psittacosis, salpingitis, urethritis, lymphogranuloma venereum (LGV).
- Rickettsial infections.
- Q fever.
- Brucellosis (doxycycline with either streptomycin or rifampicin).
- Lyme disease (*B. burgdorferi*).
- *Mycoplasma* spp. infections.
- Infective exacerbations of COPD (due to their activity against *H. influenzae*).
- Also used in acne, destructive (refractory) periodontal diseases, sinusitis, chronic prostatitis, pelvic inflammatory disease (PID), and melioidosis.

Pharmacology

- Tetracyclines are usually given PO. Absorption of tetracycline and oxytetracycline is reduced by milk, antacids, and some salts. Doxycycline and minocycline are highly bioavailable.
- They are sometimes divided into three groups on the basis of their half-lives: short-acting (tetracycline, oxytetracycline), intermediate-acting (demeclocycline), and long-acting (doxycycline, minocycline).
- Tetracyclines are widely distributed and show good tissue penetration.
- Tetracycline is eliminated in the urine. Minocycline is metabolized in the liver. Doxycycline is mainly eliminated in the faeces.

Toxicity and side effects

- Nausea, vomiting, diarrhoea, dysphagia, and oesophageal irritation are common.
- Photosensitivity reactions are common and appear to be toxic, rather than allergic.
- Prolonged minocycline administration can cause skin, nail, and scleral pigmentation.
- Deposition occurs in growing bones and teeth, so tetracyclines should not be given to children aged <12 years or pregnant/breastfeeding women.
- Hepatotoxicity due to fatty change may be fatal.
- Tetracyclines exacerbate renal impairment. All tetracyclines (except minocycline and doxycycline) should be avoided in renal failure.

Demeclocycline causes nephrogenic diabetes insipidus and is used for treatment of inappropriate antidiuretic hormone (ADH) secretion.
* Vertigo is unique to minocycline.
* Benign intracranial hypertension has been described with all tetracyclines.
* Superinfection—mucocutaneous candidiasis is common. *C. difficile* colitis may occur.
* Allergic reactions (rashes, urticaria, anaphylaxis) are uncommon.

Tigecycline

* A glycylcycline antibiotic, structurally related to tetracyclines.
* Active against Gram-positive and Gram-negative bacteria, including tetracycline-resistant organisms, and some anaerobes. It is also active against MRSA and VRE, but not against *P. aeruginosa* and *Proteus* spp.
* Reserved for treatment of complicated skin and soft tissue infections, and complicated abdominal infections caused by multidrug-resistant (MDR) organisms. The UK Medicines and Healthcare products Regulatory Agency (MHRA) and the US Food and Drug Administration (FDA) advise use only if it is known or suspected that other antibiotics are unsuitable—pooled analysis of phase 3 and 4 trials suggested higher death rates in patients receiving tigecycline, compared to those receiving comparator drugs.
* Side effects are similar to those of tetracyclines.

Sulfonamides

Prontosil was discovered in 1932, the result of 5 years of testing dyes for antimicrobial activity. It exerted its antibacterial effect through the release of sulfanilamide, an analogue of para-aminobenzoic acid (PABA). PABA is essential for bacterial folate synthesis. Although many sulfonamide drugs were developed, relatively few are in clinical use today, mainly because of their toxicity and increasing drug resistance. Those currently available in the UK include sulfamethoxazole, sulfadiazine, sulfadoxine, sulfasalazine, mafenide acetate, and sulfacetamide sodium.

Classification

Sulfonamides can be classified as follows:
* short-/medium-acting sulfonamides (e.g. sulfamethoxazole, sulfadiazine);
* long-acting sulfonamides (e.g. sulfadoxine);
* sulfonamides limited to the GI tract (e.g. sulfasalazine);
* topical sulfonamides (e.g. silver sulfadiazine, mafenide acetate, sulfacetamide sodium).

Mode of action

Sulfonamides inhibit bacterial growth by competitive inhibition of the incorporation of PABA into tetrahydropteroic acid by the enzyme tetrahydropteroic acid synthetase. They are bacteriostatic and slow to act—several generations of bacterial growth are required to deplete the folate pool. They are active against a broad spectrum of Gram-positive and Gram-negative bacteria, *Actinomyces*, *Chlamydophila*, *Plasmodium*, and *Toxoplasma* spp. Activity against enterococci (which are auxotrophic for folic acid), *Pseudomonas* spp. (possess drug efflux pumps), and anaerobes is poor.

Resistance

Resistance to sulfonamides is widespread and increasingly common; cross-resistance between different sulfonamides occurs. Resistance may be due to:

- chromosomal mutations that result in overproduction of PABA (e.g. *S. aureus, N. gonorrhoeae*) or alterations in dihydropteroate synthetase, leading to reduced affinity for sulfonamides (e.g. *E. coli*);
- plasmids that carry genes coding for the production of drug-resistant enzymes or decreased bacterial permeability.

Plasmid-mediated sulfonamide resistance is common in *Enterobacterales* and has increased greatly in recent years, often in conjunction with trimethoprim resistance.

Clinical use

They have only a limited role as single-agent antimicrobials but are still found in combination products with trimethoprim, pyrimethamine, etc. Sulfasalazine is used for its anti-inflammatory properties (e.g. in ulcerative colitis, rheumatoid arthritis)—which are probably a result of its breakdown product 5-aminosalicylic acid.

- Sulfadiazine is used in combination with pyrimethamine (➡ see Antiprotozoal drugs, pp. 128–33) for toxoplasmosis (unlicensed).
- Sulfadoxine is used in combination with pyrimethamine for treatment of falciparum malaria (➡ see Antimalarials, pp. 120–1).
- Silver sulfadiazine is used TOP to prevent/treat burn infections. Its activity is likely to owe much to the silver component.
- Sulfacetamide is used TOP in eye drops.

Pharmacology

- Usually administered PO. Sulfadiazine and sulfisoxazole are available as IV or subcutaneous (s/c) preparations.
- PO sulfonamides are rapidly absorbed. TOP sulfonamides are also absorbed and may be detectable in blood.
- Widely distributed, with high concentrations in body fluids, including the CSF.
- Metabolized in the liver and excreted in the urine. Dose modification is required in renal impairment.

Toxicity and side effects

Around 3% of people experience some form of side effect, much higher in patients with HIV. Hypersensitivity reactions are usually a class effect.

- General—nausea, vomiting, diarrhoea, rash, fever, headache, depression, jaundice, hepatic necrosis, drug-induced lupus, serum sickness-like syndrome.
- Haematological—acute haemolytic anaemia, aplastic anaemia, agranulocytosis, leucopenia, thrombocytopenia.

- Hypersensitivity reactions—drug eruption, vasculitis, erythema nodosum, erythema multiforme, Stevens–Johnson syndrome, anaphylaxis.
- Neonatal kernicterus if given in the last month of pregnancy.

Trimethoprim

Trimethoprim is a diaminopyrimidine. The other members of this class are pyrimethamine (an antiprotozoal), cycloguanil (a product of proguanil; ➔ see Antimalarials, pp. 120–1), and flucytosine (an antifungal). Trimethoprim has a fairly broad spectrum of activity against many Gram-positive bacteria and most Gram-negative rods, except *P. aeruginosa* and *Bacteroides* spp.

Mode of action

Trimethoprim inhibits the bacterial enzyme dihydrofolate reductase (DHFR), preventing the conversion of dihydrofolate to the active form of the vitamin tetrahydrofolate (➔ see Sulfonamides, pp. 63–5). It works on the pathway at a later point than sulfonamides, and their combination is synergistic. It is bactericidal or bacteriostatic, depending on the organism and drug concentration.

Resistance

Resistance is common in *Enterobacterales*. May be caused by:
- chromosomal mutations in the gene for DHFR (or its promoter), resulting in overproduction or modification of the target enzyme;
- plasmid-encoded resistance (e.g. *dfr* genes in *Enterobacterales*, producing an additional trimethoprim-resistant DHFR enzyme);
- change in cell permeability/efflux pumps;
- alterations in metabolic pathway.

More than one mechanism can occur in the same cell, resulting in higher resistance levels.

Clinical use

- UTIs—treatment and prophylaxis.
- Treatment of prostatitis and epididymo-orchitis.
- Option for PO MRSA treatment (in combination with rifampicin or fusidic acid).

Pharmacology

- Trimethoprim is given PO and is rapidly absorbed from the gut.
- Widely distributed in tissues and body fluids, including the CSF. High concentrations are achieved in the kidney, lung, sputum, and prostatic fluid.
- Sixty to 80% is excreted in the urine within 24h, with the remainder excreted as urinary metabolites or in the bile.
- Synergy with sulfamethoxazole, polymyxins, and aminoglycosides.

Toxicity and side effects

- Avoid in pregnancy, especially the first trimester (antifolate).
- Contraindicated in blood dyscrasias.
- Side effects are similar to those of co-trimoxazole, but less severe and less frequent with trimethoprim alone.
- Other side effects include GI disturbance, pruritus, rashes, and hyperkalaemia.
- Known to decrease the tubular secretion of creatinine, which can lead to rises in serum creatinine concentration that do not reflect a true fall in the glomerular filtration rate (GFR).

Co-trimoxazole

Co-trimoxazole is a synergistic combination of trimethoprim and sulfamethoxazole, in a ratio of 1:5.

Mode of action

Sequential inhibition of two enzymes (tetrahydropteroic acid synthetase and dihydrofolate reductase) in the bacterial folate synthesis pathway (➔ see Sulfonamides, pp. 63–5).

Resistance

Resistance may be due to a variety of mechanisms (for details, ➔ see Sulfonamides, pp. 63–5; ➔ see Trimethoprim, pp. 65–6). Increasing drug resistance rates have been seen in *S. aureus*, many *Enterobacterales*, and *Pneumocystis jirovecii*.

Clinical use

Apart from the following exceptions, consider using standard trimethoprim when possible—it is often as effective an antibacterial as co-trimoxazole, with fewer side effects:

- *P. jirovecii* pneumonia (treatment and prophylaxis);
- toxoplasmosis (prophylaxis and second-line therapy);
- nocardiosis (second-line therapy);
- MDR organisms (e.g. *Acinetobacter* spp., *B. cepacia*, *S. maltophilia*, *Mycobacterium marinum*, *Mycobacterium kansasii*). Seek advice from an infection specialist;
- acute exacerbations of COPD (if sensitive and no other options);
- UTIs (if sensitive and no other options);
- acute otitis media in children (if sensitive and no other options).

Pharmacology

Co-trimoxazole may be given PO or IV. PO bioavailability is around 85%. Components have different volumes of distribution, so seek advice if treating complicated cases (e.g. at an unusual site).

Toxicity and side effects

Avoid in blood disorders, infants aged <6 weeks, hepatic impairment, renal impairment, pregnancy, and breastfeeding. Side effects are mainly due to the sulfonamide component, may be more severe in the elderly, and

are more frequent in those with HIV. See also individual agents (➔ see Sulfonamides, pp. 63–5; ➔ see Trimethoprim, pp. 65–6).
- Common: nausea, vomiting, diarrhoea, anorexia, and hypersensitivity.
- Rashes: rare but can be severe, including erythema multiforme, Stevens–Johnson syndrome, and toxic epidermal necrolysis.
- Other: haematological toxicity, renal dysfunction, interstitial nephritis, hyperkalaemia, drug-induced hepatitis, pancreatitis, and hepatic failure.
- Patients with low urine output and low urine pH may be at increased risk of urinary tract crystal formation due to the sulfa component.

Quinolones

Nalidixic acid, the first quinolone antibiotic, was produced as a side product of attempts to manufacture chloroquine. The majority of quinolones now in use are fluoroquinolones (fluorine atom attached to the central molecular ring) with an expanded spectrum of activity and greater potency. In 2024 the UK MHRA issued an alert advising that this antibiotic group should only be used when others are inappropriate (https://www.gov.uk/drug-safety-update/fluoroquinolone-antibiotics-must-now-only-be-prescribed-when-other-commonly-recommended-antibiotics-are-inappropriate).

Mode of action

The only antibiotics in clinical use that directly inhibit bacterial DNA synthesis. This is via inhibition of DNA gyrase (primary target in Gram-negatives) and topoisomerase IV (primary target in Gram-positives). DNA gyrase consists of α- and β-subunits (encoded by the *gyrA* and *gyrB* genes, respectively), and is responsible for DNA supercoiling. Topoisomerase IV also consists of two subunits, encoded by the *parC* and *parE* genes, and is involved in DNA relaxation and chromosomal segregation. Quinolones bind to the complex of enzyme with DNA, blocking progress of the DNA replication enzyme and damaging bacterial DNA—they are thus bactericidal.

Resistance

The likelihood of developing resistance is related to the duration of therapy (as little as 5 days in *in vitro* conditions) and may be a result of:
- spontaneous chromosomal mutations occurring in genes that either alter target enzymes (with increasing resistance occurring by selection of resistant strains produced by sequential mutations in *gyrA*, *gyrB*, *parC*, or *parE*) or alter cell membrane permeability by mutations that reduce entry through porin channels or increase efflux. In *P. aeruginosa*, resistance has been shown to be due to overexpression of genes that encode the MexAB–OprM efflux pump;
- plasmid-encoded proteins (e.g. Qnr proteins that protect DNA gyrase from quinolone action). They have been reported in *K. pneumoniae*, *E. coli*, *Enterobacter*, and other enteric bacteria. While alone conferring only low-level resistance, they are often found in strains with additional chromosomal mutations leading to high-level MDR. Other plasmid-mediated mechanisms include efflux pumps (QepA) and antibiotic-modifying enzymes;
- acquired fluoroquinolone resistance which may be seen with MRSA and *P. aeruginosa*. They are no longer recommended for the treatment of gonorrhoea in the UK or the USA, and treatment failures are well recognized with *S. typhi* strains of decreased susceptibility.

Clinical use

- The greatest activity of quinolones is against aerobic Gram-negative bacilli (*Enterobacterales*, *Haemophilus* spp., and certain Gram-negative cocci, e.g. *Neisseria* spp.).
- Fluoroquinolones are active against non-enteric Gram-negatives (e.g. *P. aeruginosa*), staphylococci, and the common causes of atypical pneumonia (*L. pneumophilia*, *M. pneumoniae*, *C. pneumoniae*).
  - Ciprofloxacin is the most potent against Gram-negatives but has limited activity against streptococci (see Box 2.3).
  - Levofloxacin (the active *L*-racemer of ofloxacin) is more potent against Gram-positives but sacrifices some *Pseudomonas* activity.
  - Moxifloxacin has enhanced activity against anaerobes and streptococci, but further loss of activity against *P. aeruginosa* (not reliable for clinical treatment), *Proteus* spp., and *Serratia marcescens*, compared to ciprofloxacin.
  - Mycobacteria—great potential in the treatment of resistant TB (moxifloxacin has early bactericidal activity similar to that of ethambutol in patients with pulmonary TB); active against a number of NTM species (➋ see Non-tuberculous mycobacteria, pp. 397–401).
  - Delafloxacin is active against Gram-positives (including MRSA) and Gram-negatives, and is used for acute bacterial skin and skin structure infections is standard therapy is inappropriate.
- Note that activity against enterococci is marginal, and while most MSSA strains are sensitive, many MRSA strains have high-level resistance to the class as a whole.
- Not recommended for routine use in those aged <18 years (animal studies demonstrate arthropathy), but often used in those with CF and complicated UTIs, under specialist guidance.

Pharmacology

- Well absorbed, with bioavailability ranging from 50% to 100%. PO bioavailability is reduced by co-administration of antacids.
- Moxifloxacin, nalidixic acid, and norfloxacin are only given PO; ciprofloxacin and levofloxacin may also be given IV. Protein binding is low, and volumes of distribution are high. Concentrations in the prostate, lung, bile, and faecal samples may exceed plasma concentrations.
- Ofloxacin and levofloxacin, are renally eliminated. Nalidixic acid and moxifloxacin undergo hepatic metabolism. Most others are excreted by renal and non-renal pathways. Dose adjustments may be required in renal or liver disease.

Box 2.3 Indications for consideration of higher-dose ciprofloxacin

Serious infections in which antibiotic penetration may be suboptimal (e.g. septic arthritis, osteomyelitis, pseudomonal pneumonia, neurological and intraocular infections).

Toxicity and side effects

- GI—common (3–17%; e.g. nausea, vomiting, abdominal discomfort, diarrhoea—risk factor for *C. difficile* disease).
- CNS (0.9–11%; e.g. headache, dizziness, insomnia, altered mood). Rarely hallucinations, delirium, seizures (lower threshold in those prone to them, thus should not be given to epileptics), and profound muscle weakness in those with myasthenia gravis (avoid use).
- Allergic reactions—rash, photosensitivity, drug fever, urticaria, angio-oedema, vasculitis, serum sickness, interstitial nephritis.
- Arthropathy and tendon rupture (usually Achilles) in adults. Not recommended in adults with a history of tendon disorders.
- Arrhythmias—moxifloxacin is contraindicated in those with risk factors for prolonged QT, and other agents should be used with caution.
- Laboratory abnormalities (vary with agents) include leucopenia, eosinophilia, hepatitis (severe with moxifloxacin), and dysglycaemia.

Nitroimidazoles

Metronidazole

The imidazoles are remarkable in that members of the class are effective across the whole microbiological spectrum: bacteria, fungi, protozoa, and helminths. Metronidazole, a 5-nitroimidazole, was introduced for the treatment of *Trichomonas vaginalis* infections in 1959 and subsequently found to be bactericidal for most anaerobic and facultatively anaerobic bacteria (when a patient's acute ulcerative gingivitis 'spontaneously' improved while receiving therapy) and protozoa. Related compounds (e.g. tinidazole) share its properties but have longer half-lives.

Mode of action

Metronidazole has a low molecular weight and enters the bacterial cell by passive diffusion. It is a pro-drug and activated intracellularly by reduction of its nitro group by a nitroreductase under conditions achievable only in anaerobes. The highly reactive resulting compounds interact with nucleic acids and proteins, causing breakage, destabilization, and cell death.

Resistance

Resistance to metronidazole is rare, and a combination of mechanisms is required. Both chromosomally mediated and plasmid-mediated resistance have been described. Reports of resistance in *Bacteroides* spp. have been attributed to the transferable genes *nimA* and *nimD*. Metronidazole resistance in *H. pylori* is associated with mutational inactivation of the *rdxA*, *frxA*, and *fdxB* genes. Metronidazole resistance in *T. vaginalis* and *Giardia* is probably multifactorial, with reduced activation of metronidazole and/or reduced transcription of the ferredoxin gene.

Clinical use

- Parasitic infections (e.g. bacterial vaginosis, intestinal amoebiasis, giardiasis, amoebic liver abscess).
- Anaerobic infections, including *C. difficile* colitis, *H. pylori* eradication therapy, small bowel bacterial overgrowth, pouchitis (inflammatory

bowel disease (IBD)), infected leg ulcers and pressure sores, PID, dental infections, and acute ulcerative gingivitis (see Box 2.4).
• Surgical prophylaxis.

Box 2.4 Antibiotics with anaerobic cover

If your patient is on one of the following drugs, seek advice about whether it is necessary to continue metronidazole:
• co-amoxiclav;
• meropenem;
• clindamycin;
• piperacillin–tazobactam.

Pharmacology

• Metronidazole may be given PO, IV, per vagina (PV), per rectum (PR), or TOP. **It should never be taken with alcohol because of the risk of a disulfiram-like reaction (➲ see Toxicity and side effects below).**
• When given PO, it is absorbed rapidly and almost completely.
• Protein binding is low, and the drug is widely distributed in fluids and tissues. Metronidazole shows excellent penetration into abscesses.
• It is metabolized in the liver by the CYP450 enzyme system.
• Metronidazole and its metabolites are primarily eliminated by the kidneys.

Toxicity and side effects

• Metronidazole is generally well tolerated.
• Abnormal metallic taste is commonly reported.
• GI—nausea, anorexia, epigastric discomfort, vomiting, diarrhoea, constipation.
• Peripheral neuropathy occurs with prolonged treatment.
• Disulfiram-like reaction with alcohol (e.g. nausea, vomiting, flushing, tachycardia, hypotension, acute confusion/psychosis, sudden death).
• GU—transient darkening of the urine, dysuria, cystitis, incontinence.
• Allergic reactions—rash, urticaria, flushing, bronchospasm, serum sickness.
• CNS symptoms include headache, dizziness, syncope, vertigo, sleep disturbance, confusion, excitation, and depression. Cerebellar toxicity has been seen with high doses and/or prolonged therapy.
• Other—fever, mucocutaneous candidiasis, neutropenia, thrombophlebitis with IV infusion.

Nitrofurans

The nitrofuran group of antibiotics comprises nitrofurantoin, furazolidone, and nitrofurazone (the latter two are not available in the UK).

Mode of action

The mechanism of action is poorly understood but requires enzymatic reduction within the bacterial cell (like metronidazole). The reduced derivatives bind to ribosomal proteins and block translation. They also appear to directly damage bacterial DNA (like quinolones) and inhibit DNA repair. Nitrofurans are bactericidal against urinary pathogens such as *E. coli*, *Citrobacter*, group B *Streptococcus* (GBS), *Staphylococcus saprophyticus*, *E. faecalis*, and *E. faecium*. However, note that only a minority of *Enterobacter* spp. are sensitive, and most members of *Proteus*, *Providencia*, *Morganella*, *Serratia*, *Acinetobacter*, and *Pseudomonas* spp. are resistant.

Resistance

Resistance is rare. In *E. coli*, resistance may be chromosomal or plasmid-mediated, and is associated with inhibition of nitrofuran reductase activity.

Clinical use

It is rapidly excreted into the urine after PO absorption and achieves no useful blood or tissue level. It is therefore restricted to the treatment of lower UTIs in those with adequate renal function:

- acute uncomplicated cystitis (not pyelonephritis)—3 days;
- treatment of recurrent UTIs—7 days;
- prophylaxis of recurrent UTIs.

Pharmacology

- Nitrofurantoin has good PO absorption, which is enhanced by food.
- Serum concentrations are low, but urine concentrations are high.
- Activity is enhanced by acid conditions

Toxicity and side effects

- GI—nausea, vomiting.
- Pulmonary—acute hypersensitivity (fever, cough, dyspnoea, pulmonary infiltrates, myalgia, eosinophilia), chronic (pulmonary fibrosis, bronchiolitis obliterans organizing pneumonia).

Novobiocin

It acts on the β-subunit of DNA gyrase (like quinolones). It is used in the diagnostic microbiology laboratory to identify *S. saprophyticus* (coagulase-negative, novobiocin-resistant), a urinary pathogen.

Rifamycins

These are semi-synthetic derivatives of rifamycin B, one of a number of antibiotic compounds produced by *Streptomyces mediterranei*. They bind to the β-subunit of DNA-dependent RNA polymerase, resulting in inhibition and bactericidal activity against a variety of bacteria. Resistance arises readily by mutation in the *rpoB* gene (encoding the subunit), and they are therefore used in combination with other agents to suppress the emergence of resistance. They stimulate hepatic metabolism by the CYP450 enzyme system and are primarily excreted in the bile.

Rifampicin (rifampin)

This is the most important rifamycin and is widely used for the treatment of TB, leprosy, and other bacterial infections.

- Activity—bactericidal against *S. aureus* (including MRSA), GAS, *S. pneumoniae*, *N. gonorrhoeae*, *N. meningitidis*, *H. influenzae*, MTB, *M. kansasii*, *M. marinum*, *M. leprae*, *Legionella* spp., *L. monocytogenes*, and *Brucella* spp.
- Clinical use—TB, leprosy, serious or device-related infections with antibiotic-resistant staphylococci, pneumococci, *Legionella*, elimination of nasopharyngeal carriage of *N. meningitidis* and *H. influenzae*.
- Pharmacology—>90% PO absorption, widely distributed, low CSF penetration unless meningeal inflammation, metabolized in the liver (CYP450), predominantly excreted in the bile and undergoes enterohepatic circulation, some excreted in the urine. Dose reduction in renal failure.
- Interactions—enhances its own metabolism and that of other drugs (e.g. warfarin, oral contraceptives, corticosteroids, protease inhibitors (PIs)).
- Toxicity and side effects—orange discoloration of body fluids (contact lenses may discolour), skin rashes, GI upset, hepatitis, thrombocytopenia, purpura (stop drug), 'rifampicin flu' 2–3h after taking (worse with intermittent therapy than with daily regimens), 'red man syndrome' (overdose).

Rifabutin

Longer half-life and some activity against rifampicin-resistant organisms. Good *in vitro* activity against MAC.

- Clinical use—prophylaxis against MAC in uncontrolled HIV patients, treatment of NTM disease, and treatment of TB in those who cannot have rifampicin (unacceptable interactions, e.g. with certain antiretrovirals; intolerance).
- Pharmacology—12–20% PO absorption; widely distributed, with concentrations in organs being higher than in plasma.
- Interactions—clarithromycin and ritonavir inhibit CYP450, increasing rifabutin levels.
- Toxicity and side effects—skin rashes, GI upset, hepatitis, neutropenia, uveitis, and arthralgia (with higher doses).

Rifapentine

Not widely used in the UK. Similarly to rifampicin, its prolonged half-life allows once-weekly dosing for the continuation phase of TB treatment in non-cavitary, drug-susceptible, smear-negative (at 2 months) TB. It can be used weekly with isoniazid for supervised treatment of latent TB and may help improve compliance. Should not be given in HIV-infected patients, as it has high treatment failure rates.

- Pharmacology—70% PO absorption; well distributed, with tissue concentrations exceeding plasma concentrations, except in the CSF and bone.
- Interactions—potent inducer of CYP450, resulting in reduced concentrations of co-administered drugs (e.g. PIs).

- Toxicity and side effects—neutropenia, hepatitis, animal evidence of teratogenicity and fetal toxicity (avoid in pregnancy).

Other rifamycins
- Rifamide—used in staphylococcal and biliary infections (limited availability).
- Rifamycin SV—can be given parenterally or TOP (not available in the UK).
- Rifaximin—used in traveller's diarrhoea, hepatic encephalopathy (not available in the UK). May have a role in *C. difficile*-associated disease (CDAD).

Polymyxins

Polymyxins (polymyxin B, and polymyxin E or colistimethate sodium) are produced by *Bacillus polymyxa*. They were used parenterally until the development of aminoglycosides and fell into disuse in the 1980s. With the emergence of MDR Gram-negative organisms (e.g. *Pseudomonas* spp. and *Acinetobacter* spp.), injectable polymyxins began playing a greater role. Colistimethate sodium is available as colistin sulfate (TOP and non-absorbable PO products) and colistimethate sodium (IV). Polymyxin B is available TOP and as a parenteral preparation that can be given IV or IM.

Mode of action
Polymyxins are cyclic cationic polypeptide detergents. They penetrate cell membranes and interact with phospholipids, disrupting the membranes and causing cytoplasmic leakage. They are rapidly bactericidal. The effect is not very selective, explaining their toxicity. Their spectrum of action includes many GNRs (exceptions include *Proteus* spp., *S. marcescens*, *M. catarrhalis*, and *B. cepacia*). Gram-positive bacteria and Gram-negative cocci are inherently resistant. They are primarily used in the treatment of multiresistant *P. aeruginosa* and *A. baumanii*, in which acquired resistance is uncommon.

Clinical use
- Polymyxins are used for the treatment of severe infections caused by MDR Gram-negative organisms (e.g. VAP, joint infection).
- Colistin sulfate has been used for intestinal decontamination.
- Aerosolized colistimethate has been used to treat multiresistant VAP and CF patients with pulmonary colonization or infection with MDR *Pseudomonas* spp.—usually in combination with additional IV agents. There is, however, minimal evidence of outcome benefit of the nebulized route over IV when used in patients with MDR VAP.
- Greater use has seen a rise in resistance—polymyxin-resistant variants of the *K. pneumoniae* KPC clone have been reported from Greece, the UK, and other countries. The British Society for Antimicrobial Chemotherapy (BSAC) Respiratory Surveillance (2011/2012) reported 15% colistin resistance (mostly MIC >64mg/L) in *Enterobacter* spp.

Pharmacology

Not absorbed PO. Good serum levels after IV administration, but poor penetration of the CSF, biliary tract, pleural fluid, and joint fluid. Renally excreted—reduce the dose in renal impairment.

Toxicity and side effects

Dose-related nephrotoxicity and neurotoxicity (paraesthesiae, peripheral neuropathy, and neuromuscular blockade). Bronchospasm with inhalation.

Fusidic acid

Fusidic acid is a member of the fusidane class of antibiotics, derived from the fungus *Fusidium coccineum* and chemically related to cephalosporin P. The sodium salt of fusidic acid (Fucidin®) was introduced into clinical practice in 1962.

Mode of action

Bacteriostatic, inhibiting protein synthesis by blocking elongation factor G. Fusidic acid also has *in vitro* and *in vivo* immunosuppressive effects. It is active against *S. aureus*, most CoNS, β-haemolytic streptococci, *Corynebacterium* spp., and most *Clostridioides* spp. It is active against *M. leprae*, but not useful against MTB.

Resistance

Occurs by chromosomal mutations in the *fusA* gene which codes for elongation factor, and by plasmid-mediated resistance resulting in reduced permeability to the drug. This is of particular concern with long-term monotherapy, so fusidic acid is often combined with another agent.

Clinical use

Fusidic acid is mainly used for the treatment of staphylococcal infections, and many MRSA strains remain sensitive. In most clinical settings, it should be used in combination with another agent to reduce the risk of resistance developing. Useful in skin and soft tissue infections, bacteraemia, endocarditis, septic arthritis, osteomyelitis, and LRTIs in CF patients. It has been used to treat erythrasma due to *Corynebacterium minutissimum* and lepromatous leprosy.

Pharmacology

Fusidic acid may be given PO, TOP, or IV. PO absorption is rapid and almost complete. It is highly protein-bound and widely distributed in most tissues. Metabolized in the liver by CYP450 and eliminated in the bile.

Toxicity and side effects

Generally well tolerated, but the PO form may cause nausea, vomiting, and reversible jaundice (6%). The IV form is associated with thrombophlebitis and jaundice (17%). Ophthalmic preparations may cause itching or stinging. Drug-induced immune-mediated thrombocytopenia has been described.

Systemic fusidic acid should not be given with statins because of the risk of serious and potentially fatal rhabdomyolysis.

Mupirocin

Mupirocin is a pseudomonic acid, produced by *Pseudomonas fluorescens*, that is not related to any other antibiotic in clinical use. Available preparations are for external use only.

Mode of action

Bacteriostatic—inhibits bacterial RNA and protein synthesis by binding to bacterial isoleucyl tRNA synthetase, preventing the incorporation of isoleucine into protein chains in the bacterial cell wall. It is active against staphylococci and certain other Gram-positive organisms.

Resistance

Low-level resistance is due to spontaneous mutation resulting in altered access to binding sites in isoleucyl tRNA synthetase. High-level resistance is mediated on transferable plasmids by the *mupA* gene, which codes for a modified enzyme. Mupirocin resistance in MRSA has been associated with widespread use—prolonged use (>7 days) is discouraged.

Clinical use

Primarily used for skin infections (e.g. impetigo, folliculitis), and for nasal decolonization of *S. aureus* or MRSA carriage. Mupirocin has also been used for treatment of secondarily infected eczema, burns, lacerations, and ulcers.

Pharmacology

Given TOP as a cream or nasal ointment.

Toxicity and side effects

Local reactions, such as pruritus, burning sensation, rash, and urticarial, may occur, particularly if used on broken skin.

Antituberculous agents

The traditional first-line drugs (rifampicin, isoniazid, pyrazinamide, and ethambutol) remain the most effective and least toxic. Agents vary in their activity under different conditions. In classic pulmonary TB, most organisms are in cavities open to the bronchi (oxygenated, more alkaline, actively multiplying), with a smaller, less active population in necrotic tissue or inside macrophages (less oxygen and more acidic). An agent's bactericidal activity against rapidly multiplying bacteria determines the effectiveness of the early response to treatment, whereas sterilizing activity against less active persisters influences the risk of relapse after treatment finishes. Rifampicin acts against intra- and extracellular organisms, in addition to those dormant in nodules. Isoniazid and streptomycin are bactericidal against replicating tubercle bacilli in cavities. Pyrazinamide is active against intracellular organisms in acidic environments (e.g. necrosis—hence its importance in the induction phase of 'short-course' therapy). For treatment guidelines, including fixed-dose combinations, ➔ see Pulmonary tuberculosis, pp. 667–70.

Standard agents

Isoniazid (H)

• Isonicotinic acid hydrazide, synthetic agent. Penetrates rapidly into tissues and lesions.
• Mode of action—inhibits mycolic acid synthesis. Rapidly bactericidal against actively replicating MTB (MIC 0.01–2mg/L). Most other mycobacteria are resistant.
• Resistance—isoniazid resistance is one of the two most frequent forms of resistance (5.5% of isolates mono-resistant in 2014 in England). Associated with mutations in the *inhA* (mycolic acid synthesis), *katG* (catalase peroxidase), and *oryR-ahpC* genes.
• Clinical usage—treatment of all forms of TB infection, chemoprophylaxis in contacts and highly susceptible patients. LFTs should be performed before starting treatment, as a comparison for any subsequent adverse reactions.
• Pharmacology—>95% PO absorption, widely distributed, good CSF penetration (50–80% of serum levels), metabolized in the liver (*N*-acetyltransferase), excreted in the urine. Given as a single daily dose, as high peak concentrations are more important than a continuously inhibitory level. Patients may be fast or slow acetylators, depending on the genetic polymorphism—this is of clinical significance only if intermittent weekly regimens are considered. Dose reduction in renal failure.
• Toxicity and side effects—neurotoxicity (interferes competitively with pyridoxine metabolism; reduced by co-administration of the vitamin), hepatitis (potentially serious, and risk increases with age; for management, ➔ see Acute hepatitis, pp. 716–18), arthralgia, hypersensitivity, antinuclear antibody-positive lupus-like syndrome; inhibits hepatic metabolism of several drugs, increasing their plasma levels (e.g. warfarin, diazepam, phenytoin, carbamazepine).

Rifampicin (R)

(➔ See Rifamycins, pp. 71–3.)
• Highly potent and effective TB drug; 1.4% of English isolates mono-resistant in 2014, much higher (>20%) in Thailand and countries of the former Soviet Union.
• Bactericidal against actively replicating MTB and other mycobacteria (*M. kansasii*, *M. marinum*, *M. leprae*).

Pyrazinamide (Z)

• Pyrazinoic acid amide, synthetic nicotinamide analogue. Particularly effective against intracellular tubercle organisms in acidic environments (e.g. necrotic inflammatory foci) and an essential component of the first 2 months of 'short-course' (6-month) treatment regimens.
• Mode of action—unknown. Activity requires conversion to pyrazinoic acid by mycobacterial pyrazinamidase.
• Resistance—uncommon and is due to mutations in the *pncA* (pyrazinamidase) gene. *Mycobacterium bovis* is inherently resistant; consider this organism if preliminary sensitivities of a presumed TB culture indicated pyrazinamide mono-resistance.

- Pharmacology—>90% PO absorption, widely distributed, good CSF penetration. Metabolized in the liver; excreted by the kidneys. Dose reduction in renal failure. Increase the dose in dialysis patients.
- Toxicity and side effects—rare, but include GI upset, hepatotoxicity, gout (inhibits excretion of uric acid), arthralgia, and photosensitivity.

Ethambutol (E)

- Hydroxymethylpropylethylene diamine, synthetic compound.
- Mechanism of action—inhibits arabinosyl transferase enzymes (synthesis of arabinogalactan and lipoarabinomannan). Bacteriostatic and active against mycobacteria (MTB, *M. kansasii*, *Mycobacterium xenopi*, *Mycobacterium malmoense*) and *Nocardia*.
- Resistance is uncommon—develops slowly during therapy, caused by point mutations in the genes encoding the arabinosyl transferase enzyme (*embA*, *embB*, and *embC*).
- Pharmacology—75–80% PO absorption, widely distributed, 25–40% CSF penetration. Metabolized in the liver, renal excretion. Dose modification in renal failure.
- Adverse effects—optic neuritis (dose-dependent, resulting in changes in acuity and colour vision; reversible in early stages if treatment discontinued promptly; measure acuity before, and monitor during, treatment), peripheral neuropathy, arthralgia, hyperuricaemia, rashes.

Streptomycin (S)

(➔ See Aminoglycosides, pp. 52–4.)

- An aminoglycoside. Use limited by toxicity and resistance. pH-dependent activity, thus antimicrobial effect reduced in lung secretions (low pH). Bactericidal against MTB in the proliferative phase.
- Resistance emerged rapidly in the past when given as a single agent. Due to mutations in ribosomal binding protein or the ribosomal binding site (e.g. the *rpsL* gene encodes ribosomal protein S12). Primary resistance is seen in populations with a high incidence of isoniazid resistance.
- Pharmacology—not absorbed from the GI tract, administered IM. Widely distributed, but poor penetration in the CSF (better if meninges inflamed), bone, aqueous humour, and abscesses; 99% renal excretion. Monitor serum levels in those aged over 40 years.
- Adverse effects—ototoxicity is the most important problem, with vestibular damage in <30%. Perform baseline testing. Other—injection site reactions, hypersensitivity, neuromuscular blockade, peripheral neuritis, optic neuritis.

Other agents for resistant tuberculosis

Considered to have less favourable pharmacokinetic profiles, a relative lack of clinical data, or an increased incidence/severity of adverse events, compared to first-line agents. Some are considerably more expensive. They are used in cases of intolerance or resistance to first-line drugs. Treatment in these situations may be complicated, and advice should be sought from a specialist experienced in treating such patients. Certain agents are used in the treatment of atypical mycobacterial infections (➔ see Non-tuberculous mycobacteria, pp. 397–401).

Para-aminosalicylic acid (PAS)

- Mode of action—interferes with folate synthesis and iron uptake (by inhibition of the salicylate-dependent biosynthesis of iron-chelating 'mycobactins'). Bacteriostatic against MTB.
- Clinical usage—used for MDR-TB in developed countries. Cost limits use elsewhere. Evidence for its effectiveness compares unfavourably to that for cycloserine or thioamides.
- Pharmacology—incomplete PO absorption, hepatic metabolism, renal excretion (metabolites accumulate in severe renal impairment, hence contraindicated, unless no alternative).
- Adverse effects—GI upset, interferes with iodine metabolism (check thyroid function tests (TFTs) at baseline and 3-month intervals), hepatitis (check LFTs at baseline), coagulopathy.

Capreomycin

- Cyclic polypeptide antibiotic, produced by *Streptomyces capreolus*; its mode of action is unknown.
- Resistance—mechanism unknown. No cross-resistance with streptomycin, but some kanamycin/amikacin-resistant isolates are cross-resistant to capreomycin.
- Clinical usage—first-line injectable agent in MDR-TB, particularly if streptomycin-resistant.
- Pharmacology—administered IM or IV daily (lower dose for those aged over 60 years). It may be possible to reduce the frequency once the sputum is culture-negative. Renally excreted (reduce the dose and frequency in renal impairment); no useful CSF penetration. Toxicities may be potentiated by aminoglycoside use.
- Adverse effects—injection site reactions, ototoxicity, nephrotoxicity (potassium (K^+) and magnesium (Mg^{2+}) wasting, proteinuria), neuromuscular blockade. Perform baseline audiometry and vestibular testing. Monthly renal function, and K^+/Mg^{2+} and audiology testing while on therapy.

Cycloserine

- Naturally occurring amino acid that inhibits cell wall synthesis. Derived from *Streptomyces orchidaceus*. Mechanism of resistance unknown.
- Activity—broad: *S aureus*, streptococci, enterococci, *Enterobacterales*, *Nocardia* spp., *Chlamydophila* spp., and mycobacteria.
- Clinical use—usually given bd; start with a low dose, and increase as tolerated. No data to support intermittent therapy.
- Pharmacology—well absorbed PO; widely distributed, including the CSF; 50% metabolized, 50% excreted unchanged in the urine (dose modification required in renal impairment).
- Adverse events—CNS (psychosis, depression, convulsions); pyridoxine may help. Assess the neuropsychiatric status monthly.

Thioamides (ethionamide, prothionamide)

- Thioisonicotinic acid derivatives that inhibit mycolic acid synthesis. Bacteriostatic for TB, weakly bactericidal to *M. leprae*. Resistance mechanism unknown. Some isolates are resistant to both isoniazid and thioamides, which may be associated with mutations in the *inhA* gene promoter region (involved in mycolic acid synthesis).

- Pharmacology—well absorbed; widely distributed, including the CSF; metabolized in the liver, 99% excreted as metabolites in the urine (dose reduction in renal failure). Contraindicated in pregnancy.
- Adverse effects—GI upset (nausea may be severe enough to require bedtime administration with anti-emetic), hypersensitivity, hepatitis, CNS (pyridoxine may help).

Thiacetazone
- Acetylaminobenzaldehyde thiosemicarbazone.
- Mode of action—poorly understood, inhibits mycolic acid synthesis.
- Resistance—mechanism unknown. Primary and acquired resistance are common in developing countries where it has been used widely.
- Clinical usage—rarely used because of low efficacy and high rates of adverse effects. Should never be given to an HIV-infected patient.
- Pharmacology—well absorbed, 20% eliminated in the urine.
- Adverse events—rash, exfoliative dermatitis, Stevens–Johnson syndrome (especially in HIV patients), GI upset, vertigo, conjunctivitis.

Others
- Fluoroquinolones (➜ see Quinolones, pp. 67–9)—later-generation drugs (e.g. moxifloxacin) are significantly associated with cure in MDR-TB. Their use is recommended in the treatment of such patients.
- Aminoglycosides (➜ see Aminoglycosides, pp. 52–4)—kanamycin and amikacin. Ototoxic and nephrotoxic—perform baseline audiometry and vestibular testing.
- Bedaquiline—a novel agent which acts by inhibiting mycobacterial adenosine triphosphate (ATP) synthase. Approved for MDR-extensively drug resistant (XDR)-TB. For specialist use only—risk of increased mortality and prolonged QT interval.
- Delamanid—approved for MDR-XDR-TB. Blocks synthesis of mycolic acids. Limited data on effectiveness, and associated with prolonged QT.
- Drugs with limited evidence base used in the treatment of MDR-TB and XDR-TB include linezolid (increasing evidence supporting its effectiveness may see it used more routinely in resistant TB), co-amoxiclav, clarithromycin, imipenem, clofazimine, carbapenems, and thioacetazone.
- Pretomanid works in a similar way to delamanid and is used in combination with bedaquiline and linezolid (BPaL) for the treatment of MDR-TB. Given with moxifloxacin (BPaLM) this 6 month regime is now recommended by WHO for the treatment of MDR/RR-TB
- Always seek specialist advice when managing resistant TB. The British Thoracic Society (BTS) operates an online clinical advice service on the following link: ✍ mdrtb.brit-thoracic.org.uk (see also World Health Organization (WHO) TB treatment guidelines, available at: ✍ www.who.int/publications/i/item/9789240063129

Antileprotics

Introduced by the WHO in 1982, multidrug therapy (MDT) with the combination of dapsone, clofazimine, and rifampicin is the current treatment for infections with *M. leprae* (see Table 2.5). It has been very successful, with a

Table 2.5 Multidrug therapy regimens for the treatment of *Mycobacterium leprae* infections

Regimen	Drug	Duration
Paucibacillary leprosy (TT, BT)	Dapsone 100mg daily	6 months
	Rifampicin 600mg monthly	
Multibacillary leprosy (LL, BL, BT)	Dapsone 100mg daily	2 years
	Clofazimine 50mg daily and 300mg monthly	
	Rifampicin 600mg monthly	

BL, borderline lepromatous leprosy; BT, borderline tuberculoid leprosy; LL, lepromatous leprosy; TT, tuberculoid leprosy.

NB the regimens shown in this table are those of the World Health Organization. The guidance of the US National Hansen's Disease Program differs with longer treatment durations (12 months for paucibacillary, 24 months for multibacillary) and daily rifampicin dosing.

high cure rate, few side effects, and a low relapse rate. However, disability caused by leprotic neuropathy and eye damage may not be reversible.

Dapsone

Since first used to treat leprosy by Cochrane in 1947, dapsone has remained the cornerstone of treatment. The emergence of drug resistance in the 1960s led to MDT recommendations.

- Mode of action—a diaminodiphenyl sulfone which is active against many bacteria and some protozoa. It inhibits the synthesis of dihydrofolic acid. Bacteriostatic and weakly bactericidal. Resistance acquired by sequential mutations.
- Pharmacology—>90% PO absorption; widely distributed, but selectively retained in the skin, kidneys, and liver; metabolized by oxidation and acetylation; mostly renally excreted.
- Toxicity and side effects—GI upset, anorexia, headaches, dizziness, insomnia, 'dapsone syndrome' (fever, skin rash ± lymphadenopathy, jaundice, hepatomegaly), haemolysis (especially if G6PD deficiency), methaemoglobinaemia, sulfhaemoglobinaemia.
- Clinical use—leprosy, malaria (treatment and prophylaxis), toxoplasmosis (prophylaxis), *Pneumocystis* pneumonia (PCP) (treatment and prophylaxis), dermatitis herpetiformis. Patients should be screened for G6PD deficiency before treating.

Clofazimine

- Mode of action—unknown. An iminophenazine dye with anti-inflammatory properties, active against mycobacteria (MTB, *Mycobacterium scrofulaceum*, *M. leprae*, *Mycobacterium avium intracellulare* (MAI), *Mycobacterium fortuitum*, *Mycobacterium chelonae*), *Actinomyces* spp., and *Nocardia* spp. While weakly bactericidal alone, it displays pronounced synergy with dapsone. Resistance is rare.
- Pharmacology—well absorbed PO, taken up by adipose tissue and monocytes/macrophages, long half-life (10–70 days), excreted in the urine and faeces.

- Adverse effects—GI upset, skin discoloration (dose-related, reversible, and particularly pronounced in leprotic skin lesions, as the drug is lipophilic and accumulates in the organism's mycolic cell wall), small bowel oedema/subacute obstruction (prolonged use).
- Clinical use—leprosy.

Rifampicin

- Most effective antileprotic; highly bactericidal, even with monthly dosing. Renders the patient non-infectious within days of starting therapy (➔ see Rifamycins, pp. 71–3).

Alternative agents

Evidence for the use of alternative combinations is limited. Other antibiotics with bactericidal activity against *M. leprae* are shown below; all are less bactericidal than rifampicin.

- Minocycline (the only tetracycline with significant activity; ➔ see Tetracyclines, pp. 61–3);
- Ofloxacin (levofloxacin and moxifloxacin are also effective, but there are less clinical data; ➔ see Quinolones, pp. 67–9);
- Clarithromycin (the only effective macrolide; ➔ see Macrolides, pp. 54–6).

Short-course therapy

Recent research has focused on determining alternative regimens of shorter duration. A single-dose regimen of rifampicin, ofloxacin, and minocycline has been trialled for single-lesion paucibacillary leprosy and is slightly less effective.

Immunological reactions

Systemic inflammatory complications can occur before, during, or years after treatment. Symptoms include: fatigue, malaise, fever, neuritis, arthritis, and iritis. Neuritis must be treated aggressively, in an effort to avoid nerve damage and disability.

- Reversal reactions (type 1 reactions) can be treated with aspirin (if mild) or prednisolone (if moderate to severe). Up to 60mg prednisolone for 20 weeks or more may be required. Around 70% of patients improve, second-line: ciclosporin.
- Erythema nodosum leprosum (type 2 reactions) can be treated with aspirin (if mild), prednisolone, or thalidomide if severe (may require years of treatment). Clofazimine may have a role in chronic cases.

Antifungals

Antifungals: introduction

A number of antifungal agents are available:
- alkylamines that inhibit ergosterol biosynthesis by inhibiting squalene epoxidase (e.g. terbinafine);
- antimetabolites that interfere with DNA synthesis (e.g. flucytosine);
- azoles that inhibit ergosterol synthesis by blocking 14-α-demethylase (e.g. imidazoles and triazoles);
- glucan synthesis inhibitors (e.g. echinocandins);
- polyenes that bind to the fungal cell membrane and cause it to leak electrolytes (e.g. nystatin, amphotericin);
- miscellaneous agents (e.g. griseofulvin).

Fig. 3.1 shows the spectrum of activity of common antifungal agents.

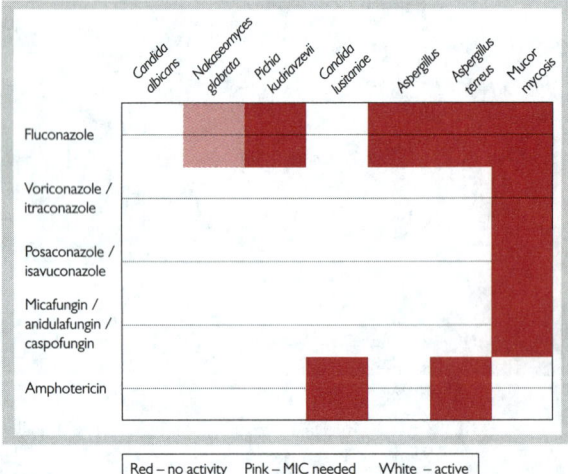

Red – no activity   Pink – MIC needed   White – active

Fig. 3.1 Spectrum of activity of common antifungal agents.

Polyenes

Polyenes have a broad spectrum of activity, including against yeasts, moulds, and mucormycosis. Two are in clinical use: nystatin and amphotericin. Neither is absorbed PO, and only amphotericin can be administered IV. Amphotericin is a cornerstone in the treatment of invasive fungal infections (e.g. disseminated candidiasis, cryptococcosis, aspergillosis), including dimorphic fungi. Organisms intrinsically resistant to amphotericin are: dermatophytes, *Aspergillus terreus*, *Fusarium* spp., *Candida guilliermondii* (now called *Meyerozyma guilliermondii*), *Scedosporium apiospermum*, *Scedosporium prolificans*, *Trichosporon beigelii*, and *Mucormycetes*.

Mode of action

Polyenes bind to ergosterol in the fungal cell membrane, resulting in increased membrane permeability. Essential cell contents leak and the cell dies.

Resistance

- *Candida lusitaniae* (now called *Clavispora lusitaniae*) may develop resistance to amphotericin B during treatment.
- Otherwise acquired resistance is rare, apart from in patients with uncontrolled HIV who have relapsing cryptococcal disease, and cancer patients with prolonged neutropenia and yeast infections.

Clinical use

Amphotericin

- Conventional IV amphotericin deoxycholate may be used to treat systemic fungal infections. It is the drug of choice for aspergillosis and also commonly used for disseminated candidiasis and cryptococcosis, either alone or with flucytosine ($\mathcal{S}$ see Other antifungals, pp. 91–2).
- Toxicity is a major problem with systemic therapy. Lipid formulations of amphotericin are better tolerated and recommended if toxicity or renal impairment precludes the use of conventional amphotericin. Other licensed indications include:
  - Abelcet® for systemic fungal infections not responding to conventional amphotericin or other antifungals (it can be given at a higher dose than the other lipid formulations);
  - AmBisome® for infections in febrile neutropenia unresponsive to broad-spectrum antibacterials, and visceral leishmaniasis.
- Amphotericin solution can be used for continuous bladder irrigation in mycotic infections.

Nystatin

- Nystatin is limited to topical treatment of mucosal infections, and *Candida* infections of the oropharynx, oesophagus, intestinal tract, and vagina.
- Nystatin cream or pessaries are used to treat vaginal candidiasis. It stains clothes yellow and damages latex condoms and diaphragms.

Pharmacology

Amphotericin is usually given IV with a carrier (e.g. deoxycholate). It is highly protein-bound and penetrates the cerebrospinal fluid (CSF) and other body

Table 3.1 Lipid formulations of amphotericin

Name	Formulation
Liposomal amphotericin (AmBisome®)	Drug encapsulated in phospholipid-containing liposomes
Amphotericin lipid complex (ABLC; Abelcet®)	Drug complexed with phospholipids to form ribbon-like structures

fluids poorly. Liver or renal impairment and dialysis have little effect on serum levels. The lipid formulations have diverse pharmacokinetics.

Toxicity and side effects

- Despite the theoretical selective toxicity to fungal cell membranes, compared to human cell membranes, conventional amphotericin is associated with infusion-related reactions (chills, fever, headache, nausea, vomiting) and nephrotoxicity. A test dose is required (because of the risk of anaphylaxis), and close supervision is necessary (monitor FBC, LFTs, renal function, and electrolytes). Prophylactic antipyretics or hydrocortisone may be tried in patients with previous acute adverse reactions, in whom ongoing treatment is essential. Toxicity has driven the development of lipid formulations (see Table 3.1) that may be preferred in well-resourced health systems.
- Additional side effects of IV amphotericin include GI symptoms (anorexia, nausea and vomiting, diarrhoea, epigastric pain), muscle and joint pain, anaemia and other blood disorders, cardiovascular toxicity (including arrhythmias, especially if infused too quickly), neurological disorders, abnormal LFTs, and rash and pain at the infusion site.

Imidazoles

Commonly used imidazoles include clotrimazole, miconazole, and ketoconazole. Other rarely used agents are econazole and tioconazole. They should be considered for topical use only; ketoconazole was previously given PO but has been implicated in fatal hepatotoxicity. Triazoles are now preferred for treating systemic fungal infections.

Mode of action

Imidazoles inhibit the synthesis of ergosterol, by inhibiting the cytochrome P450-dependent enzyme 14-α-demethylase. The damaged cell membrane becomes permeable, leading to cell lysis. Imidazoles should be considered fungistatic, although some may be fungicidal at high concentrations.

Resistance

Acquired ketoconazole resistance is rare, but there are case reports of ketoconazole resistance in patients treated for chronic mucocutaneous candidiasis and in patients with uncontrolled HIV who have mucosal candidiasis.

Clinical use

- Ketoconazole—should no longer be used PO for systemic mycoses. Topical ketoconazole can be used for tinea pedis and other fungal skin infections, vaginal and vulval candidiasis, and pityriasis versicolor.
- Miconazole—topical for treatment or prophylaxis of oral candidiasis (hold in the mouth near localized lesions, after food), vaginal and vulval candidiasis, and fungal nail infections.
- Clotrimazole or miconazole cream/pessaries are used to treat vaginal candidiasis. They can damage latex condoms and diaphragms. Topical preparations are used for many fungal skin infections (e.g. dermatophyte infections, pityriasis versicolor, and candidiasis).
- Clotrimazole solution is used for fungal otitis externa infections.

Pharmacology

- Ketoconazole should no longer be used PO due to the association with fatal hepatotoxicity.
- Miconazole is available as an oral gel for mouth infections, but systemic absorption may result in significant drug interactions. Clotrimazole is used topically.

Toxicity and side effects

With topical preparations, avoid contact with eyes and mucous membranes, and discontinue if severe local irritation or hypersensitivity reactions occur.

Triazoles

Triazoles are important agents in the treatment of systemic mycoses. They differ widely in their spectrum of activity. Varying kinetics, with potential for significant drug interactions—check product details. Avoid in pregnancy.

Mode of action

As for imidazoles. Essentially fungistatic, but voriconazole is fungicidal against *Aspergillus*. Well absorbed PO, but only fluconazole and voriconazole penetrate into the CSF in useful concentrations.

Fluconazole

- Active against yeasts, but no meaningful activity against *Aspergillus* spp. or most other moulds.
  - Useful against most *Candida* spp. (not *Candida krusei*, now called *Pichia kudriavzevii*), *Cryptococcus* spp., *Coccidioides immitis*.
  - Limited activity against *Histoplasma capsulatum, Blastomyces dermatitidis*, and *Sporothrix schenkii*.
- Resistance—*C. krusei* is intrinsically resistant to fluconazole. *Candida glabrata* (now called *Nakaseomyces glabrata*) has high fluconazole minimum inhibitory concentrations (MICs); 10–15% are resistant. Fluconazole resistance is also seen increasingly in *Candida parapsilosis*. Approximately 90% of isolates of the emerging pathogen Candidozyma auris are fluconazole-resistant. Acquired resistance to fluconazole has been reported in *C. albicans* in HIV patients. Pharmacology—available as PO and IV preparations. Well absorbed PO (90% bioavailable); CSF

levels of 60–80% of serum levels. Renal excretion; reduce the dose in impairment.
- Clinical use—treatment of oropharyngeal, vulvovaginal, and invasive candidiasis. Also used for prophylaxis in transplant patients.
- Side effects and toxicity—generally well tolerated. May cause abnormal LFTs.

Itraconazole
- Active against yeasts (including fluconazole-resistant *C. krusei* and *C. glabrata*), moulds, and dimorphic fungi.
  - Useful against: *Candida* spp., *Cryptococcus* spp., *Aspergillus* spp., *S. apiospermum*, *S. schenkii*, *H. capsulatum*, *B. dermatitidis*, *C. immitis*, *Paracoccidioides brasiliensis*, *Talaromyces* (*Penicillium*) *marneffei*, and dermatophytes. Limited against *Fusarium* spp. and mucormycosis.
- Resistance—detectable in most of the aforementioned species.
- Pharmacology—available as PO capsule, PO suspension, or IV formulation. Absorption differs between formulations and is highly variable—suspension is best, but GI upset is common. Gastric acidity and food affect absorption. Highly lipophilic; achieves high concentrations in fatty tissues and purulent exudates.
- Clinical use—treatment of yeast and mould infections, especially fluconazole-resistant *Candida* spp. and *Aspergillus* spp. Variable bioavailability limits use in the severely ill.
- Side effects and toxicity—side effects are rare and similar to those of fluconazole. Hypertension, hypokalaemia, oedema, headache, and altered mental state have been reported. Seek advice before giving itraconazole to patients at risk of heart failure (e.g. the elderly; those with cardiac disease or on negative inotropes, e.g. calcium channel blockers; those on long courses/high doses of itraconazole).
- Monitor plasma concentration in uncontrolled HIV and neutropenia, as reduced absorption in these groups.

Voriconazole
- Structurally similar to fluconazole. Inhibits P45014DM to a greater extent than fluconazole. Enhanced activity against *Aspergillus* spp.
  - Widely active: *Candida* spp. (fungistatic), *Cryptococcus* spp. (fungistatic), *Aspergillus* spp. (fungicidal), *B. dermatitidis*, *C. immitis*, *H. capsulatum*, *Fusarium* spp., and *Talaromyces* (*Penicillium*) *marneffei*. Active against fluconazole-resistant *C. krusei*, *C. glabrata*, and *C. guilliermondii*.
  - Not useful for mucormycosis, due to high MICs.
- Pharmacology—available PO or IV; 90% PO bioavailability. IV formulation contains a vehicle known to accumulate in renal failure, thus limited to those with creatinine clearance (CrCl) of >50mL/min. Non-linear pharmacokinetics, and therapeutic drug monitoring may be useful.
- Clinical use—invasive aspergillosis and invasive candidiasis; salvage therapy of *S. apiospermum* and *Fusarium* spp.
- Side effects and toxicity—dose-related, transient visual disturbance, skin rash, abnormal LFTs, visual hallucinations.

Posaconazole

- Consistent activity against mucormycosis.
  - Excellent activity against *Candida* spp. (including those with reduced fluconazole susceptibility), *Aspergillus* spp., *Fusarium* spp., *C. immitis*, *S. schenkii*, *H. capsulatum*, *B. dermatitidis*, *P. brasiliensis*, *Talaromyces (Penicillium) marneffei*, and many causative agents of chromoblastomycosis, mycetoma, and phaeohyphomycosis.
- Pharmacology—PO suspension, tablets, and IV formulation available. Tablets preferred over suspension due to higher bioavailability.
- Clinical use—prevention of invasive antifungal infections in high-risk patients with neutropenia or graft-versus-host disease (GVHD). Used as salvage therapy in patients with invasive fungal infections that failed primary therapy (usually amphotericin). Posaconazole may be effective against mucormycosis unresponsive to amphotericin.
- Toxicity and side effects—nausea, headache, rash, dry skin, taste disturbance, abdominal pain, dizziness, and flushing may occur.

Isavuconazole

- Similar spectrum of activity to posaconazole.
- Predictable pharmacodynamics, no food effect when PO formulation used, and no dose adjustment needed in renal impairment.
- Clinical use—treatment for invasive aspergillosis and invasive mucormycosis in patients in whom amphotericin B is inappropriate.
- Toxicity and side effects—well tolerated; can cause nausea, vomiting, and diarrhoea, headache, and electrolyte disturbance.

Echinocandins

This relatively new class targets the fungal cell wall and is primarily effective against *Candida* (rapidly fungicidal) and *Aspergillus* spp. (more fungistatic). Their relatively weak action against other fungi may reflect differences in fungal wall construction. Large lipopeptide molecules; all agents are administered IV.

Mode of action

Block the synthesis of glucan (a fungal cell wall component) by inhibiting the β-1,3-D-glucan synthase enzyme complex. β-glucans contribute to cell wall integrity. They account for <60% of the cell wall mass in yeasts, and depletion results in cell lysis. Filamentous fungi (e.g. *Aspergillus*) concentrate their β-glucan synthesis in the tips and hyphal branching points; thus, echinocandins merely result in impeded growth. Selective targeting results in fewer side effects, fewer drug interactions, and lack of cross-resistance with other antifungals. Agents differ in pharmacokinetics but have similar spectrums of activity.

Spectrum of activity

- *Candida*—potent activity against *Candida* spp., especially against biofilm-embedded organisms (a setting in which the MIC for amphotericin and fluconazole rises dramatically). Active against fluconazole-resistant *C. krusei* (now called *Pichia kudriavzevii*).

- Increasing resistance seen in *C. glabrata* (now called *Nakaseomyces glabrata*) (check MIC). Most isolates of the emerging pathogen *C. auris* are susceptible to echinocandins, but resistance can develop on treatment.
- *Candida albicans* and *Candida tropicalis* are highly susceptible.
- Elevated MICs seen for *C. parapsilosis* and *C. guilliermondii*.
- *Aspergillus*—growth is inhibited; most species susceptible. Rather than the 'MIC', the minimum effective concentration (MEC) end point is determined by the lowest concentration, resulting in grossly abnormal hyphal forms.
- Other—not considered useful against dimorphic fungi, mucormycosis, *Cryptococcus*, or non-*Aspergillus* moulds. No role in treatment or prevention of *Pneumocystis* (glucan synthase is expressed only during the cystic, not trophic, part of the life cycle).
- Not effective against fungal infections of the CNS.

Clinical use

All are approved for invasive candidiasis (adults) and oesophageal candidiasis. Caspofungin is also used for aspergillosis and as empirical treatment of systemic fungal infections in patients with neutropenia.

Caspofungin
- Pharmacology—protein binding is >90%. Widely distributed, with high levels in the lungs, liver, spleen, and kidneys, but low levels in the CSF. Loading dose is followed by lower daily dosing. Metabolized by the liver. Reduce the dose in moderate liver impairment. Metabolites eliminated in the urine and faeces. No dose adjustment is required in renal impairment. Dose increase may be needed with rifampicin and potent inducers of cytochrome P450.
- Clinical use—as above plus: invasive aspergillosis and empirical therapy in neutropenic patients.
- Toxicity and side effects—nausea, vomiting, abdominal pain, diarrhoea, flushing, fever, headache, and injection site reactions. Transient LFT abnormalities occur in 11–24% of patients.

Anidulafungin
- Pharmacology—loading dose necessary for rapid therapeutic concentrations. No dose adjustment for renal or liver impairment.
- Toxicity and side effects—abnormal LFTs plus others.

Micafungin
- Clinical use—as above plus prevention of *Candida* infections post-bone marrow transplantation (BMT).
- Toxicity and side effects—fever, electrolyte disturbances, abnormal LFTs.

Other antifungals

Table 3.2 shows new antifungal agents at different stages of development.

Table 3.2 New antifungal agents at different stages of development

New antifungal	Class	Mechanism of action	Spectrum of activity
Encochleated amphotericin B (oral)	Polyene	Binds to ergosterol and forms membrane pores	Broad (yeasts and moulds)
Rezafungin (given once a week)	Echinocandin	Inhibits glucan synthase	*Candida*, *Aspergillus*, and *Pneumocystis jirovecii*
Oteseconazole	Tetrazole	Inhibits 14-α-demethylase	*Candida*
Fosmanogepix	Gwt1 inhibitor	Disrupts GPI anchor synthesis biopathway	*Candida* (except *C. krusei*, now called *Pichia kudriavzevii*) *Cryptococcus* *Aspergillus*
Olorofim	Orotomide	Inhibits pyrimidine synthesis	*Aspergillus* and less common moulds
Ibrexafungerp	Triterpenoid	Inhibits glucan synthase	*Candida* and *Aspergillus*

Flucytosine

Fluorine analogue of cytosine (pyrimidine), so inhibits DNA synthesis.
- Mode of action—inhibits thymidylate synthetase. Also converted to 5-fluorouracil, which is incorporated into fungal ribonucleic acid (RNA). Active against yeasts—no useful action on filamentous fungi.
- Resistance—emerges rapidly with monotherapy, thus usually given with amphotericin (may facilitate entry of flucytosine into the cell). May be due to loss of cytosine permease (that permits entry of the drug) or loss of enzymes that convert it into its active metabolites.
- Clinical use (in combination therapy with amphotericin)— cryptococcosis, severe systemic candidiasis, severe or long-standing infections.
- Pharmacology—given IV or PO. Rapidly and almost completely absorbed. Low protein binding. CSF concentrations are 74% of plasma concentrations; 90% is excreted unchanged in the urine—dose reduction required in renal impairment.

- Toxicity and side effects—rash, diarrhoea, and abnormal LFTs. Leucopenia, thrombocytopenia, and enterocolitis may occur in patients with renal impairment—monitor FBC, renal function, LFTs, and serum flucytosine concentrations weekly during treatment. Flucytosine is contraindicated in pregnancy and dihydropyrimidine dehydrogenase (DPD) deficiency.

Griseofulvin

Previously widely used for fungal nail infections, but overall poor response rates and significant relapse rates. Given PO or topical.
- Mode of action—disruption of fungal cellular microtubules.
- Clinical use—tine pedis, tinea capitis due to *Trichophyton tonsurans*. Dermatophyte infections of skin, scalp, nails, and hair where topical therapy has failed or is inappropriate.
- Toxicity and side effects—impaired performance of skilled tasks, enhancement of effects of alcohol, headache, nausea, vomiting, and rashes. May diminish the anticoagulant effect of warfarin. Avoid in pregnancy, breastfeeding, systemic lupus erythematosus (SLE) (risk of exacerbation), and liver disease.

Terbinafine

- Mode of action—acts on squalene epoxidase, blocking transformation of squalene to lanosterol and thus inhibiting ergosterol synthesis. The intracellular accumulation of squalene also results in disruption of fungal cell membranes. Accumulates in keratin.
- Clinical use—dermatophyte and ringworm infections (including tinea pedis, cruris, and corporis) where PO therapy is appropriate. Cutaneous candidiasis. Pityriasis versicolor. Fingernail infections need a 6-week course; toenail infections usually 12 weeks. Also available topically to treat fungal skin infections.
- Pharmacology—metabolized by cytochrome P450 enzymes.
- Toxicity and side effects—abdominal discomfort, anorexia, nausea, diarrhoea, headache, rash, and urticaria. Rare events include liver toxicity and serious skin reactions (e.g. Stevens–Johnson syndrome).

Antivirals

Antivirals for herpes simplex virus and varicella-zoster virus

Alphaherpesviruses (➜ see *Herpesviridae*, pp. 437–8) possess a virally encoded enzyme called thymidine kinase (TK), which performs the initial prerequisite phosphorylation of aciclovir, the most commonly prescribed antiviral; clinical utility of this agent is thus limited to this subfamily of *Herpesviridae*.

Aciclovir

Aciclovir is a nucleoside analogue related to guanosine. It is a pro-drug that requires three phosphorylations by different kinase enzymes to produce the active antiviral derivative. Oral bioavailability can be enhanced up to 5-fold by the addition of an L-valine ester side chain to produce valaciclovir. Enzymes from herpes simplex virus (HSV)-infected host cells perform the second and third phosphorylation steps to produce aciclovir triphosphate. Notably, this lacks an essential 3′-OH group in the nucleoside molecular structure.

- Mode of action:
  - synthesis of the viral DNA chain is prematurely terminated after incorporation of the analogues due to the inability to add subsequent nucleosides;
  - acts as a competitive inhibitor of viral DNA polymerase. Additionally, chain–enzyme complex formation may irreversibly inactivate the polymerase.
- Resistance:
  - reduced/absent levels of TK (commonest);
  - altered TK activity resulting in decreased phosphorylation of aciclovir—these strains may exhibit reduced virulence;
  - decreased affinity of viral DNA polymerase for aciclovir triphosphate—emerges particularly in those receiving repeated or prolonged treatment (e.g. HIV patients).

The prevalence of aciclovir-resistant HSV is not well described, and while it increases in parallel with host immunosuppression, overall it is uncommon. Resistant HSV is seen in <1% of immunocompetent patients, increasing to 4–7% in immunocompromised patients (patients with uncontrolled HIV and transplantation patients). Aciclovir-resistant varicella-zoster virus (VZV) is even more uncommon; increased risk in chronic suppressive therapy with subtherapeutic dosage. As valaciclovir and famciclovir have similar modes of action to aciclovir, HSV may show cross-resistance to these agents and where resistance is due to TK deficiency, this may extend to ganciclovir (requires phosphorylation for activity).

- Pharmacology—oral bioavailability: aciclovir, 15–20%; valaciclovir, up to 54%. PO valaciclovir achieves total aciclovir exposure similar to that of IV aciclovir, but with lower peak plasma concentrations. Not highly bound to plasma protein, and CSF concentrations are ~50% that of plasma. Caution in pregnancy. In obese patients, weight-based dosing should be scaled down to ideal body weight to minimize toxicity. Requires dose adjustment in renal impairment. Systemic absorption from topical administration is low.

* Side effects and toxicity—topical aciclovir may cause skin irritation. Nephrotoxicity due to precipitation of aciclovir crystals can cause acute kidney injury in up to 5% of patients receiving IV aciclovir. Adequate IV hydration is preventative. Neurotoxicity (agitation, delirium, tremors, confusion, hallucinations) in 1–4% of those receiving IV aciclovir; increased incidence with underlying renal impairment.

Other agents

* Famciclovir is a pro-drug of penciclovir that is analogous to aciclovir in its mode of action. It is not in common use.
* Foscarnet (➔ see Foscarnet, pp. 96–7) and cidofovir (➔ see Cidofovir, p. 97) represent alternate choices to treat HSV infections with resistance to aciclovir (➔ see *Herpesviridae*, pp. 437–8).
* Varicella-zoster immunoglobulin (VZIG) is used as post-exposure prophylaxis (PEP) for specific immunocompromised groups (pregnancy, neonates, or those on immunosuppressive therapy) who are varicella antibody-negative. For specific indications and use, see the Green book, Chapter 34 (available at: ℘ https://www.gov.uk/government/publicati ons/varicella-the-green-book-chapter-34).
* Vaccination can reduce the incidence of VZV reactivation (shingles). Shingrix, a recombinant subunit vaccine given as a two dose schedule, has replaced Zostavax® (a high titre live attenuated vaccine) in the UK schedule as it is considered more cost effective. In the UK it is now offered at 60 years of age, and immunosuppressed individuals aged 50 and over. For details see the Green Book Chapter 28a (available at: https://www.gov.uk/gov ernm ent/publicati ons/shing les-her pes-zos ter-the-green-book-chapter-28a).

Antivirals for cytomegalovirus

The betaherpesvirus cytomegalovirus (CMV) (➔ see *Herpesviridae*, pp. 437–8) possesses different viral kinase enzymes (not TK as in HSV and VZV) (e.g. UL97). This mandates the use of different antivirals in the treatment of CMV disease. New agents with better toxicity profiles and a CMV vaccine remain highly desirable goals.

Ganciclovir

Inhibits CMV replication, in addition to that of other herpesviruses (HSV, VZV, and B virus) by disrupting viral nucleic acid synthesis. Available as a P preparation, valganciclovir (addition of an L-valine side chain analogous to valaciclovir). Toxicity is commoner than aciclovir, due to less specific inhibition of both viral and host cellular polymerases, which results in bone marrow suppression. Disseminated CMV infection itself contributes to myelosuppression, which makes differentiation between disease and toxicity difficult. Incidence and severity of marrow toxicity vary widely by patient group (advanced HIV, solid organ transplant, or haematopoietic stem cell transplant); 33% of patients receiving IV therapy interrupt or prematurely stop therapy due to marrow or CNS toxicity. Accordingly, it is restricted to life- or sight-threatening CMV infections in immunocompromised patients, or to prevention of CMV disease during immunosuppressive therapy after organ transplantation. Neither primary infection in immunocompetent hosts nor reactivation in critically ill patients usually requires treatment. Careful risk/benefit analysis must be performed before switching to less efficacious therapies (foscarnet/cidofovir). It is the preferred agent for treatment of neurological disease due to B virus.

- Mode of action—nucleoside analogue of guanosine which competitively inhibits viral polymerase activity. Initial phosphorylation occurs by a CMV viral protein kinase. Disrupts viral DNA chain elongation but does not necessarily cause chain termination (unlike aciclovir).
- Resistance—due to mutations in the protein kinase UL97 or UL54. High-level resistance seen in prolonged therapy for those with uncontrolled HIV or transplantation-related disease. Genotypic resistance testing of suspected clinical isolates is possible.
- Pharmacology—oral bioavailability: ganciclovir is very poor (6%), thus is given IV only, but valganciclovir is up to 60%. Aqueous, vitreous, and subretinal levels similar to serum levels. Requires significant dose adjustment in renal impairment.
- Interactions—concomitant use of other myelosuppressive or nephrotoxic agents increases overall incidence of toxicity.
- Adverse effects—myelosuppression (e.g. neutropenia and thrombocytopenia) occurs in 15–20% of patients with uncontrolled HIV receiving IV therapy (less in transplantation patients). Usually seen in the second week of therapy and reversible within 1 week of cessation in most cases. Recombinant granulocyte colony-stimulating factor (G-CSF) may be useful. CMV-induced marrow suppression may improve with therapy; 5–15% of cases have CNS effects—from headache to confusion and convulsions. Others—renal impairment, LFT abnormalities, rash, fever, phlebitis at IV site.
- Contraindications—pregnancy (contraception required up to 90 days after therapy cessation), breastfeeding, existing cytopenias.
- Monitoring—FBC and renal function during treatment.

Foscarnet

Its principal use is as second-line treatment of ganciclovir-resistant CMV disease and aciclovir-resistant HSV or VZV infection. It is a viral DNA polymerase inhibitor, but with a different mode of action.

- Mode of action—non-competitively binds to the pyrophosphate site in the catalytic centre of the herpesvirus DNA polymerase (and reverse transcriptase (RT) of hepatitis B virus (HBV)/HIV—not clinically useful), rendering the enzyme inactive.
- Resistance—due to point mutations in *UL54* of DNA polymerase. Not affected by mutations in *UL97* (ganciclovir) or *TK* (aciclovir) genes. Genotypic testing of suspected clinical isolates is possible.
- Pharmacology—oral bioavailability is low (8%), therefore administered IV. Almost exclusively renal elimination—most unaltered (dose-adjust in renal impairment). Removed by haemodialysis. Prolonged terminal half-life due to bone and cartilage uptake (20%). Vitreous concentrations 1.4 times higher than plasma.

- Interactions—hypocalcaemia with concomitant IV pentamidine. Renal dysfunction with concurrent nephrotoxic agents (ciclosporin, amphotericin).
- Side effects and toxicity—significant nephrotoxicity possibly due to acute tubular necrosis (one-third develop significant renal impairment—reversible within 3–4 weeks of cessation of therapy). Adequate IV hydration may reduce the incidence. Multiple electrolyte abnormalities, but mainly hypocalcaemia/hypomagnesaemia.
- Contraindications—pregnancy and breastfeeding (contraception required up to 6 months after therapy cessation for men).
- Monitoring—FBC, electrolytes, and renal function.

Cidofovir

Can be considered a broad-spectrum antiviral with activity against herpesvirus, polyomavirus (BK virus), adenovirus, and papillomavirus polymerases. Primary clinical utility is as third-line therapy of resistant CMV disease (where ganciclovir or foscarnet therapy is unsuitable). Evidence for its use in the treatment of conditions caused by the polyomaviruses JC (progressive multifocal leukoencephalopathy) or BK (BK polyomavirus-associated nephropathy) is lacking.

- Mode of action—disrupts nucleic acid synthesis by inhibiting viral polymerase activity. An acyclic monophosphate nucleotide analogue which requires only two phosphorylations by cellular kinases before incorporation into, and subsequent termination of, the viral DNA chain. Activation does not require virus-specific enzymes, therefore inhibitory for certain aciclovir- and ganciclovir-resistant HSV and CMV strains.
- Resistance—intrinsic development of resistance secondary to cidofovir therapy remains uncommon and is likely due to point mutations in the polymerase. Genotypic testing of suspected clinical isolates is possible.
- Pharmacology—oral bioavailability is low (<5%), therefore administered IV. Primarily renal elimination—80% unchanged in first 24h, but active metabolite has a prolonged half-life, allowing fortnightly dosing. Adequate IV hydration is paramount.
- Side effects and toxicity—concomitant administration with probenecid increases serum concentrations, while decreasing nephrotoxicity. Neutropenia (20%); Fanconi-like syndrome; intravitreal dosing can cause iritis/vitritis.
- Contraindications—renal impairment (creatinine clearance <55mL/min, proteinuria 2+). Pregnancy and breastfeeding (contraception required up to 90 days after therapy cessation).

Letermovir

A novel agent that targets a late stage in the CMV replication cycle. It inhibits the CMV DNA terminase complex which is required for cleavage and packaging of viral DNA into mature progeny virions. Viral genome replication is unaffected. Recently approved for prophylaxis of CMV reactivation in recipients of an allogeneic haematopoietic stem cell transplant who are donor CMV antibody-positive. Its use is attractive, as administration is PO and is remarkably less toxic than other CMV antivirals. Its clinical use in the actual treatment of CMV disease is as yet unknown but is under investigation.

Other agents

Both maribavir (inhibition of the protein product of UL97) and brincidofovir (lipid pro-drug of cidofovir) have underperformed in clinical trials. Numerous therapeutic CMV vaccines are in development.

Antivirals for influenza

The majority of uncomplicated (not requiring hospital admission) influenza infection in immunocompetent individuals is managed symptomatically. Where indicated, antiviral use with the neuraminidase inhibitors (NAs) oseltamivir and zanamivir has replaced the use of the M2 ion channel protein agents amantadine and rimantadine, due to emerged resistance. There remains ongoing debate about the extent of clinical benefit derived from the NAs; however, their use for treatment and PEP of influenza infection is advised in the UK in certain at-risk groups or those with complicated disease (UK Health and Security Agency guidance on use of antiviral agents for the treatment and prophylaxis of seasonal influenza, 2021). Annual vaccination and strict infection prevention and control (IPC) practice by healthcare staff remain the most effective ways of preventing influenza.

Neuraminidase inhibitors

The viral neuraminidase enzyme cleaves sialic acid residues that tether newly formed mature virions to the host cell surface. Their removal is crucial to the release and spread of virions within the respiratory tract. Inhibition by the NAs (acting as competitive sialic acid analogues) interferes with this late stage of the replication cycle in both influenza A and B. A decrease in viral shedding occurs rapidly after initiation of therapy, with a shortening of symptom duration by 1–3 days. Maximum benefit is derived when given within 48h of symptom onset or exposure to the index case—they may provide benefit beyond these times in severe cases or the immunocompromised. Oseltamivir and zanamivir are the primary agents used. Peramivir, another NA inhibitor, is not used in the UK currently.

Oseltamivir
- Given PO, with good bioavailability. Administered bd for 5 days (10 days if immunosuppressed) for treatment of infection, and administered od for 10 days as prophylaxis.
- The influenza neuraminidase enzyme is classified into three groups, based on active site sequence and structure. Consequently, each group will generate resistance by a different mechanism. Generally, influenza A (H1N1)pdm09 is considered higher risk for developing oseltamivir resistance than influenza A (H3N2) or influenza B. Annual epidemiological surveillance of isolates occurs to monitor circulating resistance patterns, and individual genotypic analysis can usually be arranged by discussion with local virology laboratories for suspected cases.
- Resistance results from mutations either in the active site of neuraminidase (usually drug-specific) or in haemagglutinin at the site responsible for binding sialic acid residues (resulting in broader

cross-resistance). Usually, these mutations have a deleterious effect on viral fitness and transmission.

- Overall, oseltamivir resistance is uncommon and most likely to be seen in immunocompromised patients. H275Y is the most commonly identified mutation.
  - Between 2007 and early 2009, resistance to oseltamivir became widespread among seasonal H1N1 isolates. They remained susceptible to zanamivir and adamantanes.
  - This predominantly resistant strain was replaced in the 2009 pandemic by the predominantly oseltamivir-susceptible (but adamantane-resistant) influenza A (H1N1) pdm09.
  - Global NA resistance has remained low since (<3%).
  - Resistance in influenza B is extremely rare.
- Toxicity and side effects—generally well tolerated, but most commonly reported are dizziness, GI discomfort, sleep disorders, nausea, and vertigo.
- Contraindications—few, if any, particularly if clinical benefit outweighs risk. Dose is adjusted by both weight (for paediatric use) and renal function.

Zanamivir

- Remarkably, little zanamivir resistance has been encountered. The oseltamivir resistance mutation H275Y does not affect the activity of zanamivir and so is the agent of choice for suspected cases.
- Available as a powder for inhalation or IV.
- Treatment duration is the same as for oseltamivir.
- Toxicity and side effects—GI disturbance, skin reactions, hepatocellular injury. Risk of bronchospasm when administered by inhalation (use with care in those with asthma and chronic obstructive pulmonary disease—bronchodilators should be available).
- Contraindications—few, if any, particularly if clinical benefit outweighs risk. Caution in pregnancy/breastfeeding.

Other agents

Baloxavir marboxil is administered in a single dose PO. It targets influenza's endonuclease enzyme, which performs the 'cap-snatching' process, integral to viral messenger RNA (mRNA) synthesis. It is not in widespread use, primarily due to concerns about the relative ease with which resistance appears to emerge.

A 'universal' influenza vaccine (i.e. one that covers a broad spectrum of haemagglutinin (HA) and NA subtypes), in addition to more robust antiviral drugs, remain highly desirable goals and are areas of intense research.

Antivirals for respiratory syncytial virus

Recently developed products (nirsevimab, a long acting mAb, and RSVpreF, a bivalent prefusion F matenal vaccine candidate) have not entered widespread clinical use at the time of writing.

Treatment of respiratory syncytial virus (RSV) infection is primarily supportive. There is neither a vaccine nor a generally accepted effective antiviral treatment. Two main therapies exist: a monoclonal antibody used as targeted prophylaxis in children deemed at high risk of infection, and individualized use of ribavirin in immunocompromised patients with severe disease.

Ribavirin

Considered a broad-spectrum antiviral due to wide-ranging activity in both DNA and RNA viruses *in vitro*. This has failed to be reflected *in vivo* where its clinical use is limited. The use of ribavirin in RSV infection is debated due to lack of robust efficacy data and issues with tolerability. Currently used sporadically in the treatment of severe RSV bronchiolitis and pneumonia in hospitalized immunocompromised patients; primarily lung transplant and haematopoietic stem cell transplant recipients. Used occasionally in treatment of hepatitis C virus (HCV) infection, chronic hepatitis E virus (HEV) infection, and Lassa fever.

- Mode of action—numerous and complex (can even vary by virus). Interferes with nucleotide pools, acts as a guanosine analogue (thereby interfering with nucleic acid synthesis), blocks production of viral mRNA, and has been reported to increase cytokine-mediated immune responses. Resistance in RSV infection is not well studied.
- Pharmacology—excreted renally (around 40%) and in faeces (15%), and metabolized by the liver. Its use in RSV infection is primarily by inhalation and sometimes PO. IV formulations are available.
- Toxicity and side effects—dose-related anaemia. Itch, nausea, depression, and cough. With aerosolized preparations—conjunctivitis, rash, bronchospasm.
- Contraindications—pregnancy is an absolute contradiction. Teratogenic risk continues after treatment cessation (contraception for 4 months after therapy in women and for 7 months in men). Avoid if breastfeeding. Avoid in severe cardiac disease, haemoglobinopathies, severe hepatic dysfunction, and autoimmune disease. Needs dose adjustment in renal impairment. Monitoring of blood work and ECG (cardiac history-dependent) needed throughout therapy.

Palivizumab

This is a monoclonal antibody directed against the F surface glycoprotein of RSV (responsible for virion fusing with the host cell), thereby inhibiting viral entry. Its use has been shown to reduce RSV hospitalization and morbidity in high-risk children (congenital heart disease, bronchopulmonary dysplasia, and severe combined immunodeficiency syndrome); for full usage, see the Green book, Chapter 27a (available at: ℘ https://www.gov.uk/government/publications/respiratory-syncytial-virus-the-green-book-chapter-27a). Due to its long half-life, it can be given monthly, usually at the start of the RSV season for a maximum of five doses. Except for previous anaphylaxis, there are few contraindications to its use.

Antivirals for hepatitis B

There is no cure for HBV infection (⊖ see Hepatitis B virus, pp. 465–70), but an effective vaccine and suppressive treatment options exist. The vaccine is used in two ways: pre-emptively (i.e. populations deemed high-risk of acquisition, e.g. healthcare workers) and in combination with specific HBV immunoglobulin as PEP (e.g. in prevention of vertical transmission). The aim of treatment is to suppress HBV replication, thereby reducing the risk of progressive chronic liver disease, cirrhosis, and the development of hepatocellular carcinoma (HCC). For comprehensive guidance to HBV management, see the 2017 European Association for the Study of the Liver (EASL) *Clinical Practice Guidelines on the Management of Hepatitis B Virus Infection* (available at: ✎ https://easl.eu/publication/easl-guidelines-man agement-of-hepatitis-b/).

General prescribing points

- Acute HBV infection is rarely treated, and not all cases of chronic HBV infection require treatment. Virological, biochemical, and histological criteria must be met before treatment is considered. For those who do not require treatment, regular surveillance is recommended.
- There are two main treatment strategies:
  - treatment with α peginterferon alfa (PegIFNα) for a finite period to induce long-term immunological control;
  - treatment with a nucleos(t)ide analogue to provide reliable suppressive antiviral effects in the long term.

Interferon-α

- Interferons (IFNs) are endogenously produced by cells in response to various stimuli. Their effects are multiple and incompletely understood. They are not directly antiviral but rather induce an antiviral state in the host through a myriad of immunomodulating effector actions. They upregulate numerous genes whose products block the synthesis of viral proteins, decrease viral RNA stability, and stimulate the adaptive immune response.
- PegIFNα is produced by the addition of polyethylene glycol (Peg) to IFN-α. Peg slows absorption, thereby increasing the half-life to allow weekly dosing by s/c injection. Duration is usually for 48 weeks, with early stopping rules if certain treatment targets (quantification of hepatitis B surface antigen (HBsAg) and viral load) are not met.
- PegIFNα is used in hepatitis D virus (HDV)/HBV co-infection and in young patients with HBV infection who want to avoid long-term treatment with NAs. Not all patients with HBV infection make suitable candidates for treatment, as response rates are highly variable and there are significant issues with tolerability. Predictors of success include genotype A or B, alanine aminotransferase (ALT) level 2–5 times above normal, hepatitis B e antigen (HBeAg) positivity, high inflammatory scores on liver biopsy (if available), and a lower viral load. Treatment end points, such as HBeAg loss, ALT normalization, suppression of virus, and particularly HBsAg loss, are highly desirable.
- Treatment outcomes—not a comprehensively researched area:

- HBeAg-positive patients: HBeAg loss (32%), ALT normalization (41%), HBsAg loss (3%);
- HBeAg-negative (anti-HBeAg-positive) patients: ALT normalization (59%), HBsAg loss (4%).
- Side effects—fever, chills, fatigue, myalgia, myelotoxicity (monitor FBC), impaired concentration, altered mood, exacerbation or development of autoimmune thyroid diseases, alopecia, arthralgia, hypersensitivity (rare), pulmonary infiltrates (rare).
- It should NOT be used in patients with decompensated cirrhosis or pregnancy. Also avoid if a history of suicidal tendency, active psychiatric illness, autoimmune disease, severe leucopenia, or thrombocytopenia.

Nucleos(t)ide analogues

- Nucleos(t)ide analogues inhibit the polymerase (RT) activity of HBV, thereby interfering with nucleic acid synthesis by causing chain termination after their incorporation.
- Three agents: lamivudine (nucleoside analogue of cytosine), adefovir (nucleotide analogue of adenosine), and telbivudine (thymidine nucleoside analogue) are all considered to have a low genetic barrier to resistance (in contrast to tenofovir and entecavir) and their use is no longer recommended in the treatment of HBV infection. Lamivudine resistance can be as high as 70% after 5 years.

Tenofovir

- A synthetic nucleotide analogue of adenosine. Is available as two pro-drug formulations: tenofovir disoproxil (TDF) and the newer agent tenofovir alafenamide (TAF). A tenofovir-containing regimen is recommended in HBV/HIV co-infection.
- Resistance (tenofovir)—true virological resistance is remarkably rare; most failures of viral suppression can be attributed to compliance. ~80% of HBeAg-positive and 90% of HBeAg-negative patients will have suppressed virus following a year of therapy.
- Pharmacology (TDF)—renal excretion. Dose requires adjusting in renal insufficiency—caution: consider alternate agent (TAF or entecavir).
- Side effects (tenofovir)—GI symptoms, renal impairment, lactic acidosis, and hepatic steatosis (rare).
- Due to differences in intracellular activation, TAF can be given at ~10-fold lower dose and is considered less nephrotoxic and less damaging to bone health, with equivalent antiviral activity. Consequently, it is a useful agent in these subpopulations.

Entecavir

- A nucleoside analogue of guanosine. Considered to have a high genetic barrier to resistance (similar to tenofovir).
- Drops in HIV RNA have been noted in patients receiving entecavir monotherapy, but it is not considered a clinically useful HIV antiviral. Avoid in HBV/HIV co-infection.
- Of most utility in those where bone disease or renal impairment precludes the use of TDF.
- Dosing should be decreased in those with severe renal impairment.
- Side effects—GI symptoms, lactic acidosis, hepatomegaly with steatosis, and CNS symptoms.

HBV vaccine

- The HBV vaccine is an effective and safe subunit vaccine composed of HBsAg. It does not contain live virus. For a full description, see the Green book, Chapter 18 (available at: ℜ https://www.gov.uk/gov ernment/publications/hepatitis-b-the-green-book-chapter-18).

HBV immunoglobulin

- Used where temporary, rapid passive immunity is required as part of a PEP strategy. Most commonly following high-risk needlestick injuries or in neonates in the context of maternal HBV infection where specific criteria are met (see the Green book, Chapter 18, available at: ℜ https://www.gov.uk/government/publications/hepatitis-b-the-green-book-chapter-18).

Investigational treatments

- Since curative treatments for HCV infection have become the mainstay, attention has been turned to curative therapies for HBV infection. Defining standardized end points for use in clinical trials will facilitate treatment comparisons. A sterilizing cure, defined as complete elimination of HBV in the host, with no risk of relapse/disease progression, will be extremely difficult to achieve. This is due to the formation of covalently closed circular DNA (cccDNA) and integration of viral DNA during the HBV replication cycle. Instead, agents that induce a functional cure, defined as sustained, undetectable HBsAg and serum DNA after a finite course of treatment, with resolution of residual liver injury and a decrease in risk of HCC, are being pursued.
- Numerous agents/targets in the replication cycle are in various phases of clinical trials:
  - entry inhibitor: an agent called Myrcludex B targets the hepatocyte receptor sodium taurocholate (NTCP) crucial to viral uptake;
  - cccDNA agents: compounds that degrade via the APOBEC proteins or silence transcription from cccDNA remain highly attractive, as cccDNA is the reservoir of HBV infection;
  - nucleocapsid inhibitors: these cause instability in mature virion formation, therefore interfering with HBV replication;
  - HBsAg release inhibitors: inhibit the release of mature virions and HBsAg from hepatocytes;
  - immunomodulators: boost existing immune response, similar to PegIFNα, but more targeted;
  - therapeutic vaccines: restore exhausted CD8 T-cell response.
- Hepatitis B core-related antigen (HBcrAg) is a novel serum biomarker whose levels appear to correlate with the transcriptional activity of intrahepatic cccDNA. The ability to estimate the dynamic activity/burden of cccDNA would enable more targeted treatment algorithms.

Antivirals for hepatitis C

Treatment for HCV infection (➜ see Hepatitis C virus, pp. 471–3) has transformed in the last decade—progressing from the toxicity-laden regimens of ribavirin and IFN to the present day where a myriad of well-tolerated directly acting antiviral (DAA) regimens are available. Cure rates have increased from 50% to almost 100%. Treatment success is defined by demonstration of a sustained virological response (SVR) (absence of HCV RNA) at 12 weeks post-completion of treatment (SVR12). Relapse after this is very rare, with rates of SVR12 being similar to those of SVR24. Achieving an SVR results in a decrease in all-cause mortality, liver-related death, and HCC.

General prescribing points

- PegIFNα is no longer routinely used in the management of HCV infection.
- DAA choice and availability will vary by region, so consultation with local clinical groups is necessary. For comprehensive details of treatment regimen guidelines, see EASL's *Recommendations on Treatment of Hepatitis C 2018* (available at: ➾ https://easl.eu/publication/easl-recommendations-on-treatment-of-hepatitis-c-2020/).
- Baseline assessment includes previous HCV infection treatment history, liver disease severity (presence of (de)compensated cirrhosis and Child–Pugh score), and usually the HCV genotype.
- Prior to starting DAA treatment, a full drug history to include over-the-counter, illegal, and prescribed medicines must be taken. Numerous drug–drug interactions exist, and a safety assessment can be performed with a local pharmacist (also available at: ➾ https://www.hep-druginteractions.org).
- Protease inhibitors (PIs) are contraindicated in patients with decompensated cirrhosis (Child–Pugh B/C) or compensated cirrhosis (Child–Pugh A) with previous decompensation, due to higher toxicity.
- For a simplified, genotype-free approach; in patients without cirrhosis or with compensated cirrhosis (Child–Pugh A), who are treatment-naïve or treatment-experienced (previously treated with PegIFNα, ribavirin, or sofosbuvir), treatment with sofosbuvir plus velpatasvir for 12 weeks or glecaprevir plus pibrentasvir for 8 weeks (12 weeks in treatment-experienced compensated Child–Pugh A cirrhosis) is possible (see Table 4.1).
- Resistance testing looking for resistance-associated substitutions (RAS) is only required in certain circumstances (when planning use of a particular DAA or in cases of previous failure).
- Treatment of HCV infection in certain populations requires additional expert guidance (e.g. pregnancy (not recommended), decompensated liver disease, HCC, previous DAA treatment failure, or in liver transplant patients.

Overview of directly acting antiviral treatment

- DAA treatments are primarily available as numerous fixed-drug combinations. A few key formulations will be discussed (see Table 4.1).
- There are three main classes of DAA treatments:

Table 4.1 Recommended DAA regimens for treatment-naïve/experienced[a] patients with HCV without cirrhosis[b]

Genotype	Liver status	Treatment	Sofosbuvir/ Velpatasvir	Glecaprevir/ Pibrentasvir	Grazoprevir/ Elbasvir	Sofosbuvir/ velpatasvir/ voxilaprevir
1a, 1b, 2, 4, 5, 6	Non-cirrhotic	Naïve	12 weeks	8 weeks	12 weeks (G1b only)	N/A
		Experienced		12 weeks		
	Compensated (Child–Pugh A)	Naïve	12 weeks	8 weeks	N/A	N/A
		Experienced		12 weeks		
3	Non-cirrhotic	Naïve	12 weeks	8 weeks	N/A	N/A
		Experienced		12 weeks		
	Compensated (Child–Pugh A)	Naïve	12 weeks + ribavirin[c]	8–12 weeks[d]	N/A	12 weeks[c]
		Experienced		16 weeks		

[a] Defined as patients previously treated with ribavirin and PegIFNα, PegIFNα, or ribavirin and sofosbuvir.

[b] Or compensated (Child–Pugh A) cirrhosis.

[c] If RAS testing shows absence of the NS5A Y93H mutation, then treatment with sofosbuvir/velpatasvir is recommended.

[d] There are currently insufficient data to recommend shortening to 8 weeks.

Source: data from European Association for the Study of the Liver (2020) 'EASL recommendations on treatment of hepatitis C: Final update of the series' *Journal of Hepatology* 73(5)x1170–1218.

- NS3/4A serine PIs (suffix -previr)—involved in post-translation processing (cleaving) of the large HCV polyprotein; they block a site on NS3 that is essential for effective NS3/NS4A interaction. An additional mechanism is disruption of virally induced signalling pathways that lead to impaired production of endogenous IFN. First-generation agents were considered to have a low barrier to resistance, something which has largely been overcome in subsequent generations. They vary in their degree of drug–drug interactions, and an accurate concomitant drug/medication history is crucial. Cleared by CYP3A4/5 and should not be given in conjunction with medications that are inducers (carbamazepine, phenytoin, rifampicin, certain antiretrovirals) or are highly dependent upon it for clearance (methadone, certain triazoles, non-nucleoside reverse transcriptase inhibitors (NNRTIs), etc.);
- NS5A protein inhibitors (suffix -asvir)—precise mechanism of action is not fully understood. The NS5A protein is essential for viral replication and is found extensively in viral-induced membrane vesicles called the membranous web in cellular cytoplasm. It is generally accepted that NS5A inhibitors interfere with viral replication and virion assembly, in addition to potential disruption of viral immune modulation in the host;
- NS5B polymerase inhibitors (suffix -buvir)—target is an RNA-dependent RNA polymerase crucial to HCV replication. The enzyme has a single site for nucleos(t)ide binding (which results in chain termination) and four ant more sites for non-nucleos(t)ide binding (which results in allosteric inhibition). The non-nucleos(t)ide polymerase inhibitors (e.g. dasabuvir) have not been studied in great depth due to prominence of the nucleos(t)ide agent sofosbuvir.

Sofosbuvir/velpatasvir

- This regimen is pan-genotypic with a high genetic barrier to resistance. A single tablet to be taken od with/without food. Does not require dose adjustment in renal impairment. Well tolerated. Both agents are substrates of the P-glycoprotein (P-gp) cell transporter, and so numerous drug–drug interactions must be excluded before use. Sofosbuvir should not be co-administered with amiodarone and certain statins. Increased gastric pH decreases absorption of velpatasvir and so proton pump inhibitor (PPI) use should be avoided.

Glecaprevir/pibrentasvir

- This regimen is pan-genotypic with a high genetic barrier to resistance. Three tablets to be taken od with food. Does not require dose adjustment in renal impairment. Well tolerated. Both agents are substrates and inhibitors of P-gp, breast cancer resistance protein (BCRP), and organic anion transporting polypeptide (OATP) (all cellular efflux pumps), and some drug–drug interactions exist. Administration with atazanavir, rifampicin, the oral contraceptive pill, and numerous statins is contraindicated. Contains a PI, which precludes use in some patient subgroups—previous or current decompensated liver disease.

Grazoprevir/elbasvir

- Is of most use in genotype 1b. Requires baseline RAS testing before use in genotype 1a. Does not require dose adjustment in renal impairment. One tablet od. Well tolerated. Metabolized through CYP3a and so should not be given with strong inducers/inhibitors of this enzyme (e.g. rifampicin, phenytoin, carbamazepine, some antiretroviral HIV drugs). Contains a PI, which precludes its use in some patient subgroups.

Sofosbuvir/velpatasvir/voxilaprevir

- This combination adds the NS3/4A PI voxilaprevir to the existing sofosbuvir/velpatasvir formulation in a single tablet taken with food. The regimen is pan-genotypic but is usually kept in reserve for those with previous virological failure on DAA treatment. While well tolerated, it is subject to usual drug–drug interactions and is unsuitable for those with decompensated liver disease.

Ribavirin

- Used in combination with sofosbuvir/velpatasvir for treatment in patients with decompensated liver disease or solid organ transplant recipients in whom use of a PI is precluded (➔ see Antivirals for respiratory syncytial virus, p. 100).

Antivirals for HIV

Monumental strides have been made in the treatment of HIV-1 infection (henceforth referred to as HIV) (➔ see Human immunodeficiency virus, pp. 035–6). If diagnosed and treated before significant immunosuppression occurs, life expectancy approaches that of the general population. Challenges remain: early diagnosis, global access to treatment, dependence on a daily administration schedule, concerns about long-term metabolic complications of antiretroviral therapy (ART), drug toxicity, and absence of a (functional) cure. Treatment is now recommended in all people living with HIV (PLWH), regardless of CD4 count, and there is an emerging evidence base for the use of <3 agents. Drug selection is increasingly complex; there are >20 individual agents across six main drug classes, and numerous co-formulations are now available. Drug potency has increased, such that the primary end point of an undetectable viral load (serum HIV RNA below the lower limit of standard PCR detection assay) is readily achievable, and increasing thought is directed towards avoidance of long-term, often subclinical, drug toxicity. Antiretroviral drugs (ARV) agents are also employed both as pre-exposure prophylaxis (PrEP) and PEP. PrEP dramatically reduces the risk (most 99%) of contracting HIV from sexual intercourse, which underpins the U=U campaign (undetectable=untransmissible). Guidelines for HIV treatment are particularly dynamic and updated regularly (available at: ✍ https://www.bhiva.org/guidelines and https://www.eacsociety.org/guidelines/eacs-guidelines/).

Antiretroviral therapy

ART drugs have three-letter abbreviations (e.g. lamivudine (3TC)). Prior to starting ART or any new medicine in a patient already on ART, a full drug history to include over-the-counter, illegal, and prescribed medicines must be taken. Numerous drug–drug interactions exist, and a safety assessment can be performed with a local pharmacist (see also ✍ https://hiv-druginteractions.org/checker). There are six main drug classes of HIV ART available, but only four are typically used in most regimens:

- nucleoside reverse transcriptase inhibitors (NRTIs) (➔ see Nucleos(t)ide analogue reverse transcriptase inhibitors, p. 112);
- NNRTIs (➔ see Non-nucleoside reverse transcriptase inhibitors, pp. 113–14);
- PIs (➔ see Protease inhibitors, pp. 114–15);
- integrase strand transfer inhibitors (INSTIs) (➔ Integrase strand transfer inhibitors, pp. 115–16);
- entry inhibitors and others (➔ see Entry inhibitors, pp. 116–17).

General ART prescribing points

The aim of ART is to decrease morbidity and mortality by maintaining long-term viral suppression, thereby allowing the immune system to reconstitute and function as normally as possible. Regular monitoring of both the HIV viral load (HIV RNA) and CD4 count (biomarker for immune function) is undertaken to ensure that this is taking place. Broadly speaking, contemporary ART regimens are well tolerated, with fewer side effects, compared to their predecessors. Transmitted drug resistance remains low (<20%). Analysis of genotypic resistance testing results is crucial, particularly in treatment-experienced patients or where patient care is transferred between services (available at: ✍ https://hivdb.stanford.edu). ART regimens can change over time to match evolving health requirements (e.g. new comorbidities).

When deciding on optimal HIV ART options, regimens are individualized to the patient. A few notable factors should be taken into consideration:

- results of current and past drug resistance assays;
- likelihood of the patient adhering to therapy;
- pill burden: number of tablets, desire for a single-tablet regimen;
- baseline organ dysfunction (hepatic/renal/cardiac impairment);
- concurrent opportunistic infection (OI) treatment (e.g. TB, *Pneumocystis* pneumonia (PCP));
- concurrent infections (e.g. HBV/HCV);
- HLA-B*57:01 status;
- possibility of current/future pregnancy;
- estimates of future cardiac (QRisk) and bone health (FRAX) scores.

Initial ART regimens in treatment-naïve patients with HIV

The most commonly used regimens contain an NRTI backbone (two agents) and a third agent. This third agent could be an NNRTI, a PI, or an INSTI. Treatment with dual therapy (an INSTI and an (N)NRTI or a PI and an (N)NRTI) is an area of active research. Currently, it is most commonly used in patients who have already achieved viral suppression, but use in treatment-naïve patients is likely to increase in the future.

Pre-exposure prophylaxis

The two-NRTI single-tablet formulation containing tenofovir (TDF) and emtricitabine (FTC) is used to prevent HIV acquisition in those deemed to be high risk. It can be administered either daily or in an anticipatory 'event-based' fashion (see British HIV Association (BHIVA)/British Association for Sexual Health and HIV (BASHH) guidelines on the use of HIV PrEP, 2018, available at: ℘ https://www.bhiva.org/PrEP-guidelines).

Post-exposure prophylaxis

A regimen composed of TDF/FTC and an INSTI called raltegravir (RAL) is administered as soon as possible (ideally within 24h, but up to 72h) after exposure for a total of 28 days. If the source has an undetectable viral load, PEP is not indicated. Close monitoring is required. For risk assessment, see UK guideline for the use of HIV post-exposure prophylaxis, 2021, available at: ℘ https://www.bhiva.org/PEP-guidelines) (see Table 4.2).

HIV-2

Intrinsic resistance to NNRTI and fusion inhibitors. Typically use two NRTI agents as backbone plus a PI or an INSTI as the third agent.

Table 4.2 Summary table of post-exposure prophylaxis prescribing recommendations (available at: 🌐 https://www.bhiva.org)

Recommended combination	Tenofovir disoproxil 245mg/emtricitabine 200mg [a] one tablet once daily
	PLUS raltegravir 1200mg once daily [b,c]
Alternatve	*Alternatives to tenofovir disoproxil/emtricitabine backbone*
	eGFR [d,e] 30–50 ml/min: tenofovir-alafenamide 25mg/emtricitabine 200mg one tablet once daily
	eGFR [d] <360 ml/min: seek expert advise from ID/GUM/Secual Health team
	Alternatvie to raltegravir 1200mg once daily as third agent
	Dolutegravir 50mg once daily [b,f]
	Raltegravir 400mg twice daily [b]
	Darunavir 800mg + ritonavir 100mg once daily [g]
	Atazanavir 300mg + ritonavir 100mg once daily [g]
Alternative	Elvitegravir 150mg/cobicistat 150mg/tenofovir-DF 245mg/emtricitabine 200mg FDC: one tablet once daily [g]
Combination 2	If eGFR 30–70 ml/min elvitegravir 150mg/cobicistat 150mg/tenofovir-AF 10mg/emtricitabine 200mg FDC

[a] Tenofovir disoproxil 245mg/emtricitabine 200mg FDC is the preferred agent in chronic hepatitis B virus infection.
[b] Antacids and multivitamins (products containing metal cations e.g. magnesium/aluminium, which can chelate and reduce the absorption of INSTIs) should be avoided where possible during PEP with once daily raltegravir, see appendix A. An alternative non-interacting medication may be considered. Metal cation-containing medicines must be seperated by at least 4 hours from twice daily raltegravir and dolutegravir. See appendix A for other drug-drug interactions including rifampicin.

c For women who are pregnant raltegravir 400mg twice daily is preferred as the third agent. Where accessing raltegravir 400mg twice daily is preferred as the third agent. Where accessing raltegravir 400mg might cause delay we recommend using raltegravir 600mg twice daily and switching at the earliest opportunity.

d eGFR should ideally be calculated using the Cockcroft Gault method

e Tenofovir-alafenamide/emtricitabine (Descovy®) may be preferred to tenofovir disoproxil fumarate 245mg/emtricitabine 200mg in patients with abnormal renal function at baseline. The dose of Descovy depends on the third agent chosen: Descovy® 200mg/25mg should be prescribed with dolutegravir or raltegravir. Descovy® 200mg/10mg should be prescribed with the protease inhibitors darunavir/ritonavir and atazanavir/ritonavir. Note Descovy® is more susceptible to drug interactions when combined with enzyme inducers; conduct thorough drug interaction check or seek specialist advice.

f For women who are at risk of pregnancy or under 6 weeks pregnant, we recommend avoiding the use of dolutegravir. Fror women who are more than 6 weeks pregnant, dolutegravir-based PEP can be used.

g Significant drug-drug interactions can occur with boosted protease inhibitors and elvitegravir/cobicistat; seek expert advice from an HIV specialist pharmacist, local medicines and poisons information centre or use the website ww.hiv-druginteraction.org

Swallowing difficulty – tenofovir/emtricitabine can be dissolved in 100 ml of water or orange juice and taken immediatey. Lopinavir/ritonavir can be used as an alternative to dolutegravir and is commercially available as an oral solution; the recommended dosage is 5ml twice daily with food. Where liquid firomulations are unavailable, dolutegravir tablets may be split or crushed and added to a small amount of semi-solid food or liquid, all of which shoud be consumed immediately.

Nucleos(t)ide analogue reverse transcriptase inhibitors

RT is an RNA-dependent DNA polymerase that is essential for virus replication (➔ see Human immunodeficiency virus, pp. 835–6). It enables transcription of viral RNA into DNA, which is then integrated into the host genome. NRTIs are all nucleosides, with the exception of tenofovir which is a nucleotide. Within the cell, host enzymes phosphorylate the parent drug to the active triphosphate form. NRTI inhibits viral replication by competitively binding to the viral RT, resulting in chain termination after incorporation, thereby inhibiting DNA synthesis. Akin to other NA agents, there is variable activity on host polymerases, which can cause toxicity. NRTIs are most commonly used in pairs forming the backbone of regimens, and are available as single-tablet co-formulations. The two most commonly used are TDF/FTC and abacavir (ABC)/3TC. These co-formulations are intentional, as certain pairings can be antagonistic due to competition for similar phosphorylation pathways. In general, NRTIs are well tolerated and have few drug–drug interactions. The older NRTI agents didanosine and stavudine are no longer used due to toxicity.

Resistance

- Caused by one or more mutations in the RT gene.
- Some specific mutations can confer cross-resistance to other NRTIs.
- Generally considered to have a low to medium genetic barrier to resistance.

Specific drugs

- Tenofovir (➔ see Hepatitis B virus, pp. 465–70) is available as two formulations: TDF and the newer agent TAF. A tenofovir-containing regimen is recommended in HBV/HIV co-infection. TDF is generally avoided if the estimated glomerular filtration rate (eGFR) is <60mL/min. TAF is considered to be less nephrotoxic and less damaging to bone density. Regular monitoring of renal function, including screening for proteinuria, is recommended.
- 3TC and FTC are both cytosine analogues and, due to potential antagonism, precludes co-administration. Pancreatitis (3TC) and skin pigmentation (FTC) are rare complications.
- Abacavir (ABC)—screening for HLA-B*5701 (prevalent in 5–8% of European populations, 1% in Asian/African populations) is essential prior to treatment, in order to prevent a hypersensitivity reaction. ABC is avoided in patients with, or at high risk of developing, cardiac disease. It is used with caution in those with high viral loads of >100 000 copies/mL, unless administered with the INSTI dolutegravir (DTG).
- Zidovudine (AZT, ZDV) was the first agent to demonstrate a decrease in HIV mortality. Generally less well tolerated, compared to other NRTIs, due to marrow suppression, nausea, anorexia, lipoatrophy, and dyslipidaemia. Needs bd dosing. Is available parenterally, which makes it useful in certain situations (e.g. during labour where it is given as an infusion during childbirth).

Non-nucleoside reverse transcriptase inhibitors

NNRTIs prevent nucleotides from being added to the DNA chain being synthesized by HIV RT. NNRTIs bind to a different site in RT (p66 subunit) than NRTIs, and induce a conformational change that dramatically reduces enzymatic activity. NNRTIs are not active against HIV-2.

Resistance

- Caused by one or more mutations in the RT gene.
- The first-generation NNRTIs efavirenz (EFV) and nevirapine (NVP), and to a lesser extent rilpivirine (RPV), are considered to have a low genetic barrier to resistance. It is possible that only a single mutation can confer cross-resistance to multiple agents.
- Generally speaking, NNRTIs (with notable exception of doravirine) have a long half-life (>24h). This becomes an issue if ART containing an NNRTI is not taken regularly or is stopped, as periods may arise when only the NNRTI component is present. This will promote the development of viral resistance due to the varying pharmacokinetics (faster clearance) of the other agents (the NRTI backbone). If cessation of ART is planned, then measures should be employed to avoid this (by supplementing a temporary third agent from a different class). Similarly, if ART adherence is thought to be a problem, NNRTIs should be avoided.

Specific drugs

- NVP is no longer in common use. Potentially fatal hepatotoxicity has been described in patients whose CD4 counts exceed >250 cells/mm³ (in women) or >400 cells/mm³ (in men). It is used primarily (as part of a wider regimen) in women not on ART who present in labour and in high-risk cases of neonatal PEP.
- EFV has a long-established proven track record in effective ART due to its potency and availability in a single-tablet formulation. Widespread use is now less common due to availability of agents with fewer side effects. It is an inducer of P450 enzymes and so potential drug–drug interactions must be excluded before use. While dyslipidaemia, elevated liver enzymes, and torsades de pointes have all been described, it is the potential neuropsychiatric side effects that have gathered most attention. Both short-term (vivid dreams, drowsiness, and dizziness), as well as cumulative longer-term (depression, mood changes, anxiety, and even suicidal ideation), effects have been described. It is suggested that patients who are stable on EFV-containing regimens do not necessarily need their ART changed but should be screened regularly for development of neuropsychiatric symptoms.
- RPV is available on its own or in formulations with NRTIs or INSTI. Is less potent than EFV and so is not indicated for patients with viral loads in excess of 100 000 copies/mL or CD4 counts <200 cells/mm³. Administration with food is essential, and agents that raise gastric pH require caution (PPI use is contraindicated, whereas use of H2 antagonists/antacids requires delayed administration). Neuropsychiatric

effects similar to those of EFV are described but are less common. Drug–drug interactions exist and require exclusion before use.

- Etravirine (ETV) shows a higher genetic barrier to resistance than other NNRTIs; this is, in part, due to its flexible molecular structure allowing it to bind to RT in multiple conformations. Scoring systems exist to predict response to ETV in the setting of existing NNRTI resistance mutations (Monogram or Tibotec). Accordingly, it is mainly used as salvage therapy in treatment-experienced patients in combination with other agents. The main side effect is rash (severe reactions, such as Stevens–Johnson syndrome, have been described but are rare). Numerous drug–drug interactions exist due to inducing CYP34A including to other ART agents (e.g. DTG and some PIs).
- Doravirine (DOR) is the latest NNRTI and can be administered without clinical restrictions in HIV viral load or CD4 parameters. There are no meal requirements and no contraindications to concomitant PPI use. DOR remains active in the presence of some NNRTI resistance mutations but is not as robust as ETV. Neuropsychiatric side effects are described, but not as commonly as with EFV.

Protease inhibitors

When PIs were first combined with NRTI backbones in the mid-90s, treatment of PLWH was revolutionized. Following reverse transcription and translation of the HIV genome, a long polyprotein containing all the viral gene products is produced. This large polyprotein requires cleavage by a virally encoded enzyme called protease (which targets specific *gag* and *gag–pol* regions within the polyprotein) to release the functional subunits. The PIs contain a synthetic analogue of this region and inhibit this process by binding to protease, which is detrimental towards production of mature infectious virions (active against HIV-1 and 2). PIs must be administered with a 'booster' agent—usually ritonavir (RTV) or cobicistat (COBI), both inhibitors of CYP3A4 enzyme—to increase their therapeutic half-life. Accordingly, there are multiple drug–drug interactions which require exclusion (available at: ℘ https://hiv-druginteractions.org/checker). COBI can block tubular secretion of creatinine. Several older PIs are no longer in general use due to toxicity: indinavir, nelfinavir, saquinavir, tipranavir, and fosamprenavir.

Resistance

- Caused by mutations in the protease gene. PIs are considered to have a high genetic barrier to resistance when compared to NRTIs, NNRTIs, and early INSTIs.
- Amongst the PI class, darunavir (DRV) has a particularly high genetic barrier to resistance due to a unique resistance pathway; it can retain antiviral activity despite the presence of some PI mutations. In addition to inhibition of protease catalytic activity, DRV inhibits enzyme dimerization.
- A useful class if drug adherence is thought to be problematic.

Specific drugs

- Atazanavir (ATV)—although can be unboosted, it very rarely is. ATV is a potent od treatment that was in widespread use due to better GI tolerability versus other PIs, but is now less commonly used. Unlike other PIs, it is not associated with an increase in cardiovascular disease. Absorption is dependent on an acidic gastric pH (PPI use is best avoided). An increase in the concentration of indirect bilirubin is common, but largely considered benign. It can cause nephrolithiasis and gallstone formation.
- DRV—considered the most potent PI (⊃ see Resistance above). Is associated with GI side effects (nausea and diarrhoea), dyslipidaemia, and increased cardiovascular risk, and is avoided in patients with a sulfonamide allergy (DRV contains a sulfa moiety in its structure).
- Lopinavir (LPV)—used to be widely used as the agent of choice in pregnancy and PEP. Less commonly used due to pill burden and side effects (GI, dyslipidaemia, and metabolic).

Integrase strand transfer inhibitors

The INSTIs (also known as INIs) target the third enzyme coded by, and essential for, HIV replication called integrase. After viral RNA is reverse-transcribed by RT into complementary DNA (cDNA), it is inserted into the host genome of the cell by integrase. INSTIs inhibit the strand transfer step of this process by stopping the binding of the preintegration complex (a macromolecular structure containing viral cDNA, and host and viral proteins) to cellular DNA. The integrated viral DNA serves as a reservoir of HIV infection and is crucial to viral replication. INSTIs are increasingly used due to their potency, good tolerability, lack of food requirements, and relatively few drug–drug interactions. Weight gain and nausea are the commonest side effects reported. They are useful agents in several comorbid subgroups (i.e. those with elevated cardiac risk factors or where treatment of OIs or cancer with chemotherapy is required). INSTIs are active against HIV-1 and 2.

Resistance

- Caused by mutations in the integrase gene.
- Early INSTIs, such as RAL and elvitegravir (EVG), have a relatively lower genetic barrier to resistance than later agents and cross-resistance was an issue.
- Later agents, such as DTG, are particularly potent, with virological failure rarely occurring.

Specific drugs

- Bictegravir (BIC)—only available in a co-formulation with TAF/FTC. Is well tolerated clinically.
- DTG—can be administered od for most patients (bd if previous or suspected INSTI resistance is present). Can block tubular secretion of creatinine without decreasing tubular function. CNS neuropsychiatric symptoms slightly commoner than with other INSTIs. Concerns in 2018 regarding an increased rate of neural tube defects if taken around

conception have eased with a smaller increased risk than previously thought, almost comparable to other HIV drugs.

- EVG—must be administered with a boosting agent (available as a co-formulation with COBI); this increases drug–drug interactions. Like RAL, it has a low genetic barrier to resistance.
- RAL—generally administered bd but can be given od in certain circumstances (not pregnant, absence of drug inducers, viral suppression achieved on bd RAL).
- Carbotegravir—is a new agent that is available with the NNRTI RPV as an IM injection that can be administered (bi)-monthly. Patients need to have suppressed viral loads before commencement, and due to its long half-life, promoting resistance could be an issue if adherence becomes irregular. This bypasses the archetype of daily administration of PO ART regimens and is an area of intense research.

Entry inhibitors

For HIV to successfully enter a cell, it must first bind/attach to receptors on the cell surface before the viral envelope and cellular membrane fuse together, releasing the viral capsid inside. The HIV envelope protein (composed of subunits gp120 and gp41) attaches to the cellular CD4 receptor and an additional chemokine co-receptor, either CCR5 or CXCR4. Co-receptor binding preference evolves from R5 (R5 tropic virus) in early infection (80%) to X4 (X4 tropic virus) over time (50% in late-stage disease). Attachment inhibitors are relatively new agents, and entry inhibitors as a cohort are rarely used, except for salvage therapy in treatment-experienced patients with multi-class resistance.

Attachment inhibitors

- Fostemsavir is a pro-drug that is hydrolysed to temsavir, which binds to gp120, inducing a conformational change that prevents the HIV envelope from attaching to the CD4+ receptor. It is administered bd PO, and nausea, LFT derangement, and prolonged QTc are the most commonly reported side effects.
- Ibalizumab is a monoclonal IgG4 antibody that binds to host CD4+ receptors in a different region to where HIV gp120 binds. It is referred to as a post-attachment inhibitor, as its activity takes place after the initial HIV gp120–CD4+ attachment has occurred. Upon binding, it prevents the conformational change required in the gp120–CD4+ complex that allows subsequent binding to a co-receptor. It is not affected by tropism. It is administered by IV infusion every 14 days.

CCR5 antagonist

- Maraviroc (MVC) is a receptor antagonist that prevents the binding of CCR5-tropic HIV to the CCR5 receptor on CD4+ cells. If a virus is X4-tropic, use of MVC is precluded.
- Use of MVC requires a tropism assay prior to initiating treatment, to determine if the virus is predominantly R5-tropic, combination-tropic (mixed R5 and X4), or X4-tropic. Both genotypic and phenotypic methods exist. Genotypic assays will determine the amino acid

sequence near a conserved area in the V3 loop of gp120 in the HIV envelope gene. Software can then analyse this sequence, and algorithms can predict binding capability. Phenotypic analysis is done less commonly and involves using modified laboratory virus that expresses glycoprotein derived from the patient's virus to determine tropism.

- Rarely used for initial ART regimens. Mainly used in patients who possess multi-class resistance virus. Unfortunately, this precise cohort is more likely to have X4-tropic virus, and therefore, efficacy is limited.
- Administered bd and is generally well tolerated. Drug–drug interactions with strong hepatic inducers/inhibitors need exclusion.

Fusion inhibitor

- Enfuvirtide is a 36-amino acid polypeptide that binds to the gp41 component of the HIV envelope protein, preventing fusion.
- It is administered bd as a s/c injection, which can cause local cutaneous reactions.
- It is extremely rarely used due to availability of other agents/drug classes. Its use is reserved for multi-class resistance in heavily treatment-experienced patients.

The future

- Initial goals of sustained viral suppression have been largely achieved with potent, well-tolerated regimens. Escape from a daily PO administration schedule with fewer agents remains highly desirable.
- HIV research is fast-paced, and drug development subject to intense competition. A cure remains elusive largely due to the integrated component of the viral replication cycle. Numerous investigational vaccines have yielded disappointing performance.
- New drug classes are emerging (capsid inhibitors, maturation inhibitors, and broadly neutralizing antibodies).
- Efforts to improve HIV treatment must occur simultaneously with those directed towards increasing diagnosis; too many patients are diagnosed late in their illness (50% in the European Union). Global access to treatment remains unequal.

Further reading

British HIV Association. Current guidelines. Available at: ℗ https://www.bhiva.org/guidelines

European AIDS Clinical Society (2023). *EACS guidelines 2023, Version 12.0*. Available at: ℗ https://www.eacsociety.org/guidelines/eacs-guidelines/eacs-guidelines.html

European Association for the Study of the Liver. EASL 2017 clinical practice guidelines on the management of hepatitis B virus infection. *J Hepatol*. 2017;**67**:370–98.

European Association for the Study of the Liver. EASL recommendations on treatment of hepatitis C: final update of the series. *J Hepatol*. 2020;**73**:1170–218.

i-base (2022). *U=U: Undetectable = Untransmittable*. Available at: ℗ https://i-base.info/u-equals-u/

National Institute for Health and Care Excellence (2013, updated 2017). *Hepatitis B (chronic): diagnosis and management*. Clinical guideline [CG165]. Available at: ℗ https://www.nice.org.uk/guidance/cg165

National Institute for Health and Care Excellence (2022). *Hepatitis C*. Available at: ℗ https://cks.nice.org.uk/topics/hepatitis-c/

Public Health England (2011, updated 2018). *Influenza: antiviral susceptibility surveillance and diagnosis of resistance*. Available at: ℗ https://www.gov.uk/government/publications/influenza-antiviral-susceptibility-surveillance-and-diagnosis-of-resistance

UK Health Security Agency (2013, updated 2015). *Respiratory syncytial virus: the green book, chapter 27a*. Available at: ℜ https://www.gov.uk/government/publications/respiratory-syncytial-virus-the-green-book-chapter-27a

UK Health Security Agency (2013, updated 2019). *Varicella: the green book, chapter 34*. Available at: ℜ https://www.gov.uk/government/publications/varicella-the-green-book-chapter-34

UK Health Security Agency (2013, updated 2022). *Hepatitis B: the green book, chapter 18*. Available at: ℜ https://www.gov.uk/government/publications/hepatitis-b-the-green-book-chapter-18

UK Health Security Agency (2013, updated 2023). *Influenza: the green book, chapter 19*. Available at: ℜ https://www.gov.uk/government/publications/influenza-the-green-book-chapter-19

UK Health Security Agency (2013, updated 2023). *Shingles (herpes zoster): the green book, chapter 28a*. Available at: ℜ https://www.gov.uk/government/publications/shingles-herpes-zoster-the-green-book-chapter-28a

Antiparasitic therapy

Antimalarials

Antimalarial drugs are used for both treatment and prevention of malaria (see Box 5.1). Most drugs act upon the erythrocytic stage of the parasite life cycle. Artemisinins additionally act on gametocytes—potentially reducing onward transmission—and have been shown to reduce mortality, compared to quinine. As ever, the emergence of resistance is a major threat to malaria control and treatment. Artemisinin combination therapies (ACTs) reduce the chance of resistance emerging, and the World Health Organization (WHO) has called for the banning of all PO artemisinin monotherapy.

Resistance

Resistance arises through the selection of rare naturally occurring mutants with reduced drug susceptibility. Unlike bacteria, plasmodia do not have transferable resistance mechanisms, but they are eukaryotes and can acquire or lose polygenic resistance mechanisms during meiosis. Individual mechanisms are discussed on ➜ *Plasmodium* species (malaria), pp. 556–60.

Combination therapy

Treating malaria with a suitably chosen drug combination increases efficacy, may shorten treatment duration (increasing compliance), and decreases the risk of resistant parasites arising by mutation. Drug combinations are, however, more expensive (but short-term cost is easily outweighed by

---

Box 5.1 Guidelines for prevention and treatment of malaria

Treatment
- UK guidelines:
  - Lalloo D, Shingadia D, Pasvol G, *et al*. UK malaria treatment guidelines. *J Infect* 2016;**72**(6):635–64
  - UK Health Security Agency (UKHSA). Guideline for malaria prevention in travellers from the UK 2014
  - Both available at ➜ www.britishinfection.org/guidance/published-guidelines
  - See also *British National Formulary* (*BNF*) (➜ bnf.nice.org.uk/treatment-summary/malaria-prophylaxis.html)
- US guidelines:
  - Treatment of malaria: guidelines for clinicians. Available at: ➜ www.cdc.gov/malaria/diagnosis_treatment/clinicians1.html
  - Centers for Disease Control and Prevention (CDC). *The Yellow Book*. CDC health information for international travel 2020, Chapter 4, Travel-related infectious diseases—malaria. Available at: ➜ wwwnc.cdc.gov/travel/yellowbook/2024/infections-diseases/malaria
  - World Health Organization (WHO) (2021). *WHO guidelines for malaria*. Available at: ➜ www.who.int/teams/global-malaria-programme/guidelines-for-malaria

longer-term benefits), and if there is already high resistance to one of the components (perhaps through previous monotherapy), then resistance can arise to the other.

Key prescribing points

- Uncomplicated non-falciparum malaria can be treated with chloroquine or ACTs. Chloroquine resistance in *Plasmodium vivax* is now relatively widespread, having been identified in South East Asia, Ethiopia, and Madagascar. However, chloroquine should be effective in the majority of cases, but a switch to ACTs should be considered if the parasitaemia fails to fall after 4 days of therapy.
- Where *P. falciparum* co-circulates with non-falciparum species, it is wise to treat with a falciparum-active agent.
- Following treatment of *P. vivax* or *Plasmodium ovale*, anti-relapse therapy should be given with primaquine (contraindicated in pregnancy)—the only quinoline with reliable activity on hypnozoites. It should ideally start after glucose-6-phosphate dehydrogenase (G6PD) testing and near the start of chloroquine therapy. *P. vivax* is treated with a higher dose than *P. ovale*.
- While chloroquine-sensitive falciparum malaria does occur, it should only be used for treatment when there is certainty about the region of exposure and local parasite sensitivities.
- The WHO recommends ACTs as first-line treatment for uncomplicated falciparum malaria, as they have the fastest parasite clearance times.
- Severe falciparum malaria should be treated with IV artesunate, if available (studies have demonstrated mortality benefit, compared to quinine). Artesunate has a short half-life, and monotherapy of <5–7 days has been associated with parasite recrudescence. Thus, in practice, once patients are well enough to take PO medication, they should be switched to complete a full course of ACT (usually 3 days). If IV artesunate is not available, the alternative is IV quinine (watch for hypoglycaemia), combined with a second agent (e.g. doxycycline, clindamycin), for 7 days or a complete course of ACT once well enough to swallow.

Quinolines

Quinolines (not to be confused with quino**lones**) have been the mainstay of antimalarial therapy since the seventeenth century when Peruvian Indians used the bark extracts of the cinchona tree as treatment. Chloroquine has succumbed to global resistance in *P. falciparum*. Quinine remains widely used. Primaquine is notable for its additional activity on intrahepatic forms and gametocytes.

Quinine

- A quinoline methanol derived from the bark of the cinchona tree. Inhibits the erythrocytic stages of human malaria parasites, but not all liver stages. It is active against gametocytes of *P. vivax*, *P. ovale*, and *Plasmodium malariae*.

- Mode of action—accumulates in the parasite food vacuole, forming a complex with haem. This results in the inhibition of haem polymerase and accumulation of cytotoxic free haem.
- Resistance—widespread in South East Asia where some strains are also resistant to chloroquine, mefloquine, and sulfadoxine–pyrimethamine. Cross-resistance with mefloquine in Central Africa.
- Pharmacology—well absorbed PO; IM administration more predictable than IV administration. Hepatic metabolism. Urinary clearance <20%. Give a loading dose if the patient has not received a related agent.
- Adverse effects—cinchonism (flushing, tinnitus, vomiting, diarrhoea, headache), hypoglycaemia (stimulates insulin production—monitor blood glucose level), hypotension, cardiac arrhythmias, haemolytic anaemia (blackwater fever). Cinchonism is observed in most patients; it resolves upon completion and should not prompt a change in dose.
- Use—given IV in severe falciparum malaria if artesunate is unavailable. Quinidine (a stereoisomer of quinine) was previously used, particularly in the USA, as malaria therapy but had greater cardiotoxicity and is now very rarely used in clinical practice.

Chloroquine

- A synthetic 4-aminoquinoline, active against the erythrocytic stages of all four human malaria species and gametocytes of *P. vivax*, *P. ovale*, and *P. malariae*. However, *P. falciparum* resistance is now widespread, due to increased drug efflux (mutation in the *pfmdr1* gene) and/or decreased drug uptake (mutation in the *pfCRT* gene). It remains effective for the treatment of *P. ovale*, *P. malariae*, and *P. vivax* in most regions.
- Pharmacology—80–90% PO absorption. Widely distributed. Extensive tissue binding, with high affinity for melanin-containing tissues. Extensive metabolism to active metabolite; 50% renal excretion.
- Adverse effects—pruritus (seems to particularly affect those with darker skin tones), dizziness, headache, rashes, nausea, diarrhoea. Long-term treatment may cause CNS effects and retinopathy. Rarely, photosensitivity, tinnitus, and deafness may occur.
- Use—prophylaxis and treatment of chloroquine-sensitive malaria.

Mefloquine

- A synthetic 4-quinoline methanol. Active against erythrocytic stages of *Plasmodium* spp. Effective against strains of *P. falciparum* that are resistant to chloroquine, sulfonamides, and pyrimethamine. Mefloquine has been shown to have *in vitro* activity against some bacteria (e.g. meticillin-resistant *Staphylococcus aureus* (MRSA)) and fungi.
- Resistance—increasing; 15% high-grade resistance and 50% low-grade resistance in South East Asia (primarily due to the *pfmdr1* gene as above). Cross-resistance with quinine and halofantrine. An inverse relationship has been observed with chloroquine resistance.
- Pharmacology—well absorbed PO, concentrated in erythrocytes, metabolites not active, predominantly excreted in the bile.
- Adverse effects—nausea, dizziness, fatigue, confusion, sleep disturbance, pneumonitis, QTc prolongation. Psychosis, encephalopathy, and convulsions in 1/1200–1700 patients (thus, when used as

prophylaxis, tends to be started 2–3 weeks before it is required, to assess tolerability); 1/10 000 risk of serious toxicity in prophylaxis.
- Use—prophylaxis in areas of chloroquine resistance. Treatment of uncomplicated multidrug-resistant (MDR) malaria. Commonly used for prophylaxis in pregnancy, felt to be safe in second and third trimesters, and not known to be harmful when breastfeeding.

Amodiaquine

- A 4-aminoquinoline, active against *P. falciparum* and *P. vivax*.
- Pharmacologically similar to chloroquine, with which it is cross-resistant. Elimination half-life of 1–3 weeks.
- Adverse effects appear to be related to immunogenic properties of its metabolites, rather than to direct toxicity. Severe/life-threatening adverse events have been associated with prophylaxis, including neutropenia, agranulocytosis, hepatotoxicity, and aplastic anaemia—but it is well tolerated when given as a 3-day treatment course. Adverse events increased in those with HIV infection.
- Use—treatment of falciparum malaria, in combination with artesunate. No longer available in the USA/UK due to the side effect profile.

Piperaquine

- A 4-aminoquinoline; structurally related to chloroquine, but active against chloroquine-resistant *P. falciparum*.
- Pharmacology—well absorbed PO; elimination half-life of 17 days.
- Combination with dihydroartemisinin has shown excellent tolerability and high cure rates of MDR falciparum malaria.

Primaquine

- A synthetic 8-aminoquinoline, formulated as diphosphate. Active against hepatic stages of *Plasmodium* spp., including the hypnozoite stage of *P. vivax*. Poor activity against the erythrocytic stages, but active against gametocytes. Also active against *Pneumocystis* spp., *Babesia* spp., *Leishmania* spp., and *Trypanosoma cruzi*.
- Resistance—failure rates of up to 35% reported in South East Asia in patients treated for *P. vivax*.
- Pharmacology—well absorbed PO, extensive tissue distribution, metabolized to carboxyprimaquine and methoxy and hydroxy metabolites; <4% excreted unchanged in the urine.
- Adverse effects are generally mild—abdominal cramps, anaemia, leucocytosis, methaemoglobinaemia. Haemolysis occurs in G6PD deficiency (check G6PD levels first). Contraindicated in pregnancy.
- Use—treatment of *P. vivax* and *P. ovale*. Second line for treatment of *Pneumocystis jirovecii* (in combination with clindamycin).

Tafenoquine

- An 8-aminoquinoline with activity against *P. falciparum* and the hepatic (hypnozoite) stages of *P. vivax* and *P. ovale*.
- Pharmacology—similar to primaquine, but more potent, less toxic, and longer half-life (14 days), enabling weekly or monthly administration.
- Adverse effects—methaemoglobinaemia, haemolysis in G6PD deficiency.
- Use—prophylaxis and treatment of malaria.

Lumefantrine

- Similar structure to 4-methanol quinolines. Inhibits erythrocytic stages of *Plasmodium* spp., including most chloroquine-resistant parasites. Mostly used in combination with artemether derivatives. Halofantrine is a related compound with greater cardiac toxicity.
- Worrying emerging partial resistance to artemether–lumefantrine (the most commonly used ACT) has been detected in Rwanda in 2021. Resistance has also been reported in other areas of Central and West Africa and Thailand.
- Pharmacology—widely variable absorption, bioavailability increased by a fatty meal. Not concentrated in erythrocytes; 20–30% metabolized by the CYP450 enzyme system. Little excreted in the urine.
- Adverse effects—abdominal pain, diarrhoea, pruritus. High doses are cardiotoxic, with prolongation of PR and QT intervals; mefloquine enhances these effects, and sequential use is contraindicated.
- Use—treatment of MDR falciparum malaria.

Antifolates

The antimalarial activity of biguanides (proguanil) was discovered during the Second World War. Along with diaminopyrimidines (pyrimethamine), they are referred to as antifolate drugs and are used in combination with other agents for both prophylaxis and treatment.

Proguanil

- A synthetic arylbiguanide. Its metabolite cycloguanil inhibits the erythrocytic stages of all four *Plasmodium* spp. and the hepatic stage of *P. falciparum*. Acts synergistically with atovaquone.
- Resistance arises easily by point mutation in the *DHFR* gene. Worldwide for *P. falciparum*, and reported for *P. vivax* and *P. malariae* in South East Asia.
- Pharmacology—>90% PO absorption; 75% protein-bound; concentrated in erythrocytes; 20% metabolized by the CYP450 enzyme system to cycloguanil (active metabolite). Non-metabolizers occur in Japan and Kenya, leading to resistance; 60% excreted in the urine.
- Adverse effects—GI and renal effects at high doses (>600mg/day).
- Use—antimalarial prophylaxis (with chloroquine); treatment and prophylaxis of drug-resistant falciparum malaria (with atovaquone).

Pyrimethamine

- A synthetic diaminopyrimidine. Active against *Plasmodium* spp., *Toxoplasma gondii*, and *P. jirovecii*.
- Available as a single agent or in combination with sulfadoxine (not considered combination therapy, as components act on enzymes in the same pathway), dapsone, or mefloquine and sulfadoxine.
- Resistance is due to point mutations in the *DHFR* gene and is widespread in Africa and Latin America. Sequence variations in *P. falciparum* and mutations in the *pfmdr1* gene may also be important. Sulfadoxine resistance is due to mutations in its target dihydropteroate synthase (DHPS).

- Pharmacology—well absorbed PO. Long plasma half-life (111h). CSF levels 10–25% of plasma levels. Secreted in breast milk and crosses the placenta. Hepatic metabolism.
- Adverse effects—megaloblastic anaemia, leucopenia, thrombocytopenia, pancytopenia. Very large doses in children have caused vomiting, convulsions, respiratory failure, and death. Aggravation of subclinical folate deficiency. Teratogenic in animals.
- Use—treatment of malaria in combination with other drugs; treatment of toxoplasmosis and *Pneumocystis* pneumonia (PCP).

Other agents and combination therapies

Atovaquone

- Atovaquone is a hydroxynaphthoquinone that is more active than standard antimalarials against all stages of *P. falciparum*. It is also active against *Babesia* spp., *T. gondii*, and *P. jirovecii*. It blocks complex III in the protozoal mitochondrial electron transport chain.
- Malaria resistance emerges rapidly, due to point mutations in the parasite's cytochrome bc_1 gene. It is therefore used in combination with proguanil, with which it has synergistic activity.
- Pharmacology—poor PO absorption, improved when given with meals; 99% protein-bound; poor CSF penetration (<1%). Not metabolized. Elimination half-life of 73h.
- Adverse effects—fever, nausea, diarrhoea, rash.
- Use—prophylaxis and treatment of malaria in combination with proguanil; treatment of PCP (atovaquone alone).

Tetracycline and doxycycline

- Tetracycline and doxycycline (➲ see Tetracyclines, pp. 61–3) are active against *Plasmodium* spp. via inhibition of protein synthesis in the apicoplast organelle. They are well absorbed PO, with elimination half-lives of 8h (tetracycline) and 20h (doxycycline).
- Quinine plus tetracycline has been used for treatment of MDR falciparum malaria in Thailand for years.
- Doxycycline is also used in prophylaxis of malaria in regions with chloroquine or mefloquine resistance.
- Main limitations—contraindicated in children and pregnant women; photosensitivity with doxycycline; emergence of parasite resistance to tetracycline in areas where it has been used extensively.

Clindamycin

- Clindamycin (➲ see Lincosamides, pp. 56–7) is a lincosamide antibiotic that also acts on the malaria parasite's apicoplast.
- Although numerous studies of quinine plus clindamycin have shown good efficacy and safety profiles in various populations, it has never been used widely.

Artemisinin and its derivatives

Artemisinin (qinghao) is derived from *Artemisia annua* (sweet wormwood plant). Chinese herbalists have used it for around 2000 years, but it was developed commercially as a medication since the 1970s. Artemisinin and its derivatives are metabolized to dihydroartemisinin, which is the biologically active form. They are the most effective group of antimalarial agents and act against all *Plasmodium* spp. Although widely used in the developing world to treat malaria, their use in the developed world is hampered by a lack of availability of good manufacturing practice (GMP) products. Oral use in uncomplicated malaria should always be in combination with another agent due to concerns about emerging resistance.

Mode of action

The mechanism of action of artemisinins remains unclear. They contain an unusual peroxide bridge, believed to be responsible for its action. This may disrupt redox homeostasis, resulting in the production of reactive oxygen radicals. Blood stages of *Plasmodium* spp. are rapidly killed, including gametocytes (the form infective to mosquitoes), thus leading to reduced transmission. In both uncomplicated and severe infections, artemisinins have shown faster fever and parasite clearance times than any other agent (including quinine) and are effective in cerebral malaria.

Resistance

Reduced susceptibility was reported initially in Cambodia (2008) and subsequently in Thailand (2012). Mutations to the Kelch 13 (K13) propeller domain has been associated with delayed parasite clearance and is used as a marker of resistance. Delayed parasite clearance times (>3 days) have been observed, but true treatment failure is very rare. Partial resistance is likely due to a combination of poor prescribing practices, availability of artemisinin PO monotherapy, and inadequate patient adherence. The WHO has called for the banning of all artemisinin monotherapy worldwide, to increase the barrier to resistance.

Agents

- Artemisinin—the original agent. It has poor bioavailability (improved upon in semi-synthetic derivatives; ➜ see Artemisinin combination therapies, p. 127). Concentrated in erythrocytes and hydrolysed to dihydroartemisinin. Metabolized by hepatic cytochromes. Peak concentrations after 1–3h. Elimination half-life <30min. Can be given PR. Adverse effects include drug-induced fever, reversible decrease in reticulocytes, and neurotoxicity in animal models. Also active against *T. gondii*, *Leishmania major*, and *Schistosoma mansoni* in experimental models.
- Artemether and arteether—esters of dihydroartemisinin; preparations are oil-based and can be given PO, PR, or IM. Absorbed slowly and erratically, so not suitable for severely ill patients.
- Artesunate—water-soluble hemisuccinate of dihydroartemisinin that may be given PO, PR, or IV. Widely used in the developing world. It

is not licensed in the UK or USA, but available on request from most regional infectious diseases (ID) units (and the CDC in the USA). It is the drug of choice for severe *P. falciparum* malaria, being superior to quinine in efficacy (mortality 15% versus 24%) and tolerability. Counterfeit artesunate (containing little or no active drug) has been sold in South East Asia since the late 1980s. This threatens successful treatment and may have facilitated the emergence of reduced susceptibility recently observed in Cambodia. Side effects include transient neurological abnormalities (e.g. balance) and neutropenia.

- Dihydroartemisinin—the active metabolite of artemisinin. Can be given PO and used in the treatment of uncomplicated malaria.

Artemisinin combination therapies

The best treatments for uncomplicated falciparum malaria. They combine a highly effective short-acting artemisinin with a longer-acting agent to protect against resistance, and are rapidly and reliably effective. Resistance in the partner drug limits the use of certain combinations. They are safe and well tolerated, although hypersensitivity may occasionally occur. The partner drug determines the adverse effect profiles. They should not be used in the first trimester of pregnancy (safety not established), unless there is no alternative. They are usually given as a 3-day course in a fixed-dose tablet.

- Artemether–lumefantrine—first fixed-dose combination of artemisinin derivative and another drug. It has become increasingly available in tropical countries, and is well tolerated and affordable ($1). It has been associated with irreversible hearing loss. Pharmacokinetic mismatch of components necessitates a complex 3-day dosing regimen. Widely available in the UK.
- Dihydroartemisinin–piperaquine—good tolerability, high cure rates in MDR falciparum malaria in Cambodia, Vietnam, and Thailand. The slow elimination of piperaquine determines parasitological efficacy and post-treatment prophylactic effect.
- Artesunate–mefloquine—safe, well tolerated, and highly effective. Used in Thailand, South America, and Africa. Disadvantages include its price and the pharmacokinetic mismatch of its components. However, in Thailand, resistance to mefloquine has actually decreased since its introduction.
- Artesunate–sulfadoxine–pyrimethamine—initially gave promising results in African children, but subsequent studies have been disappointing, likely due to increasing sulfadoxine/pyrimethamine resistance rates globally.
- Artesunate–amodiaquine—one African multicentre trial showed better overall efficacy than amodiaquine alone, but 6% of patients developed neutropenia. The pharmacokinetic mismatch of the components raises concerns about prolonged exposure of parasites to amodiaquine. There is increasing resistance in eastern and southern Africa.

Antiprotozoal drugs

Albendazole

(➔ See Benzimidazoles, pp. 133–4.)
- Binds to tubulin, affecting cytoskeleton function. Active against a variety of helminths and some protozoal infections, including giardiasis, microsporidiosis, intestinal worm infections, trichinosis, cutaneous larva migrans, hydatid disease, neurocysticercosis, and lymphatic filariasis.

Amphotericin

(➔ See Polyenes, pp. 85–6.)
- A polyene antifungal active against a variety of fungi and some protozoa (e.g. *Leishmania* spp., *Naegleria*, *Hartmanella*). Used in the treatment of leishmaniasis.

Antimony compounds

- Sodium stibogluconate is a pentavalent antimonial compound used in the treatment of leishmaniasis. It is active against amastigotes within macrophages. Different species vary in sensitivity. The mechanism of action is unclear.
- Acquired resistance results in poor response and high resistance rates. Relapse also common in immunosuppressed or poorly controlled HIV patients.
- Pharmacology—given IM or IV, with peak concentrations occurring after 1h. Slow accumulation in the central nervous system (CNS) and tissues. Excreted in the urine.
- Adverse effects—cough/vomiting (if infused too quickly), arthralgia, myalgia, bradycardia, abdominal cramps, diarrhoea, rash, pruritus, raised LFTs, raised creatinine levels, raised amylase levels.

Atovaquone

(➔ See Antimalarials, pp. 120–1.)
- Antimalarial, with activity against other protozoa (e.g. *Babesia* spp., *T. gondii*, *P. jirovecii*).

Benznidazole

- A synthetic 2-nitroimidazole, active against *T. cruzi* (Chagas' disease) and a member of the benzimidazole family.
- Pharmacology—well absorbed PO.
- Adverse effects—photosensitivity (50%), anorexia, nausea, vomiting, abdominal pain, disorientation, insomnia, paraesthesiae, polyneuritis, seizures.

Ciprofloxacin

(➔ See Quinolones, pp. 67–9.)
- A fluoroquinolone antibiotic with activity against *Cyclospora cayetanensis* and *Cystoisospora belli* (formerly known as Isospora belli). Used as a second-line treatment option.

Clarithromycin

(➔ See Macrolides, pp. 54–6.)
- A macrolide antibiotic with activity against *T. gondii*. A second-line treatment option.

Clindamycin

(➲ See Lincosamides, pp. 56–7.)
- A lincosamide antibiotic, with activity against some protozoa (e.g. *P. falciparum*, *Babesia* spp., *T. gondii*, *P. jirovecii*).
- Use—second-line treatment of *P. jirovecii* pneumonia; second-line treatment and secondary prophylaxis of cerebral toxoplasmosis.

Co-trimoxazole

(➲ See Co-trimoxazole, pp. 66–7.)
- A diaminopyrimidine–sulfonamide antibiotic, with useful activity against *P. jirovecii* (first line), *T. gondii*, *C. cayetanensis*, and *I. belli*.

Dapsone

(➲ See Antileprotics, pp. 79–81.)
- Sulfonamide derivative, active against *Mycobacterium leprae*, *Plasmodium* spp., *T. gondii*, and *P. jirovecii*. Main use is in the treatment and prophylaxis of *P. jirovecii* pneumonia and cerebral toxoplasmosis.

Diloxanide furoate

- Dichloromethylacetamide, active against *Entamoeba histolytica*.
- Luminal amebicide, mechanism of action unclear.
- Pharmacology—limited human data. Animal data show rapid PO absorption; hydrolysed in the gut; 75% excreted via the kidneys within 24h. No resistance reported.
- Adverse effects—nausea, vomiting, abdominal distension, flatulence, pruritus, urticaria.
- Use—treatment of intestinal amoebiasis, eradication of cysts after acute amoebiasis.

Eflornithine

- Inhibits parasite growth by inhibition of ornithine carboxylase (required for cellular replications and differentiation). Active against *Trypanosoma brucei gambiense*. *In vitro* (not used clinically) activity against *P. falciparum*, *Leishmania* promastigotes, and *Giardia lamblia*.
- Pharmacology—given IV, plasma half-life 3h, good CNS penetration, rapid renal excretion.
- Adverse effects—osmotic diarrhoea, bone marrow suppression, convulsions, hearing loss (tends to be reversible).
- Use—late-stage *T.b. gambiense* infections. NOT effective in *T.b. rhodesiense* infections. Has been used speculatively in PCP.

Fexinidazole

- Nitroimidazole derivative, which likely acts through parasite nitroreductive enzymes to generate toxic metabolites.
- Recommended for use in 2019 by the WHO for treatment of *T.b. gambiense* trypanosomiasis, particularly in the first stage of the illness. Found to have activity against *T.b. rhodesiense* and *T. cruzi*, although not currently recommended for treatment.
- Adverse reactions—GI side effects, headache, and disulfiram-like reaction with alcohol.

Fluconazole

(➔ See Triazoles, pp. 87–9.)
- Antifungal with activity against *Leishmania* spp. Used to treat cutaneous leishmaniasis.

Fumagillin

- Antibiotic derived from *Aspergillus fumigatus*. Mechanism of action not clear. Suppresses microsporidial proliferation. A second-line treatment of microsporidiosis.
- Given PO.
- Adverse effects—neutropenia, thrombocytopenia.

Furazolidone

(➔ See Nitrofurans, pp. 70–1.)
- A nitrofuran antibiotic, active against a variety of bacteria, *G. lamblia*, and *Trichomonas vaginalis*.
- Adverse effects—disulfiram reaction with alcohol. Occasionally, fever, urticaria, hypotension, arthralgia, nausea, vomiting, headache, haemolysis (G6PD deficiency).

Iodoquinol

- An 8-aminoquinoline, active against *E. histolytica* and *Dientamoeba fragilis*.
- Pharmacology—slowly and incompletely absorbed (<10%), hepatic metabolism, renal excretion.
- Adverse effects—nausea, abdominal cramps, rash, acne, optic neuritis with prolonged courses. Contraindicated if allergic to iodine.
- Use—asymptomatic or mild intestinal (non-invasive) amoebiasis.

Melarsoprol

- A trivalent arsenic-based compound, active against *T. brucei* spp. Prevents trophozoite multiplication by binding thiol groups.
- Resistance—due to reduced uptake by trypanosomes.
- Pharmacology—given IV, rapidly metabolized to melarsen oxide which crosses the blood–brain barrier, biphasic elimination.
- Adverse effects—very toxic. Fever, abdominal pain, vomiting, peripheral neuropathy; 10% risk of post-treatment encephalopathy (may be reduced by prednisolone), 2–4% risk of death secondary to treatment.
- Use—late-stage (CNS) African trypanosomiasis caused by *T.b. gambiense* and *T.b. rhodesiense*.

Mepacrine (quinacrine)

- A synthetic acridine derivative with broad antiprotozoal activity—*Blastocystis hominis*, *E. histolytica*, *G. lamblia*, *Leishmania* spp., *Plasmodium* spp., *T. vaginalis*, *T. cruzi*. Also active against tapeworms.
- Pharmacology—well absorbed PO, extensive tissue binding, concentrated in leucocytes, 10% daily dose excreted in the urine (turns it yellow).

- Adverse effects—yellow staining of skin, dizziness, headache, vomiting, psychosis, haemolytic anaemia, neutropenia, thrombocytopenia, urticaria, fever, rash.
- Use—giardiasis, prophylaxis of malaria, treatment of tapeworm, cutaneous leishmaniasis.

Metronidazole
(➲ See Nitroimidazoles, pp. 69–70.)
- A nitroimidazole antibiotic, active against anaerobic bacteria and protozoa (e.g. *T. vaginalis*, *G. lamblia*, *E. histolytica*, *Balantidium coli*, *B. hominis*).
- First line for giardiasis, intestinal/extraintestinal amoebiasis, trichomoniasis.

Miltefosine
- Hexadecylphosphocholine—mechanism of action not clear.
- Active against *Leishmania* spp., *Trypanosoma* spp., and *E. histolytica*.
- Pharmacology—well absorbed and widely distributed.
- Adverse effects—vomiting, diarrhoea, teratogenic (avoid in pregnancy).
- Use—treatment of leishmaniasis.

Nifurtimox
- A nitrofuran antibiotic, active against a variety of bacteria and *T. cruzi*.
- Adverse effects—GI symptoms (40–70%), CNS symptoms (33%), skin rash, haemolysis (G6PD deficiency).
- Use—treatment of acute *T. cruzi* infection. Little effect in chronic Chagas' disease. Used in combination with eflornithine for the treatment of African trypanosomiasis due to *T.b. gambiense*.

Nitazoxanide
- A broad-spectrum antiparasitic—mechanism of action postulated to be due to inhibition of pyruvate ferredoxin oxidoreductase (PFOR), which is required for anaerobic metabolism.
- Used in the treatment of diarrhoea due to *Cryptosporidium parvum* in children and giardiasis.
- Previously used in the treatment of HIV-associated cryptosporidiosis, but of doubtful effectiveness in this context.
- Adverse effects—GI side effects.

Ornidazole
(➲ See Nitroimidazoles, pp. 69–70.)
- A nitroimidazole antibiotic used in the treatment of giardiasis and intestinal/extraintestinal amoebiasis.

Paromomycin
(➲ See Aminoglycosides, pp. 52–4.)
- Aminoglycoside antibiotic, similar to neomycin. Poorly absorbed PO, and used as second line for non-invasive amoebiasis (oral) and for non-severe giardiasis in pregnancy when metronidazole is contraindicated. Can be used topically for cutaneous leishmaniasis and nitroimidazole-resistant trichomoniasis.

Pentamidine isethionate

- A synthetic diamidine, active against *P. falciparum*, *T. gondii*, *Leishmania* spp., *Trypanosoma* spp., *Babesia* spp., and *P. jirovecii*. The mechanism of action is unclear.
- Pharmacology—negligible PO absorption, given IV or by nebulizer, hepatic metabolism, 15–20% excreted in the urine. Poor cerebrospinal fluid (CSF) penetration (<1%). Retained in tissues (e.g. liver, kidneys, adrenals, spleen, lungs), resulting in long terminal half-life (>12 days).
- Adverse effects—phlebitis, injection site abscess, GI symptoms, hypotension, hypo-/hyperglycaemia, hypocalcaemia, neutropenia, thrombocytopenia, raised creatinine levels, raised LFTs, pancreatitis, rash.
- Use—treatment of African trypanosomiasis (early stage), prophylaxis and treatment of PCP, treatment of leishmaniasis (antimony-resistant).

Primaquine

(➔ See Antimalarials, pp. 120–1.)
- A synthetic 8-aminoquinoline, active against the hepatic stages of *P. vivax* and *P. ovale*, *P. jirovecii*, *Babesia* spp., *Leishmania* spp., and *T. cruzi*.
- Use—treatment of *P. vivax* or *P. ovale* malaria, treatment of PCP (with clindamycin).

Pyrimethamine

(➔ See Antimalarials, pp. 120–1.)
- A synthetic diaminopyrimidine, active against *Plasmodium* spp., *T. gondii*, and *P. jirovecii*.
- Adverse effects—abdominal pains, rash, folate deficiency with longer courses (folinic acid replacement is required).
- Use—treatment of malaria (in combination with sulfadoxine or dapsone), toxoplasmosis (with sulfadiazine), and PCP (with dapsone).

Spiramycin

(➔ See Macrolides, pp. 54–6.)
- A macrolide antibiotic; active against *T. gondii* and an alternative to antifolates (e.g. in pregnancy).

Sulfadiazine

(➔ See Sulfonamides, pp. 63–5.)
- Active against *T. gondii*. Used in combination with pyrimethamine.

Suramin

- A sulfated naphthylamine, active against *T. brucei* spp. and used to treat the early stages of African trypanosomiasis. First line for first-stage *T.b. rhodesiense* infection. It is effective against *T.b. gambiense* infection, but pentamidine and fexinidazole are preferred agents due to their reduced toxicity profile.
- Mode of action—binds to lipoproteins and is selectively taken up into trypanosomes by endocytosis, but intracellular mechanism of action unclear.
- Resistance—clinical relapse rates of 30–50% reported in East Africa.

- Pharmacology—poor PO absorption, given by slow IV infusion, >99% protein-bound, poor CSF penetration, plasma half-life >40 days, not metabolized, high tissue distribution (liver, kidney, adrenal glands), renal excretion.
- Adverse effects—highly toxic, especially in malnourished patients. Immediate reactions (nausea, vomiting, cardiovascular collapse) can be avoided by slow IV injection. May be followed by fever and urticaria. Anaphylaxis is rare (<1 in 2000). Delayed reactions include exfoliative dermatitis, anaemia, leucopenia, jaundice, and diarrhoea.
- Use—African sleeping sickness (early stage), onchocerciasis.

Tetracycline
(➜ See Tetracyclines, pp. 61–3.)
- A tetracycline antibiotic, active against a variety of bacteria, *Chlamydophila*, *Rickettsia*, spirochaetes, *P. falciparum*, *B. coli*, *D. fragilis*.
- Use—treatment and prophylaxis of drug-resistant falciparum malaria, treatment of *B. coli* and *D. fragilis*.

Tinidazole
(➜ See Nitroimidazoles, pp. 69–70.)
- Similar to metronidazole; used for amoebiasis, giardiasis, and trichomoniasis.

Anthelmintic drugs

Most anthelmintics were discovered and developed for use in veterinary medicine. Although no new anthelmintics have come to the market in recent years, satisfactory results can be achieved with current drugs. Exceptions to this are treatment of larval cestodes, disseminated strongyloidiasis, and guinea worm. In general, the medications are well tolerated, although allergic/anaphylactic reactions may rarely occur as a result of the death of large numbers of worms.

Benzimidazoles
- Act by binding free β-tubulin, blocking its polymerization and hence inhibiting microtubule-dependent glucose uptake.
- All cause GI side effects, and all should be avoided in pregnancy.

Albendazole
- Active against *Enterobius vermicularis*, *Ascaris lumbricoides*, *Ancylostoma duodenale*, *Necator americanus*, *Strongyloides stercoralis*, *Trichuris trichiura*, *Trichinella spiralis*, animal hookworms, microfilaria, and *Echinococcus* spp. Also active against *G. lamblia* and microsporidia.
- Pharmacology—well absorbed PO, metabolized to albendazole sulfoxide (active metabolite), half-life 8h, renal excretion.
- Adverse effects—leucopenia and raised LFTs with prolonged use. Rarely, neutropenia, pancytopenia, agranulocytosis, and thrombocytopenia.
- Use—intestinal worm infections, trichinosis, cutaneous larva migrans (topical), hydatid disease (± surgery), neurocysticercosis, lymphatic filariasis (± ivermectin), giardiasis, microsporidiosis.

Mebendazole
- Active against *E. vermicularis*, *A. lumbricoides*, *A. duodenale*, *N. americanus*, *S. stercoralis*, and *T. trichiura*.
- Pharmacology—poor PO absorption; most of the drug and its metabolites (inactive) are retained in the GI tract and excreted in the faeces (therefore of limited use in systemic infection), <2% excreted by the kidneys.
- Adverse effects uncommon due to lack of systemic absorption.
- Use—intestinal worms, trichinosis.

Flubendazole
- A benzimidazole carbamate used in some countries, instead of albendazole, for treatment of ascariasis. Less well absorbed PO.

Tiabendazole (thiabendazole)
- Active against the commonest intestinal nematodes. Poor side effect profile and now primarily used for cutaneous larva migrans (topical for single tracks, PO for multiple).

Triclabendazole
- Drug of choice for the treatment of fasciolosis. Can also be used in the treatment of paragonimiasis.
- Generally well tolerated—headaches and GI side effects reported.

Piperazine
- Active against *E. vermicularis* and *A. lumbricoides*.
- Adverse effects—transient mild GI or neurological symptoms; hypersensitivity. Avoid in epilepsy and liver or kidney disease.

Diethylcarbamazine
- A carbamyl derivative of piperazine used in the treatment of lymphatic filariasis and loiasis (*Loa loa*, *Brugia malayi*, *Wuchereria bancrofti*, *Onchocerca volvulus*).
- Mechanism of action is probably via sensitization of microfilariae to phagocytosis.
- Pharmacology—>90% PO absorption, 50% metabolized and excreted in the faeces, 50% excreted unchanged in the urine.
- Adverse effects—usually related to the microfilarial burden and may be due to the release of lipopolysaccharide (LPS) from *Wolbachia* spp. (e.g. fever, headache, dizziness, transient worsening of lymphangitis). The Mazotti reaction (itch, ocular and constitutional symptoms) may occur in onchocerciasis.

Doxycycline
Doxycycline (➔ see Tetracyclines, pp. 61–3) is active against *Wolbachia*, an endosymbiotic bacteria which resides within many species of nematodes and appears to benefit the hosts' growth, fertility, and ability to cause human pathology. Treatment with doxycycline has been shown to be effective against *O. volvulus*, *W. bancrofti*, and *B. malayi*, and is usually given for a 6-week extended course in this context.

Ivermectin

- A mixture of two semi-synthetic derivatives of avermectins, antibiotics produced by *Streptomyces avertimilis*. Active against *A. lumbricoides*, *S. stercoralis*, *O. volvulus*, *L. loa*, and *Sarcoptes scabiei*.
- Mechanism of action—binds to glutamate-gated chloride channels, leading to hyperpolarization of neurons and subsequent paralysis of susceptible helminths.
- Pharmacology—60% PO absorption, rapidly metabolized by the liver, highest concentrations in the liver and fat, excreted in the faeces.
- Adverse effects—Mazotti reactions, GI symptoms, neurological symptoms. Not recommended in pregnancy/breastfeeding.
- Use—onchocerciasis, non-disseminated strongyloidiasis. May be used for lymphatic filariasis (with albendazole) and scabies.

Moxidectin

- A milbemycin with a similar macrocyclic lactone ring to ivermectin, which has a similar mechanism of action and spectrum of activity.
- Approved in 2018 by the Food and Drug Administration (FDA) for the treatment of onchocerciasis, and clinical trials have shown moxidectin achieve a greater sustained reduction in microfilarial levels compared to ivermectin.
- Mechanism of action and range of activity similar to ivermectin.
- Adverse reactions—Mazotti reactions, orthostatic hypotension, GI side effects.

Levamisole

- Active against *A. lumbricoides* and hookworms.
- Mechanism of action—nicotinic acetylcholine receptor agonist causing contraction of muscles and subsequent paralysis.
- Adverse effects—agranulocytosis.
- An alternative to mebendazole for the treatment of ascariasis.

Praziquantel

- A synthetic pyrazinoquinoline; active against schistosomes (causes paralysis and tegumental damage), larval tapeworms, *Fasciolopsis buski*, *Metagonimus yokogawi*, *Heterophyes heterophyes*, *Nanophyetus salmincola*, *Clonorchis* spp., *Opisthorchis* spp., *Paragonimus* spp., and *Fasciola hepatica* (variable activity).
- Pharmacology—>80% PO absorption, undergoes rapid first-pass metabolism to inactive metabolites, low plasma levels, 90% excreted in the urine by 24h.
- Mechanism of action—remains uncertain.
- Adverse effects—GI symptoms, mild neurological effects during treatment of schistosomiasis; cerebral inflammation and oedema during treatment of neurocysticercosis; risk of visual impairment with ocular cysticercosis.
- Use—schistosomiasis, tapeworm infections, trematode infections (except *F. hepatica*). Resistance is emerging in schistosomes.

Niclosamide

- A synthetic chlorinated nitrosalicylanide, active against *Taenia saginata*, *Taenia solium*, *Diphyllobothrium latum*, *Hymenolepis nana*.
- Mechanism of action—inhibition of mitochondrial phosphorylation.
- Pharmacology—level of absorption uncertain, metabolized in the liver, passed in the urine and faeces (stains them yellow).
- Use—the most widely used drug for tapeworm infections. Not effective against larval worms.

Oxamniquine

- A synthetic quinoline methanol, active against *S. mansoni*.
- Pharmacology—well absorbed PO. Can be given IM.
- Adverse effects—dizziness, sleepiness, nausea, headache.
- Use—second-line treatment of *S. mansoni* infections. Higher doses required in Egypt and southern Africa for partially resistant strains.

Pyrantel

- A pyrimidine derivative; active against *E. vermicularis*, *A. lumbricoides*, *A. duodenale*, and *N. americanus*.
- Mechanism of action—induces paralysis, allowing worm expulsion.
- Pharmacology—<5% absorbed PO, metabolized, and excreted in the urine; the rest passes unchanged in the faeces.
- Adverse effects—rare due to lack of absorption; GI symptoms reported. Antagonistic with piperazine (do not use together).
- Use—single dose curative in pinworm, ascariasis, and trichostrongyliasis. Several doses required for hookworm.

Part 2

Infection Prevention and Control

Infection prevention and control

Introduction to infection control

At any one time in the UK, >10% of hospital inpatients are suffering from a nosocomial infection[1] and nosocomial infections affect up to 37% of those admitted to the intensive care unit (ICU).[2] In total, estimates suggest that 300 000 patients a year in England acquire a healthcare-associated infection (HCAI) as a result of care within the National Health Service (NHS). The top five commonest nosocomial infections are as follows:

- intravascular device-related bacteraemia;
- urinary tract infection (UTI);
- lower respiratory tract infection (LRTI);
- surgical wound infection;
- skin infection.

The socio-economic impact, in terms of increased length of stay and financial cost, is immense, as is the personal cost to each individual who acquires an essentially preventable infection.

Modelling studies suggest that there were an estimated 834 000 HCAIs in 2016/2017 in all NHS hospitals in England, costing the NHS £2.7 billion, and accounting for 28 500 patient deaths. HCAIs have triggered considerable political interest over recent years, resulting in reorganization of hospital and community infection control services and the publication of numerous documents. A 'zero tolerance' approach has been adopted. It is likely that infection prevention and control (IPC) will maintain its high political profile.

Current emphasis on infection prevention and control

The Health and Social Act came into force in April 2011. This states that *'good infection prevention and control (IPC) are essential to ensure that people who use health and social care services receive safe and effective care. Effective prevention and control of infection must be part of everyday practice and be applied consistently by everyone'*. This code of practice details 10 criteria that will be used by the Care Quality Commission (CQC) to judge how a registered provider complies with infection control. Registered providers include: primary care, primary dental care, independent sector ambulance workers, and secondary care. Key areas include:

- **High Impact Interventions (HIIs)**, published by the Department of Health and based on the care bundle approach. These are simple evidence-based tools, which reinforce the practical actions that clinical staff need to undertake to significantly reduce HCAIs. The HIIs focus on:
  - central venous catheter (CVC) care
  - peripheral IV cannula care (➲ see Intravascular line-related sepsis >, pp. 162–5);
  - renal dialysis catheter care;
  - prevention of surgical site infections (SSIs) (➲ see Surgical site infections>, p. 805);
  - care for ventilated patients (or tracheostomies, where appropriate);
  - urinary catheter care (➲ see Catheter associated urinary tract infection, pp. 165–7);

- reducing the risk of *Clostridioides difficile* infection (➔ see *Clostridioides difficile* infection, pp. 196–200);
- cleaning and decontamination of clinical equipment.
- The revised Saving Lives tools include summaries of best practice for antimicrobial prescribing and isolating patients with HCAIs.
- Important approaches include the following:
  - care bundles—these involve multiple discrete steps in the prevention of infection, and should be implemented and monitored by multidisciplinary teams;
  - a culture of zero tolerance and accountability, with adequate administrative support.

See Institute for Healthcare Improvement (available at: ✍ https://www.ihi.org).

Evidence base for infection prevention and control

Historically, there have been few controlled trials on IPC, and the evidence base for many procedures is sparse. Initiatives to rectify this include the formation of ORION (Outbreak Reports and Intervention Studies of Nosocomial Infection) and the publication of a CONSORT (Consolidated Standards of Reporting Trials) equivalent statement, in order to raise the standards of research and publication. The most recent version (available at: ✍ www.consort-statement.org/) consists of a 25-item checklist and a participant flow diagram. The full text of the ORION statement and checklist is available at: ✍ https://www.idrn.org. These guidelines have been incorporated, with others, into the EQUATOR Network (**E**nhancing the **QUA**lity and **T**ransparency **O**f health **R**esearch, available at: ✍ https://www.equator-network.org). The emphasis is on transparency to improve the quality of reporting and on the use of appropriate statistical techniques, so that the work is robust enough to influence policy and practice.

National evidence-based guidelines for preventing HCAIs in NHS hospitals in England were originally commissioned by the Department of Health and developed during 1998–2000. They were first published in January 2001 (epic) and updated in 2007 (epic2). These evidence-based guidelines are subject to timely review for new research evidence and technological advances to be identified, appraised, and, if shown to be effective for the prevention of HCAIs, incorporated into amended guidelines.

The current epic3 guidelines[3] provide comprehensive recommendations for preventing HCAIs in hospital and other acute care settings, based on the best currently available evidence. National evidence-based guidelines are broad principles of best practice that need to be integrated into local practice guidelines and audited to reduce variation in practice and maintain patient safety.

Information which will guide reading of this chapter and provide information on current practice and trials in IPC can be found in Boxes 6.1 and 6.2.

Further reading

IPC societies and resources
Healthcare Infection Society. Available at: ✍ https://www.his.org.uk
Infection Prevention Society. Available at: ✍ https://www.ips.uk.net
Society for Healthcare Epidemiology of America. Available at: ✍ https://shea-online.org

National and international policies and data

England—available at: ℘ https://www.gov.uk/government/organisations/public-health-england

Scotland—available at: ℘ https://publichealthscotland.scot/

Wales—available at: ℘ https://phw.nhs.wales/

Northern Ireland—available at: ℘ https://www.publichealth.hscni.net/

Republic of Ireland—available at: ℘ https://publichealth.ie/.

Care Quality Commission—available at: ℘ https://www.cqc.org.uk. This is the independent regulator of all health and adult social care in England.

Centers for Disease Control and Prevention. *Healthcare-associated infections (HAIs)*. Available at: ℘ https://www.cdc.gov/hai/

European Centre for Disease Prevention and Control—available at: ℘ https://www.ecdc.europa.eu/en

Health and Safety Executive—available at: ℘ https://www.hse.gov.uk

Medicines and Healthcare products Regulatory Agency—available at: ℘ https://www.gov.uk/government/organisations/medicines-and-healthcare-products-regulatory-agency

National Audit Office (2009). *Reducing healthcare associated infections in hospitals in England*. Available at: ℘ https://www.nao.org.uk/report/reducing-healthcare-associated-infections-in-hospitals-in-england/

National Institute for Health and Care Excellence (NICE)—available at: ℘ https://www.nice.org.uk

World Health Organization—available at: ℘ https://www.who.int

---

Box 6.1 Important definitions in infection control

Infection—the deposition and multiplication of organisms in tissues or on body surfaces, which usually causes adverse effects.

Colonization—organisms are present but cause no host response.

Carrier—an individual who harbours a pathogen without manifesting symptoms, thus acting as a distributor of infection. Typhoid Mary was one of the most famous carriers of all time (➲ see Enteric fever, pp. 693–5).

Nosocomial infection—hospital-/healthcare-acquired infection that was not present or incubating at the time of admission. Often an arbitrary cut-off of >48h post-admission is used. Nosocomial infections also include infections that only appear after discharge (e.g. post-operative wound infection), as well as occupational infections amongst healthcare staff.

Community infection—infection in the community. Be careful to differentiate between community-onset (may include patients recently discharged from hospitals) and community acquired (community patients with no history of direct or indirect contact with healthcare) infections.

Decontamination—a process or treatment that cleanses a medical device, an instrument, or an environmental surface to remove contaminants such as microorganisms.

Disinfection—the destruction of pathogenic and other microorganisms by physical or chemical means. Disinfection is less lethal than sterilization, because it destroys most recognized pathogenic microorganisms, but not necessarily all microbial forms such as bacterial spores (➲ see Disinfection, pp. 218–21).

Sterilization—a physical or chemical procedure that destroys all organisms, including large numbers of resistant bacterial spores (➲ see Sterilization, pp. 221–3).

Box 6.2 Infection control abbreviations used in the UK

- **AAR**—After Action Review
- **BSI**—bloodstream infection
- **CCDC**—Consultant in Communicable Disease Control
- **CDC**—Centers for Disease Control and Prevention (Atlanta, GA, USA)
- **CDSC**—Communicable Disease Surveillance Centre (now Centre for Infections (CFI))
- **COSHH**—Control of Substances Hazardous to Health
- **CQC**—Care Quality Commission
- **CSSD**—Centre for Surgical Sterilization and Disinfection (also called Theatre Supplies Unit (TSU))
- **DH**—Department of Health
- **DIPC**—Director of Infection Prevention and Control
- **ECDC**—European Centre for Disease Prevention and Control (Stockholm, Sweden)
- **EPIC**—Evidence-based Practice in Infection Control
- **HACCP**—Hazard Analysis Critical Control Points
- **HAI**—hospital-acquired infection
- **HCAI**—healthcare-associated infection
- **HELICS**—Hospitals in Europe Link for Infection Control through Surveillance
- **HICPAC**—Hospital Infection Control Practices Advisory Committee (Atlanta, GA, USA)
- **HII**—High Impact Intervention (from 'Saving Lives' programme)
- **HSE**—Health and Safety Executive
- **HTM**—health technical memorandum
- **IPC**—infection prevention and control
- **IPCC**—Infection Prevention and Control Committee
- **ICD**—infection control doctor
- **IPCN**—infection prevention and control nurse
- **IPCT**—infection prevention and control team
- **MESS**—MRSA Enhanced Surveillance System
- **MHRA**—Medicines and Healthcare products Regulatory Agency
- **PEAT**—Patient Environment Action Team, now replaced by Patient-Led Assessments of the Care Environment (PLACE)
- **PIR**—post-infection review
- **PPE**—personal protective equipment
- **RCA**—root cause analysis
- **RIDDOR**—Reporting of Injuries, Diseases, and Dangerous Occurrences Regulations
- **SICP**—standard infection control precautions
- **SUI**—serious untoward incident
- **UKAP**—UK Advisory Panel for healthcare workers infected with blood-borne viruses

References

1 Loveday HP, Wilson JA, Pratt RJ, *et al.*; UK Department of Health. epic3: national evidence-based guidelines for preventing healthcare-associated infections in NHS hospitals in England. *J Hosp Infect.* 2014;**86** Suppl 1:S1–70.
2 Guest JF, Keating T, Gould D, *et al.* Modelling the annual NHS costs and outcomes attributable to healthcare-associated infections in England. *BMJ Open.* 2020;**10**:e033367.
3 National Evidence-based guidelines for preventing healthcare associated infections in NHS hospitals in England; https://doi.org/10.1016/S0195-6701(13)60012-2

Basic epidemiology of infection

In order to introduce effective IPC measures, the basic epidemiology of an infection must be considered. The incidence and nature of an HCAI (as with any infection) depend on the:
• organism;
• host (patients and staff);
• environment;
• routes of transmission.

The organism

The organisms responsible for common nosocomial infections are listed in Table 6.1. These may be acquired endogenously or exogenously.

Endogenous infection

Infectious agents that are already present within the host cause endogenous infection. The infectious agent is usually part of the normal host flora. Antibiotics and exposure to the hospital environment can change the host's flora, promoting growth of previously suppressed infectious agents and potentially selecting resistant strains. Risk of infection may be reduced by protecting any potential sites of entry (e.g. intravascular lines).

Exogenous infection

When the infectious agent originates from outside of the host. The pathogen can be acquired through various routes (⤵ see Routes of transmission, p. 147). Within the hospital setting, environmental fomite contamination can be minimized by implementing the correct decontamination, sterilization, and infection control procedures. Cross-infection (or transmission) refers to infection acquired from another person (patients or staff). Risks can be reduced by focusing on measures to interrupt transmission (e.g. handwashing).

The host

Patient risk factors that result in an increased likelihood of acquiring an infection in hospital include:
• severity of the underlying acute illness and patient comorbidities—severely ill patients are more vulnerable to acquiring an infection and more likely to have a worse outcome;
• use of medical devices—these breach host defences and provide possible portals of entry for organisms;
• extremes of age—the elderly and very young are at higher risk;
• immunosuppression.

Table 6.1 Organisms commonly involved in HCAIs

Infection	Organism(s) involved
Urinary tract infections	Gram-negative bacteria (e.g. *Escherichia coli*, *Proteus* spp., *Klebsiella* spp., *Serratia* spp.)
	Gram-positive bacteria less common (e.g. *Enterococcus* spp.)
	Fungi are a rare cause (e.g. *Candida albicans*)
Respiratory infections (non-ventilated patients)	Bacteria (e.g. *Haemophilus influenzae*, *Streptococcus pneumoniae*, *Pseudomonas aeruginosa*, *Enterobacterales*)
	Viruses (e.g. influenza, respiratory syncytial virus, coronavirus)
	Fungi (e.g. *Aspergillus* spp.)
Wounds and skin sepsis	Bacteria (e.g. *Staphylococcus aureus*, *Streptococcus pyogenes*, anaerobes)
	Uncommon cause often reflects colonization, Gram-negative organisms (e.g. *E. coli*)
Bloodstream infections	Gram-positive bacteria (e.g. *S. aureus*, including meticillin-resistant *S. aureus*, *Enterococcus* spp., coagulase-negative staphylococci)
	Gram-negative bacteria (e.g. *E. coli*, *Proteus* spp., *Klebsiella* spp., *Serratia* spp., *P. aeruginosa*)
	Fungi (e.g. *Candida* spp.)
GI infections	Bacteria (e.g. *Clostridioides difficile*)
	Viruses (e.g. norovirus)

Staff risk factors include:
- immunosuppression (e.g. uncontrolled HIV, pregnancy);
- staff who perform exposure-prone procedures—more likely to be exposed to blood-borne viral infections;
- skin conditions (e.g. eczema)—increase prolonged carriage of organisms such as meticillin-resistant *Staphylococcus aureus* (MRSA).

The environment

The hospital environment includes all of the physical surroundings of hospital patients and staff (i.e. building, fittings, fixtures, furnishings, equipment, and supplies). The following are important environmental issues in the control of infection:
- environmental cleaning (see Box 6.3), environmental disinfection;
- decontamination of equipment;
- building and refurbishment;
- ventilation (➜ see Ventilation in hospitals, pp. 223–5);
- water management (➜ see Disinfection, Sterilisation and Box 6.10 Pseudomonas in taps in NICUs, pp. 172, 218–21, 221–3);
- clinical waste management;
- pest control;
- food services/food hygiene;
- isolation facilities/ability to cohort patients.

Box 6.3 Hospital cleaning

Patients expect hospitals to take care of them in an environment that is clean and safe. 'Dirty hospitals' are frequently reported by the media, with attention drawn to the lack of investment and poor support for hospital cleaning. Providing a clean and safe environment for healthcare is a key priority for the NHS and is a core standard in *Standards for Better Health*. Other publications, such as *Towards Cleaner Hospitals and Lower Rates of Infection*, have further emphasized this and recognize the role of cleaning in minimizing HCAIs by the physical removal of dirt, fomites, dust, and human body fluids. The National Patient Safety Agency (2007) produced guidelines for cleaning (*The National Specifications for Cleanliness in the NHS: A Framework for Setting and Measuring Performance Outcomes*). The results of Patient Environment Action Team (PEAT) assessments were calculated against these specifications, but have been replaced by Patient-Led Assessments of the Care Environment (PLACE).

Routes of transmission

The isolation precautions required depend on the likely route of transmission of the organism. The main routes are:

- airborne—when infection usually occurs via the respiratory route, with the agent carried in aerosols (<5 micrometres in diameter);
- droplet—large droplets carry the infectious agent (>5 micrometres);
- direct contact—infection occurs through direct contact between the source of infection and the recipient (i.e. person-to-person spread);
- indirect contact—infection occurs indirectly (i.e. via equipment contaminated with body fluids such as urine, faeces, and wound exudates). This route also includes contact via an environmental source (e.g. an outbreak of gastroenteritis transmitted by food);
- inoculation—infection occurs through direct inoculation (e.g. needlestick injury). Other routes include via blood products (hepatitis A, *Yersinia enterocolitica*, *Serratia*), total parenteral nutrition (*Malassezia furfur*), and other fluids (*Enterobacter*, *Burkholderia cepacia*, *Bacillus cereus*). Multidose vials should be avoided.

Infection Prevention and Control Committee (IPCC)

All NHS trusts are accountable for maintaining membership and responsibilities of the hospital infection control committee (ICC) (National Audit Office report, 2004). Thus, the chief executive and trust board are responsible for ensuring effective arrangements for infection prevention and control.

Director of Infection Prevention and Control (DIPC)

Since 2003, a DIPC has been required by all NHS care providers. DIPCs have the responsibility for ensuring strategies are implemented to prevent

HCAIs at all levels in their organization. The DIPC sits on the trust board and reports directly to the chief executive. The background of DIPCs vary, and they may be consultants, nurses, clinical scientists, or other allied health professionals (AHPs). A deputy DIPC experienced in IPC often supports the DIPC.

Responsibilities of hospital IPCC

- Endorsing all infection control policies, procedures, and guidelines.
- Providing advice and support on the implementation of policies.
- Collaborating with the infection prevention and control team (IPCT) to develop the annual infection control programme and monitor its progress.

Membership of hospital infection control committee

Membership may include the:
- DIPC;
- IPCT (➨ See Infection prevention and control team below);
- chief executive or representative;
- occupational health physician and nurse;
- senior clinical representatives;
- nurse executive director or representative;
- Consultant in Communicable Disease Control (CCDC).

Infection prevention and control team

The IPCT, led by the DIPC, includes the IPC doctor(s) and nurse(s) (and, in some centres, pharmacists and epidemiologists). The IPCT are accountable to the chief executive and trust board, and have responsibilities, including:
- ensuring advice on IPC is available on a 24h basis;
- producing the annual IPC programme in consultation with the IPCC, health professionals, and senior managers. This includes surveillance programmes and audits of compliance with selected policies;
- education and training to all hospital staff.

Management of infection control in the community

The CCDC has a key role to play in collaborating with the IPCT on the management of hospital and community outbreaks. They are responsible for advising health authorities and primary care organizations. They provide epidemiological advice and have overall responsibility for the surveillance, prevention, and control of communicable diseases and infections in the community (➨ See Management of infection control in the community, p. 148).

Infection control precautions

Standard infection control precautions (SICP) are used by all staff in all care settings at all times for all patients. It is difficult to tell which patients are infected and which are not, so all patients should be regarded as 'potentially infected'. Adherence to SICP for all patients should minimize the transmission of blood-borne viruses (BBVs) and other infectious agents. It also eliminates confusion amongst staff as to which patients are to be treated as 'infected', and will prevent any breach of confidentiality.

Main components of standard infection control precautions

- Standard precautions for preventing HCAIs are described below.
- Additional **transmission-based precautions** are required in specific circumstances (see Box 6.4; comparisons are given in Table 6.2):
- Hospital environmental hygiene. The hospital environment must be clean; cleaning levels should be increased appropriately in response to increasing rates of colonization/infection; disinfectants should be considered, and shared equipment must be cleaned and decontaminated after each use.
- Hand hygiene (➜ see Handwashing, pp. 151–4). Decontaminate hands before and after contact with patients, after gloves are removed, and after contamination with body fluids.

Box 6.4 Transmission-based precautions

Transmission-based precautions describe the PPE required, in addition to SICP measures, to safely prevent transmission from individuals colonized or infected with certain pathogens (see Table 6.2).

Contact precautions

Used to prevent and control infections that spread via direct contact with the patient or indirectly from the patient's immediate care environment (including care equipment). This is the commonest route of cross-infection transmission. Examples include MRSA or meticillin-sensitive *Staphylococcus aureus* (MSSA), vancomycin-resistant enterococci (VRE), *Clostridioides difficile* infection (CDI), and scabies. These include:

- patient placement in an isolation room;
- use of PPE, including single-use gloves and apron;
- limiting movement of the patient;
- use of disposable or dedicated patient care equipment;
- priority of cleaning rooms.

Droplet precautions

Used to prevent and control infections spread over short distances (at least 1m) via droplets (>5 micrometres) from the respiratory tract of one individual directly onto a mucosal surface or conjunctivae of another individual. Examples include pertussis, influenza, rubella, and mumps. In addition to contact precautions, these include:

- HCWs wearing a face mask when managing patients;
- patients wearing a face mask during transportation.

Airborne precautions

Used to prevent and control infection spread without necessarily having close patient contact via aerosols (≤5 micrometres) from the respiratory tract of one individual directly onto a mucosal surface or conjunctivae of another individual. Examples include TB, measles, chickenpox, and disseminated herpes zoster. In addition to droplet precautions, these include:

- placement of patients in an airborne isolation room;
- restriction of HCWs, including those with lack of immunity to infection;
- use of PPE to include respirators.

- Use of personal protective equipment (PPE). Selection of PPE must be based on risk assessment of: (1) transmission risk to patient/carer, (2) risk of contamination of healthcare worker (HCW) skin/clothing by patient body fluids, and (3) suitability of equipment for proposed use.
- Maintain integrity of skin. Clinical staff should cover all skin lesions with a waterproof dressing.
- Safe use and disposal of sharps (➜ see Management of risk: sharps injuries, pp. 213–17):
  - Never resheathe, bend, or break a needle or any other sharp.
  - Dispose of all sharps as a single unit, in a suitable sharps bin.
  - Never attempt to retrieve anything from a sharps bin.
  - Only fill a sharps bin to two-thirds full, and secure the lid before disposing of it according to local policy.
- Principles of asepsis. HCWs should be trained and be competent in aseptic techniques. Aseptic techniques should be used for any procedure that breaches the body's natural defences.
- Safe handling of linen and waste (➜ see Laundry, p. 226; ➜ Waste, pp. 227–8).

Table 6.2 Comparison of transmission-based precautions and respirators

Comparison of transmission-based precautions

	Contact precautions	Droplet precautions	Airborne precautions
Patient placement	Single room	Single room	Negative-pressure isolation room (where available)
Hand hygiene	Yes	Yes	Yes
Gloves	Yes	Yes	Yes
Clothing	Apron	Apron	Gown
Masks	Risk assessment	Surgical mask	Respirator required (FFP2/N95 or greater, see below)
Eye protection	Risk assessment	Risk assessment	Required

Comparison of respirators

	FFP2	N95	FFP3
Filter efficiency	≥94%	≥95%	≥99%
Main use	Europe	America	Europe

All respirators provide a tight-fitting seal and require fit testing. They can be valved or non-valved. The advantages of valved respirators are they allow easier exhalation and comfort. The disadvantages are that exhaled air is not filtered and the respirator may compromise fluid resistance.

- Spills:
  - Any spill of blood or other body fluids that contains blood should be treated with chlorine-releasing granules and left in place for 2min. Afterwards, this should be cleared up with paper towels, while wearing gloves and aprons. The area should then be washed with hot water and detergent.
  - If granules are not available, a solution of hypochlorite diluted to 10 000 ppm (1%) should be used in the same way.
  - Any spill of urine should be dealt with immediately using hot water and detergent.

Further reading

Loveday HP, Wilson JA, Pratt RJ, *et al.*; UK Department of Health. epic3: national evidence-based guidelines for preventing healthcare-associated infections in NHS hospitals in England. *J Hosp Infect.* 2014;**86** Suppl 1:S1–70.

Handwashing

The importance of handwashing has been recognized since the nineteenth century when Ignaz Semmelweis encouraged medical students in Vienna to wash their hands in chlorinated lime solution on the delivery unit. The maternal mortality rate from puerperal fever in patients attended to by medical students was far lower than those attended to by midwives who did not wash their hands. Today there is global recognition that hand hygiene is one of the most effective actions to reduce the spread of pathogens and prevent infections. In response, the World Health Organization (WHO) produced the first global patient safety challenge relating to hand hygiene 'Clean Care is Safer Care'. The goal of Clean Care is Safer Care is to ensure that infection control is acknowledged universally as a solid and essential basis towards patient safety. An extension of this is the annual 'SAVE LIVES: Clean your hands' campaign, a major global effort led by WHO to improve hand hygiene in healthcare by HCWs cleaning their hands at the right time in the right way.

Hand hygiene prevents the transmission of organisms residing on the hands. The skin flora can be divided into two types:

- transient organisms—these are not usually part of the normal flora and can be picked up from the patient or their environment. Examples include *Escherichia coli*, *S. aureus*, *Klebsiella* spp., and *Pseudomonas* spp. They are usually removed by washing hands with soap and water or with hand disinfection (see Box 6.4) (e.g. use of alcohol gel);
- resident organisms—these are usually found deep in the dermis. They do not usually cause infection, except if introduced during invasive procedures (e.g. line insertion or surgical procedures). Examples include coagulase-negative staphylococci (CoNS), and aerobic and anaerobic diphtheroids. They are not usually removed by a single handwashing procedure.

How to wash?

Using a good handwashing technique (see Fig. 6.1) will clean areas that are often missed (e.g. between the fingers, thumbs, fingertips, areas of the palms, and back of the hands). Make sure the hands are wet before applying soap, and rinse thoroughly before drying. If using a gel, effective decontamination only occurs when the alcohol is rubbed in until the skin is dry.

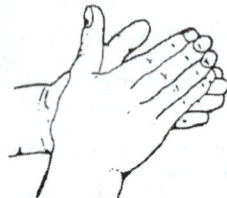

1. Palm to palm

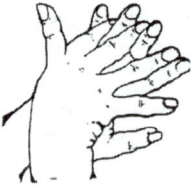

2. Right palm over left dorsum and left palm over right dorsum

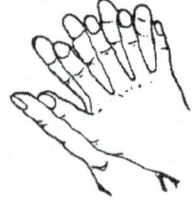

3. Palm to palm, with fingers interlaced

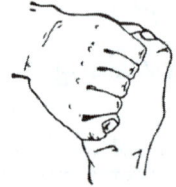

4. Backs of fingers to opposing palms with fingers interlocked

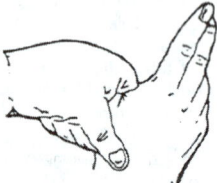

5. Rotational rubbing of right thumb clasped in left palm and vice vera

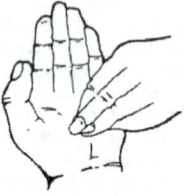

6. Rotational rubbing, backwards and forwards with clasped fingers of right hand in left palm and vice versa

Fig. 6.1 Hand decontamination.

Based on the procedure described by Aycliffe *et al.* 'A test for "hygienic" hand disinfection.' *J Clin Pathol* 1978;**31**:923.

When to wash?

- The WHO's '5 moments of handwashing' approach defines the key moments when HCWs should perform hand hygiene:
  1. before touching a patient;
  2. before clean/aseptic procedures;
  3. after body fluid exposure/risk;
  4. after touching a patient; and
  5. after touching a patient's surroundings
- These are designed to be easy to learn, to be logical and applicable in a wide range of settings, and to promote a strong sense of ownership.

What to use?

- In most clinical situations, soap and water, or an alcohol rub onto dry hands without water, are adequate for hand hygiene disinfection. The length of time and handwashing technique are more important than which soap is used. There are specifications for sinks in clinical areas. Hand lotions and creams may be used after handwashing to prevent soreness.
- Surgical scrub—this procedure aims to remove or destroy all transient flora, and reduce resident flora. There must also be a prolonged effect. Chlorhexidine, povidone–iodine, or alcohol are usually used.

Hand care in general

- Bare below the elbows—hands and arms up to the elbow are exposed and free from clothing/jewellery.
- Nail care—keep nails short and clean. False nails have been the source of HCAIs, including endocarditis, so they should not be worn.
- Jewellery and watches may harbour bacteria and hinder handwashing. Trusts often limit jewellery to a plain wedding band.
- If hands get dry and sore, as often occurs after repeated handwashing, then transient flora may become resident in skin cracks. HCWs should consult occupational health if they are concerned.

Measuring compliance with hand hygiene

At an institutional level, the gold standard for measuring compliance with handwashing is direct observation. This may, however, be subject to the Hawthorne effect, in that behaviour tends to improve when an individual is being watched. Alternative methods include devices to electronically monitor the use of soap and handwash dispensers.

The WHO has identified compliance with hand hygiene as a quality indicator for healthcare. In the UK, national audit data are collected on hand hygiene.

Changing the culture

Persisting challenges include:

- lack of sustained adherence to handwashing procedures. Average compliance of HCWs with handwashing is <50%, and the technique is often poor and rushed;
- there is no doubt that good handwashing practice reduces transmission of infections; however, to be effective, all HCWs must comply all of the time;
- research has begun to focus on how to change the culture and behaviour on the ward, and improve adherence to policies.

The main factors preventing compliance with hand hygiene are time and system constraints. Washing with soap and water can take 60–90s; therefore, many institutions have moved to alcohol-based hand rub at the point of care (i.e. at the bedside, rather than at the entrance to the ward). This is easier, takes only 15–20s, and is effective against most nosocomial pathogens—with key exceptions being *C. difficile* and norovirus.

Multifaceted approach

Evidence suggests a multifaceted approach to hand hygiene is the most efficacious way to bring about change. For example, key parameters in compliance with alcohol-based hand rubs include education of HCWs, monitoring of, and feedback to, HCWs, good administrative support, and introducing a system change (i.e. putting alcohol gel by each patient).

Cleanyourhands Campaign

In 2004, responding to increases in *S. aureus* bloodstream infection (BSI) and CDI, the Cleanyourhands Campaign was launched in England and Wales. Key elements of the campaign were:
• placing disinfectant hand rubs near to where staff have patient contact;
• displaying posters and promotional material where they will influence staff and patients;
• involving patients in improving hand hygiene.

Evaluation of the campaign in 2012 showed that increased procurement of soap was independently linked to reduced CDI, and increased procurement of alcohol hand rub was independently associated with reduced MRSA infection. The Cleanyourhands Campaign is no longer active, but the underlying principles are still relevant and used in hospitals.

Patient isolation

The use of standard precautions should minimize the need for isolation of most patients. In practice, isolation depends on a risk assessment for each patient, and on side room/facilities availability in each institute. Always act on the patient's clinical presentation, and do not wait for laboratory results to be available as it may be too late. Involve your IPCT early and consult the your Dept of Health guidance for further advice (see Box 6.5).

Effective isolation relies on all staff following the necessary procedures to ensure that transmission barriers are not breached. The simplest solution is to use single rooms, but in an outbreak, multi-bedded bays, or even whole wards, may be used.

Patients are isolated for two reasons: (1) source isolation and (2) protective isolation.

Source isolation

To minimize the chance of infecting other patients or staff (e.g. patient with open TB). Ideally the air inside the isolation room should be at negative pressure (exhaust-ventilated) compared to the air in the corridor. Patients with highly contagious infections, such as viral haemorrhagic fevers (VHFs), should be managed in a high-security isolation unit.

Box 6.5 Isolating patients with HCAIs

Guidance and summary of best practice on isolating patients with HCAIs is included in the NHS England national infection prevention and control manual. These give healthcare providers a framework to review and improve isolation practices and reduce the risk of spread of infections—the aim being a reduction in the total number of infections and safer clinical care of an individual with an infection.

Recommendations cover the following:

- single room nursing;
- cohort nursing;
- management of the patient once isolated:
  - hand hygiene and personal protective equipment;
  - cleaning and decontamination;
  - movement of the patient.

The manual is available at: https://www.england.nhs.uk/national-infect ion-prevention-and-control-manual-nipcm-for-england/1

The following measures apply to patients in source isolation:

- Limit transport to other departments (e.g. X-ray) to essential investigations only.
- If a patient does need to go to another department, brief the porters and other staff what precautions are necessary.
- Do not transfer the patient to another ward or healthcare institution without discussion with the IPCT.
- If the patient is well enough, consider sending them home.
- Keep staff caring for infected patients to a minimum. Try not to let these staff work elsewhere in the hospital.
- After the death of an infected patient, maintain infection control precautions, and consult your institution's policy for dealing with the body.

Protective isolation

To minimize the risk of a patient becoming infected (e.g. to protect susceptible or immunosuppressed patients). The air inside the isolation room should be at positive pressure (pressure-ventilated) compared to the air in the corridor. In some critical situations, such as in bone marrow transplant units, where airborne contamination with fungal spores is a problem, the efficiency of air filtration may be increased and laminar flow maintained as a barrier around the patient.

Further reading

Ayliffe GAJ, Fraise AP, Geddes AM, Mitchell K. *Control of Hospital Infection: A Practical Handbook*, fifth edition. London: Edward Arnold, 2009.

Damani D. *Manual of Infection Control Procedures*, third edition. London: Greenwich Medical Media, 2012.

Department of Health. *Health building note 04-01 (Supplement 1). Isolation facilities for infectious patients in acute settings*. London: Department of Health, 2013.

Risk assessment

Risk management is something we do every day in our personal lives—such as when crossing the road—but has recently evolved as an important science in healthcare settings. In combination with total quality management (TQM), it aims to integrate and coordinate all quality assessment activities, and focus on the identification and correction of any problems, with the ultimate goal of protecting patients and staff.

Key definitions

- **Risk management**—a systematic process of risk identification, analysis, treatment, and evaluation of potential and actual risks.
- **Hazard versus risk**—a hazard is the potential to cause harm, whereas a risk is the likelihood of harm (in defined circumstances and usually qualified by some statement of the severity of the harm).
- **Total quality management**—a management strategy aimed at embedding awareness of quality in all organizational processes. For how this applies to the diagnostic laboratory, ⊃ see Quality assurance and accreditation, pp. 258–9.
- **Controls assurance**—the need to be seen to be doing our 'reasonable best' to reduce risk by using resources effectively.
- **Clinical governance**—a framework through which NHS organizations are accountable for continually improving the quality of their services and safeguarding high standards of care, by creating an environment in which excellence in clinical care will flourish.

Risk management and economics

Health economics and cost-effectiveness play a big part in risk management. They are particularly important today because of rising healthcare costs, governmental cost containment, and adverse claims experience.

Goals of risk management

- Survival of the organization (the NHS).
- Enhanced quality and standard of care.
- Minimization of risk of medical or accidental injuries and losses.
- Improvement of programme effectiveness and efficiency through administrative direction and control.
- Coordination and integration of current policies, functions, programmes, committees, and other aspects relative to the risk management process.
- Avoidance of adverse publicity.
- Minimization of cost of risk transfer (insurance).

The risk management cycle is outlined in Fig. 6.2.

Hazard groups

In 1995, the Advisory Committee on Dangerous Pathogens (ACDP) (available at: ✆ https://www.gov.uk/government/groups/advisory-committee-on-dangerous-pathogens) classified all microorganisms into hazard groups 1–4, based on risks of exposure (hazard) and subsequent

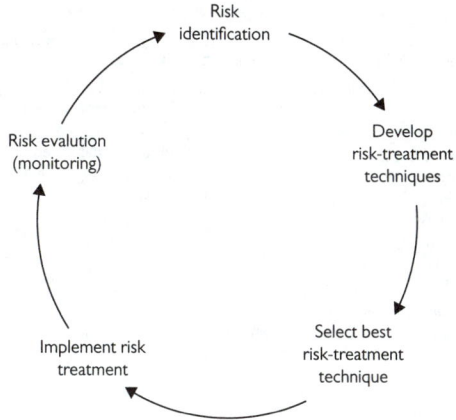

Fig. 6.2 The risk management cycle.

Table 6.3 ACDP hazard groups 1–4

Hazard group (HG)	Containment level (CL)*	Examples
Group 1 Unlikely to cause human disease	CL1	CoNS
Group 2 • May cause human disease • May be a hazard to laboratory workers • Unlikely to spread in the community • Treatment or prophylaxis available	CL2	*Staphylococcus aureus* *Salmonella enterica* serotype Enteritidis *Legionella pneumophila* *Neisseria meningitidis* Influenza, norovirus, Zika virus
Group 3 • May cause severe human disease • Serious hazard to laboratory workers • May spread in the community • Treatment or prophylaxis available	CL3	See full list in Box 6.6 Examples include: *S. enterica* serotype Typhi (*S.* Typhi); MTB; *Brucella* spp.; HIV; hepatitis B, C, and D Prion diseases

(Continued)

Table 6.3 (Contd.)

Hazard group (HG)	Containment level (CL)*	Examples
Group 4 • Severe disease • Serious hazard to laboratory workers • High risk of spread in the community • No effective treatment or prophylaxis		Haemorrhagic fevers (e.g. Ebola, Lassa fever) Note that this group only contains viruses, not bacteria

* ⤴ See Containment levels, pp. 159–61.
CoNS, coagulase-negative staphylococci; MTB, *Mycobacterium tuberculosis*.

Box 6.6 Examples of ACDP category 3 and 4 organisms

Category 3
- Bacteria:
  - *Bacillus anthracis*;
  - *Brucella* spp.;
  - *Burkholderia mallei*;
  - *Burkholderia pseudomallei*;
  - *Chlamydophila psittaci* (avian strains);
  - *Coxiella burnetii*;
  - *Ehrlichia sennetsu* (*Rickettsia sennetsu*);
  - *Escherichia coli*, verocytotoxigenic strains (e.g. O157:H7 or O103);
  - *Francisella tularensis* (type A), not type B;
  - *Salmonella* Typhi, *Salmonella* Paratyphi A, B, C;
  - *Mycobacterium tuberculosis*;
  - *Mycobacterium* (certain species);
  - *Rickettsia* spp.;
  - *Shigella dysenteriae* type 1;
  - *Yersinia pestis*.
- Viruses (certain viruses from the following groups):
  - HIV and other retroviruses;
  - hepatitis B, C, D, and E;
  - *Arenaviridae*;
  - *Bunyaviridae*;
  - *Picornaviridae*, poliovirus type 2;
  - hantaviruses;
  - phleboviruses;
  - nairoviruses;
  - caliciviruses;
  - togaviruses (e.g. chikungunya);

Box 6.6 *(Contd.)*

- flaviviruses (e.g. dengue);
- tick-borne virus group;
- poxviruses;
- rhabdoviruses (e.g. rabies and other *Lyssavirus*);
- beta-coronavirus, severe acute respiratory syndrome (SARS)- and Middle East respiratory syndrome (MERS)-related.
- Parasites (certain parasites from the following groups):
  - *Echinococcus* spp.;
  - *Leishmania* spp.;
  - *Plasmodium falciparum*;
  - *Naegleria fowleri*;
  - *Taenia solium*;
  - *Trypanosoma cruzi* and *Trypanosoma brucei rhodesiense*.
- Fungi:
  - *Blastomyces dermatitidis*;
  - *Coccidioides* spp.;
  - *Paracoccidioides brasiliensis*;
  - *Histoplasma capsulatum*;
  - *Talaromyces marneffei* (formerly *Penicillium marneffei*);
  - *Cladophialophora bantiana*.
- Prions:
  - sporadic: sporadic Creutzfeldt–Jakob disease (CJD);
  - genetic: familial CJD, Gerstmann–Sträussler–Scheinker disease;
  - acquired: variant CJD, kuru;
  - animal transmissible spongiform encephalopathies (TSFs)

Category 4
- Herpesviruses: B virus, herpesvirus simiae, macacine herpesvirus 1;
- *Filoviridae*: Ebola virus;
- *Paramyxoviridae*: Henipavirus;
- *Arenaviridae*, including Lassa virus;
- *Bunyaviridae*, including Crimean–Congo haemorrhagic fever;
- *Flavivirus*, including Far Eastern tick-borne encephalitis;
- *Poxviridae*: monkeypox, variola major and minor.

containment level (CL) requirements (see Table 6.3). The framework is based on their pathogenic potential, route of transmission, epidemiological consequences of escape, and host susceptibility. Hazard groups 1–4 are thus handled at different CLs in the laboratory, defined by Control of Substances Hazardous to Health (COSHH). ACDP category 3 organisms are listed in Box 6.6. For the complete approved list of biological agents for all categories, see ✍ https://www.hse.gov.uk/pubns/misc208.pdf.

Containment levels

The CL refers to the physical requirements necessary for working with organisms of different pathogenicity, and includes guidance about the facilities, working environment, and safety equipment and procedures (e.g. staff training). There are four different levels (CL1–CL4), and the CL of an organism usually corresponds with its categorization (e.g. all group 3 organisms must be handled at CL3). Guidance from the ACDP with detailed technical information, especially regarding CL2 and CL3, is available on the Health and Safety Executive website (available at: ℘ https://www.hse.gov.uk). This includes the legal requirements in the provision of COSHH, with particular attention to how these influence laboratory design, construction, and operation. For examples, see Box 6.7.

Summary of requirements

Containment level 1 (CL1) (i.e. low individual and community risk)
- No special facilities, equipment, or procedures are required. Standard well-designed laboratory facilities and basic safe laboratory practices suffice.
- Handwashing facilities must be provided.
- Disinfectants must be properly used.

Containment level 2 (CL2) (i.e. moderate individual risk, limited community risk)
- The laboratory should be separated from other activities, biohazard sign, room surfaces impervious and readily cleanable.
- Equipment should include an autoclave, certified high-efficiency particulate air (HEPA)-filtered class I or II biological safety cabinet for organism manipulations, and PPE to include laboratory coats worn only in the laboratory.
- All contaminated material should be properly decontaminated.

Box 6.7 Biological safety cabinets (also referred to as biosafety cabinet or microbiological safety cabinet)

- Class I—open aperture at the front, through which the operator can carry out manipulations on potentially hazardous materials. They provide operator protection by maintaining a single inward flow of air past the operator and over the work surface. Exhaust air is HEPA-filtered, but incoming air is unfiltered; therefore, this type of cabinet is not designed to offer protection to material being handled. Suitable for work with all biological agents up to hazard group (HG) 3 (not HG4 agents).
- Class II—open aperture at the front. They provide protection to both the operator and the materials being handled, as the inward airflow is diverted beneath the work surface and is HEPA-filtered before recirculation within the work area. The downward airflow onto the work surface also minimizes the possibility of cross-contamination within the cabinet. Suitable for work with all categories of biological agent, except HG4.
- Class III—completely enclosed to provide maximum protection for the operator, the work, and the environment. All inward and exhaust air is HEPA-filtered, and access to the work area is by using full arm-length gloves (gauntlets) that are sealed to ports in the front of the cabinet. Use of class III cabinets is usually restricted to work with HG4 biological agents.

Containment level 3 (CL3) (i.e. high individual risk, low community risk)

- Specialized design and construction of laboratories, with controlled-access double-door entry and body shower. All wall penetrations must be sealed. The ventilation system design must ensure that air pressure is negative to surrounding areas at all times, with no recirculation of air; air should be exhausted through a dedicated exhaust or HEPA filtration system. Minimum furnishings, all readily cleanable and sterilizable (fumigation). Laboratory windows sealed and unbreakable. Backup power available.
- Equipment must include an autoclave, certified HEPA-filtered class II biological safety cabinet for organism manipulations, and a dedicated handwashing sink with foot, knee, or automatic controls, located near the exit. PPE should include solid front laboratory clothing worn only in the laboratory, head covers and dedicated footwear, gloves, and appropriate respiratory protection, depending on the infectious agents in use.
- All activities involving infectious materials to be conducted in biological safety cabinets or other appropriate combinations of personal protective and physical containment devices.
- Laboratory staff must be fully trained in the handling of pathogenic and other hazardous material, use of safety equipment, disposal techniques, handling of contaminated waste, and emergency response. Standard operating procedures must be provided and posted within the laboratory, outlining operational protocols, waste disposal, disinfection procedures, and emergency response. The facility must have a medical surveillance programme appropriate to the agents used.

Containment level 4 (CL4) (i.e. high individual risk, high community risk)

- CL4 is the highest level of containment and represents an isolated unit that is completely self-contained to function independently. Facilities are highly specialized and secure, with an air lock for entry and exit, class III biological safety cabinets or positive pressure-ventilated suits, and a separate ventilation system with full controls to contain contamination.
- Only fully trained and authorized personnel may enter the CL4 containment laboratory. On exit from the area, personnel will shower and re-dress in street clothing. All manipulations with agents must be performed in class III biological safety cabinets or in conjunction with one-piece, positive pressure-ventilated suits.

Introduction to prevention of healthcare-associated infections

HCAIs, previously referred to as hospital-associated infections (HAIs), result in significant patient morbidity and mortality, and contribute to excess financial healthcare costs.

In high-income countries, 7% of hospitalized patients develop hospital-associated infection (HAI, now referred to as HCAI); this increases to 10% in low- and middle-income countries (LMICs). Patients on ICUs are at increased risk, and estimates suggest that 15–40% of patients will have at least one HAI. The impact varies from increased length of stay and discomfort to prolonged and permanent disability and, in some cases, death. The estimated cost to the NHS is £2.1 billion annually, doubling over the last 15 years.

It is estimated that around 15% of HCAIs are preventable through better application of 'good practice'.[4] It is difficult to calculate the financial and patient-level costs of introducing prevention methods on an institution basis, but all evidence suggests that it is more cost-effective to focus on prevention, rather than pay for costs of treating HCAIs. The National Audit Office report noted that a reduction in HAIs by 15% could save £150 million.[5] The epidemiology of HCAIs generated through UK surveillance programmes can be found at ℞ https://www.gov.uk/government/collecti ons/healthcare-associated-infections-hcai-guidance-data-and-analysis.

Prevention is everyone's business ... not just the IPC team!

There is clearly a need to change the culture and staff behaviour. This has been highlighted as one of the biggest obstacles. Evidence suggests that a variety of approaches are required, so that the individual HCW accepts personal responsibility. Training and education must be continual, and constant reminders (e.g. poster campaigns, handwashing publicity, infection awareness days) are effective. Named individuals acting as liaison representatives and role models in each specialty are beneficial. Feedback of infection rates at ward/team level is vital to engage staff, encourage a sense of ownership, and encourage continual review of practice.

Focus points on prevention

- Education and training for healthcare staff, especially doctors.
- Better compliance with hand hygiene, care of indwelling lines, catheter care, and aseptic technique.
- Good antimicrobial stewardship (AMS).
- Hospital cleanliness.
- Consultation with the IPCT on wider issues (e.g. new-build projects).

Further reading

European Centre for Disease Prevention and Control. Available at: ℞ https://www.ecdc.europa.eu
World Health Organization. Available at: ℞ https://www.who.int
Guest JF, Keating T, Gould D, Wigglesworth N. Modelling the annual NHS costs and outcomes attributable to healthcare-associated infections in England. *BMJ Open*. 2020;**10**:e033367.

References

4 National Audit Office (2000). *The management and control of hospital acquired infection in acute NHS trusts in England*. Available at: ℞ https://www.nao.org.uk/wp-content/uploads/2000/02/9900230.pdf
5 National Audit Office (2004). *Improving patient care by reducing the risk of hospital acquired infection: a progress report*. Available at: ℞ https://www.nao.org.uk/wp-content/uploads/2004/07/0304876.pdf

Intravascular line-related sepsis

Intravascular devices may be complicated by local infections (e.g. phlebitis) or systemic infections (e.g. BSI, endocarditis, osteomyelitis). The commonest organisms that cause line-related sepsis are CoNS, *S. aureus* (including MRSA), enterococci, *Enterobacterales*, *Pseudomonas* spp., and *Candida* spp. Infection may arise in numerous ways. Usually lines become contaminated by the patient's skin flora at the insertion site or by the introduction of other organisms via the cannula hub or injection port.

Always consider whether a line is absolutely necessary or whether an alternative route of administration may suffice (e.g. nasogastric (NG), rectal, s/c). Review the continued need for a line daily.

Peripheral venous catheters

Peripheral venous catheters (PVCs), or 'Venflons', are used most frequently for vascular access. Although they have a low risk of systemic complications, the overall total morbidity is high, because they are so widely used. Almost all systemic infections are preceded by visible phlebitis, which should act as a trigger for PVC removal (see Table 6.4).

Central vascular catheters

CVCs (non-tunnelled), or 'central lines', have the highest rates of catheter-related (CR)-BSIs. These are harder to prevent than PVC infections. There have been several advances in the diagnosis, prevention, and management of CVC infections (➜ see High Impact Intervention No.1; see box 6.15).[6]

Risk factors

Risk factors associated with line infections include:
* patient characteristics—age, comorbidities, immunosuppression;
* catheter characteristics—material, type, size, coating/impregnation;
* infusate and dressing type;
* experience of the person inserting the line, site preparation, anatomical insertion site, and duration of insertion;
* standard of daily line care.

Minimizing line infections

Based on epic3 guidelines for preventing infections associated with the use of intravascular access devices:
* education—HCWs caring for patients with intravascular catheters should be trained and assessed as competent in using, and consistently

Table 6.4 Visual Infusion Phlebitis (VIP) score

Score	Description
0	Site looks healthy
1	Mild pain or redness near site
2	Two of the following evident at site: redness, pain, swelling
3	All of the following evident: redness, pain along cannula site, swelling
4	All of the following evident and extensive: redness, pain along path of cannula, swelling, palpable venous cord
5	All of the following evident and extensive: redness, pain along path of cannula, swelling, palpable venous cord, and pyrexia

adhering to practices for the prevention of, catheter-related BSIs (CRBSIs);

- asepsis—prevents microbial contamination by correct hand hygiene (➲ see Handwashing, pp. 151–4) and with PPE use. Maintain a strict non-touch, aseptic technique when manipulating any part of a line or cannula. Dress using a sterile, semi-permeable, transparent dressing to allow observation of the insertion site. Documentation of date and site of insertion recorded in notes;
- cannula selection—choose the smallest possible lumen for the fluid to be infused; use a single-lumen CVC, unless multiple ports are required; consider antimicrobial-impregnated or coated CVCs if a line is needed for >3 days. Peripherally inserted central catheter (PICC) lines may be considered for patients anticipated to need vascular access for a longer time period;
- insertion site—for PVCs, look on the distal arm, away from previous sites and joint areas. For non-tunnelled CVCs, consider each case carefully, as the choice of site is important in minimizing infection. The subclavian has the lowest risk of infection;
- on insertion—use maximal sterile barrier precautions for the insertion of central venous access devices;
- skin preparation—for PVCs, use a 70% alcohol swab; for CVCs, use alcoholic chlorhexidine gluconate;
- dressing—a transparent film or sterile gauze is ideal. Write the date of insertion on the dressing. Always replace the dressing after inspecting the insertion site, or if it becomes damp, loosened, or soiled;
- continuing care—ensure all lines and associated devices are still indicated. If there is no indication, then the lines or devices should be removed. Regular observation for signs of infection, at least daily. The Visual Infusion Phlebitis (VIP) score may be useful (see Table 6.4).[7] It is the responsibility of the person completing the VIP score to act on the results of a cannula assessment. In general, a cannula should be removed if the score is 2 or greater. Use an intact, dry, adherent transparent dressing. Use aseptic techniques for line access, and swab ports or hub with alcohol prior to accessing the line or administering fluids or injections. Administration set replacement immediately after administration of blood, blood products, or lipid feeds. Replace all other fluid sets after 72h;
- catheter removal—previously maximum time limits were recommend for IV catheters. Now current guidelines recommend not to routinely replace central venous access devices to prevent catheter-related infection. Remove if there are signs of infection (e.g. VIP score ≥2). It is the responsibility of medical staff to review the need for a cannula on a daily basis and to remove it if it is no longer necessary.

Antimicrobial-coated or impregnated catheters

There has been increased interest in using antimicrobial-coated or impregnated catheters. Agents include antiseptics (e.g. chlorhexidine and silver sulfadiazine, silver, quaternary ammonium compounds) or antibiotics (e.g. minocycline and rifampicin). Ideally, compounds should be active on internal and external surfaces, and mainly target Gram-positive organisms. Evidence supports their use, but some trials were poorly designed and cost-effectiveness has been queried. Follow your hospital guidelines. One approach is to use coated or impregnated catheters if the line is likely to be in place for >3 days.

Antibiotic-containing locks

A meta-analysis has shown that vancomycin lock solutions in high-risk patients being treated with long-term central intravascular devices reduce the risk of BSIs.[8] There may be concerns regarding increasing resistance (e.g. VRE).

Further reading

epic3 guidelines. Available at: 🔗 https://www.journalofhospitalinfection.com/article/S0195–6701(13)60012-2/fulltext

References

6 Raad I, Hanne H, Maki D. Intravascular catheter-related infections: advances in diagnosis, prevention, and management. *Lancet Infect Dis*. 2007;**7**:645–57.
7 Jackson A. Infection control—a battle in vein: infusion phlebitis. *Nurs Times*. 1998;**94**:68–71.
8 Safdar N, Maki DG. Use of vancomycin-containing lock or flush solutions for prevention of bloodstream infection associated with central venous access devices: a meta-analysis of prospective, randomized trials. *Clin Infect Dis*. 2006;**43**:474–84.

Catheter-associated urinary tract infection

UTIs are one of the largest groups of HCAIs, accounting for 23% of all HCAIs.[9] The presence of a urinary catheter and the length of time it is in place are contributory factors. Estimates suggested each catheter-associated urinary tract infection (CAUTI) incurs an additional financial cost of up to £900 per patient. This report also suggested that revised urinary catheter management policies could reduce the number of UTIs. epic3 provides evidence-based guidelines for prevention of infections associated with use of short-term indwelling urethral catheters (see Box 6.8).

Risk factors

- Presence of urinary catheter/convene.
- Duration of catheterization.
- Advanced age/diabetes/immunosuppression.

Prevention

Before inserting a urinary catheter

- Is it really necessary? Review the indication for inserting a catheter in this particular patient at this particular time. Only use an indwelling urethral catheter after considering alternative options (penile sheath, incontinence pads). Suprapubic catheters, commonly used for acute retention, have a lower risk of infection.
- Choose the correct catheter type, catheter size, and drainage system. By selecting the optimum equipment, the risk of infection from recatheterization can be reduced. Use the smallest catheter possible which allows adequate drainage, and make sure the length

Box 6.8 epic3 guidelines for preventing infections associated with use of short-term indwelling urethral catheters

- Assessing the need for catheterization—only use when clinically indicated following assessment of alternative methods and discussion with the patient.
- Selection of catheter type and system—select a catheter that minimizes urethral trauma, irritation, and patient discomfort, and is appropriate for the anticipated duration of catheterization.
- Catheter insertion—via an aseptic procedure and should only be undertaken by healthcare workers trained and competent in this procedure.
- Catheter maintenance—connect a short-term indwelling urethral catheter to a sterile, closed urinary drainage system with a sampling port. Examination gloves should be worn to manipulate a catheter, preceded and followed by hand decontamination. Correct hand hygiene. Remove the catheter as soon as possible.
- Education of patients, relatives, and healthcare workers.
- System interventions for reducing the risk of infection—use quality improvement systems to support appropriate use and management of short-term urethral catheters, and ensure their timely removal.

is appropriate for ♂/♀ patients. In general, a catheter with a 10mL balloon capacity should be used, except for specific urology cases.
- Document the date of insertion, and the type and size of catheter.

Insertion of the catheter
- Use sterile equipment and an aseptic technique. Clean the urethral meatus prior to insertion by using soap and water (antiseptic preparations are not necessary). Using a sterile lubricant in both ♂ and ♀ patients should reduce urethral trauma, thus decreasing the risk of infection.
- Antibiotic prophylaxis is NOT indicated in most patients. However, in some individual cases, it may be beneficial (e.g. recent culture-positive midstream urine (MSU)).

Ongoing management of a catheterized patient
- Review the need for the catheter daily. Remove it as soon as possible.
- Empty the urinary drainage system frequently, to ensure adequate flow and prevent reflux. Use a separate container for each patient, and avoid contact between the drainage tap and the container. The drainage bag should only be changed when necessary, according to the manufacturer's instructions.
- Management of the drainage bag requires standard precautions. Wash your hands, and wear a new pair of gloves before manipulating the catheter. Always position the drainage bag below the level of the bladder (to prevent backflow). If this is not possible (e.g. when the

patient is being moved), clamp the drainage tube and ensure that the clamp is removed as soon as dependent drainage can be resumed.

- Clean the catheter urethral meatus junction daily with soap and water. Do not use antiseptic creams, as these may increase infection. Advise the patient to have a shower, rather than a bath.
- Maintain the connection between the urinary catheter and the drainage system, and only break it for good clinical reasons.
- Only flush a drainage bag if there is a clear indication (e.g. after some surgical procedures or to manage obstructive problems).
- Do not change a catheter routinely—assess each patient's needs.
- Record ongoing management in the care plan/nursing notes.

Obtaining a urine sample from a catheterized patient

Clean the sampling port with an alcohol swab, and then use sterile equipment and an aseptic, no-touch technique. If there is no sampling port available, send a sample from the drainage bag (and label it as such).

Further reading

epic guidelines for urinary catheter management, including insertion and management of short-term indwelling urinary catheters in acute care. Available at: ℘ https://www.journalofhospitalinfect ion.com/article/S0195-6701(13)60012-2/fulltext

Smith DRM, Pouwels KB, Hopkins S, et al. Epidemiology and health-economic burden of urinary-catheter-associated infection in English NHS hospitals: a probabilistic modelling study. J Hosp Infect. 2019;103:44–54.

References

9 Emmerson AM, Enstone JE, Griffin M, Kelsey MC, Smyth ET. The Second National Prevalence Survey of infection in hospitals—overview of the results. J Hosp Infect. 1996;32:175–90.

Hospital-acquired pneumonia, including ventilator-associated pneumonia

Hospital-acquired pneumonia

Respiratory infections are one of the largest contributors to HCAIs in England.[10] Approximately 1% of hospital inpatients suffer from hospital-acquired pneumonia (HAP), which results in increased length of stay (7–9 days), increased morbidity, and increased health complications. The causes of HAP are divided into those causing early-onset (<5 days after admission) and late-onset (>5 days) infections (see Table 6.5). For more detail, see recommendations from the National Institute for Health and Care Excellence (NICE), available at: ℘ https://www.nice.org.uk/guidance/ng139. ➔ See also Hospital-acquired pneumonia, pp. 167–9.

Ventilator-associated pneumonia

Pneumonia occurring during mechanical ventilation is the commonest infection in ICUs, and a leading cause of death. In the European Prevalence of Infection in Intensive Care study, ventilator-associated pneumonia (VAP) contributed to 45% of all infections in ICUs in Europe. Its incidence can vary between 9% and 68% in mechanically ventilated patients. VAP may be due to micro-aspiration of oropharyngeal secretions, aspiration of gastric contents, inhalation of infected aerosols, haematogenous spread from a distant

Table 6.5 Microbiology of hospital-acquired pneumonia

Early onset (<5 days)	Late onset (>5 days)	Others based on specific risks
Streptococcus pneumoniae	Pseudomonas aeruginosa	Anaerobic bacteria
Haemophilus influenzae	Enterobacter spp.	Legionella pneumophila
Enterobacter spp.	Acinetobacter spp.	Viruses: influenza A and B; RSV; SARS-CoV-2
	Klebsiella spp.	Moulds
	Serratia marcescens	
	Escherichia coli	
	Other GNRs	
	Staphylococcus aureus/ MRSA	

GNR, Gram-negative rod; MRSA, ethicillin-resistant S. aureus; RSV, respiratory syncytial virus; SARS-CoV-2, severe acute respiratory syndrome coronavirus 2.

site, and direct inoculation from staff (cross-infection). Predisposing factors include impaired conscious level, presence of endotracheal or NG tubes, replacement of normal flora due to prior antibiotic treatment, and severely illness and immunocompromise. About 50% of cases are defined as early VAP (i.e. within the first 5 days). VAP has significant consequences at the individual and population level:

* increased duration of ventilation;
* increased length of ICU stay and hospital stay;
* increased cost;
* possible increased mortality.

Emphasis here is on prevention of VAP; for further discussion of the pathogenesis, clinical features, diagnosis, and treatment of VAP, ➔ See Ventilator-associated pneumonia, pp. 657–8.

Prevention of ventilator-associated pneumonia

Recommendations to prevent VAP in the ICU include:
* appropriate disinfection and care of tubing, ventilators, and humidifiers to limit contamination—passive humidification and closed suction have not been shown to reduce the incidence of VAP;
* no routine changes of ventilator tubing (have not been shown to reduce incidence and may be harmful);
* avoid antacids and H_2 blockers;
* sterile tracheal suctioning;
* nurse in head-up position;
* selective decontamination of the digestive tract (SDD)—controversial (➔ see Selective decontamination of the digestive tract, p. 171).

The **Ventilator Care Bundle** was initially introduced as part of the 100 000 Lives Campaign in the USA. Its success in preventing VAP depends on all five individual steps of the bundle being performed. These five steps are:

- elevation of the head of the bed to 30–45°;
- daily 'sedation vacations' or gradually lightening the use of sedatives;
- daily assessment of readiness to extubate or wean from the ventilator;
- peptic ulcer prophylaxis;
- deep vein thrombosis (DVT) prophylaxis.

Impact of ventilator care bundle

There have been many studies on the impact of introducing ventilator bundles on ICUs, with positive outcomes overall, particularly in the reduction in ICU length of stay and mean number of ventilator days. Other benefits associated with reduced VAP include better patient outcome, shorter hospital stay, lower costs, and improved staff morale.

Further reading

British Society for Antimicrobial Chemotherapy guidelines. Available at: ℘ https://academic.oup.com/jac/article/62/1/5/844812

Centers for Disease Control and Prevention guidelines. Available at: ℘ https://www.cdc.gov/hai/vap/vap.html

References

10 Emmerson AM, Enstone JE, Griffin M, Kelsey MC, Smyth ET. The Second National Prevalence Survey of infection in hospitals—overview of the results. *J Hosp Infect*. 1996;**32**:175–90.

Infections in critical care

HCAIs complicate up to 40% of all ICU admissions. Although ICUs represent <5% of hospital beds, nosocomial infections in the ICU consume a significant amount of hospital resources.

Patients on the ICU are exposed to more broad-spectrum antibiotics (up to 60% of all patients on the ICU are on antibiotics) and medical devices and to more procedures than those on normal hospital wards. Hand hygiene, barrier precautions, cohorting of personnel, and antimicrobial policies are particularly important in preventing and controlling infection (see Box 6.9).

Organisms

- The causal organism(s) isolated depend on the length of ICU stay.
- Increasing prevalence of *Candida* infections, including non-*albicans*, which may be more drug-resistant.
- More infections with antibiotic-resistant organisms—MRSA, VRE, multiresistant Gram-negative species such as *E. coli*, *Klebsiella* spp., *Serratia* spp., *Acinetobacter* spp., *Stenotrophomonas maltophilia*, *Enterobacter* spp., and *Candidozyma auris*.

Box 6.9 Studies of HCAIs on the ICU

- Two pivotal studies relating to HCAIs on the ICU are EPIC and SENIC.
- The European Prevalence of Infection in Intensive Care (EPIC) study (1992) was a 1-day point prevalence study looking at >10 000 patients from 17 countries on all ICUs, except in paediatrics and coronary care units.[11] The infection data were linked to the patients' APACHE (Acute Physiology and Chronic Health Evaluation) score and 6-week outcome, the presence of lines, specific interventions, and demographics. Overall, 45% of patients had some sort of infection, and 20% had at least one infection acquired on the ICU. The commonest were pneumonia (47%), LRTI (18%), UTI (18%), bacteraemia (12%), and wound infection (7%). Organisms were split 50/50 into Gram-positives and Gram-negatives, with the commonest being *S. aureus*, *P. aeruginosa*, CoNS, and *Enterococcus*.
- The Study on the Efficacy of Nosocomial Infection Control (SENIC) looked at the relative change in nosocomial infection over a 5-year period.[12] Overall, when infection control measures were introduced, nosocomial infections were reduced by 32%.
- More recently, in 2016, the Infection in Critical Care Quality Improvement Programme (ICCQIP) was set up to address concerns about HCAIs in hospitals in England. Sentinel surveillance of BSIs and CVC infections across adult, paediatric, and neonatal units was instigated to characterize trends and support actions to reduce infection rates (available at: ✆ https://www.ficm.ac.uk/ICCQIP).

Patients

- Increasing population of immunosuppressed patients (e.g. uncontrolled HIV, bone marrow transplant (BMT), solid organ transplant).
- Increasing use of devices (e.g. lines, balloon pumps, pacing wires, endotracheal tubes).
- More invasive procedures (e.g. ventilator, drains).

ICU environment

- Isolating all patients with multidrug-resistant (MDR) organisms is the aim.
- As a minimum, there should be at least one side room for every six beds. There should also be sufficient space around each bed ($20m^2$), wash handbasins between every other bed, adequate ventilation, and sufficient storage space and utility space.

How to minimize infections on the ICU

- Follow evidence-based guidelines and policies.
- Good compliance with IPC measures (e.g. handwashing).
- Good AMS (e.g. specific policy based on local knowledge).
- Close liaison with infection services, pharmacy, engineers, estates, etc.
- Regular feedback of MDR organism surveillance results.

Selective decontamination of the digestive tract

This is a prophylactic technique to prevent VAP and HAP in critically ill patients by decreasing colonization of aerobic Gram-negative rods (GNRs) from the oropharynx. Regimens commonly consist of the following components:

- oropharyngeal decontamination with antiseptic (chlorhexidine);
- selective oropharyngeal decontamination with non-absorbable antimicrobials (tobramycin, colistin, and amphotericin B) applied TOP to the mouth four times daily (qds);
- selective digestive decontamination by using a liquid suspension containing the same antimicrobials given via an NG tube;
- IV antimicrobials (e.g. cefotaxime or levofloxacin) for 3 days;
- stringent IPC measures.

A systematic review and meta-analysis of >50 randomized controlled trials (RCTs) showed that SDD resulted in a significant decrease in levels of overall BSIs, Gram-negative BSIs, and overall mortality, but had no effect on Gram-positive BSIs.[13] SDD remains controversial due to concerns about the generation of MDR organisms and the risk of CDI.

Infection prevention and control in adult critical care

Recommendations for reducing the risk of infection through best practice and sustaining this reduction apply to all staff and require full engagement with best practice.

- Sustainable reductions in HCAIs require the engagement and active involvement of all staff working in the ICU, supported by the IPCT and clinical champions.
- No single action will produce effective IPC practice. This is achieved by sustained and close adherence to best practice by every member of the ICU team.
- All individuals who come into contact with ICU patients have a responsibility to ensure effective IPC afforded to them.

Infections in neonatal intensive care

Neonates often have indwelling devices, invasive procedures, and high exposure to antibiotics—and are more vulnerable to infection due to their immature skin and immune systems. More than 10% of neonates develop a neonatal ICU (NICU)-acquired infection,[14] with the commonest sites being the bloodstream (~50%), lower respiratory tract, ear, nose, and throat (ENT), and urinary tract. The commonest organisms are CoNS and enterococci. While CoNS generally exhibit low virulence, infection in neonates (e.g. with *Staphylococcus capitis*) may be associated with increased morbidity, hospital stay, and healthcare costs. Many of the principles surrounding the prevention of infection apply to neonatal and special care baby units. In addition, there have been particular issues such as the need to wash babies with sterile water after the outbreaks due to pseudomonal contamination of wash handbasin water taps (see Box 6.10).

Box 6.10 *Pseudomonas* **in taps in NICUs**

After outbreaks in neonatal units in Wales (2010) and Northern Ireland (2011/12), during which many babies suffered (and died) from invasive pseudomonal infections, there have been huge efforts to reduce the risk to vulnerable babies. The Department of Health published a review of the scientific evidence behind the contamination of hospital water supplies and outlets with *Pseudomonads*, which was followed by new IPC advice and technical guidance. These documents remind everyone to maintain high standards of IPC, and give advice on best practice to prevent *P. aeruginosa* infection in specialist care units and how to manage the risks. This includes only using the handwash station for handwashing, flushing taps regularly, and establishing a Water Safety group (Department of Health (2012). *Pseudomonas aeruginosa bacteria preventing and controlling contamination*. Available at: ℘ https://www.gov.uk/government/publications/pseudomonas-aeruginosa-bacteria-preventing-and-controlling-contamination; Department of Health (2012). *Technical guidance issued for healthcare providers on managing Pseudomonas*. Available at: ℘ https://www.gov.uk/government/news/technical-guidance-issued-for-healthcare-providers-on-managing-pseudomonas).

References

11 Vincent JL, Bihari DJ, Suter PM, *et al*. The prevalence of nosocomial infection in intensive care units in Europe. Results of the European Prevalence of Infection in Intensive Care (EPIC) Study. EPIC International Advisory Committee. *JAMA*. 1995;**274**:639–44.

12 Haley RW, Morgan WM, Culver DH, *et al*. Update from the SENIC project. Hospital infection control: recent progress and opportunities under prospective payment. *Am J Infect Control*. 1985;**13**:97–108.

13 Silvestri L, van Saene HK, Milanese M, Gregori D, Gullo A. Selective decontamination of the digestive tract reduces bacterial bloodstream infection and mortality in critically ill patients. Systematic review of randomized, controlled trials. *J Hosp Infect*. 2007;**65**:187–203.

14 Sohn AH, Garrett DO, Sinkowitz-Cochran RL, *et al*.; Pediatric Prevention Network. Prevalence of nosocomial infections in neonatal intensive care unit patients: results from the first national point-prevalence survey. *J Pediatr*. 2001;**139**:821–7.

Infection prevention and control on renal dialysis units

Outbreaks of BBV (hepatitis B virus (HBV), hepatitis C virus (HCV), HIV) infections are a well-recognized hazard for patients and staff on haemodialysis units. Adoption of standard precautions has resulted in a fall in the incidence of HBV and HCV infections in dialysis units over the last 30 years. However, increasing numbers of patients on haemodialysis, increasing numbers of immigrants, and increased foreign travel of dialysis patients may increase future risk. Other BBV (human T-cell lymphotropic virus 1 (HTLV-1)) infections are higher in dialysis patients, compared to the general population, but their clinical significance is uncertain.

The UK Kidney Association has produced NICE-accredited guidelines (2009) on the prevention of spread of BBVs in the renal unit, including issues of surveillance, segregation, and immunization (available at: ✍ https://ukkidney.org/health-professionals/guidelines/guidelines-comme ntaries).

To reduce the incidence of renal dialysis line-related BSI, a HII renal dialysis line care bundle was published as part of the NHS Saving Lives campaign. The bundle includes two sets of actions relating to line insertion and ongoing care (see Box 6.11).

Box 6.11 Saving Lives HII renal dialysis line care bundle

Insertion actions
- Dialysis line type—tunnelled dual-lumen IV catheter if dialysis treatment is expected to continue for >21 days.
- Insertion site—the internal jugular is the preferred site, and the femoral vein may be considered.
- Skin preparation—preferably use 2% chlorhexidine gluconate in 70% isopropyl alcohol, and allow to dry. If the patient has a sensitivity, use a single patient-use povidone–iodine application.
- Personal protective equipment—eye/face protection is indicated if there is a risk of splashing with blood or body fluids.
- Hand hygiene—decontaminate the hands before and after each patient contact. Use correct hand hygiene procedure.
- Aseptic technique—gown, gloves, and drapes, as indicated, should be used for the insertion of invasive devices.
- Dressing—use a sterile, semi-permeable, transparent dressing to allow observation of the insertion site.
- Safe disposal of sharps—a sharps container should be available at point of use and should not be overfilled; do not disassemble needle and syringe; do not pass sharps from hand to hand.
- Documentation—the date of insertion should be recorded in notes.

Ongoing care actions
- Hand hygiene—decontaminate the hands before and after each patient contact.
- Insertion site inspection—observe the insertion site at the beginning of each dialysis session.
- Dressing—an intact, dry, adherent transparent dressing is present.
- Catheter access—use an aseptic technique and swab ports or hub with 2% chlorhexidine gluconate in 70% isopropyl alcohol prior to accessing the line.
- Antimicrobial lock—use antimicrobial lock if indicated by local surveillance data and hospital policy.
- No routine lines replacement—malfunctioning lines should not be routinely replaced by rewiring.

Risks associated with transplants and blood transfusion

The number of organs and tissues that can be successfully transplanted is increasing. The current list of organ transplants includes the heart, kidneys, liver, lungs, pancreas, and intestine. Tissues include bones, tendons, cornea, heart valves, veins, and skin. Transplants can be individual organs or multivisceral. Rejection and infection arising from anti-rejection therapy are the main risks. Haematology and oncology patients who have received BMTs are at particularly high risk of infection. Infection in a transplant recipient may either be transmitted from the donor with the organ or arise due to the immunosuppressed state of the recipient. Depending on which organ has been transplanted, different infectious agents are commonly implicated at different time periods. Box 6.12 and Fig. 6.3 describe typical problems after a renal transplant.

Surveillance of infections amongst tissue donors

A tissue donation and banking programme is operated by NHS Blood and Transplant (NHSBT) tissue services. Donations may come from living and/or cadaveric donors, and include surgical bone (mainly femoral heads), tendons, skin, and heart valves. NHSBT also operate the National Bone Marrow Registry and a cord blood bank. All tissue donors (including stem cell and cord blood donors) are routinely tested for HIV, HCV, HBV, HTLV, and syphilis infection. The Advisory Committee on the Safety of Blood, Tissues, and Organs (SaBTO) has specific guidance on microbiological safety in transplantation.[15 4] Data concerning rates of infection are collated by UKHSA and NHSBT.

Surveillance of infections in blood donors

Every blood donation is tested for HIV, HCV, HBV, HTLV, and syphilis, and only used if all tests are negative. If an infection is detected, the donor is invited to return to the blood centre, when they will be told about their test results, asked for a repeat sample, asked to stop donating blood, and

---

Box 6.12 Example—infections post-renal transplant

Minor infections are common after a kidney transplant. Urine infections affect >50% of transplant recipients, especially if the patient has reflux nephropathy or diabetes. More serious infections in the first 6 months post-transplant include pneumonia (e.g. *Pneumocystis* pneumonia (PCP), *Pneumococcus*), cytomegalovirus (CMV), chickenpox, BK virus, and disseminated fungal infection. Each transplant unit will have guidelines for prophylaxis, which may include:
- co-trimoxazole (PCP);
- fluconazole (*Candida*);
- isoniazid for those at risk of TB;
- antibiotics (if UTIs are common);
- valganciclovir or valaciclovir if CMV-positive donor into CMV-negative recipient;
- vaccination (e.g. influenza, *Pneumococcus*).

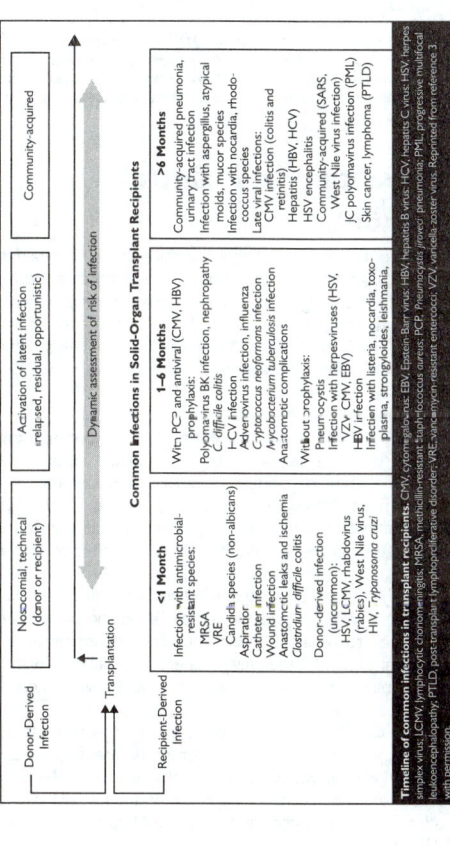

Fig. 6.3 Timeline of common infections in transplant recipients. In the absence of prophylaxis delaying illness, post-transplant infections that commonly occur develop in a predictable temporal pattern. CMV, cytomegalovirus; EBV, Epstein-Barr virus; HBV, hepatitis B virus; HCV, hepatitis C virus; HSV, herpes simplex virus; LCMV, lymphocytic choriomeningitis; MRSA, meticillin-resistant *Staphylococcus aureus*; PCP, *Pneumocystis jirovecii* pneumonia; PML, progressive multifocal leukoencephalopathy; PTLD, post-transplant lymphoproliferative disorder; VRE, vancomycin-resistant enterococci; VZV, varicella-zoster virus.

Reproduced from Fishman J A (2007) 'Infection in Solid-Organ Transplant Recipients' *N Engl J Med* 357:2601–2614, with permission from the *New England Journal of Medicine*.

referred to a specialist. In addition to ensuring our blood supply is safe, these data improve our understanding of the epidemiology of blood-borne infections. The National Blood Service and UKHSA manage a series of schemes which monitor infections in blood and tissue donor and transfusion recipients.

SHOT (Serious Hazards of Transfusion) is a scheme for reporting investigations into infections in transfusion recipients (available at: ℘ https://www.shotuk.org).

References

15 Department of Health and Social Care (2011, updated 2023). *SaBTO microbiological safety guidelines* (previously known as *Guidance on the microbiological safety of human organs, tissues and cells used in transplantation*). Available at: ℘ https://www.gov.uk/government/publicati ons/guidance-on-the-microbiological-safety-of-human-organs-tissues-and-cells-used-in-tran splantation

Infection prevention and control in the community

Community IPC refers to IPC services provided outside acute hospitals to those in another care setting such as the community or primary care setting. This covers a wide group, including nursing homes, prisons, renal patients on home dialysis, schools, and places of work. HCWs, family members, and carers are at risk of acquiring infections when caring for patients in the community. The community infection prevention and control nurse (IPCN) may have other remits such as contact tracing for TB.

It is estimated that HCAIs cost the NHS >£1 billion a year, of which £56 million are estimated to be incurred after patients are discharged from hospital. As more patients move between hospitals and the community, particularly the older and more dependent patients, the boundaries between hospital and community infections are becoming blurred. In addition, the rapid turnover of patients in acute care settings has resulted in more complex care being delivered in the community, which often involves more indwelling devices.

The clinical guideline *Healthcare-associated infections: prevention and control in primary and community care* was published by NICE and updated in 2017 (CG139). In addition to general guidance on hand decontamination, use of PPE, and disposal of waste and sharps, there is detailed information about long-term urinary catheters, enteral feeding, and vascular access devices.

- **Community-onset *C. difficile***—CDI is being increasingly recognized in the community. It is generally defined as patients who are diagnosed with CDI in the community or within 48h of hospital admission. Not all patients have been in a healthcare setting recently, and not all have received antibiotics. For further information, ➋ see *Clostridioides difficile* infection, pp. 196–200.
- **Community-acquired MRSA**—this is genetically distinct from hospital-acquired MRSA (➋ see Meticillin-resistant *Staphylococcus aureus*, pp. 264–6).

Control of antimicrobial resistance in the community

Many countries have launched campaigns to educate doctors and patients about the threat of antimicrobial resistance (AMR) and the need for AMS. In the USA, the 'Get Smart' campaign has been driven by the Centers for Disease Control and Prevention (CDC). There are many similar initiatives in the UK (for further information, ➔ see Antimicrobial stewardship, p. 34).

Further reading

National Institute for Health and Care Excellence (2012, updated 2017). *Healthcare-associated infection: prevention and control in primary and community care*. Clinical guideline [CG139]. Available at: ⌖ https://www.nice.org.uk/guidance/cg139

Overview of surveillance

Definitions

Surveillance is the continuous and systematic process of collection, analysis, interpretation, and dissemination of information for monitoring progress of key diseases and for providing epidemiological evidence to inform action to reduce them.

Surveillance may be active or passive:

- **active** surveillance—is when prospective steps are made to collect data (e.g. outbreak investigation or survey of a particular disease);
- **passive** surveillance—uses routine data that have already been collected (e.g. the UK national census).

Aims of surveillance

The aims of infection surveillance are to monitor trends (organisms, AMR markers, or clinical syndromes), provide quality outcome indicators, and identify key measures to prevent infections. All HCWs have a responsibility to collect relevant data on infection rates and to perform regular audits. Routine surveillance from the laboratory can identify new antibiotic-resistant or 'alert' organisms.

Methods of HCAI surveillance usually involve a combination of active and passive surveillance systems (➔ see Surveillance of healthcare-acquired infection, pp. 179–80). While surveillance of specific infections is mandated nationally in certain settings (e.g. UKHSA mandates surveillance of MRSA/MSSA/Gram-negative BSI, CDI), practices of monitoring non-mandatory infections vary locally within and between hospitals, and is largely dependent on the availability of staff and resources. In practice, a number of surveillance methods are used, as each provides different information. These include:

- specialty-specific—each specialty collects data on their patient risk factors, infection rates (central line-associated BSI (CLABSI), SSI, CAUTI, VAP), and IPC practices (hand hygiene). This is particularly relevant in areas such as the ICU and surgical wards;
- laboratory-based—significant culture results (BSI) or alert organisms (MRSA, *C. difficile*, VRE, MDR Gram-negatives, respiratory pathogens) are highlighted to members of the IPCT for patient review/and discussion with the patient's clinical team

- others, including review of patients with indwelling devices or those receiving broad-spectrum antibiotics (➔ see Antimicrobial stewardship, p. 34).

Evaluation of a surveillance system

- Define the event to be measured ('case definition').
- Define the population under surveillance.
- List the objectives of the system.
- Define the public health importance of the health event (e.g. number of deaths, case-fatality ratio, morbidity, economics, preventability).

Some characteristics of a surveillance system are listed in Box 6.13.

Does surveillance work?

There is good evidence that surveillance in hospitals actually reduces infection rates. The SENIC study was the first nationwide project, undertaken in the USA, to assess whether surveillance and dissemination of results reduced HCAIs.[16] The study demonstrated that hospitals with active surveillance and infection control programmes could reduce the incidence of four key nosocomial infections (UTI, pneumonia, SSI, BSI) by 32%. Other important findings of the SENIC study were the need to close the loop and present data back to the clinicians and to regularly audit practices.

References

16 Haley RW, Morgan WM, Culver DH, *et al*. Update from the SENIC project. Hospital infection control: recent progress and opportunities under prospective payment. *Am J Infect Control*. 1985;**13**:97–108.

Box 6.13 What makes a good surveillance system?

For surveillance to succeed, it should ideally have the following attributes:
- simple (well-designed reporting forms make all the difference!);
- flexible;
- acceptable to the population studied;
- sensitive;
- representative;
- timely;
- reasonable cost;
- the quality of data provided can be evaluated in terms of:
- sensitivity and specificity;
- positive and negative predictive values;
- usefulness in relation to the surveillance goals (quality indicators). It is sometimes more valuable (although usually more difficult) to focus on the outcome (e.g. the number of cases of polio), rather than on the process (e.g. the number of polio vaccinations);
- ownership is important—the ability to feed data back to those who collected them will make them more willing to help again in the future!

Surveillance of alert organisms

Local surveillance may vary between institutions, but, in most UK hospitals, the IPCT should be informed of patients suffering from the following conditions, in order to ensure appropriate IPC and public health measures are implemented:

- infectious diarrhoea (*Campylobacter*, *Salmonella*, *Shigella*, *C. difficile*, rotavirus, norovirus, etc.);
- group A *Streptococcus* (GAS) (*Streptococcus pyogenes*);
- group B *Streptococcus* (GBS) (invasive infections in neonatal or maternity units);
- meningococcal disease;
- respiratory pathogens (influenza, severe acute respiratory syndrome coronavirus 2 (SARS-CoV-2), respiratory syncytial virus (RSV), *Legionella*);
- TB;
- HIV;
- hepatitis A–E;
- severe herpes simplex;
- varicella-zoster virus (VZV) (shingles or chickenpox);
- lice/scabies.

Multidrug-resistant organisms

Practice varies across institutions, but in general, the following organisms should be reported to the IPCT. Often patients' notes and electronic records are 'flagged' if an MDR organism has been isolated in the past:

- MRSA;
- VRE;
- penicillin-resistant/non-susceptible *Pneumococcus*;
- extended-spectrum β-lactamase (ESBL)- and ampC-producing *Enterobacterales*;
- carbapenemase-producing *Enterobacterales* (CPE);
- MDR *P. aeruginosa*;
- carbapenem-resistant *Acinetobacter baumannii*;
- co-trimoxazole-resistant *S. maltophilia*;
- colistin-resistant Gram negative organisms.

Surveillance of healthcare-acquired infection

Definition

HCAIs, often referred to as nosocomial, are infections occurring in a person during (or following) healthcare that was neither present nor incubating at the time of healthcare admission, which normally manifests >48h into admission. HCAIs are preventable and associated with prolonged hospital stays, long-term disability, AMR, and excess financial costs to healthcare and unnecessary deaths. The burden of HCAIs is higher in LMICs. HCAIs also include occupational infections amongst staff.

Criteria for HCAI surveillance schemes

In order to obtain accurate and comparable results, the following criteria are important:
- agreed definitions of infection;
- accurate denominator data;
- correction of rates for risk factors (e.g. pre-existing diseases);
- identification of HCAIs post-discharge.

Brief history of national surveillance schemes

The UK's Nosocomial Infection National Surveillance Scheme (NINSS), launched in 1996, was set up to monitor HCAIs. In response to excess MRSA BSIs in 2001, this system was replaced by a mandatory laboratory-based MRSA bacteraemia surveillance. Over the last decade, the UK's national surveillance scheme has expanded to include mandatory and voluntary reporting of certain clinically relevant pathogens (see Table 6.6).

International surveillance schemes

Most other countries have established HCAI surveillance programmes, although data are often not comparable across countries/continents because of variations in definitions and methods.

The European Centre for Disease Prevention and Control (ECDC) is a European Union agency with core functions including surveillance and epidemic intelligence to strengthen Europe's defences against infectious diseases (available at: ℘ https://www.ecdc.europa.eu/en/healthcare-associated-infections).

Table 6.6 National mandatory HCAI surveillance schemes in the UK

Surveillance activity	Date	Notes
Staphylococcus aureus (including MRSA) bacteraemia	2001	Replaced by enhanced reporting in 2005 and 2011
Vancomycin-resistant *Enterococcus* (VRE) bacteraemia	2003	Mandatory reporting stopped in 2013
Clostridioides difficile infection (CDI)	2004	Annual reports initially, then quarterly, now monthly
Orthopaedic surgical site infection (four categories)	2004	Annual reports
MESS: MRSA Enhanced Surveillance Scheme— additional details of cases of MRSA bacteraemias	2005	Enhanced to include patient-level data Monthly reporting
MSSA bacteraemia enhanced surveillance	2011	Initially quarterly, now monthly
Escherichia coli bacteraemia enhanced surveillance	2011	Monthly reporting
Klebsiella spp. and *Pseudomonas aeruginosa* bacteraemia enhanced surveillance	2016	Monthly reporting

Bloodstream infection—mandatory surveillance

Overview

A laboratory-confirmed BSI is defined as one or more blood cultures yielding a viable microorganism. Key organisms causing BSIs require mandated reporting, including MRSA, MSSA, *E. coli*, *Klebsiella* spp., and *P. aeruginosa*. BSIs are categorized according to where they are detected (community or hospital) and their relationship to healthcare (healthcare- or non-healthcare-associated) (see Fig. 6.4).

Healthcare-associated infections include patients with BSI who have received healthcare in either the community or hospital in the preceding 28 days. Risk factors for healthcare-associated BSIs include: (1) vascular access devices, (2) urinary catheters, (3) invasive procedures, (4) neutropenia, (5) antimicrobial therapy within the preceding month, and (6) hospital admission within the last 28 days.

IV catheter-related bloodstream infections

Peripheral venous catheters (PVCs) are more commonly used for vascular access, but the risk of BSI is low (➔ see Intravascular line-related sepsis, pp. 162–5). BSIs are more commonly associated with CVC insertion and are a significant cause of morbidity. At present, there are no surveillance systems for CRBSI in the UK, but estimates suggest that up to 6000 patients a year in England may acquire a CRBSI and CRBSIs can contribute additional healthcare costs of up to £6000.

Intravascular infection definitions

(See Box 6.11.)

Prevention of IV catheter-related bloodstream infections

The combination of a CVC insertion guideline and a monitoring tool has been shown to significantly reduce the incidence of CRBSI in an ICU (see Box 6.15).[17] Coated catheters and antibiotic-containing locks are helpful (➔ see Antibiotic-containing locks, p. 165).

For further discussion of line-related sepsis, including the care of peripheral lines and VIP score, ➔ see Intravascular line-related sepsis, pp. 162–5.

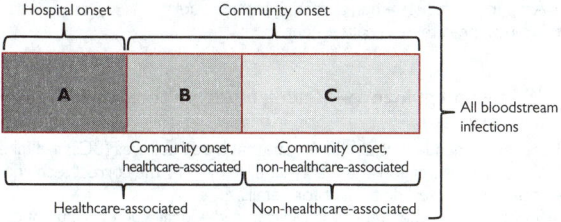

Fig. 6.4 UKHSA categorization of bloodstream infections, including hospital-onset, healthcare-associated (A); community-onset, healthcare-associated (B); and community-onset, non-healthcare-associated (C).

Box 6.14 Intravascular infection definitions

While catheter-related BSI (CRBSI) and central line-associated BSI (CLABSI) are often used interchangeably, they do have different meanings. CRBSI is a clinical definition requiring laboratory testing to identify an IV catheter as the source of BSI. It is often challenging to directly attribute the IV catheter as the cause of the BSI due to, for example, the line not removed for clinical reasons or limited laboratory resources to undertake investigations (see ⅋ https://www.gov.uk/government/publications/smi-b-20-investigation-of-intravascular-cannulae-and-associated-specimens). For epidemiological purposes, the CDC developed a simpler definition. A CLABSI is defined as a BSI identified in a patient with a central line that was present within the 48h period prior to the BSI and the infection is unrelated to another source.

A useful set of CLABSI resources can be found at: ⅋ https://www.ecdc.europa.eu/en/publications-data/directory-guidance-prevention-and-control/healthcare-associated-infections-1.

Box 6.15 'Saving Lives' High Impact Intervention No. 1: central venous catheter care

On insertion
- Catheter type—single lumen, unless indicated otherwise for patient care; consider antimicrobial-impregnated line if 1–3 weeks' duration likely and high risk of BSI.
- Insertion site—subclavian or internal jugular.
- Use alcoholic chlorhexidine gluconate for skin preparation, and allow to dry.
- Prevent microbial contamination—hand hygiene, aseptic technique.
- Sterile, transparent, semi-permeable dressing.

Continuing care
- Full documentation.
- Regular observation of line insertion site—at least daily.
- Catheter site care—intact, clean dressing.
- Catheter access.
- Aseptic techniques when accessing catheter ports.
- No routine catheter replacement.

NHS England guidance—Taking blood cultures: a summary of best practice

These recommendations aim to ensure that blood cultures (BCs) are taken for the correct indication at the correct time by using the correct technique. See the 'Saving Lives' document for details.[18]
- Only take BCs when there is a clinical need—ideally before antibiotics are started. Document the date, time, site, and indications. Do not take 'routine' cultures.
- Competence—only undertaken by trained staff.

- Always make a fresh stab—never take from peripheral lines or sites, or immediately above them. If a central line is present, time to positivity of paired peripheral and central BCs may aid diagnosis.
- Thoroughly disinfect the skin before inserting the needle.
- Once disinfected, do not touch the skin again (no-touch technique).
- Disinfect the bottle cap before transferring the sample.
- Adding an appropriate volume of blood and swift transportation to the lab both improve yield.

Further reading

American Healthcare Infection Control Practices Advisory Committee (HICPAC) guidelines - https://www.cdc.gov/infectioncontrol/guidelines/index.html

EPIC guidelines— https://www.journalofhospitalinfection.com/article/S0195-6701(13)60012-2/fulltext#seccestitle530

References

17 Berenholtz SM, Pronovost PJ, Lipsett PA, et al. Eliminating catheter-related bloodstream infections in the intensive care unit. Crit Care Med. 2004;**32**:2014–20.
18 Department of Health (2011). Taking blood cultures: a summary of best practice. Available at: ℘ http://webarchive.nationalarchives.gov.uk/20120118164404/hcai.dh.gov.uk/files/2011/03/Document_Blood_culture_FINAL_100826.pdf

Surgical site infection

Introduction

Surgical site infections (SSIs) are seen in at least 5% of patients undergoing a surgical procedure. They range from a minor wound discharge through to osteomyelitis. SSIs make up almost 20% of all HCAIs, and cause significant morbidity, increased length of stay, and increased costs. Most infections are endogenous (i.e. result from contamination of the incision by the patient's own microbes during surgery). The other route of acquisition is exogenous

Table 6.7 Factors associated with surgical site infections

Patient-related	Procedure-related
Colonization with Staphylococcus aureus	Antimicrobial prophylaxis
Corticosteroid use	Duration of procedure
Diabetes mellitus	Duration of surgical scrub
Extremes of age	Foreign material
Immunosuppression	Sterilization of instruments
Longer hospital stay	Operating room ventilation (➜) Ventilation in hospitals, pp. 223–5)
Malnutrition	Preoperative shaving
Obesity	Preoperative skin preparation
Remote infection	Skin antisepsis
Smoking	

Source: data from Mangram A J et al (1999) 'Guideline for prevention of surgical site infection, 1999. Hospital Infection Control Practices Advisory Committee' Infect Control Hosp Epidemiol **20**(4):250–78.

from the environment or other people. Factors associated with SSIs have been well defined (see Table 6.7), and multiple guidelines and recommendations have been published to aim to prevent SSIs from occurring. NICE published in 2019, and updated in 2020, best practice guidelines on prevention and treatment of SSIs (see Box 6.16).

National surveillance of surgical site infection

Mandatory reporting of SSIs in orthopaedic surgery began in 2004 for hip and knee replacements, repair of neck of femur and reduction of long bone fractures. This has shown that rates are highest in hip hemiarthroplasty—partly due to the increased risk of infection in these patients and also due to increased detection of infection, as the patients tend to have a long hospital

---

Box 6.16 NICE guideline (NG125) —SSI: prevention and treatment

Preoperative
- Showering the day before, or on the day of, surgery.
- Nasal decontamination—consider nasal mupirocin in combination with a chlorhexidine body wash before procedures in which *S. aureus* is a likely cause of a surgical site infection. See recommendations on the Healthcare Infection Society website (available at: ℘ https://www.his.org.uk).
- Hair removal—do not use hair removal routinely, to reduce the risk of SSI. If hair removal is needed, use electric clippers with single-use head on the day of surgery. Shaving with a razor is not recommended as increased risk of SSI.
- Theatre wear—patients and staff to wear appropriate theatre wear.
- Mechanical bowel preparation is not routinely required for SSI prevention.
- Prophylactic antimicrobial—where indicated, at correct timing, with appropriate agent. Remember repeat dosing in longer procedures.

Intraoperative
- Appropriate hand decontamination prior to operation.
- Appropriate PPE, incision drape use, and aseptic skin mphasizes
- Maintain homeostasis. Maintaining blood glucose level <11mmol/L has been shown to reduce wound infections in diabetic patients. Maintaining a body temperature above 36°C in the perioperative period has been shown to reduce infection rates.
- Wound irrigation/intracavity lavage is not routinely recommended.
- Cover wounds with appropriate interactive dressings.

Post-operative
- Use aseptic non-touch technique (ANTT) to change or remove dressings.
- Post-operative cleansing—patients may shower safely >48h after surgery. Use sterile saline for cleansing prior to this.
- Topical antimicrobials are not recommended.

Source: data from ℘ https://www.nice.org.uk/guidance/ng125.

stay. Most of the SSIs reported affect the superficial layers of the wound, but >25% involve deeper tissues. Annual reports are published by UKHSA; All four mandatory orthopaedic categories have shown overall decreasing 10-year trends. Voluntary surveillance is available for other surgical procedures on the UKHSA website.

Non-pharmacological measures for reducing SSI

- Appropriate hair removal.
- Appropriate operating room ventilation.
- Appropriate surgical attire.
- Glycaemic control.
- Maintenance of good oxygenation.
- Restricted foot fall in operating theatres.
- Maintaining normothermia.
- Appropriate preparation of the surgical field.

Rates of SSI in different types of operation are shown in Table 6.8.

Further reading

Healthcare Infection Society. MRSA guidelines. Available at: ℘ https://www.his.org.uk/resources-guidelines

National Institute for Health and Care Excellence (2019, updated 2020). *Surgical site infections: prevention and treatment.* Available at: ℘ https://www.nice.org.uk/guidance/ng125/chapter/Recommendations

Table 6.8 Rates of surgical site infection in different types of operation

Type of operation	SSI incidence (95% confidence interval)
Knee joint replacement	0.5% (0.4–0.5)
Hip joint replacement	0.5% (0.5–0.6)
Abdominal hysterectomy	1.8% (1.3–2.5)
Vascular surgery	2.5% (2.1–3.0)
Coronary artery bypass graft	3.0% (2.8–3.2)
Large bowel (gut) surgery	8.3% (7.9–8.7)

Data source: PHE SSI Annual report 2019/20.

Antimicrobial stewardship

AMS is a core component of IPC. Inappropriate use of antimicrobials increases the risk to patients of colonization and infection with resistant organisms and subsequent transmission to other patients. The term 'antimicrobial stewardship' is defined as an organizational or healthcare system-wide approach to promoting and monitoring judicious use of antimicrobials to preserve their future effectiveness.[19] The Chief Medical Officer (CMO) report (2011) was one of the first key documents.

The O'Neill report

In 2014, the UK Prime Minister commissioned the economist Jim O'Neill to analyse the global problem of rising AMR and propose concrete actions to tackle it internationally. Over 2 years, and with wide stakeholder engagement, in 2016, the final '*The review of AMR*' report and recommendations were published.[20] The report highlighted the escalating problem of AMR and why action is needed, and provided an overview of solutions to reduce unnecessary use and increase supply of new antibiotics. It also evaluated the role of public health campaigns, the need for improved sanitation, reduction in pollution in the environment/agriculture, improved global surveillance, and the need for rapid diagnostics and vaccines. The paper also considered funding and building political consensus.

National Action Plan

Building on the outcomes of the O'Neill report, preventing and controlling AMR has become a major political focus, with the UK government committing to leading the international fight against AMR. In addition, the UK's 20-year vision for AMR[21] and the UK's 5-year national plan to tackle AMR (2019–24)[22] focus on three key areas:

- reducing the need for, and unintentional exposure to, antimicrobials;
- optimizing the use of antimicrobials; and
- investing in innovation, supply, and access.

The plan sets out four measures of success to ensure progress towards our 20-year vision. These include targets to:

- halve healthcare-associated Gram-negative BSIs;
- reduce the number of specific drug-resistant infections in people by 10% by 2025 (note differences in primary and secondary care);
- reduce UK antimicrobial use in humans by 15% by 2024;
- reduce UK antibiotic use in food-producing animals by 25% between 2016 and 2020, and define new objectives by 2021 for 2025;
- be able to report on the percentage of prescriptions supported by a diagnostic test or decision support tool by 2024.

As well as reflecting lessons learnt during the coronavirus disease 2019 (Covid-19) pandemic, the National Action Plan was updated in 2022 to include aims to:

- improve the **surveillance** of AMR and antimicrobial use;
- improve the **availability of data** to better understand the prevalence of AMR across human health and animals, and linking of these data to enable analysis of AMR and our approach to managing infection through dashboards and research;
- explore and evaluate antimicrobial use, prescribing, new therapeutics, diagnostics, stewardship, and resistance across both **human health and animals**;
- reflect the particular role the UK is playing internationally in non-traditional and informal political groupings, including **supporting the UK Special Envoy on AMR** (currently Professor Dame Sally Davies, previous CMO for England) and taking a lead role in AMR interest groups;
- introduce **new commitments** to reducing UTIs, in support of the National Action Plan ambition to halve healthcare-associated Gram-negative BSIs by 2024.

AWaRe

AWaRe (Access, Watch, Reserve) is a classification system of antibiotics developed by WHO in 2017, and updated in 2019 and 2021, aimed at optimizing antibiotic use, taking into account what is best for patients in terms of clinical effectiveness and minimal toxicity, while minimizing the risk of developing AMR. According to this system, antibiotics can fall into one of three groups (see Table 6.9):

Table 6.9 Antibiotics classified into Access, Watch, and Reserve groups (WHO list; note UK list is different and likely to change)

AWaRe	Antimicrobials
Access	Amoxicillin
	Co-amoxiclav
	Ampicillin
	Benzathine benzylpenicillin
	Benzylpenicillin
	Cefalexin or cefazolin
	Chloramphenicol
	Clindamycin
	Cloxacillin
	Doxycycline
	Gentamicin or amikacin
	Metronidazole
	Nitrofurantoin
	Phenoxymethylpenicillin
	Procaine benzylpenicillin
	Spectinomycin
	Sulfamethoxazole and trimethoprim
Watch	Antipseudomonal penicillins with β-lactamase inhibitor (e.g. piperacillin and tazobactam)
	Carbapenems or penems (e.g. faropenem, imipenem and cilastatin, meropenem)
	Cephalosporins, third generation (with or without β-lactamase inhibitor, e.g. cefixime, cefotaxime, ceftazidime, ceftriaxone)
	Glycopeptides (e.g. teicoplanin, vancomycin)
	Macrolides (e.g. azithromycin, clarithromycin, erythromycin)
	Quinolones and fluoroquinolones (e.g. ciprofloxacin, levofloxacin, moxifloxacin, norfloxacin)
Reserve	Aztreonam
	Cephalosporins, fourth generation (e.g. cefepime)
	Cephalosporins, fifth generation (e.g. ceftaroline)
	Daptomycin
	Fosfomycin (IV)
	Oxazolidinones (e.g. linezolid)
	Polymyxins (e.g. colistin, polymyxin B)
	Tigecycline

- **access**—antibiotics with a narrow spectrum of activity and a lower potential for the development of AMR, compared to antibiotics in other AWaRe groups. They are recommended for empirical treatment of most infections and therefore should be widely available;
- **watch**—antibiotics with a higher potential for the development of AMR, with very limited recommended indications for empirical use. Their use should be carefully monitored to avoid overuse;
- **reserve**—antibiotics that should only be used when antibiotics from the other two classes cannot be used (e.g. due to infections caused by MDR pathogens).

Start Smart Then Focus

(See Box 6.17.) Originally published in 2011,[23] this evidence-based toolkit has been designed to help organizations to demonstrate compliance with

---

Box 6.17 A summary of the features of 'Start Smart Then Focus'

Start Smart
- Do not start antimicrobial therapy unless there is clear evidence of infection
- Take a thorough drug allergy history
- Initiate prompt, effective antibiotic treatment within 1h of diagnosis (or as soon as possible) in patients with severe sepsis or life-threatening infections
- Avoid inappropriate use of broad-spectrum antibiotics
- Comply with local antimicrobial prescribing guidance
- Document clinical indication (and disease severity if appropriate), drug name, dose, and route on drug chart and in clinical notes
- Include review/stop date or duration
- Obtain cultures prior to commencing therapy where possible (but do not delay therapy)
- Prescribe single-dose antibiotics for surgical prophylaxis where antibiotics have been shown to be effective
- Document the exact indication on the drug chart (rather than stating long-term prophylaxis) for clinical prophylaxis

Then Focus
- Review the clinical diagnosis and continuing need for antibiotics at 48–72h
- Document a clear plan of action—the 'antimicrobial prescribing decision'
- The five 'antimicrobial prescribing decision' options are:
  1. Stop antibiotics if there is no evidence of infection
  2. Switch antibiotics from IV to PO
  3. Change antibiotics—ideally to a narrower spectrum, or broader if required
  4. Continue and document the next review date or stop date
  5. Outpatient parenteral antibiotic therapy (OPAT)
- It is essential that the review and subsequent decision are clearly documented in the clinical notes and on the drug chart where possible (e.g. stop antibiotic)

the Health and Social Care Act 2008: Code of Practice on the prevention and control of infections and related guidance. It takes into account:

- the UK 5-Year Antimicrobial Resistance Strategy 2013 to 2018;
- the Cochrane review '*Interventions to improve antibiotic prescribing practices for hospital inpatients*';
- the English Surveillance Programme for Antimicrobial Utilisation and Resistance (ESPAUR) data;
- AMS guideline produced by NICE.

It is recommended that providers develop an action plan and monitor adherence to the Start Smart Then Focus principles regularly in all clinical areas (at least annually).

Diagnostic stewardship

- Diagnostic stewardship (table 6.10) can be described as emphasizes the right test, for the right patient, at the right time to prompt the right action.
- Traditionally, a laboratory activity focusing on optimizing specimen collection, processing, and reporting to ensure accurate test results and interpretation.
- More recently, there has been an increasing understanding that test results can strongly influence antimicrobial use.
- Newer approaches undergoing investigation include:
  - procalcitonin;
  - β-D-glucan.
- An understanding of pretest probability of infection is essential for designing diagnostic stewardship interventions that improve the usefulness of tests.

Antifungal stewardship (AFS) focuses on azoles and liposomal amphotericin B in particular, and there are key differences compared to AMS (e.g. increased drug interactions and toxicities, fewer diagnostic and monitoring tests, lack of clinician familiarity).

Behavourial science emphasizes the importance of a multidisciplinary approach to AMS. The Vanguard report (available at: ℅ https://bsac.org.uk/behavioural-science-and-amr/) focuses on three areas with potential for behavioural science interventions: 'nudging' AMS, building good hygiene habits, and leveraging market forces. The ARK (Antibiotic Review Kit) study aims to reduce antibiotic use through a package of strategies.

Further reading

Antimicrobial Resistance Collaborators (2022). *Global burden of bacterial antimicrobial resistance in 2019: a systematic analysis.* Available at: ℅ https://www.thelancet.com/journals/lancet/article/PIIS0140-6736(21)02724-0/fulltext

Public Health England (2016, updated 2017). *Antimicrobial resistance: resource handbook.* Available at: ℅ https://www.gov.uk/government/publications/antimicrobial-resistance-resource-handbook

eBNF—antibacterials, principles of therapy; considerations before starting and during therapy; superinfection; information for patients and their families/carers, in addition to syndrome- and drug-specific prescribing information. https://bnf.nice.org.uk/

UK Health Security Agency (2014, updated 2023). *Antimicrobial resistance awareness: toolkit for healthcare providers.* Available at: ℅ https://www.gov.uk/government/publications/european-antibiotic-awareness-day-resources-toolkit-for-healthcare-professionals-in-england

Department of Health and Social Care, UK Health Security Agency, Department for Environment, Food & Rural Affairs, and Veterinary Medicines Directorate (2014, updated 2023). *Antimicrobial resistance (AMR).* Available at: ℅ https://www.gov.uk/government/collections/antimicrobial-resistance-amr-information-and-resources

Table 6.10 Diagnostic stewardship

From of test	Pre-analytical	Analytical	Post-analytical
General Principles to apply to all microbiology tests	Only request a test if infection is likely (ie high pretest probability) Collect and transport samples in a way to minimise contamination and optimise yield	Use laboratory tests to try to differentiate colonisation from infection—eg quantification where relevant	Reporting of results should help guide practice, according to local guidelines
Blood Cultures (BC)	Only take BC if fever (or persistent infection / encouraged by guidelines eg IE / endovascular) Good BC technique	Rapid 4 hr MALDI may help with early identification, thus give an indication if contaminant or true pathogen. Rapid sensitivity tests undergoing trials	Interpretative comment regarding likely significance Suppress some sensitivity results
Urine Cultures	Only test if symptoms consistent with UTI, or if meets strict criteria for asymptomatic patients (eg pregnant; urological surgery) Use aseptic technique – clean the periurethral area, and take a MID-STREAM sample. If catheterised, take urine samples from catheter collection port, never from the bag.	Only culture if pyuria detected (except if meets other strict criteria eg neutropenic patients)	Interpretative comment regarding likely significance Suppress some sensitivity results
C difficile testing of stool	Only test if infection likely (see pp. 196–200) Generally avoid repeat tests or retesting equivocal samples without prior thought	Consider a testing algorithm which includes toxin immunoassay	Interpretative of equivocal results (GDH +; toxin -) as probable colonisation

Adapted from JAMA. 2017;318(7):607– 608.

References

19 National Institute for Health and Care Excellence (2015). *Antimicrobial stewardship: systems and processes for effective antimicrobial medicine use*. NICE guideline [NG15]. Available at: ℜ https://www.nice.org.uk/guidance/ng15

20 O'Neill J (2016). *Review on antimicrobial resistance*. Available at: ℜ https://amr-review.org/

21 Department of Health and Social Care (2019). *UK 20-year vision for antimicrobial resistance*. Available at: ℜ https://www.gov.uk/government/publications/uk-20-year-vision-for-antimicrobial-resistance

22 UK Government (2019). *Tackling antimicrobial resistance 2019–2024: the UK's five-year national action plan*. Available at: ℜ https://assets.publishing.service.gov.uk/government/uploads/system/uploads/attachment_data/file/784894/UK_AMR_5_year_national_action_plan.pdf

23 \UK Health Security Agency (2011, updated 2023). *Antimicrobial stewardship: start smart then focus*. Available at: ℜ https://www.gov.uk/government/publications/antimicrobial-stewardship-start-smart-then-focus

Management of outbreaks

Definition

An outbreak refers to an increase in incidence of cases of a disease where the observed number of cases unaccountably exceeds the expected number of cases. In certain circumstances, the emergence of one new infection may constitute an outbreak. Here are some examples to illustrate these definitions:

- one case of viral haemorrhagic fever in a UK hospital;
- two new hepatitis C-positive haemodialysis patients, identified by regular screening tests;
- an unusual number of cases of diarrhoea on a medical ward;
- increased number of *Campylobacter* isolates sent to the national reference laboratory, compared to the same period in previous years.

Steps in outbreak management

1. Recognition of an outbreak, either through laboratory surveillance or clinical observations, or through identification by occupational health.
2. Investigation of an outbreak.
3. Case definition.
4. Describing the outbreak.
5. Propose and test the hypothesis.
6. Control measures and follow-up.
7. Communication.

Management of hospital outbreaks

Outbreaks of HCAIs must be identified and thoroughly investigated, because of their importance in terms of morbidity and mortality. Also there is a need to identify any breakdown in a process and to prevent spread or future recurrences. The declaration of an outbreak is a decision that should be made by the IPCT, in conjunction with senior members of staff from the affected area. The declaration of an outbreak can have a significant impact on patient care and bed pressures, as well as political and financial implications. Before an outbreak is declared, there is often a 'period of increased incidence' (PII).

Period of increased incidence

This situation may result from an increase in the number of sporadic cases (the same organism is isolated, but the organisms are found to be unrelated, e.g. CDI where the ribotypes are all different). During a PII, a formal outbreak meeting does not need to be held. However, a full investigation (➔ see Outbreak management, pp. 192–3) should be performed, as the PII may become an outbreak. There are often no formal criteria for declaring an outbreak, but it is dependent on a number of factors, including: the pathogenicity of the organism, whether the number of cases continues to rise, or if transmission is confirmed. Transmission is usually confirmed once organism typing results have been obtained. If the organisms are highly related or identical, then a transmission event amongst patients is confirmed and the cases are highly unlikely to be sporadic.

Outbreak management

The main aim of outbreak (and PII) management is to limit and control the spread of infection by identifying and addressing any breakdown in IPC practices. A meeting will be held to review information and decide whether to declare an outbreak (which is the responsibility of the DIPC or their representative). If an outbreak is called, an outbreak control team (see Box 6.18) will be formed and steps 2–7 (➔ see Steps in outbreak management, p. 191) will be addressed. Outbreak meetings are usually chaired by the DIPC or their representative and allow documentation of decisions and actions taken in response to the outbreak. Particular attention is paid to reviewing:

- patients—identify those affected and those who have been in contact with the infected patient(s) and are at risk of developing disease (➔ see Contact tracing, pp. 194, 740). The length of time for which

---

Box 6.18 Outbreak management

Core members of an outbreak control team should include:
- infection prevention and control (IPC) doctor;
- medical microbiologist/virologist;
- IPC nurse;
- senior nurse/midwife;
- divisional management team representative;
- clinician;
- occupational health service representative (if staff are affected);
- site operations manager;
- facilities manager;
- estates manager;
- clinical governance representative;
- Consultant in Communicable Disease Control;
- communications team;
- administrator (coordinates meetings, minutes).
  In the event of a major outbreak, additional members may include:
- Director of Infection Prevention and Control;
- medical director;
- director of nursing;
- director of public health;
- regional epidemiologist;
- environmental health officer.

someone remains a contact will depend on the incubation period of the infection;
- staff—identification of potential staff involvement. Support will be required from occupational health;
- hand hygiene—review hand hygiene audits, and perform ad hoc audits when necessary. Any deficiencies should be dealt with in real time, with educational sessions for staff. Commonly, assessments of non-touch technique practices are also undertaken;
- ward cleaning—audits are usually performed regularly to review practice. Deficiencies should be addressed, and decisions made regarding enhanced cleaning. Enhanced cleaning can include increased frequency of cleaning of the entire ward or certain areas at greatest risk of causing transmission (e.g. high-touch surfaces);
- ward equipment—the same pieces of equipment have the potential to be used throughout the ward, and they should be properly cleaned, maintained, and stored (e.g. commodes). All equipment used in patient areas should be examined;
- the ward environment—determine if there are potential reservoirs in the environment. Remedial building work should be carried out (e.g. repairing cracks in walls or broken ceiling tiles). Rarely, environmental screening is required but should be considered;
- antibiotic prescribing—antibiotic prescribing can add a selection pressure in favour of the infecting organism;
- communications—with internal agencies (clinical governance, comms), external agencies (Health Protection, Integrated care board), patients, and relatives.

A key strategy for controlling an outbreak or a PII is restricting the movement of patients by ward closure, patient isolation, and assessing the risk to contacts.

The frequency of outbreak meetings will be determined at the initial meeting and reviewed at each subsequent meeting. It is common practice for daily meetings in the event of ward closure.

Bay and ward closure

To control and prevention spread of infection, it may be necessary to restrict admission to, and transfers from, ward bays and even entire wards. This is referred to as ward or bay closure. The decision to close a ward (or even a single bay!) can have a significant impact on the functioning of the entire hospital. The decision to close bays or the ward is based on a number of factors, including:
- geographical spread of the patients affected—if the infected cases are currently located within the same bay, then the bay can be closed, and admissions to, and transfers from, this bay restricted. However, if the infected cases are distributed throughout the ward, it is more practical to close the ward than to manage multiple bay closures;
- rate of acquisition of new cases—a rapid increase in the number of new cases suggests control will be challenging without initial broad restrictions;
- staff members affected—staff will interact with patients throughout a ward and also socialize with other members of staff. Therefore, staff

involvement in outbreak may potentially result in large numbers of contacts. Defining limited areas where staff work can help;
- the nature of the ward—closure of an ICU has enormous implications for patient safety, operating lists, and pressures for the ICU in neighbouring hospitals. Therefore, the decision to close an ICU requires major planning and involvement of senior management;
- the pathogenicity of the organism—for example, any hospital-acquired cases of *Legionella* will often result in closure of that unit until water quality can be assessed and the source determined.

Patient isolation and cohorting

In outbreaks, a key challenge is to balance appropriate measures to prevent further transmission with limiting patient movement. Ideally, all infected patients and their contacts should be isolated promptly (preferably in the same ward area). This is often impractical due to the lack of side room facilities. Patients who are already symptomatic should be prioritized for isolation. It is often pragmatic for contacts sharing a similar risk of exposure to be cohorted into the same bay. In a complex outbreak, symptomatic patients may need to be cohorted into one bay, their contacts in another, and unaffected patients in another. When cohorting patients, admission to, and transfer from, their bay is restricted to reduce the risk of exposure of uninfected patients to contacts and developing (symptomatic or asymptomatic) infection. Patients should only be transferred out of that bay if they are moving to a side room or being discharged home, or if they remain asymptomatic beyond the incubation period of the infection to which they were exposed.

Contact tracing

Another key element of controlling an outbreak or a PII is identifying contacts of the infected patients. A contact is someone who has had exposure to the route of transmission of a particular infection and so potentially may be infected (e.g. all patients in a bay where a patient with norovirus has vomited). All patients who are a contact should be observed and appropriately isolated for the incubation period of the illness. If they do not manifest symptoms following the incubation period, then they are highly unlikely to be infected. As part of an outbreak/PII, it is essential to identify and appropriately isolate/cohort all contacts of the index case. Remember, staff can also be contacts if they have been exposed and not wearing appropriate PPE!

Hospital outbreaks of diarrhoea and vomiting

Most outbreaks of diarrhoea and vomiting in hospitals are caused by viruses (norovirus/small round structured virus (SRSV)/winter vomiting virus). However, remember to exclude other important causes, such as *C. difficile*, *Salmonella* spp., and *Shigella* spp., although these bacteria predominantly cause diarrhoea, rather than vomiting.

Preventing spread

In cases of viral diarrhoea, IPC precautions apply from when the diarrhoea first starts until 48h after symptoms have settled. If an alternative cause for the diarrhoea is found, enteric precautions are required for different lengths of time, so seek advice from the IPCT.

- As soon as the diarrhoea starts, move patients to single rooms, if available. Do not wait for faecal culture/PCR results to come back. Ideally, each patient with diarrhoea or vomiting should have their own toilet, commode, or bedpan. If isolation is not feasible, clean equipment after use with a detergent hypochlorite solution (1000ppm).
- Clean the bed space from which the patient has moved with a detergent hypochlorite solution (1000ppm).
- Staff and visitors should wear enteric precautions when managing patients.
- Visiting may be restricted to exceptional circumstances if a bay/ward is closed.
- Careful handwashing is vital after each contact with the patient. Use soap and water, followed by alcohol gel.
- Masks may be considered only if there is a risk of droplets or aerosol generation.
- Prompt decontamination of soiling and spillages should take place. The area should be cleaned with a neutral detergent and hot water, followed by 0.1% hypochlorite (1000ppm available chlorine).
- Some products have been developed which both clean and disinfect at the same time.
- Aerosols from vomiting are an important route of transmission in viral gastroenteritis.
- During an outbreak, clean all toilets on the ward with a disinfectant hypochlorite solution (1000ppm) at least twice a day. Pay particular attention to toilet flush handles, toilet seats, and door handles.
- Dispose of used linen as infected laundry.
- No special treatment is needed for washing crockery or cutlery.

Controlling outbreaks of infection

Outbreaks can occur readily. Liaising with your IPCT is key in coordinating outbreaks. Specific points to consider in relation to outbreaks involving diarrhoea and vomiting are given below.

Patients

- Identify all patients.
- Identify patient contacts of the index case (usually those in the same bay within 48h prior to onset of diarrhoea/vomiting).
- Notify the IPCT immediately if any contacts (or non-contacts) develop symptoms.
- Patients may need to be cohorted in bays if there is a lack of individual side rooms. Ideally, symptomatic patients and asymptomatic contacts should be cohorted separately.
- For each symptomatic patient, send one faecal sample for virology, culture, and *C. difficile* toxin.

- Involve the UKHSA regional laboratory. Patients must be asymptomatic for 48h, before they can be transferred to another healthcare setting or nursing home.
- Patient contacts who have not yet developed symptoms should not be transferred elsewhere without consulting the IPCT, as they may be incubating the infection.
- Patients may be sent home at any time, even if they still have symptoms.

Staff
- Staff should pay particular attention to handwashing.
- No food or drink should be consumed in clinical areas.
- If symptoms develop, staff should stop work immediately and inform the line manager and occupational health, as appropriate to their institution. They can return to work 48h after symptoms have settled.
- Staff must not work in any other clinical area without consulting occupational health.

Environment
- The ward should be cleaned at least twice daily with a neutral detergent and hot water, followed by disinfection with hypochlorite solution at 1000ppm available chlorine. This includes the environment around symptomatic patients, toilets/commodes/bedpans, bathrooms and showers, and sluice (especially the macerator/bedpan washer).
- Terminal cleaning/environmental decontamination is important.

Further reading

Public Health England (2012). *Norovirus: managing outbreaks in acute and community health and social care settings*. Available at: ℛ https://www.gov.uk/government/publications/norovirus-manag ing-outbreaks-in-acute-and-community-health-and-social-care-settings

Clostridioides difficile infection

C. difficile was originally defined as the cause of antibiotic-associated colitis in 1978 and continues to have a significant impact on patient morbidity and mortality. Recently, the genus was changed from *Clostridium* to *Clostridioides*. On average, patients with CDI have an increased length of stay of 21 days, with all the consequent costs. The political profile is high, with compulsory reporting of *C. difficile* rates by acute trusts. For epidemiology, clinical features, pathogenesis, diagnosis, and management of CDI, ➔ see *Clostridioides difficile* diarrhoea, pp. 698–701.

Diagnosis

In 2012, the Health Protection Agency (HPA) published the results of a large prospective observational diagnostic study to determine the best testing strategy for *C. difficile*.[24] There are three main categories of laboratory tests:
- glutamate dehydrogenase (GDH) enzyme-linked immunoassay (EIA), which detects whether the organism is present in the gut. Some

institutions may use GDH PCR or nucleic acid amplification test (NAAT), both of which are approved alternative tests;
- toxin EIA detects whether the organism is producing toxin. Toxin production is a classic feature of CDI;
- toxin gene NAAT or PCR determines whether the organism has the gene encoding the toxin and therefore has the potential to produce it.

The study found that *C. difficile* toxin EIA was not suitable as a stand-alone test for the diagnosis of CDI. A combination of tests, one of which should detect GDH (by EIA or PCR if available) and the other should be a sensitive toxin test, must be used. The results are interpreted as follows.
- If GDH EIA is positive and toxin EIA is positive (positive predictive value of 91.4%), then CDI is highly likely.
- If GDH EIA is positive and toxin EIA is negative, then *C. difficile* is present, but not producing toxin. These patients are considered to be 'excretors' or 'carriers' of the organism. Therefore, the diarrhoea may have a cause other than CDI. Many laboratories are employing a third test at this stage and use toxin gene PCR. If the toxin gene PCR is positive, then this suggests the organism has the potential to produce toxin. If the patient has worsening diarrhoea, this may suggest the organism has 'switched on' toxin production and the patient may now have CDI. However, if the toxin gene PCR is negative, then the organism has no potential to produce toxin; therefore, some laboratories will class this as an overall negative result, which will be reflected in the report.
- If GDH EIA is negative and toxin EIA is negative (negative predictive value of 98.9%), then CDI is very unlikely and this is effectively a negative result.

Other tests infrequently used include vero-cell culture for cytopathic effect and examination under fluorescent light after culture on specific agar (cefoxitin cycloserine fructose agar (CCFA) or cefoxitin cycloserine egg yolk (CCEY)).

Policies for testing samples vary; in some hospitals, tests for *C. difficile* must be specifically requested, whereas elsewhere all unformed faeces will be tested. It is usual practice not to repeat the test within 28 days, once a patient has a positive result. Previous views on the requirement of three negative results needed to exclude CDI have been largely abandoned due to improved sensitivity of current tests.

Reporting

Patients testing positive after 48h of admission (hospital onset), or within 48h but have had preceding healthcare admission within the last 28 days (community onset), are classed as healthcare-acquired and must be reported. There are targets relating to the number of cases an institution is allowed before measures are undertaken (previously including financial penalties). The number is determined by the DH, based on the previous year's total.

Typing

Various typing techniques have recently been placed in order of decreasing discriminatory ability. These are (most discriminatory first): multiple locus variable-number tandem repeat analysis (MLVA), restriction endonuclease analysis (REA), pulsed-field gel electrophoresis (PFGE), surface layer protein A gene sequence typing (slpAST), PCR ribotyping, multiple locus sequence typing (MLST), and amplified fragment length polymorphism (AFLP).[25] The commonest technique used in the UK is PCR ribotyping, which is coordinated by the *Clostridium difficile* Ribotyping Network (CDRN) Service. Further DNA fingerprinting using MLVA can be carried out to investigate clusters, to identify closely related isolates and probable transmission. Antimicrobial susceptibility testing surveillance (metronidazole and vancomycin) is performed on selected isolates.

Control of infection

CDI is transmitted by spores, which are shed in large numbers by infected patients and are capable of surviving for long periods in the environment. Enteric precautions should be followed, as outlined in ➡ Hospital outbreaks of diarrhoea and vomiting, pp. 194–6.

General guidance on CDI is contained in the document '*Clostridium difficile infection: how to deal with the problem*', published by the NHSE (see Box 6.19). There are key recommendations for providers and commissioners, aimed at reducing cases. These include use of the SIGHT protocol when managing suspected potentially infectious diarrhoea (see Box 6.20). Public Health England issued updated management and treatment guidance in 2013, emphasizing the importance of a multidisciplinary team review of all CDI patients.[26]

Box 6.19 *C. difficile:* **how to deal with the problem?**

NHSE produced evidence-based guidance (updated in 2019) on prevention and control of *C. difficile* infection, including:

- surveillance (➡ see Surveillance, pp. 177–8);
- management (➡ see *Clostridioides difficile* diarrhoea, pp. 698–701);
- AMS—prudent antibiotic prescribing, as per local policy. Minimize use of broad-spectrum agents; review prescription daily; include stop dates;
- patient isolation—always use a single room, if available; cohort patient care should be applied if a single room is not available;
- environmental cleaning and disinfection—use chlorine-based disinfectants to reduce environmental contamination with *C. difficile* spores, as per local policy. Deep-clean and decontaminate a room after a CDI patient has been discharged;
- hand hygiene—wash hands with soap and water before and after each patient contact;
- PPE—always use disposable gloves and an apron when handling body fluids and when caring for CDI-infected patients.

Box 6.20 The SIGHT protocol

To support control of *C. difficile* infection, clinicians should apply the following mnemonic protocol (SIGHT) when managing suspected potentially infectious diarrhoea:

* **S**—Suspect that a case may be infective where there is no clear alternative cause for diarrhoea;
* **I**—Isolate the patient and consult with the IPCT, while determining the cause of the diarrhoea;
* **G**—Gloves and aprons must be used for all contacts with the patient and their environment;
* **H**—Handwashing with soap and water should be carried out before and after each contact with the patient and the patient's environment;
* **T**—Test the faeces for toxin by sending a specimen immediately.

C. difficile infection

Management of the patient

NICE recommendations on antimicrobial prescribing in CDI were published in 2021 (available at: ⅋ https://www.nice.org.uk/guidance/ng199). They recommend the following:

* Review the need to continue treatment with concurrent antibiotics, proton pump inhibitors (PPIs), or drugs which impact GI activity;
* First episode (mild/moderate/severe) is PO vancomycin for 10 days. Second line if vancomycin is ineffective is fidaxomicin (➔ see Fidaxomicin, pp. 51–2) for 10 days. Third line is higher-dose vancomycin ± IV metronidazole.
* Relapse within 12 weeks should be treated with fidaxomicin (if >12 weeks, consider vancomycin instead).
* Life-threatening infection requires urgent advice, which may include surgery. Treat with 500mg vancomycin PO qds, with IV metronidazole.
* There is no benefit of adding rifampicin to metronidazole.
* Bezlotoxumab (a monoclonal antibody) is not recommended as it is not cost-effective.
* Faecal microbiota transplantation has been used successfully in relapse cases but usually require undertaking at a dedicated centre.
* Areas of research include pre- and probiotics (not currently recommended due to limitations in data availability), alternative antibiotics such as fusidic acid, nitazoxanide, teicoplanin, rifampin, rifaximin, bacitracin, cadazolid, surotomycin, ridinilazole (no superiority identified to date), IV immunoglobulin (IVIG), recolonization with non-toxogenic strains, bile acids (natural and synthetic), anion-binding resins to absorb toxins, monoclonal antibodies, hyperimmune bovine colostrum, and bacteriophage therapy.

Prevention of infection

* Contact precautions must continue until the diarrhoea resolves. Patient isolation can discontinue when they have had 48h without diarrhoea and passed formed faeces. If in doubt, seek advice from the IPCT.

Note that faecal samples may remain positive for *C. difficile* toxin for a considerable time afterwards, so microbiological clearance and repeat specimens are not required.

- *C. difficile* spores survive in the environment. Disinfect all furniture and horizontal surfaces with dilute hypochlorite solution (1000ppm). Many institutions are now using hydrogen peroxide vapour (HPV) to clean side rooms, as the coverage of the gas is much greater than physical surface cleaning. However, environmental cleaning is required prior to HPV use, and it is expensive and has practical implications (staff training, necessity of room sealing, etc.).
- When enteric precautions are discontinued, the curtains around the patient's bed must be laundered or discarded.
- Alcohol handwash does **not** reliably remove spores.
- Handwashing—by washing with soap and water, the dilutional effect of the water and friction through rubbing the hands may help to remove some of the spores. The only way to reduce transmission is to wear gloves, but overall the environment is more important in transmission.
- Probiotics/yoghurt drinks are used in some hospitals to try to prevent CDI, but firm evidence is lacking.
- *C. difficile* vaccines and anti-toxin immunoglobulins are still in research/ development stages.
- There is no evidence that giving 'pre-emptive' metronidazole or vancomycin, when a patient starts broad-spectrum antibiotics, is beneficial.

Epidemiology

The epidemiology of CDI is changing and there are large regional variations. The *C. difficile* ribotype 027, associated with excess severe disease in the 2000s, is no longer prevalent. With high all-cause mortality associated with ribotype 027, the reduction in prevalence may be associated with reductions in case fatality observed at present (see Fig. 6.5).

Further reading

National Institute for Health and Care Excellence (2021). *Clostridioides difficile infection: antimicrobial prescribing*. NICE guideline [NG199]. https://www.nice.org.uk/guidance/ng199

References

24 Department of Health and Social Care (2012). *Clostridium difficile: updated guidance on diagnosis and reporting*. Available at: ℘ https://www.gov.uk/government/publications/updated-guidance-on-the-diagnosis-and-reporting-of-clostridium-difficile

25 Killgore G, Thompson A, Johnson S, *et al*. Comparison of seven techniques for typing international epidemic strains of *Clostridium difficile*: restriction endonuclease analysis, pulsed-field gel electrophoresis, PCR-ribotyping, multilocus sequence typing, multilocus variable-number tandem-repeat analysis, amplified fragment length polymorphism, and surface layer protein A gene sequence typing. *J Clin Microbiol*. 2008;**46**:431–7.

26 Public Health England (2019). *Updated guidance on the management and treatment of Clostridium difficile infection*. Available at: ℘ https://assets.publishing.service.gov.uk/government/uploads/system/uploads/attachment_data/file/321891/Clostridium_difficile_management_and_treatment.pdf

Clostridioides difficile infection: antimicrobial prescribing

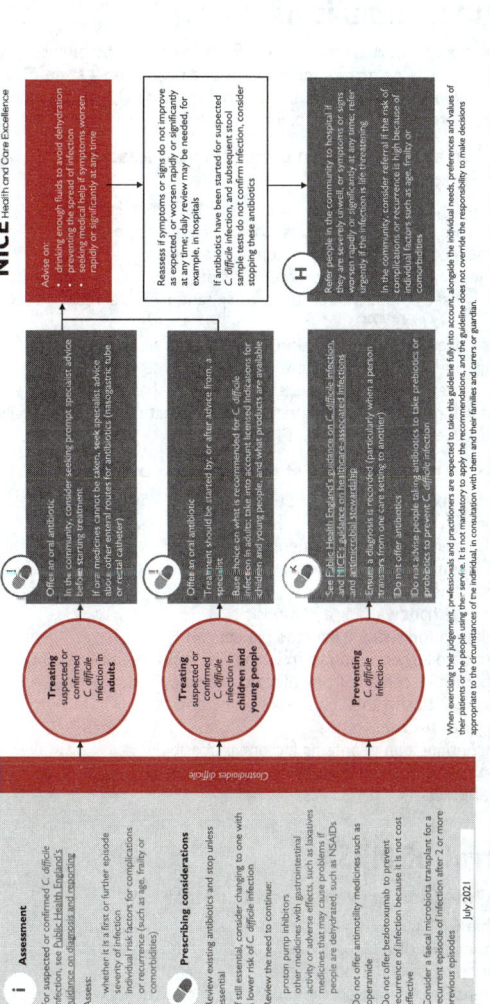

NICE National Institute for Health and Care Excellence

Assessment

For suspected or confirmed C. difficile infection, see Public Health England's guidance on diagnosis and reporting.

Assess:
- whether it is a first or further episode
- severity of infection
- individual risk factors for complications or recurrence (such as age, frailty or comorbidities)

July 2021

Prescribing considerations

Review existing antibiotics and stop unless essential.

If still essential, consider changing to one with a lower risk of C. difficile infection.

Review the need to continue:
- proton pump inhibitors
- other medicines with gastrointestinal activity or adverse effects, such as laxatives
- medicines that may cause problems if people are dehydrated, such as NSAIDs

Do not offer antimotility medicines such as loperamide.

Do not offer bezlotoxumab to prevent recurrence of infection because it is not cost effective.

Consider a faecal microbiota transplant for a recurrent episode of infection after 2 or more previous episodes.

Treating suspected or confirmed C. difficile infection in adults

Offer an oral antibiotic.

In the community, consider seeking prompt specialist advice before starting treatment.

If oral medicines cannot be taken, seek specialist advice about other enteral routes for antibiotics (nasogastric tube or rectal catheter).

Treating suspected or confirmed C. difficile infection in children and young people

Offer an oral antibiotic.

Treatment should be started by, or after advice from, a specialist.

Base choice on what is recommended for C. difficile infection in adults; take into account licensed indications for children and young people, and what products are available.

Preventing C. difficile infection

See Public Health England's guidance on C. difficile infection and NICE's guidance on healthcare-associated infections and antimicrobial stewardship.

Ensure a diagnosis is recorded (particularly when a person transfers from one care setting to another).

Do not offer antibiotics.

Do not advise people taking antibiotics to take prebiotics or probiotics to prevent C. difficile infection.

Advice on:
- drinking enough fluids to avoid dehydration
- preventing the spread of infection
- seeking medical help if symptoms worsen rapidly or significantly at any time

Reassess if symptoms or signs do not improve as expected, or worsen rapidly or significantly at any time; daily review may be needed, for example, in hospitals.

If antibiotics have been started for suspected C. difficile infection, and subsequent stool sample tests do not confirm infection, consider stopping these antibiotics.

H

Refer people in the community to hospital if they are severely unwell, or if symptoms or signs worsen rapidly or significantly at any time; refer urgently if the infection is life threatening.

In the community, consider referral if the risk of complications or recurrence is high because of individual factors such as age, frailty or comorbidities.

When exercising their judgement, professionals and practitioners are expected to take this guideline fully into account, alongside the individual needs, preferences and values of their patients or the people using their service. It is not mandatory to apply the recommendations, and the guideline does not override the responsibility to make decisions appropriate to the circumstances of the individual, in consultation with them and their families and carers or guardian.

Fig. 6.5 Summary algorithm for antimicrobial prescribing in the first case of *Clostridioides difficile* infection (National Institute for Health and Care Excellence).
Reprinted from *Clostridioides difficile* infection: antimicrobial prescribing NICE guideline [NG199] Published: 23 July 2021 ℗ https://www.nice.org.uk/guidance/ng199/resources/visual-summary-pdf-9194639149.

Principles of managing multidrug-resistant organisms

In this section, the management of MDR organisms will be discussed at the population level. For management of specific organisms → see Meticillin-resistant *Staphylococcus aureus*, pp. 261–4 and → carbapenemase-producing enterobacteriaceae, p. 43.

Detection and prevention of multidrug-resistant organism spread

The main steps in preventing outbreaks of MDR organisms are:
- risk factors for MDR organisms (travel, hospital exposure);
- screening of patients for asymptomatic carriage;
- IPC measures to control potential spread;
- AMS (→ see Antimicrobial stewardship/antimicrobial resistance, pp. 6–8, 34, 177, 274);
- surveillance of invasive infection and new acquisition to monitor trends, identify outbreaks, and facilitate key performance indicators;
- communication—record results in hospital databases for further hospital admissions and update the general practitioner (GP) usually via discharge letters.

Control of multidrug-resistant organism outbreaks

The main steps in controlling an outbreak of MDR organisms are:
- identifying reservoirs:
  - colonized and infected patients;
  - environmental contamination (fomites, water).
- halting transmission:
  - improve handwashing and asepsis;
  - isolate colonized and infected patients;
  - eliminate any common source, and disinfect the environment;
  - separate susceptible from infected and colonized patients;
  - consider closing the unit to new admissions.
- modifying host risk:
  - discontinue compromising factors, if possible;
  - control antibiotic use (consider rotation, restriction, or discontinuing antibiotics).

Control of MRSA

MRSA infection prevention and control

(See Table 6.11.)
The principles of IPC for reducing spread of MRSA include:
- attention to careful hand hygiene
- adherence to contact precautions for care of patients with known MRSA infection
- surveillance
- effective environmental cleaning
- Antimicrobial stewardship
- screening and suppression.

Table 6.11 UK guidelines for management of MRSA

Publication	Reference	Notes
Implementation of modified admission MRSA screening guidance for NHS (2014)	Department of Health Expert Advisory Committee on Antimicrobial Resistance and Healthcare Associated Infection (2014)	Outlining a more focused 'cost-effective' MRSA screening policy, reflecting the overall decline in MRSA
UK standards for microbiology investigations: investigation of specimens for screening for MRSA	Public Health England (2014)	Reliable detection of MRSA colonization
Guidelines for the control and prevention of meticillin-resistant *Staphylococcus aureus* (MRSA) in healthcare facilities	Coia JE, Duckworth GJ, Edwards DI, *et al. J Hosp Infect.* 2006;**63** Suppl 1:S1–44	Infection control guidance and strategies for preventing spread of MRSA or infection with MRSA

MRSA screening and suppression

This consists of performing screening cultures (usually the nares, oropharynx, and/or perineum) to identify asymptomatic colonized patients, with the goal of intervening with suppressive therapy to minimize the likelihood of spread to other patients and staff.

Screening

In 2009/10, the UK Department of Health introduced mandatory MRSA screening of all elective and emergency hospital admissions, with the aim of preventing MRSA infections. It was subsequently noted that settings without universal screening (e.g. Wales) also saw marked falls in MRSA infection, and the NOW study was commissioned.[27] This demonstrated poor compliance with screening and big falls in MRSA prevalence (often <1%) that meant compliance was unlikely to be cost-effective. Cost-effectiveness increases with increasing prevalence. At current prevalence levels, it is considered cost-effective to screen only high-risk specialties. It is common practice to screen:

- all elective admission pre-admission;
- all emergency admissions at the time of admission;
- all patients in high-risk areas on a regular basis, including critical care units, neonates, haematology, oncology, and dialysis outpatients. Daycase surgery/procedures and paediatrics are not usually screened.

Suppression

Also referred to as decolonization (see Box 6.21). The optimal regimen and duration of decolonization are uncertain (see Box 6.22). The best-studied regimen consists of 4% rinse-off chlorhexidine for daily bathing or showering, 0.12% chlorhexidine mouthwash bd, and 2% nasal mupirocin bd, all administered for 5 days twice per month for 6 months.[28]

Box 6.21 MRSA suppression versus decolonization

Opinions differ on whether to use the terms 'MRSA suppression' or 'MRSA decolonization'. They are often used interchangeably. Suppression suggests decreasing the bacterial load, whereas decolonization suggests eradication of carriage.

Box 6.22 MRSA suppression of nasal/ extranasal colonization

- Likely to be beneficial:
  - mupirocin nasal ointment.
- Unknown effectiveness:
  - antiseptic body washes;
  - chlorhexidine–neomycin nasal cream;
  - mupirocin nasal ointment for 5 days (compared with >5 days);
  - systemic antimicrobials.
- Unlikely to be beneficial:
  - tea tree preparations.

Further reading

Department of Health and Social Care (2014). *Who to screen for MRSA?* Available at: ℘ https://www.gov.uk/government/publications/how-to-approach-mrsa-screening

Gemmell CG, Edwards DI, Fraise AP. Guidelines for the prophylaxis and treatment of methicillin-resistant *Staphylococcus aureus* (MRSA) infections in the UK. *J Antimicrob Chemother.* 2006;**57**:589–608.

References

27 Fuller C, Robotham J, Savage J, *et al.* The national one week prevalence audit of universal meticillin-resistant *Staphylococcus aureus* (MRSA) admission screening 2012. *PLoS One.* 2013;**8**:e74219.

28 Huang SS, Singh R, McKinnell JA, *et al.* Decolonization to reduce postdischarge infection risk among MRSA carriers. *N Engl J Med.* 2019;**380**:638.

Control of carbapenemase-producing organisms

The UK has seen a rapid increase in the incidence of infection and colonization by organisms resistant to carbapenems such as *Enterobacterales*, *Pseudomonas*, and *Acinetobacter*. Carbapenemases are enzymes that destroy carbapenem antibiotics, conferring resistance. There are different types of carbapenemases, of which KPC, OXA-48, NDM, and VIM are the commonest in the UK (➲ see Section X, p. 44). While some Gram-negative bacteria possess intrinsic carbapenem resistance, acquired carbapenemases are particularly concerning as they are usually located on mobile genetic elements (plasmids) and can be transferred vertically (within a strain) or horizontally (between strains, species, and genera). Organisms expressing these resistance mechanisms are extremely difficult to treat.

Enterobacterales

Major risk factors for CPE carriage include in the last 12 months:
- previous colonization or infection with CPE;
- being an inpatient in any hospital, in the UK or abroad;
- having multiple hospital treatments (e.g. dialysis-dependent);
- had known epidemiological link to a known carrier of CPE.

Patients who fall into an at-risk group must be isolated immediately and screened, with strict adherence to standard IPC precautions.

In 2020, Public Health England published '*Framework of actions to contain CPE*',[29] an update of their CPE toolkit. The key to controlling the spread is early detection and prompt isolation. The framework sets out eight areas of evidence-based recommendations.

Screening

Patient screening should be based on local prevalence in specific populations or on risk factors. Do not wait for screening results before isolating a patient. Screening is done using a rectal swab, and for an effective screen, faeces must be visible on the swab. Contacts should only be screened when the index case is confirmed.

Rescreening

There are limited data relating to how long humans remain colonized with CPE. Therefore, how long to consider a patient is colonized and when to rescreen are matters for debate. All institutions should produce their own infection control guidance relating to the management of patients colonized with CPE.

Surveillance

Surveillance systems are needed to rapidly detect and monitor patients colonized or infected with CPE and acquisition in healthcare settings.

IPC precautions

Isolate the patient in a side room, ideally with en-suite facilities. Standard IPC precautions must be strictly adhered to. Risk assessment is required for the need to use contact precautions.

Antimicrobial stewardship

Antimicrobial usage and audit data should be reviewed at regular intervals by local AMS committees. Specific actions should be taken where there are early signals of increasing AMR or antimicrobial consumption trends, particularly broad-spectrum agents including carbapenems. There is no evidence for skin or gut decolonization.[30]

Cleaning and decontamination

Enhanced cleaning of the environment must take place during the patient's stay, including high-touch surfaces. Following discharge, the isolation room must be deep-cleaned. Some institutions include adjunctive hydrogen peroxide cleaning after enhanced cleaning.

Outbreaks and clusters

(➔ see Management of outbreaks, pp. 191–4.)

Prompt response following detection of CPE in healthcare settings is required to minimize onwards transmission. Environmental samples should only be taken when epidemiologically indicated.

Organizational responsibilities

Organizational leadership should support the IPC programme by providing organizational and administrative support.

What about multidrug-resistant *Pseudomonas* and *Acinetobacter*?

Compared to CPE, carbapenem-resistant *Pseudomonas* spp. and *Acinetobacter* spp. differ in epidemiology, microbiology, transmission, and environmental persistence. Some CPE interventions may be common. In 2017, the WHO produced detailed guidance on IPC of these organisms in healthcare settings.[31]

References

29 UKHSA Framework of actions to contain carbapenemase-producing *Enterobacterales*. Available at: ℘ https://www.gov.uk/government/publications/actions-to-contain-carbapenemase-producing-enterobacterales-cpe

30 Tacconelli E, Mazzaferri F, de Smet AM, *et al.* ESCMID-EUCIC clinical guidelines on decolonization of multidrug-resistant Gram-negative bacteria carriers. *Clin Microbiol Infect.* 2019;**25**:807–17.

31 World Health Organization (2017). *Guidelines for the prevention and control of carbapenem-resistant Enterobacteriaceae, Acinetobacter baumannii and Pseudomonas aeruginosa in health care facilities.* Available at: ℘ https://apps.who.int/iris/bitstream/handle/10665/259462/978924 1550178-eng.pdf;jsessionid=D086CBA35BEEC6590A5CB0B52988238D?sequence=1

Control of tuberculosis in hospitals

While most TB infections are acquired in the community, healthcare-associated TB can occur in patients and staff. Most healthcare-acquired TB cases result from delayed diagnosis of TB, inadequate treatment of latent TB, or lack of appropriate isolation. Understanding the routes of TB transmission is fundamental to preventing the spread of infection. Person-to-person transmission of TB occurs via inhalation of droplet nuclei (airborne particles, 1–5 micrometres in diameter). Coughing and singing facilitate formation of droplet nuclei. An important distinction to make in the risk assessment of a patient suspected of having TB is their risk of infectiousness to others (see Box 6.23):

- **pulmonary TB**—refers to those with primary lung infection. Patients not on treatment who have 'smear-positive' sputum (i.e. sputum microscopy has detected acid-fast bacilli (AFB)) are at increased risk of transmitting TB and must be isolated. They are frequently referred to as having 'open-pulmonary' TB.
- **non-pulmonary TB**—refers to infection at any site other than the lung. Non-pulmonary TB has a low risk of transmission, and patients can be nursed in the open bay. However, if they have a procedure that may aerosolize the organism (see Box 6.24), then they must be isolated during the procedure and appropriate respiratory precautions must be used. Immunocompromised patients with extrapulmonary TB should be presumed to have pulmonary TB until proven otherwise.

Box 6.23 Factors associated with risk of TB transmission

- Presence of active untreated pulmonary or laryngeal TB
- Presence of cavitary disease
- Presence of sputum with positive nucleic acid amplification test (NAAT) result for *Mycobacterium tuberculosis* (MTB) complex
- Presence of sputum with positive smear for acid-fast bacilli (AFB)
- Presence of sputum with positive MTB culture (even if the sputum is AFB smear-negative)
- Short time (<9 days) to positive MTB culture

Box 6.24 Procedures associated with increased risk of TB transmission in healthcare settings

- Endotracheal intubation
- Bronchoscopy
- Sputum induction
- Chest physiotherapy
- Administration of aerosolized drugs
- Irrigation of a tuberculous abscess
- Post-mortem on a cadaver with untreated TB disease

Transmission of tuberculosis

From patients

Successful control and prevention of TB in hospitals are achieved through three main approaches:[32]

- airborne PPE – in the UK, FFP3 masks are only specifically recommended by NICE for patients with suspected/known MDR-TB and extensively drug-resistant (XDR)-TB or for aerosol generating procedures (e.g. bronchoscopy). All masks must be fit-tested. For further information, see NICE clinical guidelines (2011; available at: ✆ https://www.nice.org.uk/guidance/ng33/chapter/Recommendations#infection-control);
- early investigation and diagnosis of those suspected to have TB—all patients suspected of having pulmonary TB must be isolated promptly, while appropriate investigations are carried out. Contact tracing should be initiated as soon as possible to identify secondary cases of active and latent TB;
- patient isolation and the extent of IPC precautions—are dependent on whether the patient is at risk of MDR- or XDR-TB. Risk factors include: history of prior treatment or treatment failure, known contact, birth in a country with a high incidence of TB, HIV co-infection, residence in London, ♂, age 25–44 years. All patients suspected of having TB must be risk-assessed and isolated appropriately for MDR-/XDR-TB, pending culture results:
- High-risk patients must be isolated in a negative-pressure side room throughout their admission. All contacts with the patient must involve

airborne precautions with using an FFP3 respirator, regardless of whether they are of an aerosol-generating nature or not. Smear-positive material can be rapidly assessed for rifampicin resistance genes by PCR to aid in the diagnosis.
- Low-risk patients can be nursed in a standard side room under normal atmospheric pressure. Respiratory precautions only to be used during aerosol-generating procedures. Following 2 weeks of appropriate treatment, the patient is considered low risk of transmission and can be moved out of isolation. However, despite low risk of infectivity, they must not be moved into the same bay as an immunocompromised patient (e.g. HIV, oncology patient).

From healthcare workers

When a HCW develops TB, this may lead to expensive, time-consuming, large-scale contact investigations to determine the extent of transmission and prevent further spread. The incidence of acute and latent TB is higher amongst foreign-born HCWs. Difficulties arise in the interpretation of tuberculin skin tests (TSTs) in this group. Management of HCWs with TB is usually shared by occupational health, IPC, and clinical teams. For advice on screening all new NHS employees who will have contact with patients or their samples, see NICE clinical guidelines (2020; available at: ℘ https://www.nice.org.uk/guidance/ng33/).

Further reading

National Institute for Health and Care Excellence (2016, updated 2019). *Tuberculosis*. Available at: ℘ https://www.nice.org.uk/guidance/ng33/chapter/Recommendations#drug-resistant-tb

References

32 Humphreys H. Control and prevention of healthcare-associated tuberculosis: the role of respiratory isolation and personal respiratory protection. *J Hosp Infect*. 2008;**69**:91–2.

Control of transmissible spongiform encephalopathies, including Creutzfeldt–Jakob disease

Transmissible spongiform encephalopathies (TSEs) include Creutzfeldt–Jakob disease (CJD), which may be sporadic, familial, iatrogenic, or variant CJD (vCJD), variably protease-sensitive prionopathy, and Gerstmann–Sträussler–Scheinker (GSS) syndrome (⊕ see Gerstmann–Sträussler–Scheinker syndrome, p. 505). The prion proteins associated with TSEs are unusually resistant to inactivation by heat and chemicals, requiring specific decontamination procedures. Cases of iatrogenic CJD have been transmitted by contaminated pituitary-derived hormones, dura mater grafts, neurosurgical instruments, corneal transplantation, organ transplantation, and blood transfusion. Current challenges faced are early detection and diagnosis of vCJD, therapy and support for those affected, and understanding of transmission risks.

Variant CJD and new variant CJD

vCJD was first reported in the UK in 1996 and subsequently linked to bovine spongiform encephalopathy (BSE). It has a distinct clinical presentation

(➋ see Creutzfeldt–Jakob disease (CJD) and variant CJD, pp. 208–11, 505–6), tending to affect a younger age group than classical CJD. Following the decline of BSE and the introduction of dietary protective measures, vCJD has become extremely rare, but the total number of predicted cases is a topic of debate. In vCJD, prion proteins have been detected in systemic lymphoid tissue before the patient is symptomatic, and the infectious agents are more resistant to inactivation than previously observed. Therefore, the greatest risk of cross-infection comes from potential contamination and subsequent failure to remove the prions from clinical equipment. Thus, there are widespread consequences in IPC procedures such as traceability of endoscopes and quarantining of surgical instruments. Quarantining of equipment can have significant financial implications for the hospital.

Risk assessments

All patients admitted for surgery should have a risk assessment performed. The IPC measures are dependent on the risk status of the patient and the nature of the surgery. Patients at increased risk of CJD or vCJD include:

• those who are symptomatic with a neurological condition that is consistent with CJD;
• individuals who have had one or more blood relatives affected by CJD or who have been shown by genetic testing to be at risk;
• those who have received blood products, organs, or tissues from someone who developed vCJD, or who have donated blood and the recipient subsequently developed CJD;
• those who received hormones derived from human pituitary tissue;
• those who have received >300 blood products since 1990.

Patients who fall into one or more of these groups are at risk. The risk of the surgery should then be stratified. This is effectively dependent on whether the surgery involves at-risk tissue (see Box 6.25).

Classification of risk and outcomes

If the patient is considered to be at risk and the surgery involves medium- to high-risk tissue, the options are:
• quarantining the equipment for reuse exclusively in the same patient;
• using single-use equipment;
• destroying the equipment.

If the surgery involves an at-risk patient and low-risk tissue, then no special equipment processing is required.

Box 6.25 Tissue infectivity risk of CJD/vCJD

• **High-risk tissues** (all types of CJD)—brain, spinal cord, cranial nerves, cranial ganglia, posterior eye, pituitary gland.
• **Medium-risk tissues** (all CJD types other than vCJD)—spinal ganglia, olfactory epithelium.
  • For vCJD, the following tissues are medium risk: tonsil, appendix, spleen, thymus, adrenal gland, lymph nodes, and gut-associated lymphoid tissue.
• **Low-risk tissues**—any not mentioned above.

Prevention of transmission of CJD

Always consult your institution's CJD policy, and involve the IPCT. Some general principles are advised for the processing of instruments (see Box 6.26) and in blood transfusion (see Box 6.27), in order to minimize transmission of CJD. Guidance for care of symptomatic or at-risk patients is detailed in Box 6.28. There have been five cases of blood transfusion-associated CJD in the UK. The blood products were all donated when the donor was in the preclinical stage of the disease, and none were leucodepleted. There is no evidence of any UK clinical case of vCJD being linked to a blood transfusion given after 1999. All clinical specimens from known, suspected, or at-risk patients should be handled at CL3 in the microbiology laboratory, as the agent of CJD is in hazard group 3.

Box 6.26 Precautions regarding processing of instruments exposed to low-risk tissue to minimize transmission of CJD

- Staff should practise standard IPC precautions.
- Clean all surgical instruments to remove organic matter before sterilization.
- Consider using single-use instruments, whenever possible. Never reprocess single-use kits—throw them away immediately. Use single-use kits for all lumbar punctures.
- High-vacuum, porous-load autoclaving at 134–137°C for 18min for six cycles can reduce infectivity.
- The following methods are ineffective for prions: autoclaving at 134°C for 3min, alcohol, ethylene oxide, glutaraldehyde, and formalin.
- Record the unique identification number of all flexible endoscopes every time they are used, and ensure all instruments are traceable through the audit trail.
- Research in mice has suggested that dental tissue may be infective; thus, instruments used for root canal work should be single-use.

Box 6.27 Precautions regarding blood transfusion to minimize transmission of CJD

- Blood donors who have themselves received a blood transfusion or tissue donation are now excluded (2005).
- Leucodeplete all blood donations—this will reduce infectivity but will not eliminate it.
- Plasma for use in those aged <16 years is purchased from outside the UK.
- Note that screening tests are being developed to detect the prion protein in blood products, but none are currently in use.

Box 6.28 Care of symptomatic or at-risk patients

All patients should be subject to standard IPC precautions. There is no evidence to suggest CJD is spread from person to person by close contact. Patients known to have CJD do not require special nursing precautions or special precautions for management of sharps injuries, exposure to blood and body fluids, used and infected linen, and disposal of clinical waste. However, particular care must be taken to adhere to institution policy for the following:

- collection, labelling, and transport of clinical specimens—use 'Danger of Infection' stickers, and provide adequate clinical information for laboratory staff to undertake a risk assessment;
- CNS and lymphoid tissue biopsies—these procedures should be performed by experienced staff using disposable equipment. Gloves, goggles, and aprons should be worn, and any contaminated objects should be incinerated.

Further reading

Advisory Committee on Dangerous Pathogens Spongiform Encephalopathy Advisory Committee (2015). *Transmissible spongiform encephalopathy agents: safe working and the prevention of infection.* Available at: ℘ https://www.gov.uk/government/uploads/system/uploads/attachment_data/file/260961/report.pdf

Public Health England (2003, updated 2015). *Infection prevention and control of CJD and variant CJD in healthcare and community settings.* Available at: ℘ https://www.gov.uk/government/uploads/system/uploads/attachment_data/file/427854/Infection_controlv3.0.pdf

Management of risk to healthcare workers

Staff management requires close liaison with members of the occupational health team.

IPC practices are in place to reduce the risk of HCWs acquiring infections from their patients. However, HCWs (including laboratory staff) do become infected at work, with organisms ranging from the relatively benign infectious diarrhoea to life-threatening conditions. Infection control procedures for patients infected with HIV, HBV, or HCV may be considered together because routes of acquisition are similar. The main risk of transmission is from accidental inoculation of blood (➔ see Management of risk: sharps injuries, pp. 213–17). While challenges remain in identifying all carriers of BBVs, standard infection control precautions and barrier nursing are required for all patients.

Blood-borne viruses

For transmission of HIV and HBV, the following from patients with BBVs are potentially infectious: blood, CSF, peritoneal fluid, pleural fluid, pericardial fluid, synovial fluid, amniotic fluid, breast milk, semen, vaginal secretions, and saliva in the context of dentistry. The following are **not** regarded as infectious, unless visibly contaminated with blood: faeces, nasal secretions, saliva (except in dentistry), sputum, sweat, tears, urine, and vomit.

The risk of HCV transmission to HCWs from occupational contact with blood or with body fluids containing blood is thought to be around 0.3%.

Care of patients with HIV or hepatitis B or C

Patients known to be positive for these viruses (or likely to be positive as a result of certain risk factors) should have a risk assessment performed. This should include the likelihood of exposure of staff or other patients to the patient's body fluids, and whether that body fluid is likely to be infectious. The risk assessment should fully respect patient confidentiality. Medical and nursing care of infected patients depends on local hospital policy, but here are a few practical suggestions:

- single-room isolation—is only usually required if uncontrolled bleeding or loss of other body fluids is likely, or if the patient has another condition requiring isolation (e.g. diarrhoea, open pulmonary TB, salmonellosis, herpes zoster). On vacation of the room, terminal cleaning is necessary if contamination with blood or body fluids has occurred;
- HBV/HCV-positive patients—should not be nursed in close proximity to patients who require haemodialysis/haemofiltration.;
- disposal of sharps—if the patient needs single-room isolation, sharps must be disposed of in a sharps bin inside the room;
- spills—any spills of blood/body fluids should be covered immediately with chlorine-releasing granules or hypochlorite (10 000ppm available chlorine);
- equipment disinfection and sterilization—use single-use/disposable items, whenever possible;
- PPE—depends on the likelihood and degree of exposure to the patient's blood and body fluids. Apron and gloves must be worn when dealing with blood or bloodstained body fluids. Masks and eye protection are required wherever there is a possibility of aerosolization/splashing;
- linen from patients in isolation or contaminated with blood or body fluids should be regarded as 'infected linen' (➔ see Laundry, p. 226);
- toilet/bathroom facilities—patients may use ward facilities, except if there is bleeding (or risk of bleeding) in which case toilet/bathroom facilities must be reserved for this patient only (or use of a commode);
- crockery—standard cleaning methods are adequate, and disposable crockery is rarely required. If there is excessive bleeding from the mouth, the patient can retain their own crockery and cutlery, which they or the nursing staff wash up;
- waste—clinical waste and disposable items must be placed in yellow bags (➔ see Waste, pp. 227–8), with double-bagging if leakage of body fluids is possible.

Other infections

Other infections can be transmitted to HCWs, but the following are recognized more frequently or have more significant consequences:
- viral gastroenteritis;

- *Neisseria meningitidis*—HCWs who intubate the patient or perform mouth-to-mouth resuscitation;
- MTB;
- VZV;
- respiratory pathogens, including influenza, severe acute respiratory syndrome (SARS), and SARS-CoV-2;
- others, including pertussis, diphtheria, rabies, and VHFs.

Further reading

Health and Safety Executive. *Sharps injuries*. Available at: ℜ https://www.hse.gov.uk/healthservices/needlesticks/

Health and Safety Executive. *Risk to healthcare workers*. Available at: ℜ https://www.hse.gov.uk/biosafety/blood-borne-viruses/risk-healthcare-workers.htm

Management of risk: sharps injuries

The main infectious risks associated with needlestick and other sharps injuries are transmission of BBVs. With significant inoculation of blood through a hollow-bore needle, the rates of transmission to the recipient are:

- up to 30% if the donor is HBsAg-positive (the risk ranges from 30% if the patient is HBeAg-positive to 3% if HBeAb-positive);
- ~3% if the donor is hepatitis C antibody-positive;
- ~0.3% if the donor is HIV-positive (the risk will vary, depending on the level of detectable viral load).

There is also the risk of emerging or unknown agents.

Prevention of sharps injuries

Good clinical practice is essential in preventing needlestick injuries, such as:

- safe handling and disposing of needles and other sharps;
- never resheathing needles;
- using a sharps bins as indicated.

Action in the event of sharps injury

- Immediate first aid—encourage bleeding of the area; wash with soap under running water, and cover with waterproof dressing. If eye splash, irrigate well with running water. If splash into the mouth, do not swallow, and rinse out the mouth several times with cold water.
- Report the incident to the senior person in that area. Complete an incident form.
- Management will require involvement from occupational health and infection clinicians (e.g. microbiology/infectious diseases (ID)).
- Risk assessment—consider the hazard (potential to cause harm) and risk (likelihood that harm will occur), based on the injury, the source, and the recipient (see Box 6.29).

Management of a 'needlestick' injury

(See Table 6.12.)

- Always involve occupational health and infection specialists (microbiology or ID) immediately. They will support the risk assessment of severity of the injury.

Box 6.29 Risk assessment

Consider the injury, the source, and the recipient.
- Injury:
  - extent and depth of injury;
  - size and type of needle;
  - visible contamination with blood;
  - site.
- Source (usually the patient undergoing the procedure, but this may be unknown):
  - hepatitis B and C, HIV status (if known);
  - viral load/stage of illness if HIV-positive.
- Recipient:
  - hepatitis B vaccine status/antibody level;
  - any conditions that may affect treatment (e.g. pregnancy).

Table 6.12 Summary flow chart for needlestick injury

- Check basic first aid has been performed.
- Discuss with occupational health/infectious diseases/microbiology.
- Risk assessment to determine significance of injury.

Was there a significant injury?
- Deep and penetrating injury.
- Visibly bloodstained device.
- Needle involved has been in the source patient's artery or vein.

No	Yes
• Occupational health referral for routine assessment • Recipient sample for LTS and anti-HBs if unknown • Encourage HBV vaccination if not done	• Recipient sample for long-term storage (LTS) and anti-HBs if unknown • Request source sample for urgent testing for HIV, HBsAg, and HCV, LTS • Unknown source: gather as much information as possible to make a risk assessment
	Further risk assessment: • Known or highly likely to be HIV +ve—URGENT: infection expert will consider PEP • Known or highly likely to be HBV +ve—URGENT: infection expert will consider HBIG and accelerated vaccine/booster, depending on the recipient's anti-HB status/vaccine history • Known or highly likely to be HCV +ve—no immediate intervention. Infection expert will check HCV RNA in source if known anti-HCV +ve donor. Follow up recipient at 6 and 12 weeks (PCR), and at 12 and 24 weeks (anti-HCV)

- If this is a significant injury, then a member of the team looking after the donor (but not the recipient of the injury) should explain the event to the donor and request consent to test for HIV, HBsAg, and HCV antibody. For management of sharps injury from an infected donor, see Table 6.13.
- The source patient may decline to be tested, and this will not affect their medical care.
- Provide patient information leaflets, as appropriate.
- General Medical Council (GMC) guidance offers advice on difficult situations (e.g. if there is conflict between the needs of the recipient and the wishes of the source, or if the source patient is unconscious or has died). Decisions about testing an incapacitated patient must take account of the current legal framework governing capacity issues and the use of human tissue. Consult local occupational health services and infection experts. Currently, blood should not be tested for BBVs from an unconscious patient if it is not in the medical interests of that patient.
- If the injury was significant, then blood will be taken from the recipient for storage. The hepatitis B vaccination history of the recipient should be taken, and a course of vaccination or a booster dose considered, as appropriate. With a high-risk patient, HIV PEP and/or hepatitis B immunoglobulin (HBIG) may be considered. Management of exposure to hepatitis B is discussed in Table 6.14.

Reporting

All injuries should be reported to the senior on duty and recorded on an incident form/accident book. If the injury was with a used needle or instrument, advice should be sought from infection experts/occupational health. A review of equipment/procedures should occur, led by a senior member of the department.

Table 6.13 Management of sharps injury from an infected patient

Patient known positive or likely positive	Action
HIV	**URGENT**. Discuss with an infection expert who will consider PEP. The risks associated with PEP versus the risk of acquiring HIV will be explained to the recipient. PEP usually consists of a 3-day starter pack of antiviral therapy, with plans for ongoing counselling/treatment, depending on results.
HBV	**URGENT**. Discuss with an infection expert who will consider HBIG and accelerated vaccination or booster(s), as shown in Table 6.14.
HCV	No immediate intervention. If donor anti-HCV-positive, they will be tested for HCV RNA to determine whether they are viraemic (greater risk)—HCV RNA tested in the recipient by PCR at 6 and 12 weeks, and anti-HCV tested at 12 and 24 weeks. If signs of infection in the recipient, the test will be confirmed, and the patient will be referred for specialist assessment as soon as possible

Table 6.14 Management of significant exposure to HBV

In addition to percutaneous inoculation (needlestick, scratch, bite, etc.), this may result from contamination of mucous membranes (e.g. spillage into the eyes or mouth) or contamination of non-intact skin (open wounds, dermatitis, eczema). For management of HBV exposure, see UK Health Security Agency (2013). *Hepatitis B: the green book, chapter 18* (available at: ⚹ https://www.gov.uk/government/publications/hepatitis-b-the-green-book-chapter-18). **Below is a summary table of HBV prophylaxis for reporting exposure incidents.**

HBV status of person prior to exposure	Significant exposure			Non-significant exposure	
	HBsAg-positive source	Unknown source	HBsAg-negative source	Continued risk	No further risk
Unvaccinated	Accelerated course of HepB vaccine plus HBIG with first dose	Accelerated course of HepB vaccine	Consider course of HepB vaccine	Initiate course of HepB vaccine	No HBV prophylaxis. Reassure
Partially vaccinated	One dose of HepB vaccine and finish the course	One dose of HepB vaccine and finish the course	Complete course of HepB vaccine	Complete course of HepB vaccine	Complete course of HepB vaccine
Fully vaccinated with HepB primary course	Booster dose of HepB vaccine if last dose ≥1 year ago	Consider booster dose of HepB vaccine if last dose ≥1 year ago	No HBV prophylaxis. Reassure	No HBV prophylaxis. Reassure	No HBV prophylaxis. Reassure
Known non-responder to HepB vaccine (anti-HBs <10mIU/ mL 10-2 months post-immunization)	HBIG Booster dose of HepB vaccine A second dose of HBIG should be given at one month	HBIG Consider booster dose of HepB vaccine A second dose of HBIG should be given at one month	No HBIG Consider booster dose of HepB vaccine	No HBIG Consider booster dose of HepB vaccine	No HBIG Reassure

Reproduced from *Hepatitis B: the green book*, chapter 18 under the Open Government Licence v3.0.

Health and safety law applies to risks from sharps injuries, just as it does to other risks from work activities. Relevant legislation includes:
- Health and Safety at Work etc. Act 1974;
- COSHH 2002;
- Management of Health and Safety Regulations 1999;
- Reporting of Injuries, Diseases, and Dangerous Occurrences Regulations (RIDDOR) 1995.

Management of risk from healthcare workers infected with blood-borne viruses

Staff infected with BBVs are usually managed by the occupational health department. Please note that up-to-date guidance from the UKHSA should be consulted (available at: ℘ https://www.gov.uk/government/publications/bbvs-in-healthcare-workers-health-clearance-and-management).   The information provided in this section is a guide.

Hepatitis B-infected healthcare workers
- For HCWs who will perform exposure-prone procedures (EPPs)/work in an exposure-prone environment or perform clinical duties in renal units:
  - New HCWs who are HBsAg-positive must have their current viral load established; those with HBV DNA >200IU/L require restriction from procedures where there is a risk that injury to themselves will result in their blood contaminating a patient's open tissues (i.e. they should not perform EPPs).
  - HCWs living with HBV with DNA <200IU/L (either natural suppression or 12 months after stopping treatment) require annual DNA testing.
  - Those HCWs on continuous antiviral therapy with DNA <200IU/L should have their DNA viral load tested every 12 weeks.
  - If viral load ≥200IU/L, HCWs should cease EPPs immediately, pending repeat test and further management.
  - HBeAg is no longer included in the assessment of HBV-infected HCWs.

Hepatitis C-infected healthcare workers
- For HCWs who will perform EPPs/work in an exposure-prone environment:
  - All HCWs who are HCV RNA-positive should be restricted from carrying out EPPs and referred for consideration of antiviral treatment.
  - Test HCV RNA 3 months after stopping treatment. If detected, then ongoing restriction from EPPs continues. If RNA is undetected, the HCW can return to perform EPPs, with 3-monthly RNA tests.

HIV-infected healthcare workers
The risk of a HCW infecting a patient during an EPP is very low. Worldwide, there are very few reported cases of transmission from HCWs to patients.

These transmissions occurred during high-risk procedures and the HCWs were not on therapy.

Current guidance recommends:

- all HCWs who undertake EPPs should be tested for HIV antibody;
- HIV-infected HCWs can perform EPPs if they are on effective antiretroviral therapy (ART) and have a plasma viral load of <200 copies/mL on serial tests taken at least 12 weeks apart;
- HIV-infected HCWs (including elite controllers) undertaking EPPs must have their plasma viral load monitored every 12 weeks, be jointly managed by a physician and occupational health, and be registered with the UK Advisory Panel (UKAP) (see Box 6.30). If the viral load is >200 copies/mL, the HCW must stop performing EPPs immediately;
- patient notification exercises following patient exposure to blood/bodily fluids from HIV-infected HCWs, in general, would only be done if the HCW had a viral load of >1000 copies/mL and is on treatment. However, all exposure incidents should be risk-assessed locally;
- patients who are exposed to blood from an infected HCW would only be considered for PEP and HIV testing if the viral load was >200 copies/mL. Otherwise, no action is taken.

Further advice is shown in Box 6.30.

> ### Box 6.30 Further advice from UK Advisory Panel (UKAP) for healthcare workers infected with blood-borne viruses
>
> Although this was originally set up to consider individual cases of HIV-infected healthcare workers, the UKAP now considers other blood-borne viruses, in particular hepatitis B and C viruses. They can provide advice for specific situations, as well as general policies (available at: https://www.gov.uk/government/groups/uk-advisory-panel-for-healthcare-workers-infected-with-bloodborne-viruses).

Disinfection

Disinfection is the process of killing microorganisms by physical or chemical means. It does not imply complete inactivation of all viruses or removal of bacterial spores (as occurs in sterilization).

A disinfectant is defined as a chemical used to destroy microorganisms. These agents only act on surfaces (environmental surfaces, equipment, or body surfaces) and do not penetrate layers of dirt or grease. Thus, disinfection is not a substitute for cleaning. Disinfectants do not usually have a persistent effect.

Use of disinfectants

Disinfectants fall into two main groups:

- environmental (see Table 6.15)—often too toxic for use on skin; may require protective clothing. Hypochlorite is most commonly used. The environmental use of disinfectants is usually restricted to accidental

Table 6.15 Environmental disinfectants

Class	Examples	Use	Notes
Hypochlorite (bleach)	Hypochlorite powder (e.g. Titan® sanitizer), detergent hypochlorite (liquid or tablet) (e.g. Domestos®, Presept®)	Best general-purpose disinfectant available. However, not suitable for particularly dirty situations. Generally use a solution of 1000ppm (parts/mL) available chlorine, but increase concentration to 1ppm if need to destroy hepatitis viruses (e.g. dialysis units). Use hypochlorite granules for spillage of body fluids, except urine	Sodium hypochlorite acts by the release of chlorine on contact with organic matter, so rapidly destroys all bacteria and viruses. However, some agents are unstable, and disinfecting properties may be lost by the rapid release of chlorine on contact with blood, faeces, or textiles. Strong solutions are corrosive to aluminium and other metals
Phenolics	Black fluids (e.g. 'Jeyes' fluid', white fluids (e.g. 'Izal®'), clear phenolics (e.g. 'Stericol®')	Not for routine environmental cleansing or disinfection; used in laboratory and post-mortem rooms	Derived from coal tar, and in common use in hospitals for over a century. Reasonable in visibly dirty situations. However, many bacteria and viruses are resistant, and prolonged exposure is needed for effective action. Also toxic, so handle with special precautions
Chloroxylenols	'Dettol®'	Household disinfectant	Said to combine some of the properties of phenolics with those of hypochlorites. Less effective at killing Gram-negatives than phenolics, and expensive

Table 6.16 Skin disinfectants

Class	Examples	Use	Notes
Alcohols	Ethyl alcohol (available as industrial methylated spirit (IMS)); isopropyl alcohol (e.g. 'Mediswabs')	Often used as a base for other skin disinfectants (e.g. iodine or chlorhexidine)	Ethyl alcohol (70%) effectively kills organisms on the skin, but this effect ceases after evaporation. Isopropyl alcohol evaporates less rapidly but is thought to be less effective against some viruses
Iodine	Huge variety of products (e.g. Betadine®)	Surgical scrubs, shampoos, etc.	Iodine dissolved in 70% alcohol is less popular, as it is messy and may be an irritant
Chlorhexidine	Hibitane®, Hibiscrub®	Surgical scrubs, popular disinfectant in hospitals and laboratories	Often marketed with other disinfecting agents and in alcoholic or aqueous solution. Some hospital organisms show resistance to it, but this is not a problem when using the alcoholic solution
Quaternary ammonium compounds (QACs)	Cetrimide	Trauma wounds and other special situations, not used in routine wound cleaning	Ineffective against some hospital organisms (e.g. *Pseudomonas* spp.)

spills or build-up of infected material in areas where this may be a hazard to patients or HCWs;

• skin (also called antiseptics) (see Table 6.16)—often have limited range of action, so are inappropriate for environmental disinfection, and usually relatively expensive. Chlorhexidine is the preferred agent. Alternatives are alcohol (inferior) and iodine (irritant).

Other disinfectants may be used to sterilize instruments, but heat treatment is usually preferred (➔ see Sterilization, pp. 221–3).

Selection of disinfectants

Different disinfectants have different properties; many are corrosive and toxic, and the speed of action is highly variable. Most are highly selective and only kill a limited range of organisms. Considerations include the following:

- Which organisms do you want to destroy?
- What is the object to be disinfected?
- Does the object need cleaning first?
- What concentration of disinfectant is required?

For equipment, please refer to the manufacturer's instructions.

As part of the Saving Lives campaign, a HII care bundle was introduced to improve the cleaning and decontamination of clinical equipment (available at: ⌖ https://webarchive.nationalarchives.gov.uk/20120118165100/http://hcai.dh.gov.uk/whatdoido/high-impact-interventions/). Two separate sets of actions are detailed, depending on the HCAI status of the patient. Recommendations include:

- location of cleaning activity;
- hand hygiene—use of WHO's '5 moments of hand hygiene';
- PPE;
- cleaning and decontamination;
- storage;
- documentation.

Sterilization

Sterilization is the process by which transmissible agents are killed or eliminated. These include fungi, bacteria, viruses, and spores, but not prions. There are two main types of sterilization:

- physical sterilization—this includes heat sterilization and radiation (e.g. electron beams, X-rays, γ rays);
- chemical sterilization.

Cleaning of instruments

Whichever sterilization process is deemed most appropriate, thorough cleaning is essential; otherwise, any dirt or biological matter may shield any organisms present. Physical scrubbing with detergent and water is recommended. Cool water is needed to clean organic matter from instruments, as warm or hot water may cause coagulation of organic debris. Alternative cleaning methods include ultrasound or pulsed air.

Physical sterilization: heat

This can be either dry heat or moist heat sterilization.

- **Dry heat** sterilization uses hot air that is free (or almost free) from water vapour, so any moisture plays no role in the process of sterilization. Methods include hot air oven, radiation, and microwave. Dry heat coagulates proteins in any organism and causes oxidative free radical damage and drying of cells.

- **Moist heat** (steam under pressure) sterilization uses hot air heavily laden with water vapour. Moist heat destroys microorganisms by irreversible denaturation of enzymes and structural proteins. Water vapour has a very high penetrating property and also causes damage through formation of oxidative free radicals. Methods include autoclaving, pressure cooking, pasteurization of milk, boiling, and steam sterilizing (steam at atmospheric pressure for 90min).

Autoclaves—steam sterilization using autoclaves is commonly used in hospitals and provides an inexpensive means of sterilizing large numbers of surgical instruments. To achieve sterility, a holding time of >15min at 121°C, or 3min at 134°C, is required. Liquids and instruments packed in cloth may take longer to reach the specified temperature, so they usually need more time. Autoclave treatment inactivates all bacteria, fungi, viruses, and spores. Certain prions may be eradicated by autoclaving at 121–132°C for 60min or 134°C for >18min, but this process is not 100% reliable for CJD (see Box 6.26). Monitoring an autoclave cycle is important and involves recording the temperature and pressure over time. To ensure adequate conditions have been met, most hospitals use indicator tape which changes colour. Bioindicators (e.g. based on spores of *Bacillus stearothermophilus*) are also used to independently confirm autoclave performance. These indicators should be positioned to ensure that steam penetrates the most difficult places. Note that autoclaving is often used to sterilize medical waste prior to disposal.

Chemical sterilization

Chemical sterilization is generally used when heat methods are inappropriate (e.g. for sterilizing heat-sensitive materials such as plastics, paper, biological materials, fibreoptics, and electronics). Options include:
- ethylene oxide (EO) sterilization is very common, particularly for disposable medical devices. Sterilization is usually carried out between 30°C and 60°C for objects that are sensitive to higher temperatures (e.g. plastics, optics). EO gas penetrates well and is highly effective, killing all viruses, bacteria, fungi, and spores. However, it is highly flammable, takes longer than any heat treatment, and produces toxic residues. *Bacillus subtilis* spores are used as a rapid biological indicator for EO sterilizers;
- ozone is used to sterilize water and air in industrial settings, and as a surface disinfectant. It can oxidize most organic matter but may be impractical, because it is toxic and unstable and it must be produced on site;
- chlorine bleach will kill bacteria, fungi, viruses, and most spores. Household bleach (5.25% sodium hypochlorite) is usually diluted to 1/10 before use. To kill MTB, it should only be diluted 1/5, and to inactivate prions, it should be diluted 1/2.5 (1 part bleach and 1.5 parts water). For full sterilization, bleach should be allowed to react for 20min. It is highly corrosive (including to some stainless steel surgical instruments);
- glutaraldehyde and formaldehyde are volatile liquids, which are only effective if the immersion time is long enough. It can take up to 12h to kill all spores in a clear liquid with glutaraldehyde, and even longer

with formaldehyde. Both liquids are toxic if inhaled or if they come into contact with skin. Glutaraldehyde is expensive and has a shelf life of <2 weeks. Formaldehyde is cheaper, but much more volatile (in fact, it may be used as a gaseous sterilizing agent);
- ortho-phthalaldehyde has many advantages over glutaraldehyde—it shows better mycobactericidal activity, kills glutaraldehyde-resistant spores, is more stable, less volatile, and less irritating, and acts faster. However, it is more expensive, and stains skin and proteins grey;
- hydrogen peroxide is a non-toxic chemical at low concentrations and leaves no residue. It can be used to sterilize endoscopes, either in low-temperature plasma sterilization chambers or mixed with formic acid. It can also be used at a concentration of 30–35% under low pressure conditions in the dry sterilization process (DSP). This process achieves bacterial reduction of 10^{-6}–10^{-8} in >6s, and the surface temperature is increased by only 10–15°C.

Guidelines on decontamination of endoscopes are available at:
- ✍ https://www.gov.uk/government/publications/management-and-decontamination-of-flexible-endoscopes
- ✍ https://www.bsg.org.uk/wp-content/uploads/2019/12/Guidance-for-Decontamination-of-Equipment-for-Gastrointestinal-Endoscopy_-2017-Edition-3.pdf

Ventilation in hospitals

Different ventilation systems

Effective ventilation is important to prevent spread of infection to staff and patients. Ventilation can be natural or mechanical.

Natural ventilation refers to the use of natural forces (e.g. wind) to introduce and distribute outdoor air into and out of a building. Most ward areas are naturally ventilated, providing around 5–6 air changes per hour (ACH). Opening windows can increase the rates of ACH. Natural ventilation is frequently the only form of ventilation in resource-limited settings, often confounded by hot and humid conditions.

Mechanical ventilation is used in ward areas and operating theatres. There are two types of mechanical ventilation:
- **positive-pressure ventilation**—used to prevent the entry of microorganisms, usually for patients who are susceptible to infections. For rooms under positive pressure, the air inside the room is maintained at a higher pressure than outside, so air leaves the room without recirculating. Air is filtered through a HEPA filter before entering a sealed room. HEPA filters can remove almost all airborne particles of 0.3 micrometres in diameter (e.g. *Aspergillus* spores). There is usually an anteroom to facilitate the donning of protective clothing. Require a minimum of 12 ACH;
- **negative-pressure ventilation**—negative-pressure isolation rooms are used to prevent pathogens (e.g. TB) from an infected patient from infecting other patients or HCWs in the hospital. Lower air pressure inside the rooms draws air into the room and prevents recirculation into the external environment. Rooms are sealed, except for a small gap

under the door through which air enters. The direction of airflow can be confirmed by a smoke test (hold a smoke tube >5cm in front of the bottom of the door, and, if the room is at negative pressure, the smoke will travel under the door and into the room). Require a minimum of 12 ACH.

In addition, **neutral-pressure isolation rooms** are being increasingly used. They have positively pressured ventilation lobbies, providing a barrier to airborne infection originating: (1) within the isolation room (equivalent to negative pressure) and (2) in the corridor (equivalent to positive pressure). In turn, there is no difference in pressure between the room and the corridor (hence neutral pressure).

Operating theatres

To prevent acquisition of infection during surgery via airborne routes, ventilation in operating theatres requires a higher level of air filtration. Two broad systems are used.

Plenum ventilation

This is the most frequently used system in general-purpose operating theatres. Atmospheric air is filtered in two stages:
- coarse filter to remove dust and debris;
- bacterial filter of >2 micrometres in pore size, with 95% efficiency, used inside the inlet grill.

Some air may recirculate within the suite. An exhaust system removes the air to the outside. There are >20 ACH.

Laminar flow

Laminar flow is used in orthopaedic theatres to reduce the number of microorganisms present. This is of particular value in preventing prosthetic joint infections (PJIs). A continuous flow of filtered air recirculates under positive pressure into the operating field, and any contaminants generated under surgery are removed from the site. There are >300 ACH, which should result in <10 colony-forming units (cfu)/m³. Different systems include introduction of air horizontally or vertically, in an enclosed, semi-enclosed, or open manner.

National guidance on ventilation

Health Technical Memorandum (HTM) 03-01 provides guidance on design and management of specialist ventilation in healthcare premises (part A covers design and validation, and part B covers operational management and performance ventilation). This is a set of standard schemes for ventilation of conventional and ultraclean ventilation (UCV) operating theatres. There are four main sections:
- management policy—management responsibilities/legal issues;
- design requirements;
- validation/verification—commissioning (i.e. when a new theatre is built or after major constructional changes), performance tests, handover;
- operative management—day-to-day issues such as minimum standards, maintaining performance, routine maintenance, etc.

For a discussion of practices in operating theatres, see Box 6.31.

Air sampling

Microbiological tests are needed to complement the physical monitoring systems, although few studies have demonstrated a link between microbiological air quality and wound infections. For details of performing air sampling and testing infection control rooms, see Walker et al. (2007),[34] and for operating theatres, see HTM 03-01(➜ see National guidance on ventilation, p. 224). Separate guidance is given for empty and in-use theatres.

- If an empty theatre fails the air sampling tests, check the technique and repeat sampling. If it fails again, discuss the findings with the IPCT, engineers, or other experts. Consider testing the particle penetration of filters and/or the air velocity.
- If an in-use theatre fails the air sampling tests, check the technique, and repeat sampling when the theatre is empty.

References

33 Woodhead K, Taylor EW, Bannister G, Chesworth T, Hoffman P, Humphreys H. Behaviours and rituals in the operating theatre. A report from the Hospital Infection Society Working Party on Infection Control in Operating Theatres. J Hosp Infect. 2002;**51**:241–55.

34 Walker JT, Hoffman P, Bennett AM, et al. Hospital and community acquired infection and the built environment—design and testing of infection control rooms. J Hosp Infect. 2007;**65** Suppl 2:43–9.

Box 6.31 Rituals and behaviours in operating theatres

All operating theatres should have their own up-to-date IPC policy. This should include standard precautions for every invasive procedure, and outline the need for an additional risk assessment for each patient, to see if other specific precautions are required. There are many 'rituals and behaviours' that have crept into 'standard practice' in many operating theatres—some of which are beneficial and some harmful. The standard of evidence varies, but a few practical pointers are listed below (for further discussion, ➜ see Surgical Site Infection, p. 805):[33]

- patients' clothes—it may not be necessary to change (e.g. for cataract surgery). Jewellery only needs to be removed (for infection control purposes) if near the site of operation;
- shaving—should be avoided;
- hand hygiene—scrubbing brushes should not be used on the skin;
- drapes—there is no evidence for adhesives around the edge of wounds;
- gloves—needle puncture is not an indication to change gloves; if necessary, a second pair should be worn on top;
- masks—there is no good evidence that masks reduce infection rates; however, they are recommended to protect the surgeon. The scrub team should wear masks and hats for implants, and the mask should be changed for each procedure. Non-scrubbed staff in plenum ventilated theatres do not require masks or hats;
- linen—should be waterproof and disposable (European standard).

Laundry

Hospital linen should be processed so it is not an infection risk to future users. The laundry should remove evidence of previous use, including organisms, but cannot be expected to kill bacterial spores.

HTM 01-04 provides guidance on decontamination of linen for health and social care. NHS Executive guidance (HSG(95)18) differentiates used (soiled or fouled) and infected linen, and describes a framework to reduce risk to staff (porters, laundry staff, etc.), as is shown in Table 6.17. Washing temperature requirements vary between countries. In the UK, the cycle temperature should reach 65°C for at least 10min or 71°C for at least 3min. Heat-labile laundry that would be damaged at high temperatures can be washed at 40°C with sodium hypochlorite to give a final concentration of 150 ppm available chlorine to the final rinse. Monitoring of critical points is important under hazard analysis and critical control point (HACCP). These include temperature and exposure times, treatment of rinse water (if potentially contaminated), in-use detergent concentrations, and drying temperatures.

Curtains should be laundered:
- if visibly soiled;
- after an outbreak of viral gastroenteritis;
- if around the bed of a patient who has been barrier-nursed (e.g. MRSA, *C. difficile*)—they should be washed on patient discharge;
- routinely (3 months minimum).

Table 6.17 Categories of linen

Linen category	Definition	Bag colour
Soiled	All used linen that is not fouled or infected	White nylon bag
Fouled	Contaminated with any bodily fluid	White or clear plastic bag, then white linen outer bag
		Treat as potentially infected, so wear gloves and aprons when handling it
Infected	Linen from patient with, or suspected to have, infection with enteric organism (e.g. diarrhoea and/or vomiting, *Campylobacter*, viral gastroenteritis, *Salmonella*, *Shigella*, hepatitis A, etc.)	Red alginate bag, then red nylon outer bag, labelled with point of origin
	Bloodstained linen from patient with HIV/hepatitis B or C infection	
	Linen visibly contaminated with sputum from patient with open TB	

Waste

Disposal of waste is subject to strict legislation set out by the Department of Health, Department of the Environment, the Health and Safety Commission Advisory Group, and the amended European Communities Framework Directive on Waste. This legislation places a duty of care on anyone handling clinical waste, including porters and incineration staff. Thus, hospital guidelines apply not only to clinical areas, but throughout the hospital. There is a move towards a unified approach for disposal of infectious and medicinal waste, and to operate the same category codes throughout Europe. HTM 07-01 provides guidance on safe management of healthcare waste. Apart from direct environmental benefits, this guidance[35] presents opportunities for introducing cost savings, safer working practices, and reducing carbon emissions related to managing waste.

Clinical waste

Clinical waste is always incinerated and is defined as:
- all human tissue and body fluids, and related items (e.g. dressings, incontinence pads, stoma bags, urine containers);
- sharps and contaminated sharps items (e.g. glass);

Table 6.18 National colour-coded system for waste disposal containers

Type of waste	Container	Notes
Clinical waste	Yellow plastic bags (orange/red in some hospitals)	Make sure bags are only two-thirds full. Tie them securely, and label each bag with the ward of origin before sending for incineration. If there is a chance that body fluids may leak from a single yellow bag, then use double-bagging
Non-clinical waste	Black plastic bags	
Sharps	Yellow rigid plastic boxes	Do not overfill these boxes. Never resheathe needles or separate needles from a syringe, unless using an approved safe method. Put IV giving sets into these boxes too
Glass (larger items)	Black dustbins	
Central sterile services department (CSSD)	Brown bags marked 'CSSD'	
Confidential or cytotoxic waste	Local policies apply	

CSSD, Centre for surgical sterilization and disinfection.

- certain pharmaceutical products and their containers;
- potentially infected laboratory waste.

Table 6.18 summarizes other types of waste, the national colour-coded system, and recommendations for disposal.

References

35 Department of Health (2013). *Health technical memorandum 07-01: safe management of healthcare waste*. Available at: ⌖ https://www.gov.uk/government/publications/guidance-on-the-safe-management-of-healthcare-waste

Part 3

Systematic Microbiology

Bacteria

Basic principles of bacteriology

Taxonomy

Taxonomy is the organizing structure underpinning biology, based on evolutionary relationships between organisms. With respect to bacteria, it refers to two concepts:

- classification—the division of organisms into related groups based on similar phenotypic and genotypic characteristics. Species is the most definitive level of classification. 'genetic relatedness) becomes available;
- nomenclature—the naming of groups and members of a group. This is governed by the International Committee on Systematics of Prokaryotes (available at: ℘ https://www.the-icsp.org). The most recent revision of the International Code of Nomenclature of Prokaryotes was published in 2019. Amendments are published in journal form (*International Journal of Systematic and Evolutionary Microbiology*). The basic rules for naming are outlined in Boxes 7.1 and 7.2.

Identification

Taxonomy is dynamic and dependent on the techniques of organism identification available. Originally reliant on phenotypic characteristics, more recent methods of determining the genetic 'relatedness' (phylogenetics) of a group of organisms should lead to a more stable classification, with fewer

---

Box 7.1 Microorganism nomenclature rules

- Each organism should have only one correct name. Where >1 exists, the oldest legitimate name takes precedence.
- Confusing names should be abandoned.
- Regardless of origin, all names are in Latin or are latinized.
- The genus (first word) always starts with a capital letter.
- The species (second word) is always in small letters.
- The genus and species name are italicized when printed.
- Up-to-date organism nomenclature can be found at:℘ https://www.bacterio.net/

Box 7.2 The naming hierarchy

- Order—names ending in *-ales*
- Families—names ending in *-aceae*
- Tribes—names ending in *-eae*
- Genus—groups of closely related species
- Species—a collection of strains sharing common characteristics
- Strain—a bacterial culture derived from a pure isolate

revisions in the future. Changes are overseen by the Judicial Commission of the International Union of Microbiological Societies.

- Phenotypic characteristics—cellular morphology, staining (e.g. Gram or acid-fast; see Box 7.3), motility, growth characteristics (speed, requirements, colonial appearance), biochemical characteristics (e.g. acid from specific carbohydrates), serology, analysis of metabolic end products).
- Phylogenetic identification—nucleic acid hybridization (denaturation of double-stranded DNA (dsDNA) into single strands and assessing their ability to anneal to the single strands of another related organism), 16S rRNA sequence analysis. While valuable, these are largely being replaced by whole-genome sequencing (WGS).

For identification purposes, simple phenotypic characteristics continue to be used, which often (but not always) correlate with genotypes. These methods of phenotypic characterization have been developed and codified over years to facilitate laboratory identification of organisms (collected in texts such as Bergey's Manual of Systematic Bacteriology).

Bacterial structure and function

Bacteria are prokaryotic—they have a single chromosome that is not enclosed in a nuclear membrane. They are around 0.2–2 micrometres wide by 1–6 micrometres long, and exist in four basic shapes: cocci (spheres), bacilli (rods), spirillia (spirals), and vibrios (comma-shaped).

Cytoplasm

Cytoplasm is a gel containing enzymes, ions, subcellular organelles, and energy reserves of an organism. Prokaryotes lack mitochondria (cf. eukaryotes) and instead produce energy (adenosine triphosphate (ATP)) on their cell surface membranes. Ribosomes are the sites of protein synthesis. Bacterial ribosomes are 70S (the 'S' referring to a unit of sedimentation on ultracentrifugation) and are formed from two subunits: 30S (which contains 16S RNA) and 50S. Ribosomes are formed from specific ribosomal proteins and ribosomal RNA (rRNA) (they account for 80% of total cell RNA). They complex with a messenger RNA (mRNA) transcript from DNA to form polyribosomes (polysomes). Within the cytoplasm is the single circular dsDNA molecule. Additional extrachromosomal DNA is often found within the cytoplasm in the form of plasmids. These are covalently closed dsDNA circles and capable of replication, and are inherited by progeny cells. They may contain genetic information encoding structure or functions relating to bacterial virulence (antibiotic resistance, adhesions, toxins, etc.).

Cytoplasmic membrane

The cytoplasm is surrounded by the cytoplasmic membrane, a phospholipid bilayer into which various proteins are inserted. The membrane is involved in the synthesis and secretion of enzymes and toxins, and active transportation of materials into the cytoplasm.

Bacterial cell wall

This provides rigidity and a physical barrier to the outside world. Peptidoglycan provides strength and is found in all bacterial species, except *Mycoplasma* and *Ureaplasma* spp. and cell-wall deficient variants (L-forms). It comprises a carbohydrate backbone cross-linked by short peptides. Variations in the peptide linkages are responsible for different cell wall properties (see Box 7.3).

Box 7.3 The Gram stain

Named after Hans Christian Gram, the Danish bacteriologist who devised it in 1884, the Gram stain remains a pivotal test in any bacteriology laboratory. The fundamental principle exploits differences in the structure of the bacterial cell wall. The procedure is simple:

- Cells are stained with crystal violet.
- Then they are treated with iodine, forming a crystal violet/iodine complex in the cell.
- Next they are washed with an organic solvent (acetone–alcohol).
- Then they are stained with a red counterstain (e.g. safranin).
- Gram-positive organisms retain the crystal violet/iodine complex within the cell, because of the thick peptidoglycan cell wall, and appear dark purple. In Gram-negative organisms, the stain is leached from the cell, due to disruption of the lipid-rich outer membrane by the organic solvent, and they appear pink.

Gram-positive cell walls

These are composed of several layers of peptidoglycan, within which are trapped a variety of proteins, polysaccharides, and teichoic acids (polymers of glycerol or ribitol), which stabilize the cell wall and maintain its association with the cell membrane, as well as have roles in cellular interaction and growth. They are antigenic in some organisms. Certain organisms will possess cell wall structures that confer virulence characteristics (e.g. M protein of Group A *Streptococcus* (GAS)).

Gram-negative cell walls

These are thinner, yet more complex, than those of Gram-positive organisms. Outside the cytoplasmic membrane is a periplasmic space. The outer part of this is bounded by a single peptidoglycan layer, beyond which lies the outer membrane—a phospholipid bilayer within which lie other large molecules. Lipoproteins link this membrane to the peptidoglycan below. Unique to Gram-negative bacteria are the lipopolysaccharides (LPS) in the outer membrane. These are key surface antigens and endotoxins of Gram-negative organisms. They are composed of lipid A (principally responsible for the endotoxin activity), attached to a core polysaccharide, with side chains which vary within a species and confer the serological identity (O antigen) of individual strains. Other components of the outer membrane include porin proteins (allow entry to the periplasmic space from the outside) and non-porin proteins (such as penicillin-binding proteins (PBPs)).

'Acid-fast' cell walls

Mycobacterium spp. and *Nocardia* spp. have a modified Gram-positive cell wall. They have a higher lipid content which is due to mycolic acids, which can confer virulence characteristics. Acid-fast organisms are so-called because, once stained with red carbol fuchsin dye, they are resistant to decolorization with acid-alcohol—a property conferred by the cell wall lipids.

Bacterial surface structures

Capsules

Certain bacteria possess a capsule around their cell wall, usually composed of polysaccharide, but occasionally of polypeptide. They are manufactured at the cell membrane. They serve to protect cells from toxins, desiccation, complement proteins, and antibodies, and play a role in adherence (e.g. the glucan capsule of *Streptococcus mutans* forms the matrix of dental plaque). Capsules are antigenic and can be used to identify certain organisms (e.g. *Haemophilus influenzae* type b), and may be detectable in body fluids.

Flagellae

These are long, thin appendages that are anchored in the cytoplasmic membrane and extend through the cell wall into the surrounding medium; they are responsible for cellular motility. They are usually found on Gram-negative rods (GNRs), but motile Gram-positive organisms also exist (e.g. *Listeria* spp.). Flagellar number and arrangement vary from single (monotrichous) to multiple over the whole surface (peritrichous). These filaments are composed of multiple flagellin proteins, which have the capacity to self-assemble. The cell membrane-anchored base rotates as part of an energy-dependent reaction, causing the rigid flagella to rotate. They are antigenic, and several genera (e.g. *Salmonella* spp.) are able to alter their antigenic type of flagella they produce (phase variation) by the differential expression of the genes encoding various flagellin proteins.

Fimbriae

These are smaller appendages (~15–20 micrometres in length), composed of fibrillin and found on many Gram-negative bacteria. They form hollow tubes and are involved in attachment to cells or mucosal surfaces (also called adhesins). Different adhesins display different binding properties (e.g. mannose), which are partly responsible for the tissue tropism seen with certain species of bacteria. They are also involved in bacterial conjugation and the exchange of DNA from one cell to another. The term 'pili' is given to the fimbriae used by Gram-negative bacteria for DNA transfer in conjugation, such as the F pilus in *Escherichia coli*.

Bacterial genetics

Bacterial DNA

Bacterial genetic information is encoded in the cell's DNA, of which there are two types:

- chromosomal DNA—prokaryotic organisms have a single, covalently closed, circular chromosome of dsDNA. It lies in a supercoiled state within the cytoplasm, not enclosed, but attached to the bacterial cell membrane at certain points. Individual genes are arranged linearly. Depending on species, bacterial chromosomes commonly contain between 2 and 5 million bp. DNA replication and transcription to mRNA occur continually (unlike in eukaryotes);
- extrachromosomal DNA—plasmids are small DNA molecules consisting of circular dsDNA. Replication is autonomous and occurs independently of the host cell. Multiple copies of the same plasmid and many different plasmids can coexist in the same cell. Plasmids pass to daughter cells, and some are capable of transferring to other bacteria of the same (or other) species. They code for many different functions and structures (e.g. antibiotic resistance).

Genetic material can move between plasmids and from plasmid to chromosome (and vice versa) via transposons. These are DNA sequences that can copy themselves to a new site, carrying associated genes with them.

In manufacturing proteins, single-stranded 'messenger' RNA (mRNA) is synthesized from dsDNA during transcription by a DNA-dependent RNA polymerase, using the 'sense' strand of the DNA as a template. The mRNA forms a complex with several ribosomes (a polysome–mRNA complex). The mRNA is translated as transfer RNA (tRNA) molecules bearing the appropriate amino acid, and its 'sense' bases associate with the mRNA 'antisense' bases.

Genetic variation

Genetic variation can occur by mutation or direct gene transfer.

Mutation

This occurs when one or more bases in the DNA sequence changes. It is permanent (barring re-mutation to the original sequence) and will be inherited by any progeny. Such changes may alter the amino acid sequence of the encoded protein or may change the circumstances in which a normal protein is produced (transcription changes). Mutations can be by:

- deletion—losing a base will cause a frameshift mutation, changing the amino acids represented by the sequence from the point of mutation onwards. Deletions can involve several bases;
- insertion—additional base or bases will also cause a frameshift;
- substitution—change of a single base to one of the other three changes the amino acid represented by the code.

Gene transfer

This is the main means by which bacteria achieve their rapid genetic variability. There are three mechanisms:

- transformation—the uptake of free bacterial DNA from the surrounding environment into recipient cells. Cells able to take up and incorporate free DNA are termed 'competent'. This state is usually transient, occurring towards the late exponential phase of growth, with the expression of surface receptors for DNA. DNA that enters can only be incorporated into the genome if there are homologous regions with which it can integrate (only DNA from related species is likely to achieve it), and requires the presence of the *recA* gene;

- transduction—the exchange of genes by bacteriophages (often simplied to 'phages'). Phages are viruses that infect only bacteria. Certain phages integrate their genetic material into the bacterial host DNA. During phage replication, excision of a viral sequence from the host DNA may result in fragments of bacterial DNA becoming enclosed within the viral particle. When this particle infects a new bacterial cell, the DNA fragment recombines into the chromosome of the second bacterium. Transduction may be generalized (random accidental host DNA is transferred) or specialized (specific host genes are transferred, as the phage DNA integrates at specific sites). Phage conversion refers to the phenomenon of phage DNA becoming integrated into the bacterial chromosome and bringing about a change in the bacterial phenotype (e.g. toxin production in *Corynebacterium diphtheriae*). This is due to phage DNA precipitating the expression of otherwise unexpressed bacterial genes;

- conjugation—the only mechanism that requires cell-to-cell interaction, and the major means by which bacteria acquire additional genes. Gram-negative cells achieve this by means of the sex pilus, which is encoded on a specific plasmid (the F plasmid). The pilus establishes contact with another cell and is the tube through which DNA is passed. Some organisms integrate the F plasmid into chromosomal DNA—such cells are termed Hfr (high-frequency recombination) cells. Gram-positive cells achieve conjugation by aggregating in response to the production of pheromones by the donor bacterium.

Bacterial growth and metabolism

Bacterial growth requires materials for the manufacture of cell components and a source of energy.

Materials

Some bacteria can synthesize all they require from simple raw materials. However, most pathogenic bacteria require a ready made supply of the organic compounds they need for growth. Most of these nutrients diffuse freely across the cell membrane to enter the cell. Some are required at high concentration, and uptake is energy-dependent. Enzymes involved in these processes may be inducible (produced in the presence of the substrate) or constitutive (produced constantly and independent of the substrate).

Carbon

Lithotrophic bacteria are able to use carbon dioxide (CO_2) as the sole source of carbon, and use it as the basis of their organic metabolites. Thus, the only other materials needed are water, inorganic salts, and energy. Organotrophic bacteria require organic carbon such as glucose—thus, their energy source is also used in the synthesis of materials. Different bacterial species can utilize different organic carbon sources, with *Pseudomonas* spp. being amongst the most versatile.

Nitrogen

Ammonium ions (NH_4^+) provide the nitrogen required by bacterial cells. This is turned into glutamate and glutamine, which, in turn, are processed into certain amino acids, purines, etc. Certain bacterial species (predominantly soil-dwelling organisms) and blue-green algae can make NH_4^+ directly from atmospheric nitrogen—certain human pathogens, such as *Klebsiella* and *Clostridium* spp., can also 'fix' nitrogen in this manner. Other organisms produce their NH_4^+ by nitrate reduction or from deamination of amino acids released from proteins.

Growth factors

Substances such as B vitamins, minerals, certain amino acids, purine, and pyrimidines are required by many bacteria, although not all are capable of synthesizing their own. An organism is described as prototrophic for a growth factor if it is capable of synthesizing it and does not require an exogenous source. All bacteria need certain inorganic ions such as magnesium and calcium, and some need zinc and copper, amongst others.

Environmental conditions

As well as water and CO_2, bacteria have specific optimal environmental requirements for growth, including temperature and pH. Oxygen requirements are discussed in ➋ Energy below.

Energy

- Bacterial metabolism is a balance between biosynthesis (anabolism) and degradation (catabolism). Catabolic reactions power the biosynthetic processes, as hydrolysis of substances being broken down liberates energy which is captured in the formation of the phosphate bonds of ATP.
- An organism's ability to utilize certain carbohydrates (e.g. sucrose, mannose) and convert them to glucose (the starting point for both aerobic and anaerobic catabolism) for metabolism is a useful feature for characterizing bacteria. Historically, many tests in clinical microbiology detect the acidic end products of bacterial metabolism in controlled conditions.
- The oxygen requirement of a specific organism reflects the means it uses to meet its energy needs:
  - obligate anaerobes—grow only in conditions of high reducing intensity, and oxygen is toxic;
  - aerotolerant anaerobes—anaerobic metabolism, but not killed by the presence of oxygen;
  - facultative anaerobes—can grow in anaerobic and aerobic conditions;
  - obligate aerobes—need oxygen to grow;
  - microaerophilic organisms—best growth is seen at low oxygen levels; high levels may be inhibitory.

Anaerobic metabolism

Glucose use in anaerobic conditions is through fermentation. This occurs via glycolysis, producing pyruvate and two molecules (net) of ATP per glucose molecule. Pyruvate can then enter several different pathways, producing different end products (e.g. lactic acid, acetaldehyde, ethanol, etc.)

Aerobic metabolism

Glucose use in aerobic conditions is through respiration. Pyruvate forms in glycolysis, as in anaerobic conditions, but then enters the Krebs cycle. Complete oxidation of glucose via these pathways results in 38 molecules (net) of ATP per glucose molecule. The Krebs cycle also produces precursors for several other important cellular components such as purines, pyrimidines, amino acids, and lipids. Aerobes produce a free radical superoxide (O_2^-), which is reduced to oxygen and hydrogen peroxide (H_2O_2). Catalase enzymes convert the latter to water and oxygen.

Bacterial growth phases

Bacterial growth occurs as the mass of cellular constituents increases. Cell division starts once a critical mass is reached, occurring by binary fission. In liquid media, bacteria display a uniform growth curve (see Fig. 7.1):

- lag phase—the cell synthesizes new enzymes and cofactors, and imports nutrients from the media;
- increasing growth phase—enzymatic reaction rates approach steady state, and cell growth begins;

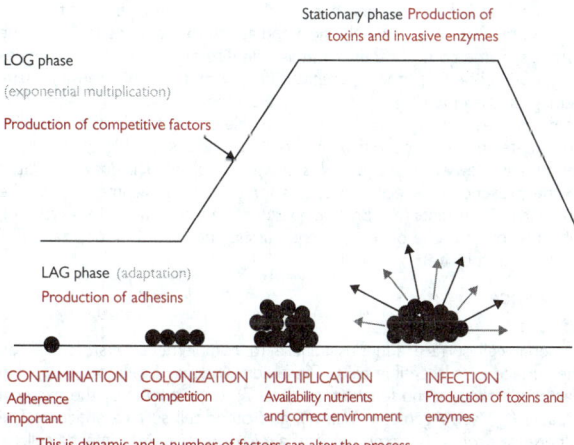

Stationary phase Production of toxins and invasive enzymes

LOG phase

(exponential multiplication)

Production of competitive factors

LAG phase (adaptation)
Production of adhesins

CONTAMINATION	COLONIZATION	MULTIPLICATION	INFECTION
Adherence important	Competition	Availability nutrients and correct environment	Production of toxins and enzymes

This is dynamic and a number of factors can alter the process

Fig. 7.1 Typical bacterial growth curve in batch culture (i.e. bacteria placed in a nutritionally supportive growth medium and allowed to grow uninterrupted in optimum growth conditions). The infectious process (depicted as contamination, colonization, multiplication, and infection) is represented below the growth curve at the respective stages. Adapted from Edward-Jones V (2016) '*Essential Microbiology for Wound Care*' Oxford University Press, with permission from Oxford University Press.

- logarithmic growth phase—cell growth and division are at maximum. This is influenced by temperature, the carbon source, oxygen, nutrient availability, and so on;
- declining growth phase—nutrients are exhausted, and growth slows;
- stationary phase—new organisms produced equal those dying;
- death phase—cells die off.

Bacterial virulence and pathogenicity

Definitions

Pathogenicity is defined as the ability of an organism to cause disease, whereas virulence is the degree of pathogenicity within a group of organisms. Virulence is determined by several factors related to the organism and the host, most particularly the infectivity of the bacteria and the severity of the condition it produces. To be considered pathogenic, organisms will have strains of varying degrees of virulence.

Pathogenicity

Infection of the host is the necessary first step—infection does not, however, equate with disease. We are all asymptomatically colonized with many bacteria. These, however, only become disease-causing in certain situations.

The organism must enter the host and attach to the mucous membrane surfaces. Some go no further than this, and disease is caused by exotoxins (e.g. *Vibrio cholerae*); others penetrate deeper and multiply, causing tissue damage and eventually gaining access to blood and potentially disseminating. Some species, such as mycobacteria, are able to reside within cells, taking up long-term residence within the host. Still others are highly specific in the organs they will infect (e.g. *Neisseria gonorrhoeae*). This may be related to the presence of specific receptors for bacterial attachment or to the presence of nutrients (e.g. *Brucella abortus* has a requirement for erythritol, which is found in the bovine placental tissue and results in localization of infection to this site).

Virulence factors

Adhesins

Bacterial cell surface adhesins adhere to complementary structures on the surface of susceptible cells. These adhesins may be fimbriae (➔ see Bacterial structure and function, pp. 235–7), components of the bacterial capsule (➔ see Aggressins below), and other cell surface antigens. The adherence process is a prerequisite if a microorganism is to infect a cell.

Aggressins

These substances allow the cell to evade host defence mechanisms. These may act to prevent an initial immune attack and phagocytosis, or to enable the cell to survive once phagocytosed (with the added benefit that, once settled within a phagocytic cell, they are safe from continued exposure to antibody and complement). They include:

- **capsules**—enable organisms to avoid phagocytosis by preventing interaction with the bacterial cell surface and the phagocytic cell, or by concealing surface antigens. Specific antibodies against the capsular material will opsonize the organism and allow its ingestion. Examples include *Streptococcus pneumoniae* and *H. influenzae* type b. Mycobacteria have components in their cell wall that prevent lysosome/phagosome fusion, once ingested;

- **extracellular slime substances**—these are surface proteins or carbohydrates (polysaccharides). Examples include the M protein of GAS (*Streptococcus pyogenes*) which impairs complement function, protein A of *Staphylococcus aureus* which binds IgG by the Fc region, interfering with the phagocytosis of opsonized organisms, and LPS of Gram-negative bacteria which may delay or blunt the acute inflammatory response;

- **enzymes**—some bacteria produce proteases which can hydrolyse and inactivate IgA, aiding mucosal colonization. *Listeria monocytogenes* secretes enzymes that inhibit destruction by the myeloperoxidase system of phagocytic cells. *S. aureus* produces hyaluronidase, an enzyme that depolymerizes hyaluronic acid (responsible for cell-to-cell adhesion), thereby easing the spread of the organism. GAS produce streptokinases that lyse fibrin clots; *Clostridium perfringens* produces collagenases, contributing to its ability to produce necrotizing skin infection;

- **siderophores**—molecules produced by most pathogenic bacteria, which scavenge iron from the host. Iron is required for virulence by several bacteria, and siderophores seem to protect bacteria from the killing effects of human serum;

- **plasmids**—although these are not conventional virulence factors, they may code for a wide range of additional features promoting virulence such as antibiotic resistance, sex pili, and chromosomal mobilization (allowing the transfer of genetic material encoding antibiotic resistance or toxins to other cells).

Toxins

Exotoxins are amongst the most potent biological toxins and are mainly produced by Gram-positive organisms. They are usually heat-labile proteins, and many can be inactivated by proteolytic enzymes or neutralized by specific antibodies. The effects are highly varied; for example, the clinical manifestations of tetanus, botulism, and diphtheria are all due to toxins. Some toxins are secreted in the active form, whereas others require cleavage to become active (e.g. *C. diphtheriae*): some strains that contain a lysogenic bacteriophage (β-corynephage) are able to produce the toxin. The toxin genes exist on the phage genome.

Endotoxins are only produced by Gram-negative bacteria and consist primarily of LPS. They are heat-stable and are only partly neutralized by specific antibodies. They are generally less toxic than exotoxins. They can cause fever, hypotension, haemorrhage, and disseminated intravascular coagulation (DIC), and stimulate cytokine release from macrophages.

Microbiological specimens

This is a brief overview of specimen collection. For full details, consult your hospital guidelines, laboratory handbook, and the UK Standards for

Microbiology Investigations (SMIs) (available at: www.rcpath.org/profess
ion/publications/standards-for-microbiology-investigations.html).

A laboratory will perform different tests on different samples, depending
on the site, clinical setting, and nature of the specimen. It is therefore important to consider whether the sample you are planning to send will help
answer your clinical question, particularly when sending from a site that is
not normally sterile. For example, a skin swab may be useful for screening
for meticillin-resistant *S. aureus* (MRSA) but is unlikely to identify the cause
of an abscess. Conversely, any growth from a CSF sample is likely to be
important. Provide full clinical information, including specific organisms in
which you may be interested if they are not routinely included.

Blood cultures

Blood cultures (BCs) are taken to identify patients with bacteraemia. They
usually comprise two bottles (aerobic and anaerobic) in adults, but practice
may vary. BC bottles typically contain growth media, anticoagulant, and resin
for binding antibiotics. Single 'paediatric' bottles are available and include
additives to optimize growth of organisms affecting children. Haematology
patients may have a third fastidious antibiotic neutralization (FAN) bottle.
BACTEC™ and BacT/Alert automated systems provide continual monitoring for growth via fluorescence technology. Recommendations from the
UKHSA aim to keep the BC contamination rate to <3% (➔ see Chapter 6).

Urine samples

Urine samples, including midstream urine (MSU), clean-catch urine
(CCU), catheter specimen of urine (CSU), bag urine in infants, suprapubic
aspirate (SPA), and nephrostomy fluid, are taken to investigate suspected
urinary tract infections (UTIs). Should be sterile. Laboratory practice varies
in terms of which samples have dipstick (➔ see Chapter 17, Introduction,
p. 725), microscopy (white cells, red cells, epithelial cells), culture (e.g.
chromogenic agar), level of speciation, and antibiotic susceptibilities.
Epithelial cells usually indicate contamination. Automated urine analysers
(e.g. sediMAX) are increasingly available.

Respiratory samples

Respiratory samples (e.g. sputum, bronchoalveolar lavage (BAL), tracheal aspirate, induced sputum, bronchial washings, nasopharyngeal aspirate (NPA)) are taken to investigate a suspected respiratory infection,
along with samples for virology and serology. Laboratory methods may
include Gram staining (rarely performed), routine bacterial culture (plus
Legionella on BAL), *Pneumocystis* antigen detection/PCR, *Aspergillus* antigen
(galactomannan), acid-fast bacilli (AFB) smear, and culture if indicated.
Clinical details are critical; for example, patients with cystic fibrosis (CF) require additional investigations for *Burkholderia*, etc. (➔ see Cystic fibrosis,
pp. 663–5).

Tuberculosis samples

TB samples include sputum, urine, bronchial washings, tissue/biopsy specimens, and others, as relevant (CSF, bone marrow, fluids, etc.). Smears
may be stained with auramine–phenol or Ziehl–Neelsen (ZN) (➔ see
Mycobacterium tuberculosis, pp. 391–5). Lowenstein–Jensen slopes have

been largely replaced by the automated Mycobacteria Growth Indicator Tube (MGIT) system.

Faecal samples

Faecal samples are usually taken to investigate diarrhoea. Routine culture includes *Salmonella*, *Shigella*, *Campylobacter*, *E. coli* O157, and sometimes stains for cryptosporidia. Clinical history is important in terms of parasitology. TCBS (thiosulfate–citrate–bile salts–sucrose) plates for *Vibrio*, etc. *Clostridioides difficile* testing should be specifically requested.

Biopsies

Biopsies, including tissue, bone, and pus, can come from most body sites. Pus is always preferable to a swab because of the higher culture yield, especially for anaerobes. These samples usually have Gram staining and routine bacterial culture, with additional culture and tests as indicated by the clinical picture.

Fluids

Fluids (ascitic, pleural, joint, etc.) should be sterile. Gram staining and culture performed as indicated by the clinical picture. More than 250 white cells in ascitic fluid may indicate spontaneous bacterial peritonitis (SBP).

Swabs

Swabs (wound/ulcer, conjunctiva, ear, nose, throat, vaginal, genital) have different culture plates, dictated by the site and suspected infection. Always thoroughly clean a wound first, to avoid colonizing the flora. Culture results need careful interpretation to determine the significance of organisms, and remember that superficial swabs are poor predictors of deep/invasive infection.

Cerebrospinal fluid

The **CSF** will undergo total white and red cell counts and Gram staining. If raised, differential leucocyte counts are provided (polymorph = neutrophil, mononuclear = lymphocyte). CSF protein and glucose levels are usually performed in biochemistry. Gram and special stains, such as ZN and India ink, as indicated by the clinical picture. Antigen tests (e.g. cryptococcal antigen), culture, and PCR are available. CSF samples from neurosurgical shunts require careful interpretation due to potential colonization or contamination.

Intravascular catheter line tips

Intravascular catheter (IVC) line tips—not all laboratories process IVC tips. Using a quantification technique, such as the Maki roll, >15cfu is usually regarded as significant, but these need to be interpreted within the clinical context.

Serum or EDTA blood samples

Serum or EDTA blood samples are required for serological and molecular tests, respectively. Consult your local laboratory guidelines.

Bacterial culture media

Selective media enable certain organisms to grow, while inhibiting other organisms; for example, adding an antibiotic to an agar will select for organisms which are resistant to that agent.

Differential media help distinguish different organisms growing on the same media by virtue of their different biochemical behaviours. For example, those organisms that can ferment lactose will do so if it is present in the media, producing acid. pH indicators (neutral red in MacConkey agar) will thus help identify lactose fermenters. There are a number of commercial chromogenic agar available, designed to facilitate rapid identification (e.g. for uropathogens).

Enriched media contain specific nutrients required by certain organisms, including fastidious ones (i.e. *H. influenzae*).

Specific media include:

- blood agar (BA)—an enriched differential media used to demonstrate haemolysis and isolate fastidious organisms. It contains 5–10% sheep or horse blood;
- MacConkey agar—selects for Gram-negatives. Contains bile salts (to inhibit most Gram-positives), crystal violet (inhibits certain Gram-positives), lactose, peptone, and a dye (neutral red) that is turned pink by lactose fermenters. Sorbitol MacConkey (S-MAC) helps differentiate enteropathogenic *E. coli*, such as O157, as most are non-sorbitol fermenters;
- CLED (cystine, lactose, electrolyte-deficient) agar is used to isolate and differentiate Gram-negatives, as it inhibits *Proteus* swarming and can differentiate between lactose fermenters (yellow) and non-fermenters (colourless/white);
- chocolate agar—enriched with heat-treated blood (40–45°C). Particularly good for isolating *S. pneumoniae* and *H. influenzae*;
- Hektoen enteric (HE) agar—Gram-negative selective used for distinguishing between *Salmonella* and *Shigella*. It contains peptone, as well as various other sugars. *Salmonella*/*Shigella* cannot use the latter but can use the former, alkalinizing the agar and turning the pH indicator blue. Other enteric bacteria use the latter in preference, producing acidic products and turning the pH indicator yellow/red. In addition, the presence of thiosulfate produces a black precipitate in the presence of hydrogen sulfide (H_2S)—which *Shigella* does not produce (appears green), but *Salmonella* does (appears black);
- xylose–lysine–deoxycholate (XLD) agar—also facilitates discrimination of *Salmonella* from *Shigella*, utilizing thiosulfate (as under HE agar) and differential use of the sugar xylose (*Shigella* appears red; *Salmonella* appears red with black centres; coliforms appear yellow/orange);
- mannitol salt agar (MSA)—a high level of salt (7.5–10%) selects Gram-positives, such as staphylococci, which are 'halophilic' (i.e. salt-loving). The presence of mannitol helps to separate *S. aureus* (can ferment mannitol, turning phenol red to yellow) from other staphylococci (small pink/red colonies);
- buffered charcoal yeast extract (BCYE) agar—selects for *Legionella pneumophila*;

- Thayer–Martin agar or New York City (NYC) agar—used to isolate pathogenic *Neisseria* spp. (*N. gonorrhoeae* and *Neisseria meningitidis*).
- Mueller–Hinton agar—contains beef infusion, peptone, and starch, and is used primarily for antibiotic susceptibility testing. It is non-selective and non-differential, and facilitates the diffusion of antibiotic from testing discs;
- cetrimide agar—used for selective isolation of *Pseudomonas aeruginosa*;
- Tinsdale agar—contains potassium tellurite, which can isolate *C. diphtheriae*. Löeffler's and Hoyle's tellurite agar are also useful for *C. diphtheriae*;
- Sabouraud agar—used to culture fungi. Its low pH (5.6) inhibits the growth of most bacteria. It contains dextrose and peptones. Chloramphenicol is commonly added for the purpose of inhibiting Gram-negative organisms. The growth of fungal structures, such as whiskers in the case of *Candida albicans*, facilitates identification.

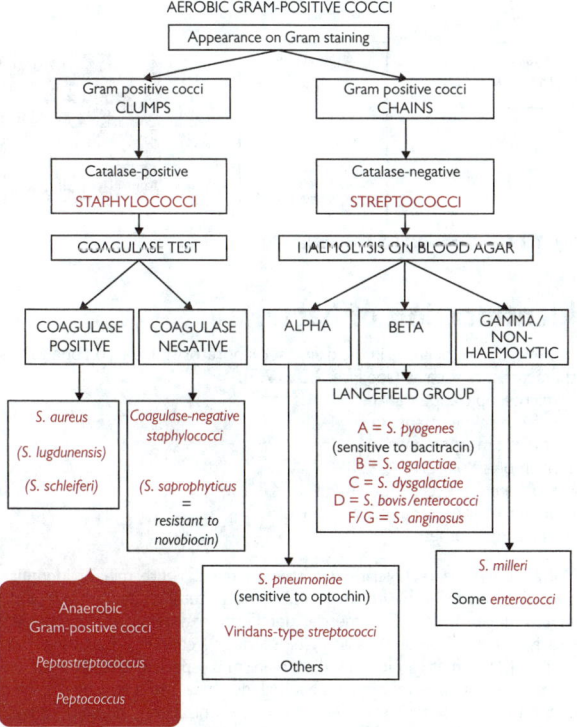

Fig. 7.2 Identification of Gram-positive cocci.

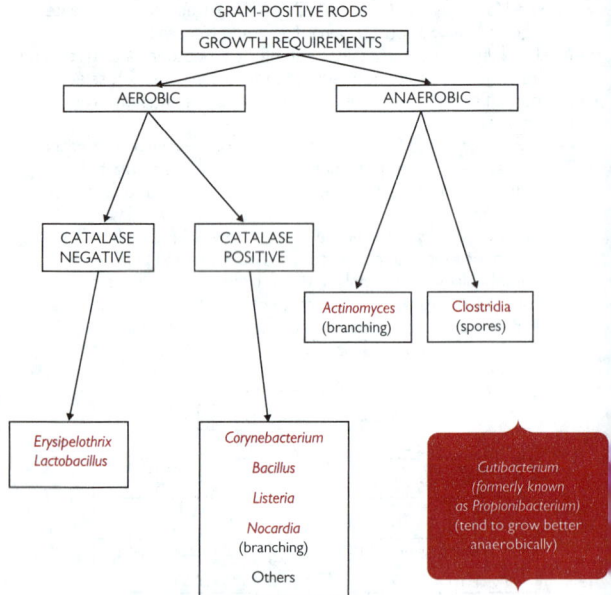

Fig. 7.3 Identification of Gram-positive rods.

Identification of bacteria

Identification of bacteria in the diagnostic laboratory is based on phenotypic characteristics such as (see Figs. 7.2 to 7.5):

- microscopic appearance;
- growth requirements;
- colonial morphology;
- haemolysis pattern;
- biochemical tests;
- antimicrobial susceptibility patterns;
- mass spectrometry.

Many laboratory technicians are able to make a preliminary identification to genus level, based on clinical data, cultural characteristics, and a limited range of tests. Commercial identification systems, such as the API® (Analytical Profile Index) system (bioMérieux), contain a battery of biochemical tests that can identify the organism to species level. The last few years have seen a revolution in bacterial identification, following the introduction of matrix-assisted laser desorption ionization time-of-flight mass spectroscopy (MALDI-TOF).

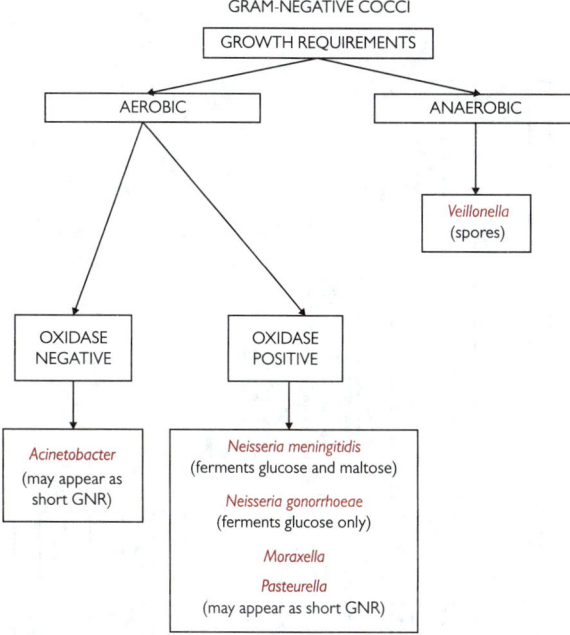

Fig. 7.4 Identification of Gram-negative cocci.

Microscopy

Staining and microscopic examination of samples or cultures reveal the size, shape, and arrangement of bacteria and the presence of inclusions (e.g. spores). The following stains are commonly used (for full details, see the UKHSA SMI 'Staining procedures', available at: ℘ www.gov.uk/governm ent/publications/smi-tp-39-staining-procedures

- **Gram stain**—a fixed slide is flooded with crystal violet (30s), followed by Lugol's iodine (30s), followed by rinsing with 95–100% ethanol or acetone, followed by counterstaining with 0.1% neutral red, safranin, or carbol fuchsin (2min). Gram-positive organisms stain deep blue/purple, and Gram-negative organisms stain pink/red.
- **Auramine stain**—this is used to identify mycobacteria in clinical specimens. It is considered more sensitive than the ZN stain. A heat-fixed slide is flooded with auramine–phenol (1:10) for 10min. It is rinsed with water and then decolorized with 1% acid–alcohol for 3–5min (until no further stain seeps from the film). It is rinsed and stained with 0.1% potassium permanganate for 15s. It is rinsed and allowed to air-dry before examination under fluorescence microscopy. AFB appear bright yellow/green against a dark background.
- **ZN stain**—this is used to identify mycobacteria in cultures and provides better morphological detail than an auramine stain.

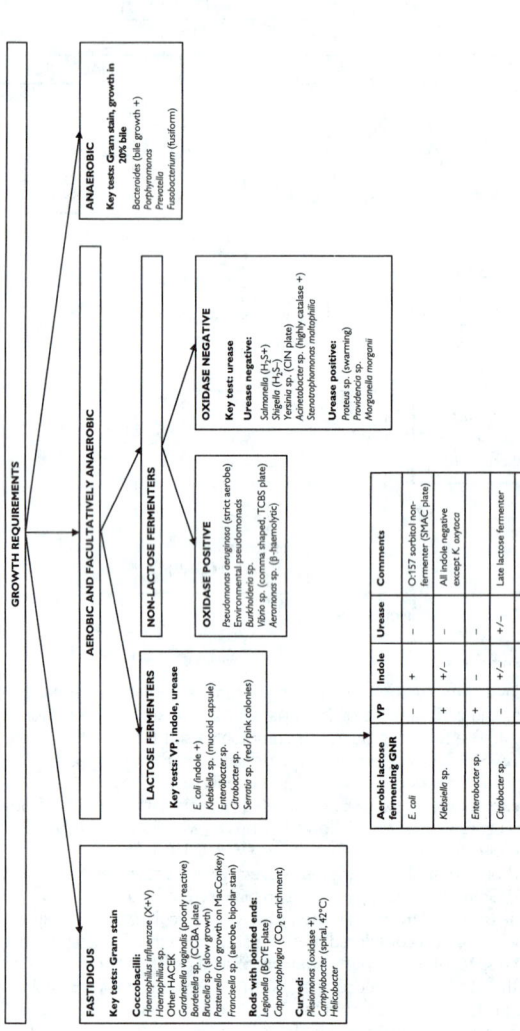

GROWTH REQUIREMENTS

GRAM-NEGATIVE RODS

FASTIDIOUS

Key tests: Gram stain

Coccobacilli:
Haemophilus influenzae (X+V)
Haemophilus sp.
Other HACEK
Gardnerella vaginalis (poorly reactive)
Bordetella sp. (CCBA plate)
Brucella sp. (slow growth)
Pasteurella (no growth on MacConkey)
Francisella sp. (aerobe, bipolar stain)

Rods with pointed ends:
Legionella (BCYE plate)
Capnocytophaga (CO₂ enrichment)

Curved:
Plesiomonas (oxidase +)
Campylobacter (spiral, 42°C)
Helicobacter

AEROBIC AND FACULTATIVELY ANAEROBIC

LACTOSE FERMENTERS

Key tests: VP, indole, urease

E. coli (indole +)
Klebsiella sp. (mucoid capsule)
Enterobacter sp.
Citrobacter sp.
Serratia sp. (red/pink colonies)

NON-LACTOSE FERMENTERS

OXIDASE POSITIVE

Pseudomonas aeruginosa (strict aerobe)
Environmental pseudomonads
Burkholderia sp.
Vibrio sp. (comma shaped, TCBS plate)
Aeromonas sp. (β-haemolytic)

OXIDASE NEGATIVE

Key test: urease

Urease negative:
Salmonella (H₂S+)
Shigella (H₂S−)
Yersinia sp. (CIN plate)
Acinetobacter sp. (highly catalase +)
Stenotrophomonas maltophilia

Urease positive:
Proteus sp. (swarming)
Providencia sp.
Morganella morganii

ANAEROBIC

Key tests: Gram stain, growth in 20% bile

Bacteroides (bile growth +)
Porphyromonas
Prevotella
Fusobacterium (fusiform)

Aerobic lactose fermenting GNR	VP	Indole	Urease	Comments
E. coli	−	+	−	O:157 sorbitol non-fermenter (SMAC plate)
Klebsiella sp.	+	+/−	+	All indole negative except K. oxytoca
Enterobacter sp.	+	−	−	
Citrobacter sp.	−	+/−	+/−	Late lactose fermenter
Serratia sp.	+	−	+	Late lactose fermenter

Fig. 7.5 Identification of Gram-negative rods.

A heat-fixed slide is flooded with strong carbol fuchsin and heated gently until it is just steaming. It is left to cool (3–5min), rinsed with water, and decolorized with a 3% acid–alcohol solution (5–7min, until the slide is faintly pink). The slide is rinsed with water and counterstained with 1% v/v methylene blue or malachite green (30s). It is allowed to air-dry before examination under oil immersion light microscopy. AFB appear red on a blue or green background. A modified ZN stain is used for identification of *Nocardia* spp. and cryptosporidia.

- **Nigrosin (India ink) stain**—this stain is used to identify *Cryptococcus neoformans* in clinical specimens. A drop of India ink is put on the slide, followed by a drop of the specimen, and mixed together. A coverslip is applied, and the slide is examined under light microscopy. *C. neoformans* is identified by a clear zone (capsule) around the organism.

Growth requirements

These can vary considerably and include:

- **atmosphere**—organisms can be divided into categories, according to their atmospheric requirements:
  - **strict aerobes**—grow only in the presence of oxygen;
  - **strict anaerobes**—grow only in the absence of oxygen;
  - **facultative organisms**—grow aerobically or anaerobically;
  - **microaerophilic organisms**—grow best in atmospheres with reduced oxygen concentration (e.g. 5–10% CO_2);
  - **capnophilic organisms**—require additional CO_2 for growth.
- **temperature**—organisms can also be differentiated by their temperature requirements:
  - **psychrophilic organisms**—grow at temperatures of 10–30°C;
  - **mesophilic organisms**—grow at temperatures of 30–40°C;
  - **thermophilic organisms**—grow at temperatures of 50–60°C;
  - most clinically encountered organisms are mesophilic.
- **nutrition**—some organisms grow readily on ordinary nutrient media, whereas others have particular nutritional requirements (e.g. *H. influenzae* requires specific growth factors such as factor X (haemin) and factor V (NAD)). Halophilic organisms require high salt concentrations.

Colonial morphology

Bacterial colonies of a single species, when grown on specific media under controlled conditions, are described by their characteristic size, shape, texture, and colour. Colonies may be flat or raised, smooth or irregular, and pigmented (e.g. *P. aeruginosa* is green/blue, *Serratia marcescens* is pink) or non-pigmented. Experienced laboratory technicians can often provisionally identify an organism using colonial appearance alone.

Haemolysis

Some organisms produce haemolysins that cause partial or complete lysis of red blood cells (RBCs) in blood-containing media. This haemolysis may be:

- β-haemolytic—a clear zone of complete haemolysis around the colony;
- α-haemolytic—a green zone of incomplete haemolysis due to reduction of haemoglobin in RBCs;
- non-haemolytic.

This feature is often used in the initial identification of streptococci.

Further information

For information on the identification of bacteria, see the UK SMIs, which are a comprehensive referenced collection of recommended algorithms and procedures for clinical microbiology (web search for 'UK SMI').

Biochemical tests

A variety of biochemical tests may be used for the identification of bacteria in the diagnostic laboratory. These may be performed manually, as part of a multi-test commercial kit (e.g. API®), or more commonly are performed via automated identification systems.

Catalase test

Catalase is an enzyme that facilitates the breakdown of H_2O_2 into water and oxygen. Many aerobic and facultatively anaerobic organisms are catalase-positive, whereas streptococci and enterococci are catalase-negative. H_2O_2 solution is drawn up into a capillary tube, and the tip is then touched onto a colony. Vigorous bubbling indicates the presence of catalase. NB media containing blood may produce a false-positive result.

Coagulase test

Coagulase is an enzyme that enables breakdown of fibrinogen to fibrin. This test is used to differentiate staphylococci. Coagulase exists in two forms: bound coagulase/clumping factor (detected by the slide coagulase test) and free coagulase (detected by the tube coagulase test).

Slide coagulase test

A colony is emulsified in a drop of distilled water on a slide. A loop or wire is dipped into plasma and then mixed into the bacterial suspension. A positive test result occurs if agglutination is seen within 10s.

Tube coagulase test

A colony is emulsified in a tube containing plasma and incubated at 37°C for 4h. A visible clot indicates a positive result. If negative at 4h, the tube should be reincubated overnight (MRSA can give a negative result at 4h).

Deoxyribonuclease (DNase) test

DNase is an enzyme that enables the degradation of DNA. This test is used to identify pathogenic staphylococci (e.g. *S. aureus*, *Staphylococcus schleiferi*) that produce large quantities of extracellular DNase. A colony is streaked onto a DNase plate and incubated at 37°C for 18–24h. The following day, the plate is flooded with hydrochloric acid—unhydrolysed DNA is precipitated, producing a white opacity in the agar. Cultures surrounded by a clear zone (hydrolysed DNA) are DNase-positive. NB some strains of MRSA are DNase-negative, and *Staphylococcus epidermidis* may be weakly positive.

Optochin test

This test is used to differentiate *S. pneumoniae* (optochin-sensitive) from other α-haemolytic streptococci (optochin-resistant). Optochin (ethylhydrocupreine hydrochloride) is a chemical that causes lysis of the cell wall of *S. pneumoniae*. An optochin disc is placed in the centre of the bacterial inoculum and incubated at 37°C in 5% CO_2 for 18–24h. A zone of inhibition of ≥5mm indicates a positive result.

Aesculin hydrolysis test

This test is used to differentiate enterococci (aesculin-positive) from streptococci (aesculin-negative). It tests the ability of the organism to hydrolyse aesculin to aesculetin and glucose in the presence of 10–40% bile. Aesculetin combines with ferric ions in the medium to form a black complex. The organism is inoculated onto a bile aesculin plate or slope, and incubated at 37°C for 24h. The presence of a dark brown or black halo indicates a positive result.

Indole test

The indole test is used to differentiate *Enterobacterales*. It detects the ability of an organism to produce indole from the amino acid tryptophan. A coloured product is obtained when indole is combined with certain aldehydes. There are two methods.

Spot indole test

A piece of filter paper is moistened with the indole reagent, and a colony is smeared onto the surface. A green/blue colour indicates a positive result.

Tube indole test

The organism is emulsified in a peptone broth and incubated at 37°C for 24h. A volume of 0.5mL of Kovac's reagent is added; a pink colour in the top layer indicates a positive result.

ONPG (β-galactosidase) test

This test is used as an aid to differentiate *Enterobacterales* (see Box 7.4). Two enzymes—permease and β galactosidase—are required for lactose fermentation. Late lactose fermenters do not possess permease but do have β-galactosidase. Tubes containing *o*-nitrophenyl-β-*D*-galactopyranoside (ONPG) are inoculated with the organism and incubated at 37°C for 24h. If present, β-galactosidase hydrolyses ONPG to produce galactose and *o*-nitrophenol, a yellow compound.

Urease test

This test is used to differentiate urease-positive *Proteus* spp. from the other *Enterobacterales*. Some strains of *Enterobacter* and *Klebsiella* spp. are urease-positive. Inoculate a slope of Christensen's medium with the test organism at 37°C for 24h. A pink/purple colour indicates a positive result.

Oxidase test

This test determines if an organism has the cytochrome oxidase enzyme and is used as an aid in the differentiation of *Pseudomonas*, *Neisseria*, *Moraxella*, *Campylobacter*, and *Pasteurella* spp. (oxidase-positive). Cytochrome oxidase catalyses the transport of electrons from donor compounds (e.g. NADH) to electron acceptors (usually oxygen). The test reagent *N, N, N′, N′* -tetramethyl-*p*-phenylenediamine dihydrochloride acts as an artificial electron acceptor for the enzyme oxidase. The oxidized reagent forms the coloured compound indophenol blue.

Box 7.4 Nomenclature of enteric Gram-negative rods

These were previously referred to as *Enterobacteriaceae*, but as they make up seven different families, the correct nomenclature is *Enterobacterales* as this refers to the order. In practice, both terms are still used interchangeably. Do not confuse with the species *Enterobacter*.

Further information

For information on the identification of bacteria, see the UK SMIs, which are a comprehensive referenced collection of recommended algorithms and procedures for clinical microbiology (web search for 'UK SMI').

Automated diagnostics

Automated identification systems allow rapid identification ± antibiotic susceptibility testing of organisms. Different methodologies have strengths and weaknesses. Selection for use in a diagnostic laboratory depends on factors such as assay throughput, turnaround times, labour, and compatibility with existing systems. The benefits include reduction in labour, faster reporting, and reduced human transcription errors (systems can link directly to laboratory databases). Problems include inoculum preparation (over-/under-inoculation or missing a mixed culture), the ability to test only a certain range of organisms (slow-growing, fastidious, or heavily mucoid organisms may need to be processed manually), culture conditions, and data entry. Currently available methods include the following.

VITEK® 2 (bioMérieux)

The unknown organism is automatically placed in suspension at an appropriate dilution and inoculated onto a small card that has 64 microwells. Each well contains identification biochemical substrates or antimicrobial dilutions. After inoculation and incubation, the system measures turbidity and colour changes within the card wells. Results are available within 4–24h. There are several caveats to the interpretation of certain organism/antibiotic combinations, but overall the system is accurate, rapid, and safe.

Phoenix™ (Becton Dickinson)

Panels are inoculated manually and thus may require a specific organism dilution for accuracy. It uses a colorimetric oxidation–reduction indicator for susceptibility testing, and several fluorometric and colorimetric indicators for identification. Results are available in 4–16h.

MALDI-TOF

MALDI-TOF is a novel technique used for the identification of bacteria or fungi. The organism is mixed with a suitable matrix material and irradiated with a laser pulse. The resulting hot plume is accelerated in an electric field and enters the flight tube, in which different molecules are separated according to their mass-to-charge ratio, reaching the detector at different times. The mass spectra generated are analysed and compared with stored profiles of known organisms. It is normal practice in a routine laboratory to set a 'cut-off' for acceptable identification. Some species are difficult to distinguish, notably α-haemolytic streptococci. Mixed cultures can be challenging, and *Shigella* cannot be differentiated from *E. coli*. Despite these limitations, MALDI has been a significant advance in diagnostic bacteriology.

Next-generation sequencing

(➔ See Molecular typing methods, pp. 256–8.) The cost and speed of DNA sequencing are falling rapidly. Although still largely a research tool, it is certain that next-generation sequencing (NGS) will begin to replace traditional culture-based diagnostics for many purposes in the near future.

Molecular organism identification

Real-time or quantitative PCR

Real-time or quantitative PCR (qPCR) is used to amplify and simultaneously quantify a targeted DNA/RNA molecule, as the reaction progresses. The process involves extraction, amplification, and detection. Detection is either by non-specific fluorescent dyes that intercalate with any dsDNA or by fluorescent marker-labelled DNA probes specific to the reaction concerned. The DNA/RNA quantity is inferred either by reference to a standard control curve (absolute) or relative to an internal control within the reaction (e.g. the target is present at four times the quantity of the internal control).

Multiplex PCR

Multiplex PCR allows the detection of multiple PCR targets in a single reaction. Multiplex reactions have been developed for specific clinical syndromes (e.g. respiratory panel for influenza A (H1N1, swine flu), influenza B, respiratory syncytial virus (RSV), human metapneumovirus, parainfluenza 1–3, Legionella).

16S rRNA PCR

16S rRNA PCR—16S rRNA is a component of the 30S subunit of the bacterial ribosome. The genes coding it are highly conserved but contain hypervariable genus- or species-specific regions. Thus, 'universal' primers allow gene amplification. This is then sequenced and compared to known sequences for genus/species-level identification. Advantages include diagnosis of fastidious or unculturable organisms (e.g. *Tropheryma whipplei*), or identification of a pathogen after antibiotic therapy. 16S rRNA PCR may be negative on a culture-positive specimen—this may be due to low levels of the organism below the detection threshold of the assay or the presence of PCR inhibitors. Certain bacteria can be difficult to identify, because they share most of their 16S sequences (e.g. *E. coli* from *Shigella*, members of the *Streptococcus milleri* complex, *S. pneumoniae* from *Streptococcus oralis*).

18S rRNA PCR

18S rRNA PCR (pan-fungal PCR)—18S rRNA is the eukaryotic homologue of 16S rRNA in prokaryotes. PCR of 18S sequences allows the classification of most *Candida* spp. and many other fungi.

Molecular typing methods

Epidemiological typing of bacteria facilitates infection control investigations and surveillance (i.e. to monitor vaccine effectiveness). Traditional methods are based on phenotypic characteristics (e.g. antibiogram, serotype, phage type). The development of a variety of molecular typing methods has enabled genetic comparison of strains, providing improved discrimination.

Pulsed-field gel electrophoresis

Pulsed-field gel electrophoresis (PFGE) has been considered the gold standard method for typing bacterial isolates and is still widely used. A highly purified genomic DNA sample is cleaved with a restriction endonuclease that recognizes infrequently occurring restriction sites in the genome of bacterial species. The resulting restriction fragments can be separated on an agarose gel by 'pulsed-field' electrophoresis, in which the orientation of the electric field across the gel is changed periodically. The separated DNA fragments can be visualized on the gel as bands. Limitations—technically demanding, labour-intensive, time-consuming, may lack the resolution to distinguish bands of nearly identical size, and analysis of results is prone to subjectivity.

Amplified fragment length polymorphism

Genomic DNA is cut with two restriction enzymes, and double-stranded adaptors are ligated to the sticky ends of the restriction fragments. A subset of the fragments are amplified by PCR, using primers complementary to the adaptor sequence, the restriction site sequence, and a number of additional nucleotides from the end of the unknown DNA template. Amplified fragments are separated and visualized on gels. Analysis enables the determination of genetic relatedness amongst bacterial isolates. Amplified fragment length polymorphism (AFLP) is at least as discriminatory as PFGE, and is reproducible and portable. However, its major limitations are that it is labour-intensive and expensive.

Random amplification of polymorphic DNA and arbitrarily primed polymerase chain reaction (RAPD PCR)

Random amplification of polymorphic DNA (RAPD) does not require any specific knowledge of the DNA sequence of the target organism. Short arbitrary primers (usually 10 bases) are used in a reaction conducted at low, non-stringent annealing temperatures, allowing the hybridization of multiple mismatched sequences. If the distance between two primer binding sites is within 0.1–3kb, an amplicon may be generated. The number and positions of primer binding sites are unique to a particular strain. Amplicons can be analysed by gel or DNA sequencing. RAPD is less discriminatory than PFGE but is widely used, because it is simple, inexpensive, and rapid. The main limitation is low intra- and inter-laboratory reproducibility (due to very low annealing temperatures, and differences in reagents, protocols, and machines).

Repetitive element polymerase chain reaction (rep-PCR)

This method uses primers that hybridize to non-coding intergenic repetitive sequences scattered across the genome. DNA between adjacent repetitive elements is amplified using PCR, and multiple amplicons can be produced. The sizes of these amplicons are then electrophoretically characterized, and the banding patterns are compared to determine the genetic relatedness between the isolates. It is quick, cheap, and discriminatory. Limitations— lacks reproducibility, which may result from variability in reagents and gel electrophoresis systems.

Multiple locus variable-number tandem repeat analysis

Bacterial genomes possess many regions with nucleotide repeats. Variable-number tandem repeats (VNTRs) are repeating patterns of one or more nucleotides occurring adjacent to each other (e.g. ATTCATTCATTC) and show variations between species. Multiple locus variable-number tandem repeat analysis (MLVA) types an organism by differences in the number of tandem repeats at different loci. PCR of the VNTR loci is followed by sizing of the PCR products, allowing calculation of the number of repeats at each locus, creating an MVLA profile.

Single locus sequence typing

Single locus sequence typing (SLST) uses sequence variation within a single gene to distinguish bacterial isolates (e.g. spa typing (*S. aureus* protein A) for *S. aureus*). Not as discriminatory as other methods such as PFGE or multilocus sequence typing (MLST).

Multilocus sequence typing

A total of 450–500bp of 7–8 housekeeping genes are amplified by PCR and sequenced. For each locus, unique sequences (alleles) are assigned arbitrary numbers. Based on the combination of alleles, the sequence type is determined. MLST is unambiguous and reproducible, and has an internationally standardized nomenclature. Allele sequences and sequence typing profiles are available in central databases (⌗ https://pubmlst.org). Main disadvantages of MLST—costly, labour-intensive, and may not be sufficiently discriminatory for outbreak investigations.

Comparative genomic hybridization

A collection of DNA probes attached in an ordered fashion to a solid surface (microarray) is hybridized to DNA extracted from a pathogen. The probes on the array may be PCR amplicons (>200bp) or oligonucleotides (up to 70 mers). Successful hybridization events are measured by a scanner. Routine application of this technique is hindered by the high costs of materials and the specialized equipment needed for the tests.

Whole-genome sequencing

WGS sequences the entire (or near entire) genome of organisms much more rapidly and at a much lower cost than traditional sequencing methods. Millions of short-sequence reads (35–700bp in length) are produced, and either mapped to a reference genome or assembled to generate the genome. This enables genomic comparison at a nucleotide level and is much more discriminatory than other typing methods. Analysis includes:
- evolution of strains over time to determine the mutation rate, or the molecular clock;

- comparison of strains to determine the level of genetic similarity. This will vary between different organisms, depending on their molecular clock;
- interrogation of individual genomes to identify the presence/absence of genes associated with antimicrobial resistance or specific clinical phenotypes.

WGS has been used to investigate outbreaks of infections in both hospital and community settings, and rapidly diagnose multidrug-resistant (MDR) organisms (e.g. extensively drug-resistant (XDR)-TB). Cost limits routine clinical use, but this is falling rapidly. It is likely that this technology will replace many of the previously discussed typing methods in the near future.

Quality assurance and accreditation

A total quality management (TQM) system ensures that microbiology laboratories provide a prompt, quality-assured, and clinically appropriate service to its users. This is done through a process of quality planning, which is the part of quality management focused on setting quality objectives and specifying necessary operational processes and related resources to fulfil quality objectives. The main components of a quality management system are:
- written quality objectives consistent with the quality policy;
- a quality manual which is reviewed and updated as required;
- a quality manager responsible for implementation and maintenance of the quality management system;
- document control;
- control of process and quality records, according to current regulations;
- control of clinical material, according to current regulations;
- an annual review of the laboratory's quality management system by the laboratory management.

Quality assurance

The total process whereby the quality of laboratory reports can be guaranteed. A comprehensive quality assurance system includes provision and control of standard operating procedures (SOPs)—education and training, planned maintenance and calibration of equipment, and monitoring of turn-around times.

Internal quality control

The processes carried out to check that media, reagents, and equipment are performing within specifications.

Internal quality assurance

Internal quality assurance (IQA) is usually measured by routine reprocessing of a sample. By assessing two results from the same sample, any discrepancies can be investigated, and, if necessary, practice can be changed to improve the consistency of that particular laboratory test. Part of the laboratory internal quality control (IQC) procedures.

External quality assessment

Provision by an external body of a specimen of known, but undisclosed, content for analysis. External quality assessment (EQA) is not a substitute for other components of the quality system, and, in particular, EQA cannot replace IQC. The National External Quality Assessment Service for Microbiology (NEQAS; available at: ℘ https://ukneqasmicro.org.uk) was established in 1971 and is recognized as a major contributor to quality assurance in clinical diagnostic microbiology. The scheme provides participants with a wide range of specimens and constructive feedback. Participants can monitor the effectiveness of their quality assurance measures, and detect and remedy problems, thus allowing continuing quality improvement.

Laboratory accreditation

Clinical Pathology Accreditation (CPA) (UK) Ltd was established by various professional organizations, such as the Institute of Biomedical Science (IBMS) and the Royal College of Pathologists, together with the private health sector and the DH. CPA is now a subsidiary of United Kingdom Accreditation Service (UKAS; available at: ℘ https://www.ukas.com) and is managing the transition of all CPA-accredited laboratories to the internationally recognized ISO 15189:2012 standard.

Pathology networks

Lord Carter of Coles published his Independent Review of Pathology Services for the DH in 2008. His recommendations suggested that the standard district general hospital with a full range of services would be increasingly unsustainable. He proposed consolidation of acute trust pathology services into managed pathology networks. Arrangements for this 'hub-and-spoke' model vary by specialty and by region, with some 'spoke' microbiology laboratories retaining 'hot labs' for tests needed within 4h, but with many having no on-site microbiology laboratory. Whereas the last few years have seen some service aggregation (e.g. single laboratories for multi-site hospital trusts, within London where hospitals are closely located), there has been nothing like the scale of consolidation originally envisioned.

Overview of Gram-positive cocci

Gram-positive cocci (GPC) are commonly isolated from clinical specimens. They are widely distributed in the environment and are found as commensals of the skin, mucous membranes, and other body sites. Because of their ubiquitous nature, recovery of these organisms from specimens should always be interpreted in the context of the clinical presentation. The two medically most important groups are staphylococci and streptococci. Please see Fig 7.2 for identification of Gram-positive cocci.

Classification

The classification of GPC is based on a combination of phenotypic and genotypic characteristics, and has changed over time as a result of genetic sequencing data. The current classification of some medically important GPC is as follows:

- family *Staphylococcaceae*, genus *Staphylococcus*;
- family *Streptococcaceae*, genus *Streptococcus*;
- family *Enterococcaceae*, genus *Enterococcus*;
- family *Leuconostocaceae*, genus *Leuconostoc*;
- family *Micrococcaceae*, genus *Micrococcus** and genus *Rothia*;
- family *Lactobacillaceae*, genus *Pediococcus*;
- family *Aerococcaceae*, genus *Aerococcus* and genus *Abiotrophia*;
- family *Carnobacteriaceae*, genus *Alloiococcus*;
- family *Peptococcaceae*, genus *Peptococcus*;
- family *Peptostreptococcaceae*, genus *Peptostreptococcus*;
- other anaerobic cocci (e.g. genus *Anaerococcus*, genus *Finegoldia*, genus *Parvimonas*, and genus *Peptoniphilus*).

Staphylococci

- Staphylococci are non-motile, non-spore-forming, catalase-positive GPC.
- They occur as single cells, pairs, tetrads, or grape-like clusters (commonest).
- Most species are facultative anaerobes, except *S. aureus* subspecies *anaerobius* and *Staphylococcus saccharolyticus*, which are anaerobic.
- Staphylococci are normally found on the skin and mucous membranes of animals. In some cases, their location may be very specific (e.g. *Staphylococcus capitis* subspecies *capitis* on the scalp or *Staphylococcus auricularis* in the external auditory canal).
- *S. aureus*, *S. epidermidis*, *Staphylococcus lugdunensis*, and *Staphylococcus saprophyticus* are the main human pathogens.
- They may be differentiated on the basis of the coagulase test (see Fig. 7.2) into coagulase-positive (e.g. *S. aureus*) and coagulase-negative (coagulase-negative staphylococci (CoNS), e.g. *S. epidermidis*).
- In addition, *S. aureus* produces DNase, whereas other staphylococci are usually DNase-negative.
- There are around 50 species of CoNS.

Streptococci

- Streptococci are non-sporing, non-motile organisms, and catalase-negative GPC that grow in pairs and chains.
- Some species are capsulated.
- They are facultative anaerobes and may require enriched media to grow.
- Streptococci are subdivided on the basis of their 'classic' appearance on horse BA into α-, β-, and non-haemolytic streptococci.
- The α-haemolytic streptococci (incomplete haemolysis on BA, resulting in a greenish tinge) include *S. pneumoniae* (➜ see *Streptococcus pneumoniae*, pp. 273–5) and the viridans streptococci.

---

* NB some *Micrococcus* have been renamed Kocuria (➜ see Micrococcus species and Kocuria, p. 271).

- The β-haemolytic streptococci (complete haemolysis/clear zone on BA) are grouped on the basis of their Lancefield carbohydrate antigens. The medically important ones are groups A, B, C, F, and G.
- The enterococci (*Enterococcus faecalis* and others; ➔ see Enterococci, pp. 275–7) were originally called *Streptococcus faecalis* and often react with Group D antisera, but are now a separate genus.
- Non-haemolytic streptococci make up the remainder and include the viridans (*Streptococcus mutans*, *Streptococcus salivarius*, *Streptococcus anginosus*, *Streptococcus mitis*, and *Streptococcus sanguinis* groups), and anaerobic and nutritionally variant streptococci.
- For a comprehensive review of taxonomic and nomenclature changes of the streptococci, see Facklam (2002).[1]

Other Gram-positive cocci

These include: *Peptococcus*, *Peptostreptococcus*, *Leuconostoc*, *Pedioccoccus*, *Abiotrophia*, *Micrococcus*, and *Stomatococcus*.

References

1 Facklam R. What happened to the streptococci: overview of taxonomic and nomenclature changes. *Clin Microbiol Rev.* 2002;**15**:613–30.

Staphylococcus aureus

S. aureus is a facultatively anaerobic, non-motile, non-spore-forming, catalase-positive, coagulase-positive, Gram-positive coccus. It is a major human pathogen and can cause a wide variety of infections, ranging from superficial skin infections to severe life-threatening conditions (e.g. toxic shock syndrome (TSS)).

Epidemiology

S. aureus is a skin colonizer and is found in the anterior nares of 10–40% of people. Chronic carriage is associated with an increased risk of infection (e.g. in haemodialysis patients). Nasal carriage has contributed to the persistence and spread of MRSA.

Pathogenesis

S. aureus possesses a wide array of virulence factors, including:

- **ability to form a biofilm**—this is an extracellular polysaccharide network produced by staphylococci (and other organisms) that results in colonization and persistence on prosthetic material. Polysaccharide intercellular adhesin (PIA) is synthesized by the *ica* operon and forms a key part of the biofilm, alongside teichoic acids and extracellular DNA (eDNA);
- **capsule**—>90% of *S. aureus* isolates have a capsule which interferes with function of phagocytic cells. Eleven serotypes have been reported;
- **surface adhesins** (also known as microbial surface components recognizing adhesive matrix molecules (MSCRAMMs))—enables the organism to adhere to host extracellular matrix. These include protein A, clumping factors A and B, collagen-binding protein, fibronectin-binding protein, serine aspartate repeat protein, plasmin-sensitive protein, and surface proteins A to K;

- **peptidoglycan**—is the scaffold for anchoring the MSCRAMMs. It also triggers the release of cytokines. Modification of peptidoglycan synthesis is associated with antimicrobial resistance;
- **techoic and lipotechoic acids**—these are components of the cell wall. Lipotechoic acids trigger release of cytokines by macrophages;
- **coagulase**—an enzyme which converts fibrinogen to fibrin in the plasma, which interferes with phagocytic function of immune cells. S. aureus also produces several enzymes which aid in migration through tissues, including **hyaluronidase** and **staphylokinase**, which dissolve hyaluronic acid and fibrin, respectively;
- **exotoxins**—enzymes secreted by S. aureus, which contribute to its virulence. They include **haemolysins** (α, β, γ, δ), which lyse erythrocytes by inducing a pore in the cell membrane;
- **Panton–Valentine leucocidin** (PVL)—is a further haemolysin encoded by two genes (lukS and lukF) that are carried on a mobile phage (φSLT). PVL-producing strains are associated with furunculosis and severe haemorrhagic pneumonia.
- **exfoliative toxins** (ETs)—ETA and ETB are encoded by the eta and etb genes, respectively. They are proteases which cause skin desquamation such as in staphylococcal epidermal necrolysis (also known as staphylococcal scalded skin syndrome (SSSS)) (➔ see Staphylococcal epidermal necrolysis, pp. 856–7);
- **superantigens**—this group includes TSS toxin (TSST)-1 and staphylococcal enterotoxins (SEs). These toxins bind non-specifically to T cells, resulting in non-selective activation and release of proinflammatory cytokines. TSST-1 is associated with TSS, whereas SEs are associated with food poisoning;
- **pathogenicity (genomic) islands**—these are part of the genome acquired by horizontal gene transfer, and harbour virulence and drug resistance genes. They vary in size from 15 to 70kb—examples include SaPI1 and SaPI2, which carry the gene for TSST-1;
- **small colony variants**—slow-growing subpopulations with atypical colony morphology and unusual biochemical characteristics (e.g. coagulase tube test positive only after 18h, thus harder to identify). They can be less susceptible to antibiotics, and implicated in persistent infections by downregulating genes for metabolism and virulence, while upregulating those for persistence and biofilm formation.

Clinical features

S. aureus can cause a wide spectrum of clinical infections, including:
- skin and soft tissue infections (e.g. impetigo, folliculitis, hidradenitis, mastitis, wound infections, erysipelas, cellulitis, pyomyositis, necrotizing fasciitis);
- bone and joint infections (e.g. septic arthritis, osteomyelitis, discitis);
- systemic infections (e.g. bacteraemia, endocarditis, meningitis);
- prosthetic device-related (e.g. IVC-associated, pacemaker infections, prosthetic joint infections (PJIs), etc.);
- toxin-mediated disease (e.g. food poisoning, staphylococcal epidermal necrolysis, TSS).

Diagnosis

- In some cases (e.g. skin and soft tissue infections), the diagnosis is clinical. In others, appropriate samples (e.g. pus, tissue, blood) should be submitted to the laboratory for microscopy, culture, and sensitivity (MC&S).
- **Gram staining**—GPC in clusters.
- **Culture on BA or liquid media**—growth usually occurs within 18–24h on simple media where they may appear grey or golden yellow. Prolonged incubation may detect small colony variants.
- **Biochemical tests**—catalase-positive, coagulase-positive, DNase-positive, and novobiocin-sensitive.
- **Identification**—API® Staph and automated methods (i.e. VITEK®, MALDI). Selective agar, such as MSA, can encourage growth of staphylococcal species (fermentation of mannitol by staphylococci turns the agar yellow—due to the indicator phenol red).
- Typing methods can be useful in epidemiological studies or suspected outbreaks. Methods include PFGE, MLST, or spa typing.
- Molecular diagnosis (e.g. 16S rRNA PCR, or *mecA* gene (for meticillin resistance) and PVL gene PCR).

Treatment

- Treatment depends on the type of infection and drug susceptibility of the organism. Control and removal of any source are vital (e.g. cannula).
- Flucloxacillin IV should be used as first choice for MSSA bacteraemia. Alternatives include cefazolin in patients with a non-anaphylaxis hypersensitivity.
- Vancomycin or daptomycin IV for suspected *S. aureus* infections where MRSA is a possibility or in penicillin anaphylactic patients. Vancomycin is associated with poorer outcomes in MSSA bacteraemia when compared to β-lactams.
- Other active agents include clindamycin, teicoplanin, and linezolid.
- *S. aureus* bacteraemia should be evaluated for a source. Echocardiography is advised, as 20–30% of bacteraemias are associated with endocarditis. Clearance BCs are recommended to ensure microbiological cure.
- Aminoglycosides exhibit synergism with β-lactams; however, routine combination with flucloxacillin or vancomycin for treatment of *S. aureus* endocarditis is not recommended. Unlike streptococcal endocarditis, studies have shown little clinical benefit—and an increased incidence of renal dysfunction.
- Duration of treatment depends on the source—7 days for skin and soft tissue infections, and up to 6 weeks for endocarditis. For short-lived bacteraemia with a removable source (e.g. IVC), 2 weeks of treatment after source control is adequate, presuming no further growth of *S. aureus* on subsequent BCs.

The ARREST trial

(See Box 7.5.)

> **Box 7.5 The ARREST trial**
>
> The adjunctive rifampicin for *Staphylococcus aureus* bacteraemia (ARREST) trial was a multicentre, double-blind randomized controlled trial published in 2018. It showed that there was no benefit from adjunctive rifampicin in meticillin-sensitive *S. aureus* (MSSA) or MRSA bacteraemias without a deep focus with standard backbone antibiotics (usually flucloxacillin and vancomycin, respectively) in terms of mortality or duration of bacteraemia. There was a modest, but statistically significant, reduction in recurrence of *S. aureus* bacteraemias with deep foci with adjunctive rifampcin, though its overall clinical significance is uncertain.

Prevention

- Prevention of *S. aureus* infections is based on bacterial decolonization of carriers with local antiseptics (e.g. nasal mupirocin and chlorhexidine soap). This is routinely performed on MRSA carriers. MSSA decolonization is performed in some high-risk settings (e.g. dialysis units). Vaccines—a subject of ongoing research, with the aim of reducing bacteraemia rates in those at high risk (e.g. haemodialysis patients). None in use outside of clinical trials.

Meticillin-resistant *Staphylococcus aureus*

MRSA was first detected in 1961, a few months after meticillin was introduced into clinical practice. However, it was not until the 1980s that endemic strains of MRSA with MDR became a global nosocomial problem.

Mechanism of resistance

MRSA strains are resistant to all β-lactams due to alteration to PBP2 (penicillin-binding protein 2). PBPs are peptidase enzymes which catalyse the final transpeptidation reactions during cell wall synthesis. The resistance is due to the *mecA* gene that encodes the PBP2 protein, which has a low-affinity for β-lactams (known as PBP2a). *mecA* is usually located on a mobile genetic element (MGE) called SCC-*mec* (staphylococcal cassette chromosome). It is believed the *mec* gene was acquired from CoNS—some MRSA strains have also acquired other virulence and resistance genes from CoNS. There are at least 12 major SCC-*mec* clones that have been identified, defined by the class of the *mecA* gene and the type of *Ccr* (cassette chromosome recombinase) complex. SCC-*mec* types I to III are usually found in healthcare settings, whereas types IV and V are commoner in the community. The community variants used to be sensitive to alternative antibiotic classes, but they have become increasingly resistant in recent years.

Epidemiology

- Risk factors for MRSA include recent hospitalization (particularly intensive care unit (ICU) stay), long-term facility residence (including nursing home residents and prisoners), recent surgery, indwelling catheters (particularly hamodialysis patients), increasing age, prior antibiotics, HIV infection, and IV drug use.
- Healthcare-acquired MRSA (HA-MRSA) rates vary in different parts of the world. During the 1990s, the UK saw an emergence of two epidemic MRSA strains (EMRSA 15 and 16), resulting in a year-on-year increase in MRSA bacteraemias. These strains were also resistant to erythromycin and ciprofloxacin. In 2002, between 25% and 50% of *S. aureus* bacteraemias were due to MRSA in the UK, Ireland, France, Italy, and Portugal. Finland, Denmark, and the Netherlands had very low rates (<5%). MRSA rates in the UK fell to <10% of *S. aureus* bacteraemias in 2013/14, as a result of good infection control practice and national mandatory surveillance, though rates have been relatively static since then. In 2017/18, ~7% of *S. aureus* bacteraemias were caused by MRSA.
- Community-acquired MRSA (CA-MRSA) is a significant issue in the USA, due, in part, to the widespread dissemination of a specific clone USA300. While this has been identified in a number of European countries, it exists only at low levels. Its success in the USA relates to its transmissibility and the presence of other virulence factors such as PVL.

Clinical features

- HA-MRSA (defined as that occurring >48h after hospital admission) and community onset HA-MRSA (that occurring within 12 months of exposure to healthcare, e.g. dialysis, residence in a care home) cause similar infections to MSSA (➜ see *Staphylococcus aureus*, pp. 261–4). However, patients have higher mortality and longer inpatient stays, and thus cost the healthcare system more than those with MSSA infection (➜ see Chapter 6).
- CA-MRSA was originally seen in people with a previous history of hospitalization or who were related to healthcare workers (HCWs). The emergence of the USA300 clone in the USA was associated with a rise in skin and soft tissue infections in young, healthy individuals. There have also been community outbreaks of CA-MRSA in settings such as sports teams, day-care centres, prison inmates and guards, and men who have sex with men (MSM). CA-MRSA has evolved from community MSSA, rather than HA-MRSA, and is often PVL toxin-positive.

Laboratory diagnosis of MRSA

- Conventional methods—chromogenic selective MRSA agar is recommended if direct plating of screening samples is used. A presumptive positive result is available after 24h of incubation but should be confirmed as MRSA due to relatively low specificity (see below). There are multiple commercial chromogenic products available. Enrichment in 2.5% sodium chloride (NaCl) nutrient broth prior to plating on selective media may increase the diagnostic rate but increases the time for diagnosis.

- Molecular detection of the *mecA* gene—commercial systems are available that can detect MRSA directly from screening swabs within 2–3h via PCR. Some may fail if there are polymorphisms in the conserved regions of the SCC-*mec* region.
- Detection of a presumptive MRSA strain should be followed by full identification by *S. aureus* and resistance testing. Oxacillin-susceptibility disc testing tends to be affected by test conditions; thus, cefoxitin disc testing is considered the most accurate phenotypic test as it is also a more potent inducer of *mecA* expression. Criteria for meticillin resistance (European Committee on Antimicrobial Susceptibility Testing (EUCAST))—oxacillin minimum inhibitory concentration (MIC) >2mg/L or cefoxitin MIC >4mg/L.
- Isolates with suspected toxin-mediated diseases (e.g. PVL) should be submitted to a reference laboratory for PCR.

Treatment of MRSA

- UK isolates are so far susceptible to glycopeptides (e.g. vancomycin, teicoplanin). There are concerns about an upward 'creep' in vancomycin MIC (attributed to a thicker cell wall), and serum levels should be monitored during therapy, with current practice tending towards a target vancomycin trough of >15mg/L (particularly for *S. aureus* bacteraemia).
- Daptomycin has evidence for its use in complicated skin/soft tissue infections, right-sided endocarditis, and MRSA bacteraemia. It should not be used for pneumonia (it is inhibited by pulmonary surfactant). Daptomycin MIC may increase during therapy, which can lead to microbiological failure—repeat susceptibility testing is important, if therapy is prolonged and there is evidence of persistent infection.
- There is variable susceptibility to trimethoprim, rifampicin, tetracycline, doxycycline, fusidic acid, aminoglycosides, and nitrofurantoin (treatment of UTIs only). These may provide alternative treatment choices if PO therapy or a second agent is required.
- Linezolid has activity against MRSA and may be used to treat MRSA pneumonia. It also has anti-toxin effects for PVL infection (➔ see Staphylococcus aureus, pp. 261–4).
- New cephalosporins have activity against MRSA such as ceftaroline.

Infection control issues

The main strategies to control MRSA infection are screening and decolonization, isolation/cohorting of patients, appropriate hand hygiene by HCWs, and effective cleaning of shared equipment.

Glycopeptide resistance in *Staphylococcus aureus*

Mechanism of resistance

The mechanisms of vancomycin resistance in *S. aureus* are:
- an increase in cell wall turnover that leads to an increase of non-cross-linked D-alanyl-D-alanine side chains that bind vancomycin outside the cell wall and inhibit binding to target peptides;

- transfer of the enterococcal *vanA* determinant from *Enterococcus* spp. to *S. aureus*. This allows synthesis of an alternative terminal peptide in the cell wall (D–ala–D–lac) in preference to D–ala–D–ala, which inhibits vancomycin binding.

Intermediate resistance

Strains of *S. aureus* with reduced susceptibility to glycopeptides have been reported in several countries. These organisms have been termed vancomycin-intermediate (VISA) or resistant *S. aureus* (VRSA). The Clinical and Laboratory Standards Institute (CLSI) breakpoints, upon which the definitions are based, were reduced in 2006, in response to reports of treatment failures in infections due to strains with MIC of 2 micrograms/mL:

- susceptible ≤2 micrograms/mL;
- intermediate 4–8 micrograms/mL (VISA);
- resistant ≥16 micrograms/mL (VRSA).

EUCAST recommends reporting all strains with MIC >2 micrograms/mL as resistant on the basis that glycopeptides should not be used to treat such organisms, even at increased doses.

Heteroresistance

A much commoner situation is for a strain to yield a small proportion of daughter cells (1 in 10^5) able to grow in the presence of 8 micrograms/mL of vancomycin. Such heterogeneously resistant strains are called hetero-VISA, and there is considerable debate about their clinical significance.

Vancomycin resistance

The first VISA infection occurred in 1995 in France in a child with leukaemia and catheter-associated MRSA bacteraemia.

The first clinical VRSA infection was reported in the USA in 2002. VRSA (vancomycin MIC >128mg/L, teicoplanin MIC 32mg/L) was isolated from a haemodialysis catheter tip and a chronic foot ulcer of a patient in Michigan. Vancomycin-resistant *E. faecalis* was also isolated from the ulcer, and the transfer of the *vanA* determinant was confirmed by PCR. The first VRSA in Europe was reported from Portugal in May 2013. Once again, *vanA*-positive, vancomycin-resistant *E. faecalis* was co-isolated, suggesting sporadic transfer from one to the other. Worldwide, 52 VRSA isolates have been reported to date.

Laboratory detection

The detection of glycopeptide resistance in *S. aureus* is problematic, as both VISA and hetero-VISA isolates appear susceptible to vancomycin by routine disc diffusion tests. Furthermore, there have been conflicting recommendations regarding methods of detection. Current advice from the British Society for Antimicrobial Chemotherapy (BSAC) (March 2020) is as follows.

- MIC by broth dilution should be used, as disc diffusion methods are known to be unreliable and variability has been reported using MIC gradient strips.

- Laboratories should target testing to invasive or serious infections, or cases of treatment failure. This is supported by the rarity of resistant isolates in the UK (0.2% in BSAC bacteraemia surveillance).

Infection control issues

MRSA is known to be highly transmissible in healthcare settings, and it seems reasonable to assume that VISA and VRSA will be likewise highly transmissible. Although infection control experience with VRSA is limited, implementation of rigorous infection control procedures is crucial for containing an outbreak of VRSA.

Prevention

Appropriate use of antimicrobials, especially vancomycin, is paramount in preventing the continued emergence of VISA and VRSA. Several studies have shown that vancomycin is frequently used for inappropriate reasons. Strategies to reduce inappropriate vancomycin use are essential (e.g. minimizing the use of temporary CVCs, diagnostic techniques to avoid prolonged empirical use of vancomycin, prompt removal of *S. aureus*-infected prosthetic devices).

Panton–Valentine leucocidin-associated *Staphylococcus aureus*

PVL is a toxin associated with around 2% of *S. aureus* isolates in the UK. The majority of isolates in the UK have been MSSA but can be associated with MRSA strains, particularly the USA300 clone in the USA. PVL is haemolysin which is encoded by two genes (*lukS* and *lukF*) that are carried on a mobile phage (φSLT). The toxin forms pores in the membranes of leucocytes, which result in their lysis.

Epidemiology

Panton–Valentine leucocidin-associated *S. aureus* (PVL-SA) is associated with skin-to-skin contact or sharing of contaminated objects such as towels, with compromised skin integrity an additional risk factor. Several settings have been associated with PVL-SA, including institutions such as prisons, military training camps, and gyms, alongside transmission within individual households.

Clinical features

- PVL-SA predominantly causes skin and soft tissue infections like other *S. aureus* clones. Infections with PVL-SA often manifest as recurrent boils (furunculosis). These often have an area of necrosis and may display pain and erythema out of proportion to the clinical findings. PVL-SA has also been associated with osteomyelitis and septic arthritis.
- Necrotizing pneumonia secondary to PVL-SA is well described. It is often associated with a preceding 'flu-like' illness and is associated with significant haemoptysis and often toxic shock. Leucopenia (secondary

to the PVL toxin), C-reactive protein (CRP) >200, and multilobar infiltrates on chest X-ray (CXR) are suggestive—only 25% patients have concurrent skin lesions. It often affects young people and has a high mortality rate.

Laboratory diagnosis

- PVL toxin detection is performed via PCR on suspected *S. aureus* isolates. In the UK, the reference laboratory is the Bacteriology Reference Department at Colindale.

Treatment

- Boils/small abscesses—incision and drainage may be sufficient treatment. Larger abscesses and cellulitis require antistaphylococcal antibiotics, such as flucloxacillin or clindamycin, for 5–7 days. If PVL-MRSA is suspected, consult national guidelines—one option is rifampicin with doxycycline for those over 12.
- There is limited evidence for empirical treatment for suspected PVL-SA pneumonia, but agents that inhibit toxin production via interruption of protein synthesis are recommended. Linezolid and clindamycin are suggested initially. If clinically deteriorating, the addition of rifampicin or intravenous immunoglobulin (IVIG) can be considered.
- Decolonization with TOP chlorhexidine and nasal mupirocin should be offered to primary cases. Close contacts should undergo a risk assessment, and decolonization given as appropriate.[2]

References

2 Health Protection Agency (2008). *Guidance on the diagnosis and management of PVL-associated Staphylococcus aureus infections (PVL-SA) in England.* Available at: https://assets.publishing.serv ice.gov.uk/government/uploads/system/uploads/attachment_data/file/322857/Guidance_ on_the_diagnosis_and_management_of_PVL_associated_SA_infections_in_England_2_Ed.pdf

Staphylococcus argenteus

Staphylococcus argenteus is an emerging pathogen whose species was only differentiated from *S. aureus* in 2009. It was first described in Australia, but sporadic infections have been reported around the world since then, particularly in South East Asia. It has an association with skin and soft tissue infections, but otherwise causes a similar spectrum of disease to *S. aureus*. There are conflicting reports about its relative pathogencity.

Due to the lack of the yellow pigment staphyloxantin, it does not have the 'golden' appearance of *S. aureus* on agar and instead has a 'silvery' appearance. It can be correctly identified by most MALDI-TOF libraries. *S. argenteus* has a similar antibiotic sensitivity profile to *S. aureus*, but there are limited data on optimal therapy.

Coagulase-negative staphylococci

CoNS may present as culture contaminants or as true pathogens. Infection is often associated with the presence of prosthetic material (e.g. IVCs, cardiac valves, joint prostheses). Infections are often indolent, but treatment may require removal of the foreign material. These organisms are frequently resistant to multiple antibiotics, which can make therapy difficult.

Epidemiology

CoNS are ubiquitous and are natural inhabitants of the skin. *S. epidermidis* is the commonest species, accounting for 65–90% of all isolates, followed by *Staphylococcus hominis*. *S. saprophyticus* is a urinary pathogen in young, sexually active women. *S. saccharolyticus* is the only strict anaerobe. Other less frequent species include *Staphylococcus haemolyticus*, *Staphylococcus warneri*, *Staphylococcus xylosus*, *Staphylococcus cohnii*, *Staphylococcus simulans*, *S. capitis*, *S. auricularis*, *S. lugdunensis* (coagulase-positive), and *Staphylococcus schleiferi* (coagulase-positive).

Pathogenesis

Plasmid-mediated antibiotic resistance to a wide variety of antibiotics is known to occur and may be transferred by conjugation to other organisms. CoNS also produce PIA, resulting in biofilm formation, particularly on prosthetic devices. This biofilm protects the organisms from antibiotics and host defence mechanisms. *S. saprophyticus* produces a number of substances that enable it to attach and invade the uroepithelium.

Clinical features

- Nosocomial device-related bacteraemia (commonest cause).
- Prosthetic valve endocarditis.
- CSF shunt infections.
- Peritoneal dialysis catheter-associated peritonitis.
- UTIs (*S. saprophyticus*).
- Bacteraemia in immunocompromised patients.
- Sternal osteomyelitis (post-cardiothoracic surgery).
- PJIs.
- Vascular graft infections.
- Neonatal nosocomial bacteraemias (particularly *S. capitis*).
- Endophthalmitis (after surgery or trauma).

Diagnosis

Appropriate samples (e.g. blood, pus, tissues) should be submitted to the laboratory. The following tests may be performed:
- Gram staining for GPC in clusters;
- **cultures on BA**—appear as white or grey colonies;
- catalase-positive, DNase test-negative/weakly positive;
- coagulase-negative (exceptions: *S. lugdunensis*, *S. schleiferi*);
- **antimicrobial susceptibility testing**—*S. saprophyticus* is novobiocin-resistant;
- **biochemical tests**—for example, API® Staph, automated methodologies (i.e. VITEK®, MALDI).

Treatment

Infections usually require the removal of prosthetic material, if present. CoNS are often resistant to multiple antibiotics; >80% are resistant to meticillin. CoNS may be sensitive to vancomycin, linezolid, and daptomycin. Sensitivity to teicoplanin is variable, and a teicoplanin MIC must be checked before use. Note that *S. haemolyticus* frequently demonstrates reduced susceptibility to teicoplanin. *S. saprophyticus* UTIs may be treated with trimethoprim, nitrofurantoin, or a fluoroquinolone.

Staphylococcus lugdunensis

S. lugdunensis was first described in 1988 and was differentiated from other CoNS via DNA relatedness and a positive slide coagulase (but negative tube coagulase) result. Like other CoNS, it ranges from a harmless skin commensal to a life-threatening pathogen. Unlike other CoNS, it can cause virulent infections similar to *S. aureus*, such as aggressive native valve infective endocarditis (IE), which has a high associated mortality rate. It also has a propensity for formation of biofilm and therefore has been implicated in PJIs, prosthetic valve IE, and implantable device infections. It is susceptible to most antibiotics tested, and penicillin is the drug of choice if proven sensitive.

Micrococcus species and *Kocuria*

Both these species are aerobic GPC and are often arranged in tetrads. They are skin commensals and cause a similar disease spectrum to other CoNS species, and are common contaminants in BCs. Based on phylogenetic and chemotaxonomic analysis, many micrococci (except *Micrococcus leteus* and *Micrococcus lylae*) have been reclassified as *Kocuria* spp. *Micrococcus* spp. are oxidase- and catalase-positive, with *M. luteus* producing bright yellow colonies. *Kocuria* spp. are also oxidase- and catalase-positive, and can produce colourful colonies on agar, depending on the species. Both species are readily speciated via MALDI-TOF.

Rothia mucilaginosus

Formerly known as *Micrococcus mucilaginosus* or *Staphylococcus salivarius*, these facultative anaerobes are weakly catalase-positive and are similar to the other CoNS species clinically.

Streptococci—overview

For an introduction to streptococci, ➲ see Overview of Gram-positive cocci, pp. 259–61. For classification of streptococci, see Table 7.1.

Table 7.1 Classification of streptococci

Species name	Lancefield group	Haemolysis	Common clinical syndromes
Streptococcus pyogenes	A	β	Invasive (necrotizing fasciitis, Group A staphylococci toxic shock syndrome, bacteraemia, etc.), tonsillitis, skin infections
Streptococcus agalactiae	B	β	Neonatal meningitis and bacteraemia. Adults: bacteraemia, skin and soft tissue infections, urinary tract infection
Streptococcus dysgalactiae subspecies *dysgalactiae*, *S. dysgalactiae* subspecies *equisimilis*, *Streptococcus equi* subspecies *equi*, *S. equi* subspecies *zooepidemicus*	C/G	β	Sore throat, cellulitis, bacteraemia, skin and wound infections
Streptococcus bovis group; *Streptococcus gallolyticus*, *Streptococcus lutetiensis*, *Streptococcus infantarius*, and *Streptococcus pasteurianus* and enterococcal species such as *Enterococcus faecalis* and *Enterococcus faecium*	D	β or γ	*S. bovis* bacteraemia, endocarditis, *Streptococcus suis* bacteraemia and meningitis
Streptococcus anginosus group *Streptococcus constellatus*, *Streptococcus intermedius*, and *Streptococcus anginosus*	Variable—F, A, C, or G. May not group	β or γ	Infective endocarditis, abscesses

Table 7.1 *(Contd.)*

Species name	Lancefield group	Haemolysis	Common clinical syndromes
Streptococcus pneumoniae	Does not group	α	Pneumococcal pneumonia, bacteraemia, meningitis, otitis media, sinusitis
Viridans streptococci	Does not group	α	Dental caries, endocarditis, abscesses

Types of haemolysis

α-haemolytic—a green zone of incomplete haemolysis.

β-haemolytic—a clear zone of complete haemolysis around the colony.

γ-haemolytic (or non-haemolytic)—no haemolysis present.

Lancefield grouping

A system of classifying catalase-negative, Gram-positive cocci by the carbohydrate composition of bacterial antigens found on their cell wall, originally described by Rebecca Lancefield. It is usually performed by using a commercial latex agglutination test and gives a rapid indication of possible species of an isolate.

Streptococcus pneumoniae

S. pneumoniae was first isolated in 1881 by Sternberg in the USA and Louis Pasteur in France. It became recognized as the commonest cause of lobar pneumonia and was given the name pneumococcus. *S. pneumoniae* is an important bacterial pathogen of humans, causing a range of infections as below. It is a Gram-positive coccus that grows in pairs (diplococci) or chains. It produces pneumolysin that causes α-haemolysis (green discoloration due to breakdown of haemoglobin) on BA.

Epidemiology

- *S. pneumoniae* colonizes the nasopharynx of 5–10% of healthy adults, and 20–40% of healthy children. The rate of colonization is seasonal, with an increase in winter.
- The rate of invasive pneumococcal disease is 15/100 000 persons/year. The incidence is up to 10-fold higher in certain populations (e.g. African-Americans, Alaskans, Australian aboriginals). Invasive pneumococcal disease is commoner at the extremes of age (<2 years or >65 years).
- Risk factors for pneumococcal infection include antibody deficiencies, complement deficiency, neutropenia or impaired neutrophil function, asplenia, corticosteroids, malnutrition, alcoholism, chronic diseases (liver, renal, diabetes, asthma, chronic obstructive pulmonary disease, and overcrowding).
- Antimicrobial resistance is increasing. Penicillin resistance rates are high in certain European countries (e.g. Spain, Portugal, Hungary, Iceland) and in Asia (e.g. Thailand, Hong Kong, Vietnam, Korea). The major

source of resistance is the worldwide geographic spread of a few clones that harbour resistance determinants. Rates of resistance in Europe correlate with the total consumption of β-lactams in that country.

Pathogenesis

A number of virulence factors have been identified:

- capsular polysaccharide (>90 serotypes; prevents phagocytosis, activates complement), cell wall polysaccharide (activates complement, cytokines);
- pneumolysin (activates complement and cytokines);
- pneumococcal surface protein A (PspA) (blocks deposition of complement, inhibits phagocytosis);
- pneumococcal surface protein C (PspC) (inhibits phagocytosis by binding complement factor H);
- pneumococcal surface adhesin A (PsaA) (mediates adherence);
- autolysin (causes release of bacterial components, resulting in trigger of cytokine cascade);
- neuraminidase (possibly mediates adherence).

Antimicrobial resistance

- β-lactam resistance is mediated by alterations in PBPs. Lower-level β-lactam resistance may be overcome by higher concentrations of the antibiotic. Site of infection and route of administration determine MIC breakpoints that should be used for penicillin (➔ see Treatment below).
- Macrolide resistance is mediated by acquisition of the *ermB* (ribosomal methylase) and *mefA* (efflux pump) genes.

Clinical features

S. pneumoniae may cause infection by direct spread of the organism from the nasopharynx to contiguous structures (e.g. middle ear, lungs) or by haematogenous spread (CNS, heart valves, joints). Unusual infections in young people should prompt investigation for HIV. Clinical syndromes include otitis media, sinusitis, exacerbation of chronic bronchitis, pneumonia, meningitis, endocarditis, septic arthritis/osteomyelitis, pericarditis, epidural/cerebral abscess, and skin/soft tissue infections.

Diagnosis

- BC bottles may flag positive, but no organisms are seen on Gram staining due to autolysis of the pneumococcus. The blood may be lysed (and appear chocolate brown), and the pneumococcal antigen test directly on blood is often positive.
- **Grows on routine media**—causes α-haemolysis of BA. May see central autolysis of colonies (draughtsmen), occasionally mucoid.
- Gram-positive lanceolate diplococci, often with visible capsule.
- **Identification**—catalase-negative, optochin-sensitive, soluble in 10% bile salts. Commercial identification tests (e.g. API® Strep, latex agglutination tests, serotyping tests) are available. MALDI-TOF identification used to be unreliable in distinguishing between *S. pneumoniae*, *S. mitis* group, and *Streptococcus pseudopneumoniae*, but has improved as libraries have been updated.
- Benzylpenicillin MIC should be determined for invasive isolates.

Treatment

- The original MIC thresholds for determining penicillin resistance were in the setting of meningitis and levels of drug needed in the CSF. Thus, individual breakpoints for β-lactams are listed in EUCAST for meningitis and indications other than meningitis.
- EUCAST recommends that if an oxacillin zone ≥20mm or benzylpenicillin MIC ≤0.06mg/L, this excludes all β-lactam resistance mechanisms and all indications can be treated with benzylpencillin.
- Oxacillin ≥8mm—benzylpenicillin should be reported as resistant, but sensitive to amoxicillin and ceftriaxone.
- Oxacillin <8mm—breakpoints for individual β-lactams should be sought for the treatment site and alternative agents should be considered. Vancomycin ± rifampicin is a preferred alternative for meningitis; other agents that can be considered for extrapulmonary sites include later-generation fluoroquinolones, carbapenems, macrolides, and tetracyclines, but seek expert advice.
- Pneumococcal meningitis benefits from adjunctive corticosteroids, unlike other bacterial pathogens (excluding TB), and is recommended by National Institute for Health and Care Excellence (NICE) and Infectious Diseases Society of America (IDSA) (➔ see Bacterial meningitis p. 764). Dosing is 10mg/kg qds in adults and 0.15mg/kg qds, up to a maximum of 10mg/kg qds, in children aged 3 months to 16 years for 4 days if pneumococcal meningitis is confirmed.

Prevention

- The 7-valent pneumococcal conjugate vaccine (PCV7) was introduced into the UK childhood immunization schedule in 2006, and replaced by a 13 valent product in 2010. Before 2020, three doses were given. Now two doses are given at 3 months and 12 months.
- The 23-valent unconjugated polysaccharide vaccine (PPV23) is given to adults aged 65 years and 'at-risk' groups (e.g. homozygous sickle-cell disease, asplenia or severe splenic dysfunction, chronic renal disease or nephrotic syndrome, coeliac disease, immunodeficiency or immunosuppression due to disease or treatment, including HIV infection, chronic diseases (cardiac, respiratory, liver, renal), diabetes mellitus, patients with cochlear implants). It is also recommended for those with CSF leak.
- Children at special risk (e.g. sickle, asplenia) should have PCV13, followed by PPV23 after their second birthday (web search 'UK Green book pneumococcal' for full details).
- Prophylaxis—PO phenoxymethylpenicllin is recommended for prevention of pneumococcal disease in asplenic patients, but not for CSF leaks.

Enterococci

Enterococci are environmental organisms that are found in the soil, water, food, and the GI tract of animals. They are GPC that occur singly, in pairs, or in short chains, and thus resemble streptococci. Until fairly recently, they were classified amongst the Lancefield group D streptococci. In the

1980s, they were reclassified as a separate genus *Enteroccoccus*, because of different pathogenic, biochemical, and serological profiles. At least 12 different species exist. *E. faecalis* is the commonest clinical isolate (80–90%), followed by *E. faecium* (5–10%). Others include *Enterococcus avium*, *Enterococcus casseliflavus*, *Enterococcus durans*, *Enterococcus gallinarum*, *Enterococcus hirae*, and *Enterococcus raffinosus*.

Epidemiology

Enterococci are part of the normal gut flora and can cause endogenous or exogenous infections, both in and out of hospital. In the hospital setting, enterococci are readily transmissible between patients and institutions. Risk factors for nosocomial enterococcal infections include GI colonization, severe underlying disease, prolonged hospitalization, prior surgery, renal failure, neutropenia, transplantation, urinary or vascular catheters, ICU admission, and prior antibiotic use.

Pathogenesis

- Enterococci are less intrinsically virulent than organisms such as S. *aureus* and GAS. They do not have classical virulence factors but are able to adhere to heart valves and renal epithelial cells. Several extracellular molecules play an important role in colonization and adherence (e.g. aggregation factor and extracellular surface protein). Other virulence factors include extracellular serine protease, gelatinase, and haemolysins.
- Enterococci are frequently found in cultures of intra-abdominal and pelvic infections—their role in this setting is unclear.
- Enterococcal bacteraemia carries high mortality (42–68%), but it is not clear whether this is due to the organism itself or a marker of severe debilitation. However, epidemiological studies have calculated an attributed mortality of ~30% in patients with enterococcal bacteraemia.
- The intrinsic resistance of enterococci to many antibiotics enables them to survive and multiply in patients receiving broad-spectrum agents, and accounts for their ability to cause nosocomial infections.

Clinical features

UTIs (commonest), bacteraemia and endocarditis, intra-abdominal and pelvic infections, skin and soft tissue infections, meningitis (associated with anatomical defects, trauma, or surgery), neonatal sepsis, device-related infections (i.e. prosthetic valve endocarditis and CNS shunt infections), and respiratory infections (rare).

Diagnosis

- **Gram staining**—elongated GPC ('cigar-shaped'), often in pairs and short chains.
- **Culture**—facultative anaerobes that can grow under extreme conditions (e.g. 6.5% NaCl, pH 9.6, temperatures of 10–45°C).
- **Biochemical tests**—enterococci hydrolyse aesculin.
- Often agglutinate with Group D with Lancefield grouping kits.
- Intrinsically resistant to aminoglycosides (low levels), cephalosporins, ciprofloxacin, lincosamides (low level), and co-trimoxazole (*in vivo*).

- Isolates should be tested for susceptibility to nitrofurantoin (UTIs), ampicillin, gentamicin, vancomycin, teicoplanin, linezolid, chloramphenicol, and daptomycin.

Treatment

- Enterococci are intrinsically resistant to many agents (e.g. cephalosporins, ciprofloxacin) and readily acquire new resistance mechanisms.
- Ampicillin is the usual first-line agent for *E. faecalis* infections, with vancomycin as an alternative. *E. faecium* is usually resistant to ampicillin.
- When bactericidal therapy is needed (e.g. endocarditis, meningitis), combination synergistic therapy of a cell wall agent plus an aminoglycoside may be considered.
- Ciprofloxacin may be active *in vitro* but is not usually recommended clinically. Newer fluoroquinolones are said to be more active against enterococci, but not against ciprofloxacin-resistant strains.
- For details of vancomycin resistance mechanisms, ➔ see Glycopeptides, pp. 47–50. *E. gallinarum* and *E. casseliflavus* are intrinsically resistant to glycopeptides (pentapeptide terminates D-alanine-D-serine) (see Box 7.4). High-level resistance to aminoglycosides and vancomycin resistance (vancomycin-resistant *Enterococcus* (VRE)) are significant problems, particularly on renal and haematology units.
- VRE bacteraemia has a worse prognosis than vancomycin-sensitive enterococcal bacteraemia, but this may be related to comorbidity and delay in receiving appropriate antibiotic therapy. Agents which may be active against VRE include linezolid, tigecycline, and daptomycin. Linezolid resistance has been detected in enterococci in the UK and is potentially transferable. Choice of agent depends on the source of infection.

Streptococcus bovis group, including *S. gallolyticus*

S. bovis group includes four major species that all agglutinate with Group D antisera. These are *Streptococcus gallolyticus* (*S. bovis* biotype I), and *Streptococcus lutetiensis*, *Streptococcus infantarius*, and *Streptococcus pasteurianus* (*S. bovis* biotype II). *S. bovis* group bacteraemia and endocarditis are associated with GI disease (primarily colonic malignancy). *S. gallolyticus* subspecies *gallolyticus* biotype I has a stronger association with colo-rectal cancer and endocarditis (71% and 94%, respectively, in one study) than *S. bovis* biotype II. The others (*Streptococcus equinus*, *S. infantarius*, *Streptococcus alactolyticus*, *Streptococcus gallolyticus* subspecies *pasteurianus* and subspecies *macedonicus*) are old biotype II, which have a much lower incidence of endocarditis and are much less likely to be associated with colonic malignancy. This group tends to be associated with other GI sources, and occasionally skin/soft tissue or CNS infection.

Pathogenesis

It is not clear whether *S. bovis* group organisms are a marker for malignancy or have an aetiological role. In some cases, *S. bovis* group bacteraemia is the only pointer to the GI disease. There are also reports of the malignancy being found up to 2 years after the initial *S. bovis* group infection. There seems to be an increase in faecal carriage of *S. bovis* group in patients with malignancy or pre-malignancy, compared to healthy subjects. Biotype I has a type-specific adherence mechanism, which may assist adherence to both cardiac valves and abnormal colonic mucosa.

Clinical features

The main clinical infections due to *S. bovis* group organisms are bacteraemia and endocarditis. Occasionally, *S. bovis* group organisms cause other infections such UTIs, meningitis, or neonatal sepsis. The GI tract is the usual portal of entry for bacteraemia. Most patients with endocarditis have an underlying valve abnormality or prosthetic valve. They tend to have a subacute course, indistinguishable clinically from endocarditis due to the *Streptococcus viridans* group, but studies suggest *S. bovis* group endocarditis has a higher mortality rate (45%), compared to non-*S. bovis* group endocarditis (25%).

Previously, all patients with *S. bovis* group bacteraemia were advised to have a comprehensive workup to exclude colonic malignancy and endocarditis. Advice is changing, to recommend transthoracic echocardiography (TTE)/transoesophageal echocardiography (TOE) and colonoscopy for *S. gallolyticus* subspecies *gallolyticus* (old biotype I), but not necessarily for biotype II (depending on the history, risk factors, source of infection, etc.; see Table 7.2).

Table 7.2 Clinical infections of *Streptococcus bovis* group organisms

Genotypic name	Phenotypic name	Synonym	Clinical recommendations
S. gallolyticus	Biotype I	*S. gallolyticus* subspecies *gallolyticus*	High incidence of IE/colonic malignancy, therefore TTE/TOE and colonoscopy for all patients
S. lutetiensis	Biotype II.1	*S. infantarius* subspecies *coli*	Consider history, other risk factors, and source of infection before workup for IE/colonic malignancy
S. infantarius	Biotype II.1	*S. infantarius* subspecies *infantarius*	
S. pasteurianus	Biotype II.2	*S. gallolyticus* subspecies *pasteurianus*	

IE, infective endocarditis; TOE, transoesophageal echocardiography; TTE, transthoracic echocardiography.

Diagnosis

- *S. bovis* group organisms may be misidentified as enterococci or viridans streptococci.
- **Biochemical tests**—*S. bovis* group organisms share a number of properties with enterococci; for example, they agglutinate with Group D antisera, hydrolyse aesculin, and are bile-tolerant.
- **Identification**—the API® Rapid Strep reliably identifies *S. bovis* and differentiates it to the biotype level, which is important for association with malignancy and endocarditis. Automated methods (i.e. VITEK® and MALDI-TOF) can reliably identify *S. bovis* group organisms. A PCR to differentiate the biotypes has been developed.

Treatment

Penicillin is the treatment of choice for *S. bovis* group infections; vancomycin is an alternative in β-lactam-allergic patients.

Viridans streptococci

The viridans streptococci, sometimes known as the oral streptococci, are important in dental caries, endocarditis, bacteraemia, and deep-seated infections (abscesses). They include *S. sanguinis*, *S. mutans*, *S. mitis*, and *S. salivarius*. This heterogeneous group has been reclassified into five distinct groups, on the basis of 16S rRNA analysis:

- *S. mutans* group—now divided into seven species and collectively known as the 'mutans streptococci'. The commonest are *S. mutans* and *Streptococcus sobrinus*;
- *S. sanguinis* group—now divided into *S. sanguinis*, *Streptococcus gordonii*, and *Streptococcus parasanguinis*;
- *S. anginosus* group—now divided into three species: *Streptococcus constellatus*, *Streptococcus intermedius*, and *S. anginosus*—also called the *Streptococcus milleri* group;
- *S. mitis* group—includes *S. mitis*, *Streptococcus cristatus*, and *S. oralis*;
- *S. salivarius* group—includes *S. salivarius* and *Streptococcus vestibularis*.

Epidemiology

The viridans streptococci are commensals of the human upper respiratory tract, ♀ genital tract, and GI tract, with large numbers present in the mouth. Each species has its own particular ecological niche.

Pathogenesis

These organisms seem to possess few virulence factors.

- The ability to produce acid, especially by *S. mutans*, is thought to be important in dental caries.
- Production of various carbohydrates, which aid in adherence to tooth enamel and gums, is important in colonization.
- Extracellular dextran production is important in adherence of organisms to heart valves and in resistance to antimicrobial therapy.
- Fibronectin production also mediates adherence to heart valves.

Clinical features
- Endocarditis (common cause in patients with abnormal valves).
- Bacteraemia (may cause severe sepsis in neutropenic patients).
- The *S. anginosus* group has an association with pyogenic abscesses (particularly brain abscesses, empyemas, and hepatic abscesses).
- Other clinical manifestations are rare but include pericarditis, peritonitis, sialadenitis, odontogenic infections, endophthalmitis, meningitis, and pneumonia.

Diagnosis
- Facultatively anaerobic GPC, catalase-negative.
- Most are α-haemolytic on BA; some are non-haemolytic.
- Resistant to optochin and lack bile solubility (unlike pneumococci).
- Unable to grow in 6.5% NaCl (unlike enterococci).
- Can be identified by biochemical tests, API® Strep, or automated methods.
- The *S. anginosus* group variably agglutinates with Lancefield grouping kits. Group F is the commonest agglutinating antigen, but A, C, and G are also possible. They often have a characteristic caramel odour in the laboratory.

Treatment
- Community-acquired infections are usually sensitive to penicillin—the treatment of choice.
- Other β-lactams (e.g. ceftriaxone) also have good *in vitro* activity against viridans streptococci.
- Nosocomial infections are associated with increased resistance to penicillin and other β-lactams.
- Some strains (e.g. *S. sanguinis*, *S. gordonii*) exhibit tolerance—that is, they are inhibited at low concentrations of antibiotic, but high levels are required for bactericidal activity.
- Often resistant to aminoglycosides (when traditional breakpoints are applied) but exhibit synergy in combination with β-lactam antibiotics. This principle underlies combination treatment for bacterial endocarditis.
- Vancomycin is used in penicillin-allergic patients and penicillin-resistant infections.

Group A *Streptococcus*

GAS, also known as *S. pyogenes*, is responsible for a variety of conditions—pyogenic (pharyngitis, cellulitis, necrotizing fasciitis), toxin-mediated (scarlet fever), or immunological (glomerulonephritis).

Epidemiology
GAS are upper respiratory tract commensals in 3–5% of adults and in up to 10% of children. Transmission is mainly via droplet spread. Some people develop pharyngitis/tonsillitis; others are asymptomatic, and a handful will become carriers of GAS in the throat. In the 1990s, the number of reports of invasive GAS increased globally, probably due to a re-emergence of more virulent strains. Risk factors for sporadic disease include people

>65 years old, those with recent varicella-zoster virus (VZV) infection, HIV-positive individuals, those with diabetes, heart disease, and cancer, people who inject drugs (PWID), or those on high-dose steroids. Over time, the epidemiology of GAS infection, in terms of clinical manifestation of disease, has changed—for example, acute rheumatic fever has become less common, and TSS commoner, over the last few decades. Since an upsurge in 2013–14, there has been a steady decline in the annual incidence of scarlet fever cases.

Pathogenesis

GAS possess a number of virulence factors:

- somatic constituents—hyaluronic capsule (resists phagocytosis), M protein (evasion of phagocytosis, inhibits binding of antibody with opsonin), serum opacity factor, lipotechoic acid, fibronectin-binding proteins;
- extracellular products—streptolysin O and S (α-haemolysis on BA), DNases A to D, hyaluronidase (facilitates spread through tissues), streptokinase (catalyses conversion of plasminogen to plasmin), streptococcal pyrogenic exotoxins (SpeA, SpeB, SpeC, SpeF—superantigens that induce fever), C5a peptidase, streptococcal superantigens (SSAs);
- immune-mediated disease (e.g. immune cross-reactions between components of the glomerular basement membrane and cell membranes).

Clinical features

- Pharyngitis—commonest infection. Suppurative complications include tonsillitis, peritonsillar abscess, retropharyngeal abscess, suppurative cervical lymphadenitis, mastoiditis, sinusitis, otitis media.
- Soft tissue infection—impetigo, erysipelas, cellulitis, necrotizing fasciitis, pyomyositis.
- Scarlet fever—notifiable disease. Pharyngitis associated with scarlatinal rash due to erythrogenic toxin production. The rash usually starts in the axillae and groins, and extends round the trunk and may subsequently desquamate. May be associated with a 'strawberry tongue' with erythema and red papillae. Around 90% of cases occur in children under 10 years of age.
- Rheumatic fever—may occur 1–5 weeks after pharyngitis. The Revised Jones Criteria are often used for diagnosis; they were updated in 2015 and are stratified depending on whether the patient is from a high- or low-risk population (➲ see Chapter 21).
- The five major criteria are:
  - arthritis (often migratory);
  - carditis and valvulitis;
  - CNS involvement (Sydenham's chorea);
  - rash (erythema marginatum); and
  - subcutaneous nodules.
- The four minor criteria are:
  - arthralgia;
  - fever;

- elevated acute phase reactants (CRP/erythrocyte sedimentation rate (ESR)); and
- prolonged PR interval.
- Two major manifestations and one minor are sufficient for a diagnosis of acute rheumatic fever after proven GAS infection, but there are exceptions. The majority of manifestations of rheumatic fever resolve without sequelae, apart from cardiac abnormalities. Around 10% of patients may develop severe carditis after the initial episode of rheumatic fever. A further 60% of patients go on to develop rheumatic heart disease, which can occur 10–20 years after initial infection. This tends to manifest as valvulitis, with or without signs of valvular dysfunction. Management of rheumatic fever involves symptomatic relief by using non-steroidal anti-inflammatory drugs (NSAIDs) (historically aspirin, but increasingly other agents such as naproxen), eradication of GAS with antibiotic therapy (usually with a penicillin for 10 days' therapy), and advice to the family/close contacts (➔ see Prevention below). Prophylactic antibiotics to prevent progression to rheumatic heart disease is controversial but is recommended by the American Heart Association (AHA).
- Post-streptococcal glomerulonephritis—may occur after throat infections (commonly M types 12, 1, 25, 4, and 3) and skin infections (commonly M types 49, 52, 53–55, and 57–61).
- Invasive GAS (iGAS) (e.g. bacteraemia)—recent increase in GAS bacteraemia in previously healthy adults. A small proportion of invasive GAS infections start with a skin or respiratory tract infection. Other risk factors—burns, trauma, uncontrolled HIV, PWID, alcoholism, immunosuppression, diabetes mellitus, and malignancy. ❶ iGAS is a notifiable disease.
- Streptococcal TSS—fulminant disease with high mortality; is mainly associated with types M1 and 3, but types 12 and 28 are also implicated. It involves rapidly progressive symptoms, with low blood pressure and multi-organ failure.
- Others—meningitis, osteomyelitis, puerperal sepsis, and septic arthritis.

Diagnosis

- Facultative anaerobic, catalase-negative GPC, which tend to form long chains when observed on Gram staining. They are non-sporing, non-motile, and usually non-capsulated.
- Culture on BA produces smooth, circular colonies, 2–3mm in diameter, usually β-haemolytic (large zone), and may be mucoid. Strains that produce haemolysin O, and not haemolysin S, will only demonstrate β-haemolysis when cultured anaerobically. Usually sensitive to bacitracin.
- Serology is used to diagnose immunological complications (e.g. rheumatic fever). A rise in anti-streptolysin O titre (ASOT) is suggestive of recent GAS disease but may cross-react with Group C and G streptococci, and may be falsely negative in skin disease. Anti-DNase B is more sensitive for recent GAS disease, and titres remain elevated longer than ASOT.
- All invasive isolates (i.e. found in a sterile body site) and scarlet fever should be notified to the local health protection unit.

Treatment

- The treatment of choice is PO phenoxymethylpenicillin (mild infections) or IV benzylpenicillin (severe infections). Pharyngitis is treated for 10 days, and invasive disease for at least 14 days.
- In penicillin-allergic patients, options include azithromycin (comparative clinical and bacteriological response rates to penicillin, but higher GI side effects) or erythromycin. Clindamycin may be used.
- It is common practice to treat bacteraemia with IV penicillin and clindamycin. There is no synergistic effect *in vitro*, but clindamycin is associated with a better outcome (perhaps due to protein synthesis inhibition) if the organism is found to be sensitive.
- Urgent surgical debridement is required in necrotizing fasciitis. There may be a role for IVIG in those with invasive infection and shock.

Prevention

- Infection control—GAS can spread from infected patients to close contacts, so isolate patients with invasive disease; use droplet precautions, and involve the infection prevention and control team (IPCT) early. The available evidence suggests that routine administration of prophylactic antibiotics for close contacts of invasive disease is not justified, but all household contacts should be informed of clinical manifestations of invasive disease and instructed to seek medical attention immediately if they develop any symptoms. Antibiotics are only given to certain 'high-risk' groups (e.g. mother/neonate contact).
- Hospital outbreaks of GAS have been described in the literature, whereas outbreaks in schools, nurseries, and institutions, such as prisons, are well described.
- The main difficulties associated with the development of a GAS vaccine are the widespread diversity of circulating GAS strains and M protein types, the immunological cross-reactivity between epitopes in the M protein and several human tissues, and the lack of a relevant animal model.

Guidelines

The UKHSA has a number of useful resources available for both managing contacts and outbreaks (available at: ℘ https://www.gov.uk/government/collections/group-a-streptococcal-infections-guidance-and-data).

Group B *Streptococcus*

Group B *Streptococcus* (GBS, *Streptococcus agalactiae*) was first reported as causing puerperal sepsis in 1938. By the 1970s, GBS had become the main cause of neonatal sepsis in infants aged <3 months.

Epidemiology

- In the UK, ~25% of women are colonized with GBS (genital tract or lower GI tract), which may be intermittent.
- Colonization of neonates usually occurs via the mother's genital tract. Risk factors—African ethnicity, diabetes.

- **Early-onset neonatal GBS disease** (<7 days)—risk factors include GBS genitourinary (GU) or GI colonization, premature rupture of membranes (PROM), delivery <37 weeks, intrapartum fever or amnionitis, and prolonged rupture of membranes. Affects around 1 in 2000 births in the UK and Ireland.
- **Late-onset neonatal GBS disease** (7–90 days)—risk factors include overcrowding, poor hand hygiene, and increased length of stay.
- Over the past 20 years, there has been an increase in invasive GBS disease in non-pregnant adults, most of whom had underlying medical conditions. The strongest risk factors identified are obesity and diabetes. Other risk factors include malignancy, uncontrolled HIV, corticosteroid use, splenectomy, liver cirrhosis, and chronic kidney disease.

Pathogenesis

Bacterial virulence factors that influence the outcome between exposure and development of colonization/invasive disease include the polysaccharide capsule (in particular, high amounts of sialic acid and type III virulent strains).

Clinical features

- Early-onset neonatal disease (defined as systemic infection in the first 6 days of life, mean age of onset 12h, pneumonia or meningitis) tends to result from vertical transmission *in utero* or at the time of delivery.
- Late-onset neonatal disease (onset 7 days to 3 months of age, mean 24 days, bacteraemia) likely arises from horizontal transmission either from the mother or nosocomial transmission. Incidence is not affected by intrapartum antibiotic prophylaxis.
- GBS infection in adults and older children, especially those with an underlying disease such as diabetes, includes bacteraemia, post-partum infections, pneumonia, endocarditis, meningitis, arthritis, osteomyelitis, otitis media, conjunctivitis, UTI, skin and soft tissue infections, and meningitis.

Diagnosis

- GBS are facultative anaerobic, catalase-negative GPC. They form long chains on Gram staining, and are non-sporing, non-motile, and usually capsulated.
- Culture on BA produces smooth, circular colonies of 2–3mm diameter, usually surrounded by a very small zone of β-haemolysis.
- **Identification**—Lancefield Group B, resistant to bacitracin, do not hydrolyse aesculin, production of CAMP factor (results in synergistic haemolysis with the β-lysin of *S. aureus* on sheep BA plate). Identified using API® Strep or via automated methods such as MALDI.
- **Typing**—GBS may be classified as serotypes I–VIII, based on the capsular polysaccharide and surface protein antigens. Other typing methods—MLST, PFGE.

Treatment

- Newborns with signs of sepsis should be treated with broad-spectrum antibiotics that cover GBS such as penicillins, cephalosporins, or vancomycin.
- Confirmed neonatal infections are usually treated with IV benzylpenicillin. Ten days of therapy are usually sufficient for an uncomplicated bacteraemia, whereas 14 days of therapy are given in uncomplicated meningitis.
- Adult bacteraemias are treated preferentially with β-lactams. GBS is variably sensitive to tetracyclines and macrolides. Duration depends on the source of the bacteraemia.
- Intrapartum prophylaxis should be offered if GBS is detected incidentally during pregnancy and to women with a previous baby with neonatal GBS disease (IV penicillin until delivery, clindamycin if penicillin-allergic) or women with GBS bacteruria. Observe the infant for 24–48h if well and no risk factors (PROM, chorioamnionitis, etc.)

Prevention

Routine screening for antenatal carriage is controversial and varies in different countries. Systematic screening is not recommended in the UK, following a further review in March 2017 for the following reasons.

- The impact of screening on mortality and morbidity is not proven.
- Screen-positive women may no longer be carriers at the point of delivery.
- Many thousands of low-risk women would receive IV antibiotics during labour.
- The incidence of early-onset neonatal GBS disease in the UK (0.5/1000 births) is similar to that seen in the USA (which has a universal screening and treatment programme), despite similar vaginal carriage rates.
- Antenatal antibiotic treatment of GBS carriage, if detected incidentally, is not recommended, as it does not reduce the chance of colonization at the time of delivery.
- Vaccines—capsular polysaccharide vaccines are under development. One of the difficulties is the existence of a multiplicity of serotypes with different geographical distributions.

For more information, web search 'RCOG green-top guideline 36'.

Other β-haemolytic streptococci

- Group C/G streptococci—there are four species in this group: *Streptococcus dysgalactiae* subspecies *dysgalactiae*, *S. dysgalactiae* subspecies *equisimilis*, *Streptococcus equi* subspecies *equi*, and *S. equi* subspecies *zooepidemicus*. They are primarily animal pathogens (*S. equi* causes strangles in horses), with *Streptococcus equisimilis* being the primary human pathogen. The commonest problem in humans is outbreaks of tonsillitis, especially in schools and institutions. Group C streptococci can cause syndromes similar to GAS such as post-partum sepsis, septicaemia, meningitis, pneumonia, and skin and wound infections, but Group C infections are usually less severe. Bacteraemias

have a strong association with endocarditis. Group C streptococci are usually sensitive to penicillin.
• Group F streptococci—this antigen is found on members of the *Streptococcus anginosus* group (*S. constellatus*, *S. intermedius*, and *S. anginosus*—also called the *S. milleri* group), which have a characteristic caramel odour when cultured in the laboratory (➲ see Viridans streptococci, pp. 279–80).

Other Gram-positive cocci

Leuconostoc

Leuconostoc are catalase-negative GPC or coccobacilli, which occasionally cause opportunistic infections. They are usually found on plants and vegetables, or rarely in dairy products and wine. There are only a few case reports of human infections, including bacteraemia (± indwelling line infection), meningitis, and dental abscess.

Note that *Leuconostoc* are intrinsically resistant to glycopeptides (see Box 7.6), because the pentapeptide cell wall precursors terminate in D-alanine-D-lactate. The usual agent of choice for these infections is penicillin or ampicillin, but they are generally susceptible to most agents with activity against streptococci.

Box 7.6 Gram-positive organisms resistant to glycopeptides
• *Leuconostoc*
• *Lactobacillus*
• *Pediococcus*
• *Erysipelothrix rhusiopathiae*
• *Nocardia*
• *S. haemolyticus* (resistant to teicoplanin)
• *E. gallinarum* and *E. casseliflavus*—both carry VanC, which is not transferable, and are considered intrinsically resistant to vancomycin

---

Abiotrophia defectiva

Abiotrophia defectiva is a member of **nutritionally variant streptococci** (NVS), alongside the closely related *granulicatella* spp. These organisms have previously been classified in various ways, but 16S rRNA sequencing defined the new genus *Abiotrophia* to be distinct from the streptococci. NVS are defined by the need for pyridoxal or thiol group supplementation for growth, and thus appear as satellite colonies around bacteria such as *S. aureus*. Gram staining tends to show pleomorphic variable-staining cells.

A. defectiva is the major pathogenic species, and is resistant to optochin and susceptible to vancomycin. Because it grows poorly on solid media, it can be easily overlooked if not cultured in broth or subcultured appropriately (e.g. with a *S. aureus* streak or onto selective media). *Abiotrophia* are normal flora in the upper respiratory, urogenital, and GI tract, and are clinically important as they cause >5% of cases of endocarditis. *Abiotrophia* endocarditis responds less well to antibiotics, and has higher morbidity and mortality, compared to endocarditis due to other streptococci. Correlation of *in vitro* antibiotic susceptibility testing and clinical outcome is a specialist field, and the general recommendation is for long-term combination therapy (e.g. penicillin and gentamicin for 4–6 weeks). Bacteriological failure and relapse rates are high.

Granulicatella spp.

Granulicatella spp. are further members of the nutritionally variant streptococci (NVS). *Granulicatella adiacens* is the predominant pathogenic species in humans. It is part of normal upper respiratory flora and is very similar to the closely related *A. defectiva* in terms of its growth requirements and strong association with endocarditis.

Anaerobic Gram-positive cocci

Anaerobic GPC have undergone multiple taxonomic changes. There are several genera that may be isolated from humans: *Peptostreptococcus*, *Peptoniphilus*, *Parvimonas*, *Finegoldia*, and *Anaerococcus*. The majority of human isolates are *Peptostreptococcus*, *Peptoniphilus*, and *Anaerococcus*. Less common isolates include *Atopobium parvula*, *Coprococcus* spp., *Ruminococcus* spp., and *Sarcina* spp.

Anaerobic GPC are part of the normal flora of the mouth, upper respiratory tract, GI tract, vagina, and skin. They can cause abscesses (e.g. brain abscess, often associated with otitis media, mastoiditis, chronic sinusitis, and pleuropulmonary infections), anaerobic pleuropulmonary disease, and bacteraemia (notably due to oropharyngeal, pulmonary, and ♀ genital tract sources). When mixed with other bacteria, they may be involved with serious soft tissue infections such as necrotizing fasciitis. Anaerobic GPC also cause osteomyelitis and arthritis at all sites, including bites and cranial infections. Little is known about virulence factors or pathogenesis of infection. Regarding treatment, anaerobic GPC are often mixed with aerobes and other anaerobes on culture plates. Obtaining appropriate specimens may be difficult; culture can be prolonged, and anaerobic sensitivity testing can also be challenging. Usually, a combination of surgery (e.g. drainage/debridement) and antibiotic therapy is required (e.g. metronidazole, penicillin, clindamycin).

Aerococcus

- *Aerococcus viridans* and *Aerococcus urinae* are catalase-negative GPC. They tend to form tetrads and may resemble staphylococci on Gram staining, but their biochemical and growth characteristics are more similar to α-haemolytic streptococci.
- *A. viridans* is generally considered a contaminant on culture but occasionally may be implicated in bacteraemia and endocarditis. It is a low-virulence organism and only causes systemic infections in the immunocompromised. Optimal treatment of such cases is unclear, so consult an infection specialist.
- *A. urinae*, first reported in 1989, has been implicated as a cause of ~0.5% of UTIs. Most patients were elderly with predisposing

conditions. It has also been found in patients with urogenic bacteraemia/septicaemia with or without endocarditis. *A. urinae* does not grow on CLED, and is usually susceptible to penicillin and resistant to sulfonamides and aminoglycosides.

Overview of Gram-positive rods

Gram-positive rods (GPRs) can be divided into three groups, based on growth characteristics and/or morphology (see Table 7.3 and Fig 7.3):

Table 7.3 Laboratory features of selected Gram-positive rods

Group	Species	Laboratory features
Aerobic	*Bacillus* spp.	Colonial appearances depend on species. Large, rod-shaped bacilli, often with rounded or square ends. Often β-haemolytic (except *Bacillus anthracis*). Endospores may be visible
	Corynebacterium spp.	Black colonies on tellurite media. Small bacilli, often occur in palisades on microscopy, known as 'Chinese lettering'. All species are catalase-positive
	Listeria spp.	β-haemolytic translucent colonies on blood agar. Short bacilli, may appear coccobacillary. Display tumbling motility at 25°C. All species are catalase-positive and oxidase-negative
	Erysipelothrix rhusiopathiae	Colonial appearance is variable and depends on the media used. Small straight or slightly curved bacilli. May appear in V shapes, or short or long chains. Catalase-negative
	Rhodococcus equi	Salmon-pink mucoid colonies on standard media. May appear coccobacillary. Catalase-positive
	Arcanobacterium haemolyticum	β-haemolytic colonies which 'pit' agar when removed. Small, thin bacillus, which may be slightly curved and pleomorphic. Catalase-negative

Table 7.3   *(Contd.)*

Group	Species	Laboratory features
Anaerobic	*Cutibacterium* spp. (formerly known as *Propionibacterium*)	Colonial appearance varies, depending on species. Small bacilli, may appear singly or in branching structures. Catalase-positive (except *Cutibacterium propionicum*)
	Clostridium spp.	Large straight or slightly curved bacilli with rounded or square ends. Commonly pleomorphic. May have endospores visible, which can be central or subterminal, depending on the species. Catalase- and oxidase-negative
Branching	*Actinomyces* spp.	Colonies may have 'molar teeth' appearance on agar (depending on the species). Highly filamentous long bacilli, morphologically indistinguishable from *Nocardia*. Facultatively anaerobic, weakly acid-fast, unlike *Nocardia*
	Nocardia spp.	Colonies may be brightly coloured and chalky in appearance. Highly filamentous long bacilli, morphologically indistinguishable from *Actinomyces*. Strictly aerobic, not acid-fast, unlike *Actinomyces*
	Actinomadura and *Streptomyces* spp.	Amongst causative species of actinomycetoma.

- aerobic GPRs (e.g. *Bacillus*, *Corynebacterium*, *Arcanobacterium*, *Listeria*, *Erysipelothrix rhusiopathiae*, *Rhodococcus equi*);
- anaerobic GPRs (e.g. *Clostridium* (see Table 7.4), *Cutibacterium* (formerly known as *Propionibacterium*));
- branching GPRs (e.g. *Actinomyces*, *Nocardia*, *Actinomadura*, *Streptomyces*).

Bacillus species

Bacillus spp. are environmental saprophytes that are found in water, vegetation, and soil. They are Gram-positive (or Gram-variable) aerobic or facultatively anaerobic rods with rounded or square ends. They form endospores that tolerate extremes of temperature and moisture. The ubiquitous nature of *Bacillus* spp. means that isolation from clinical specimens may represent contamination. Members of the group include:

- *Bacillus anthracis* (➲ see *Bacillus anthracis*, pp. 291–3);
- *Bacillus cereus*;
- *Bacillus circulans*;
- *Bacillus licheniformis*;
- *Bacillus megaterium*;
- *Bacillus pumilis*;
- *Bacillus sphaericus*;
- *Bacillus subtilis*;
- *Bacillus stearothermophilus*.

MALDI continues to identify new organisms which were previously in the *Bacillus* group, such as those from the *Paenibacillus* family. Isolation from sterile samples should be correlated with clinical presentation.

Clinical features

- Food poisoning—*B. cereus* is the commonest *Bacillus* causing food poisoning, followed by *B. licheniformis* and *B. pumilis*. Symptoms occur within 24h of ingestion of the preformed toxin in food and usually resolve in 24h. The emetic form presents after 1–5h, with nausea, vomiting, and abdominal cramps. The diarrhoeal form occurs 8–24h after ingestion of food. Production of a heat-labile toxin results in profuse diarrhoea and abdominal cramps (fever and vomiting are rare). Bacteraemia is often associated with the presence of an IVC. Bacteraemia or endocarditis may occur in people who inject drugs.
- Disseminated infection has been reported in neonates and young children. Neonatal infection is acquired perinatally. Multisystem involvement may occur. Immunocompromise (e.g. neutropenia) is associated with severe, and sometimes fatal, infections.
- CNS infections may occur, following trauma or neurosurgery, or in association with a CSF shunt. Removal of prosthetic material is required. Lumbar puncture may result in *Bacillus* spp. meningitis.
- Eye infections—endophthalmitis may occur, following trauma, eye surgery, or haematogenous dissemination. *B. cereus* is the commonest cause. Keratitis may occur after corneal trauma.
- Soft tissue and muscle infections may occur after injuries or wounds (e.g. road traffic accidents or after orthopaedic surgery).

Diagnosis

Bacillus spp. grow readily on routine culture media at environmental temperatures (25–37°C). All species may form spores, but they vary in their colonial morphology, motility, and nutritional requirements. Microscopically, they are large bacteria and usually Gram-positive (older cultures may be Gram-variable or Gram-negative). Most non-*anthracis Bacillus* spp. are β-haemolytic and motile (unlike *B. anthracis*). They also lack the glutamic acid capsule (thus negative with McFadyean's stain). *B. cereus* grows as characteristic peacock blue colonies on PEMBA agar.

Treatment

- There is no specific treatment for food poisoning syndromes, and most cases settle in 24h.

- For IVC- or prosthetic device-related infections, removal of the catheter or device is required for source control.
- Most *Bacillus* spp. isolates are susceptible to vancomycin, clindamycin, fluoroquinolones, aminoglycosides, and carbapenems. They are usually penicillin-resistant.
- Serious infections are usually treated with vancomcyin or clindamycin ± an aminoglycoside.

Bacillus anthracis

The name anthrax is derived from a Greek word for coal and refers to the eschar seen in cutaneous anthrax. Anthrax occurs most commonly in wild and domestic animals in Asia, Africa, South and Central America, and parts of Europe. *B. anthracis* readily produces spores, and these can remain dormant for years before germinating once in contact with a host. Human disease is rare, but the route of transmission is through handling, ingesting, injecting, or inhaling spores. This tends to be in the context of contact with anthrax-infected carcasses, wool, hair, meat, or bones, but there have also been outbreaks of injectional anthrax amongst drug users (2009–10 in Glasgow) and cases associated with animal-hide drums. Anthrax was used as an agent of bioterrorism in the USA in 2001 when *B. anthracis* spores were sent in contaminated letters (see Bioterrorism, pp. 882–3).

Pathogenesis

B. anthracis has a number of virulence factors:
- **capsule**—under anaerobic conditions, a polypeptide capsule consisting of poly-D-glutamic acid is produced. Synthesis of the capsule is by three enzymes encoded by the *capA*, *capB*, and *capC* genes on the pX 02 plasmid. A fourth protein, encoded by the *dep* gene, catalyses the formation of polyglutamates that inhibit phagocytosis;
- **toxin**—two binary toxins (o)edema factor (EF) and lethal factor (LF) bind a third toxin component protective antigen (PA), before entering the target cell. The three toxin components are also encoded on plasmid pX-01. LF is a zinc-dependent metallopeptidase that inhibits dendritic cell function. EF converts adenosine monophosphate (AMP) to cyclic AMP (cAMP), resulting in dysregulation of water and ions.

Clinical features

There are four forms of human disease:
- **cutaneous anthrax**—>95% of cases, usually acquired by direct contact with infected animals/animal products. The incubation period is 1–12 days. The initial pruritic papule gradually becomes a vesicular or bullous lesion, surrounded by extensive non-pitting oedema. The central part becomes necrotic and haemorrhagic, and may develop satellite vesicles. Finally, there is a classic black eschar which falls off in 1–2 weeks, unless systemic disease ensues;
- **injectional anthrax**—anthrax outbreaks have occurred with heroin contaminated with anthrax spores. An eschar may not occur at the site of injection, but significant local oedema, alongside swelling and erythema, and eventual skin necrosis are typical. This may progress to necrotizing fasciitis in around 30% of cases;

- **GI anthrax**—accounts for <5% of cases. Oropharyngeal anthrax presents with fever and neck swelling due to cervical adenopathy and soft tissue oedema after ingestion of contaminated meat. Intestinal anthrax is commoner, and presents with fever, syncope, and malaise, followed by abdominal pain, nausea, and vomiting. Examination shows abdominal distension and a mass in the right iliac fossa or periumbilical area. The third phase is characterized by paroxysmal abdominal pain, ascites, facial flushing, red conjunctivae, and shock;
- **inhalational anthrax**—very rare. Occurs after inhalation of spores. The incubation period is <1 week. It presents as a flu-like illness, with non-productive cough, haemorrhagic mediastinal lymphadenopathy, and multilobar pneumonia ± pleural effusions. CXR typically shows a widened mediastinum. High mortality rate (45–85%);
- **systemic disease (fulminant phase)**—can occur with all forms of anthrax, but particularly associated with injectional and inhalational anthrax. Rapidly progressive hypoxaemia and shock. Almost uniformly fatal despite intensive care support;
- **CNS disease**—rare, but associated with disseminated disease from injectional anthrax. Presents with haemorrhagic meningoencephalitis; 95% mortality.

Diagnosis

- *B. anthracis* is an Advisory Committee on Dangerous Pathogens (ACDP) category 3 organism.
- **Specimens**—*B. anthracis* may be isolated from wound swabs (if cutaneous disease), tissue, nasal swabs, and BCs.
- **Microscopy**—GPRs in 'box car', or cigar-shaped chains. The spore is oval-shaped, and central or subterminal. McFadyean's stain shows capsulated, dark, square-ended bacilli in short chains.
- **Culture**—*B. anthracis* grows readily on ordinary media (optimal incubation temperature 35°C) after 2–5 days' incubation. Colonies are white or grey-white, with a characteristic 'medusa head' appearance. In contrast to most other *Bacillus* spp., *B. anthracis* is non-haemolytic, non-motile, and penicillin-sensitive.
- **Identification**—*B. anthracis* can be identified by PCR or MALDI. However, if *B. anthracis* is suspected, no further identification should be **performed**—the case should be discussed with the reference laboratory urgently.

Treatment

- Cutaneous anthrax without systemic disease—ciprofloxacin or doxycycline. Duration is 60 days for bioterrorism-related cases and 7–10 days for naturally acquired cases.
- Systemic anthrax with meningitis—ciprofloxacin and meropenem with either linezolid or clindamycin.
- Systemic anthrax without meningitis—ciprofloxacin with either linezolid or clindamycin.
- Obiltoxaximab, a monoclonal antibody directed against protective antigen, was approved by the Food and Drug Administration (FDA) in 2016 for use in anthrax treatment, though efficacy has only been shown in animals.

- Anthrax immunoglobulin has also been trialled in animal studies and has been shown to be safe in human volunteers.

For full details, see Hendricks et al., 2014.[3]

Prevention

Anthrax is a notifiable condition.
- Pre-exposure prophylaxis—human and animal vaccines are available to prevent anthrax. Vaccination is recommended for workers at risk of cutaneous anthrax such as those who work with leather, textiles, or animals. For details, see *Anthrax: the green book* (available at: ✆ www. gov.uk/government/publications/anthrax-the-green-book-chapter-13).
- Post-exposure prophylaxis (PEP)—vaccination is recommended post-exposure to inhalational anthrax. In addition, antibiotic prophylaxis (PO ciprofloxacin or doxycycline) is indicated for PEP of inhalational anthrax.

References

3 Hendricks KA, Wright ME, Shadomy SV, *et al.* Centers for Disease Control and Prevention Expert Panel Meetings on prevention and treatment of anthrax in adults. *Emerg Infect Dis.* 2014;**20**:e130687.

Corynebacterium diphtheriae

The name for *C. diphtheriae* is derived from the Greek '*korynee*' meaning club and '*diphtheria*' meaning leather hide (for the leathery pharyngeal membrane It provokes). The organism spreads via nasopharyngeal secretions, and can survive for months in dust and contaminated dry fomites. Incidence is highest In young children (>3–6 months old) when protective maternal antibodies wane. Diphtheria is rare in the UK (previously 10 cases reported in England and Wales each year) but remains a problem in developing countries and the former Russian states. In 2008, an unimmunized boy in London died from *C. diphtheriae* var. *mitis*, but there have been no deaths since in England, with only one case identified in 2020.

Pathogenesis

C. diphtheriae produces a potent exotoxin, the result of the infection with a lysogenic bacteriophage. It consists of two fragments: fragment A (which inhibits polypeptide chain elongation at the ribosome) and fragment B (which helps transport fragment A into the cell). Inhibition of protein synthesis probably accounts for the toxin's necrotic and neurotoxic effects, which are mainly on the heart, nerves, and kidneys. Cell death accounts for the characteristic pharyngeal membrane. It is important to note that other toxigenic *Corynebacterium* strains may cause diphtheria (e.g. *Corynebacterium ulcerans*). Milder infections without toxin production do occur and resemble streptococcal pharyngitis, and the pseudomembrane may not develop. Asymptomatic carriers are important for transmission. Immunity—whether vaccine or natural—does not prevent carriage.

Clinical features

- **Respiratory tract**—asymptomatic upper respiratory tract carriage is common in endemic countries and is an important reservoir of infection. Anterior nasal infection presents with a serosanguinous or seropurulent nasal discharge, often associated with a whitish membrane. Clinical features include fever, malaise, sore throat, pharyngeal injection, and development of a pseudomembrane, which is initially white, then grey with patches of green or black necrosis. Cervical lymphadenopathy may result in a characteristic 'bull neck' and inspiratory stridor.

- **Cardiac disease**—myocarditis occurs after 1–2 weeks, usually as the oropharyngeal disease is improving. Patients should have cardiac monitoring for ST segment changes, heart block, or arrhythmias. Clinical features include dyspnoea, cardiac failure, and circulatory collapse.
- **Neurological disease**—local paralysis of the soft palate and posterior pharynx leads to nasal regurgitation of fluids. Cranial nerve palsies and ciliary muscle paralysis may follow. Peripheral neuritis occurs 10–90 days after onset of pharyngeal disease and presents with motor deficits.
- **Skin infections**—in the countries where public hygiene is poor, cutaneous diphtheria is the predominant presentation, causing chronic non-healing ulcers with grey membranes. Outbreaks have been described in homeless alcoholics in the USA. Cutaneous diphtheria can be caused by toxigenic and non-toxigenic strains.
- **Invasive disease**—endocarditis, mycotic aneurysms, septic arthritis, and osteomyelitis may be caused by non-toxigenic strains.

Diagnosis

- **Culture**—nasopharyngeal, throat, or skin swabs should be immediately transported to the laboratory and cultured on suitable culture media (e.g. Löeffler's, Hoyle's tellurite, Tinsdale media). The colonies are black on tellurite media. *C. diphtheriae* shows a halo effect on Tinsdale agar.
- **Microscopy**—Gram staining of *C. diphtheriae* shows characteristic palisades, resembling Chinese letters. The beaded appearance obtained with Neisser or Albert stain, whereby the volutin/metachromatic granules are dark purple, compared to brown/green counterstain, is characteristic.
- **Identification**—*C. diphtheriae* is a non-motile, non-sporing, and non-capsulated GPR. It is catalase-positive and can be reliably identified with API® Coryne or MALDI. Isolates should be submitted to the reference laboratory at UKHSA Colindale for toxigenicity testing. Several methods are available—PCR has replaced the Elek plate or rapid enzyme-linked immunoassay (EIA).
- **Biotyping**—colonial appearance on tellurite and also biochemical tests (e.g. Hiss serum sugars) subdivide *C. diphtheriae* into the biotypes var. *gravis*, *intermedius*, and *mitis*. These biotypes correspond to clinical severity. *Gravis* and *intermedius* (and some *mitis*) biotypes are usually toxigenic. The fourth biotype var. *belfanti* is rare and cannot produce the lethal exotoxin.

Treatment

- Antibiotics—if high clinical suspicion, treat immediately with IV penicillin for 14 days. Alternatives—erythromycin, azithromycin, or clarithromycin. Confirm elimination by nasopharyngeal swab; if cultures are positive, give a further 10 days of antibiotics.

- Anti-toxin may be given at different doses, depending on site severity and patient age (➜ see Guidelines below). First, test the patient with a trial dose to exclude hypersensitivity to horse serum. This can be obtained from the UKHSA Colindale laboratory.
- Infection control—isolate and barrier-nurse the case. Identify close contacts; take nose and throat swabs, and arrange clinical surveillance for 7 days. Provide prophylactic antibiotics (single dose of benzylpenicillin or 7 days of erythromycin) and booster vaccination for close contacts.
- Diphtheria is a notifiable disease—contact your local health protection unit (HPU).

Prevention

Diphtheria toxoid is part of the triple vaccine DTP (diphtheria, tetanus, polio), given at 2, 3, and 4 months as part of the UK immunization schedule. As a result of vaccination, toxigenic strains lose their selective advantage and become less prevalent, with reduced transmission to unvaccinated individuals. There is no reduction in non-toxigenic carriage. Note that diphtheria can occur in immunized individuals, but disease is less severe.

Guidelines

- Bonnet JM, Begg NT (1999). Control of diphtheria: guidance for consultants in communicable disease control. World Health Organization. *Commun Dis Public Health*. 1999;**2**:242–9.
- UK Health Security Agency (2023). *Public health control and management of diphtheria (in England): 2023 guidelines*. Available at: ➜ https://assets.publishing.service.gov.uk/media/654944a9bdb7ef000d4af91c/diphtheria-guidelines-version19-November2023.pdf

Non-diphtheria corynebacteria

Corynebacteria are also known as coryneforms or diphtheroids. They are environmental organisms found in water and soil, and commensals of the skin and mucous membranes of humans and other animals. In the hospital environment, they may be cultured from surfaces and equipment. Thus, corynebacteria are frequently considered contaminants but may cause severe disease in hospitalized or immunocompromised patients.

Classification

Corynebacteria are classified, according to cell wall composition and biochemical reactions, into the following groups:
- non-lipophilic fermentative (e.g. *C. ulcerans*, *Corynebacterium pseudotuberculosis*, *Corynebacterium xerosis*, *Corynebacterium striatum*, *Corynebacterium minutissimum*, *Corynebacterium amycolatum*, *Corynebacterium glucuronolyticum*);
- non-lipophilic, non-fermentative (e.g. *Corynebacterium pseudodiphtheriticum*);
- lipophilic (e.g. *Corynebacterium jeikeium*, *Corynebacterium urealyticum*).

Clinical features

Infections may be classified into two groups:

- **community-acquired** (e.g. pharyngitis, native valve endocarditis, GU tract infections, periodontal infections);
- **nosocomial** (e.g. IVC-associated bacteraemia, endocarditis, prosthetic device-related infections, surgical site infection (SSIs)).

Diagnosis

- **Microscopy**—club-shaped GPRs. Cells demonstrate variable size and appearance, from coccoid to bacillary forms, depending on the stage of their life cycle. Corynebacteria typically aggregate to form 'Chinese letter' arrangements when viewed on Gram staining.
- **Culture**—grow readily on BA and BC media. Thioglycolate broth may be used for wound cultures. Special media used for species identification include tryptic soy agar, with or without 1% TWEEN® 80, to assess lipid-enhanced growth.
- **Identification**—catalase-positive, can be identified to species level by the API® Coryne system or MALDI-TOF.
- The CAMP test (named after Christie, Atkins, and Munch–Petersen) was used historically. A streak of β-lysin-producing S. aureus is plated onto BA, with the test strain streaked perpendicular. A positive reaction is seen if CAMP factor (a haemolysin secreted by some corynebacteria) enhances the haemolysis produced by S. aureus.
- Susceptibility testing is problematic, but isolates are usually sensitive to vancomycin, teicoplanin, and daptomycin.

Infections caused by various corynebacteria

- *C. ulcerans* is primarily a cause of bovine mastitis. However, it has the potential to produce diphtheria toxin and cause an exudative pharyngitis, indistinguishable from *C. diphtheriae*. Several reported outbreaks of diphtheria have been found to be due to *C. ulcerans*.
- *C. pseudotuberculosis* is an animal pathogen that causes caseous lymphadenitis in sheep. Human disease is rare, but granulomatous lymphadenitis has been seen in farm workers and vets.
- *C. xerosis* is a commensal of the human nasopharynx, conjunctivae, and skin. It may cause invasive disease in the immunocompromised.
- *C. striatum* is a commensal of the skin and mucous membranes. It can rarely cause severe invasive disease in hospitalized patients.
- *C. minutissimum* is a skin commensal which was previously thought to cause erythrasma. Bacteraemia and endocarditis may occur in patients with indwelling catheters or immunocompromise.
- *C. amycolatum* is another skin commensal. There are case reports of invasive disease.
- *C. glucuronolyticum*—normal flora of the GU tract. May cause UTI and prostatitis.
- *C. pseudodiphtheriticum*—normal flora of the upper respiratory tract. Primarily associated with respiratory tract infections in the immunocompromised.
- *C. jeikeium* colonizes the skin of hospitalized patients. It may cause severe nosocomial infections (e.g. bacteraemia, endocarditis, meningitis,

CSF shunt infections, PJIs). Risk factors include immunocompromise (malignancy, neutropenia, poorly controlled HIV), indwelling devices, prolonged hospital stay, broad-spectrum antibiotics, and impaired skin integrity. *C. jeikeium* is resistant to many antibiotics, and vancomycin is the treatment of choice.

- *C. urealyticum* colonizes the skin of hospitalized patients. It causes chronic and recurrent UTIs in the elderly or immunosuppressed.

Listeria

L. monocytogenes is the main pathogen in this genus, and affects pregnant women, neonates, the immunocompromised (especially if impaired cell-mediated immunity), and the elderly. *Listeria ivanovii* occasionally causes human infection. Generally, *Listeria innocua*, *Listeria welshimeri*, and *Listeria seeligeri* are non-pathogenic to humans. Around 1–3% of healthy adults carry *Listeria* spp. in the gut, with the primary reservoir being soil and decaying vegetable material. *Listeria* infections are rare in the general population but can cause life-threatening bacteraemia and meningoencephalitis in susceptible groups.

Epidemiology

Disease is mainly sporadic but may be part of an epidemic associated with contaminated foodstuffs such as pâté, unpasteurized milk, chicken, or soft cheese. Hospital outbreaks have been reported. Vets or farmers may become infected through direct animal contact. Human–human transmission occurs vertically (i.e. mother to baby). Cross-infection in neonatal units has been reported. There was a dramatic rise in non-pregnancy-associated listeriosis between 2001 and 2010 in the UK, especially in those aged >60 years, the reasons for which are unclear. Annual incidence has remained relatively static since then.

Pathogenesis

Animal studies have identified listeriolysin O—this is important for bacterial survival after phagocytosis, and its production is related to extracellular iron. In rodents, T lymphocytes are important in protective immunity, rather than as antibodies. T cells attract monocytes to the infection, activate them, and destroy the *Listeria*, resulting in granuloma. The organisms themselves show tropism for the brain, particularly the brainstem and meninges. In humans, GI disease (e.g. low gastric pH or disrupted normal flora) may help establish *Listeria* infection in the bowel.

Clinical features

- **Pregnancy**—maternal listeriosis is rare before 20 weeks' gestation. After this, infection may be asymptomatic or present with mild symptoms (fever, back pain, sore throat, headache). Fever may result in reduced fetal movements, premature labour, stillbirth, abortion, or early-onset neonatal disease (➜ see Chapter 23).
- **Neonate**—(1) early neonatal disease occurs <5 days post-delivery, usually presents with septicaemia, and has a mortality of 30–60%;

20–40% of survivors develop long-term sequelae such as lung disease or CNS defects; (2) late neonatal disease occurs >5 days post-delivery, usually presents as meningitis, and may be hospital-acquired; mortality in late disease is lower (<10%).

- **Adults**—the main syndromes are gastroenteritis (generally self-limiting), meningitis, and bacteraemia ± endocarditis. Rare manifestations include other CNS disease (e.g. encephalitis, cerebritis, CNS abscesses), arthritis, hepatitis, endophthalmitis, continuous ambulatory peritoneal dialysis (CAPD) peritonitis, and pneumonia. Risk factors include age, immunosuppression due to steroids, cytotoxic therapy, and poorly controlled HIV. Mortality is high—CNS 20–50%, bacteraemia 5–20%, endocarditis 50%. Up to 75% of survivors of CNS infection have sequelae such as hemiplegia.

Diagnosis

- **Microscopy**—*Listeria* are short intracellular GPRs. However, in clinical specimens, they may appear Gram-variable and look like diphtheroids, cocci, or diplococci.
- Note that, in *Listeria* meningitis, a high lymphocyte count in the CSF is not always seen. Gram staining is often negative for organisms, but *Listeria* may be cultured from the CSF ± blood.
- **Culture**—*Listeria* grow on BA and is usually β-haemolytic, so it can be mistaken for streptococci. Selective media are available such as those containing aesculin.
- **Identification**—*Listeria* are non-sporulating, catalase-positive, aesculin-positive, and oxidase-positive. They show tumbling motility at 25°C and grow optimally at 30–37°C, but better than most bacteria at 4–10°C (refrigeration temperature). *L. monocytogenes*, *L. ivanovii*, and *L. seeligeri* show enhanced haemolysis in the presence of *S. aureus* (positive CAMP test, as described in ➔ Non-diphtheria corynebacteria, pp. 295–7). Species can also be differentiated by API® Listeria/Coryne and MALDI-TOF.
- Typing techniques in current use include serotyping and WGS with single-nucleotide polymorphism (SNP) analysis.

Treatment

IV ampicillin ± gentamicin is the usual regimen for meningitis, with co-trimoxazole or meropenem as an alternative in penicillin-allergic patients. There are no randomized controlled trials (RCTs) to establish the most effective drug or duration of therapy. In meningitis, antibiotics are usually given for at least 14 days (21 days in the immunocompromised). Most other clinical syndromes should be treated with ampicillin, with consideration given to adding gentamicin for synergy. Vancomycin may be given for bacteraemia but has been associated with relapse of disease. Cephalosporins should never be used to treat listeriosis due to inherent resistance.

Prevention

Invasive listeriosis is a notifiable condition. Health education and dietary advice to pregnant women, the immunocompromised, and others who are at risk of disease.

Erysipelothrix rhusiopathiae

E. rhusiopathiae is a thin, pleomorphic, non-sporing GPR. It was first isolated in mice by Robert Koch in 1878 and from swine by Louis Pasteur in 1882. It was identified as a human pathogen in 1909.

Epidemiology

E. rhusiopathiae is found in a variety of animals and invertebrates, and transmission to humans is by direct contact. Most human cases associated with occupational exposure (e.g. fishermen, fish handlers, farmers, vets, butchers, abattoir workers).

Clinical features

There are three clinical presentations:

- **erysipeloid**—localized cutaneous infection. The organism enters the skin by trauma, and after an incubation period of 2–7 days, pain and swelling of the affected digit occur. The lesion is well defined, slightly raised, and violaceous. It spreads peripherally, with central fading. Regional lymphadenopathy and lymphangitis may occur;
- **diffuse cutaneous infection**—this is rare and caused by progression of the primary lesion. Fever, arthralgia, and lymphadenopathy may occur. Recurrence is common;
- **bacteraemia**—this is rare, but often associated with endocarditis.

Diagnosis

- **Microscopy**—*E. rhusiopathiae* is a straight to slightly curved GPR (1–2.5 micrometres); it decolorizes readily and may appear Gram-negative. Rods may be arranged singly, or in V-shaped pairs, short chains, or non-branching filaments.
- **Culture**—colonial and microscopic appearances vary with the medium, pH, and incubation temperature. Incubation in 5–10% CO_2 improves growth.
- **Identification**—*E. rhusiopathiae* is catalase-negative and oxidase-negative. Automated methods, such as MALDI-TOF, have been used successfully to identify the organism.
- **Drug susceptibility**—*E. rhusiopathiae* is usually susceptible to penicillins, cephalosporins, clindamycin, carbapenems, and ciprofloxacin. It is resistant to vancomycin, teicoplanin, sulfonamides, co-trimoxazole, and aminoglycosides.

Treatment

- Penicillin is the treatment of choice.
- Alternatives include ampicillin, cephalosporins, and ciprofloxacin.
- *Erysipelothrix* is intrinsically resistant to vancomycin.

Rhodococcus equi

R. equi (previously known as *Corynebacterium equi*) was identified in 1923 as an animal pathogen causing pneumonia in horses. Since then, it has been found in a wide variety of animals. The first human case was reported in 1967—but since the 1980s, the increase in immunosuppressed patients

(HIV, transplantation, etc.) has been mirrored by an increase in *R. equi* infections. Contact with soil contaminated with herbivore manure is felt to be a significant mode of transmission.

Clinical features

- Necrotizing pneumonia is the commonest clinical presentation (80%) and is characterized by cavitation on CXR. BCs are positive in 50% of HIV patients and in 25% of solid organ transplant recipients.
- Extrapulmonary infection may occur with or without pulmonary disease—the commonest manifestations are brain and subcutaneous abscesses.
- Isolated bacteraemia may also occur, usually associated with IV catheters with concurrent neutropenia.

Diagnosis

- *R. equi* is a Gram-positive obligate aerobe that is non-sporing and non-motile.
- **Microscopy**—it may appear coccoid or bacillary on Gram staining, depending on growth conditions. It can be acid-fast.
- **Culture**—*R. equi* grows optimally at 30°C, and colonies may appear salmon-pink. Selective media include colistin–nalidixic acid (CNA) agar, phenyl ethanol agar (PEA), and ceftazidime–novobiocin agar.
- **Identification**—*R. equi* is catalase-positive and oxidase-negative. It differs from other coryneforms by its lack of ability to ferment carbohydrates or liquefy gelatin. It can be identified using API® Coryne or via automated methods such as MALDI.

Treatment

Optimal treatment has not been determined by clinical trials. *R. equi* is susceptible to vancomycin, erythromycin, fluoroquinolones, rifampicin, carbapenems, and aminoglycosides. A combination of a macrolide or fluoroquinolone with rifampicin has been suggested until antimicrobial susceptibility results are available. Extended courses of therapy (up to 2 months) have been used due to a high relapse rate.

Arcanobacterium haemolyticum

Arcanobacterium haemolyticum is a β-haemolytic, catalase-negative GPR, which may be pleomorphic and slightly curved. It also often pits the agar when a colony is removed. Identification can be confirmed by API® Coryne or via automated methods. It causes acute pharyngitis, particularly in adolescents, and can be difficult to distinguish from GAS pharyngitis. A rash occurs in 50% of patients, which, in contrast to the rash associated with GAS, occurs on the extensor surfaces of the arms and does not desquamate. Erythromycin is felt to be the treatment of choice as *in vitro* resistance to pencillin has been shown.

Cutibacterium

Cutibacterium (formerly *Propionibacterium*) are facultatively anaerobic GPRs, which form part of the normal flora of human skin and sebaceous glands. They possess relatively few virulence factors and therefore only cause disease in a limited number of settings, particularly of indwelling prosthetic material. The majority of infections are caused by *Cutibacterium acnes*, though infections with *Cutibacterium granulosum*, *Cutibacterium avidum*, and *Cutibacterium propionicum* have been described.

Clinical features

- *Cutibacterium* tend to cause infections of indwelling prosthetic devices, in particular PJIs (especially shoulder prostheses) and infections of pacemakers and other implantable cardiac devices and CNS shunts. They tend to present indolently and rarely cause fulminant infection. Rarely, *Cutibacterium* have been implicated in native joint infections, particularly following shoulder arthroscopy and post-operative vertebral osteomyelitis.
- *C. acnes* has been implicated in the pathogenesis of acne, though its precise role remains unclear.

Diagnosis

Cutibacterium appear as small anaerobic Gram-positive bacilli on Gram staining, which may occur singly or in groups and may appear to form branching structures. They grow readily on several agars but may require prolonged incubation. They are catalase-positive (with the exception of *C. propionicum*) and are identifiable via automated methods such as MALDI or commercial identification kits. A major difficulty with the diagnosis of *Cutibacterium* infections is distinguishing contamination from true infection. Multiple positive specimens from the same site and/or positive deep tissue specimens (particularly involving prosthetic material) should raise suspicion.

Treatment

Removal of the infected prosthetic device, where present, is key—*Cutibacterium* possess multiple adherence factors and readily form biofilms. Antibiotic treatment alone is often unsuccessful with the prosthesis *in situ* (➔ see Prosthetic joint infections, pp. 824–7). *Cutibacterium* are usually sensitive to multiple antibiotics such as β-lactams, clindamycin, tetracyclines, vancomycin, and linezolid.

Clostridium botulinum

C. botulinum is widespread in the soil and environment. It produces one of the most potent toxins known, which causes botulism (see Table 7.4).

Pathogenesis

Toxins A to G have identical pharmacological effects, despite possessing different antigens. All can cause human disease, but A, B, and E are most common. Note that type-specific antibody must be given to a patient with suspected botulism (➔ see Clinical features below).

Table 7.4 Diseases caused by *Clostridium* spp.

Organism	Clinical syndrome	Toxin production
*Clostridium botulinum**	Botulism	Neurotoxin
*Clostridium tetani**	Tetanus	Neurotoxin
Clostridioides difficile	Antibiotic-associated diarrhoea/ pseudomembranous colitis	Toxin A and B
*Clostridium perfringens**	Type A causes gas gangrene	Histiotoxic
*Clostridium novyi**	Type A causes gas gangrene	Histiotoxic
Clostridium sporogenes	Debate regarding pathogenicity	
Clostridium septicum	Gas gangrene	Histiotoxic
Clostridium histolyticum	Gas gangrene	Histiotoxic
Clostridium sordellii	Gas gangrene	Histiotoxic

* Clusters in people who inject drugs in Europe.

Clinical features

- **Food-borne botulism**—the preformed toxin is ingested from food (hams, sausages, tinned fish, meat, and vegetables, particularly home-preserved, and honey). The food itself may not appear spoilt. Botulinum toxin is absorbed from the human GI tract and blocks the release of acetylcholine, mainly in the peripheral nervous system. Initial symptoms include nausea and vomiting, diplopia, and bilateral ptosis (due to oculomotor muscle involvement), followed by progressive descending motor loss with flaccid paralysis. Speech and swallowing become difficult, but the patient maintains consciousness and has normal sensation. Botulism is fatal in 5–10% of cases. Death is usually due to cardiac or respiratory failure.
- **Wound botulism**—causes a similar clinical picture but is due to toxin release secondary to growth of the organism. Outbreaks and ongoing sporadic cases occur in PWID.
- **Intestinal botulism**—is also due to organism proliferation in the gut and toxin production *in vivo*.
- **Infant botulism**—presents as hypotonia, usually in babies <6 months old, as the gut is not yet resistant to colonization.

Diagnosis

If there is a suspected clinical case, involve experts and always alert laboratory staff, as the toxin is dangerous. Blood (taken prior to administration of anti-toxin), faecal samples, vomit, and food samples should be tested for the organism and toxin. *Clostridium botulinum* is a motile, strictly anaerobic rod, with optimal growth at 35°C, but some strains are able to grow at as low as 1–5°C. The oval subterminal spores are very hardy—some spores persist, despite boiling at 100°C for several hours. Moist heat at 120°C for 5min usually destroys spores.

Treatment

Involve the ICU as the patient is likely to need organ support. A polyvalent anti-toxin is available to neutralize unfixed toxin and is effective at reducing the severity of symptoms, if given early in the course of disease. In food-borne disease, any unabsorbed toxin should be removed from the stomach and GI tract. In wound botulism, give benzylpenicillin and metronidazole and request surgical debridement (reduces organism load and ongoing toxin production). Antibiotics are not recommended for food-borne or intestinal botulism.

Prevention

- Avoid home canning. Do not give honey to infants.

Clostridium tetani

Tetanus is a vaccine-preventable disease. Despite this, it is a cause of considerable morbidity and mortality in the developing world and cases occur every year in developed countries. Tetanus is a notifiable disease.

Pathogenesis

Resilient spores survive in soil and the GI tract of horses and other animals. Transmission usually occurs via introduction of spores into open wounds (particularly in PWID), patients with recent abdominal surgery, patients with ear infections (otogenic tetanus), and neonates after cutting of the umbilical cord (tetanus neonatorum). *C. tetan* produces the exotoxins tetanospasmin (powerful neurotoxin which diffuses to the CNS and causes localized or generalized disease) and tetanolysin (oxygen-labile haemolysin).

Clinical features

Localized tetanus involves muscle rigidity and painful spasms near the wound site. The symptoms of generalized tetanus are summarized by ROAST (rigidity, opisthotonus, autonomic dysfunction, spasms, trismus).

Diagnosis

Tetanus is a clinical diagnosis. These microbiological tests support the diagnosis:

- isolation of *C. tetani* from the infection site by culture or PCR. *C. tetani* is a Gram-variable, motile, obligate anaerobe, which classically produces 'drumstick' terminal spores. Due to the motility by peritrichous flagella, it produces a thin spreading film on enriched BA;
- presence of tetanus toxin in serum (performed at the Gastrointestinal Bacteria Reference Unit, Colindale);
- low/no antibody levels to tetanus toxin (serum must be taken prior to immunoglobulin being administered).

Treatment

Involve the ICU early. Give tetanus immunoglobulin, wound debridement, and antimicrobials, including metronidazole or penicillin. Vaccination with tetanus toxoid following recovery is important to prevent future episodes (see Table 7.5).

Table 7.5 Recommendations for vaccination

Immunization status	Clean wound	Tetanus-prone wound	
	Vaccine	Vaccine	Tetanus immunoglobulin
Full (i.e. five doses)	No	No	Only if high risk
Primary immunization complete, boosters incomplete but up to date	No	No	Only if high risk
Primary immunization incomplete/boosters not up to date/never immunized/status unknown or uncertain	Yes—one dose and plan to complete schedule	Yes—one dose and plan to complete schedule	Yes—one dose in a different site

Tetanus-prone wound risk factors

Any wound where there is a risk of introduction of tetanus spores is considered tetanus-prone. These include puncture wounds in a contaminated environment, burns, compound fractures, presence of foreign bodies, presence of sepsis, and certain animal bites. A tetanus-prone wound is then considered high risk if there is (not an exhaustive list):

- heavy contamination with soil or manure;
- a significant degree of devitalized tissue;
- any wound with a delay of >6h before surgical treatment.

Prevention

Tetanus immunization, introduced in the UK in 1961, now involves the combined tetanus/low-dose diphtheria vaccine (Td) (previously single-antigen vaccines (T) were given). Five doses of tetanus toxoid are considered to give lifelong immunity (usually three as DTP, as part of childhood immunizations, and two doses of Td later) (see *Tetanus: the green book*, available at: ℘ www.gov.uk/government/publications/tetanus-the-green-book-chapter-30).

Other Clostridia

These anaerobic Gram-positive, spore-forming organisms are responsible for a variety of conditions, many of which involve exotoxin production (see Table 7.3). The rods are pleomorphic, but typically large, straight, or slightly curved, with rounded ends.

- *C. perfringens* type A causes gas gangrene. It is occasionally isolated from BCs and may be associated with food poisoning (enterotoxin production), endocarditis, or a contaminant. In developing countries, it may cause enteritis necroticans ('pig bel').
- *Clostridium histolyticum* and *Clostridium sordellii* may also cause gas gangrene.

- *Clostridium novyi* gas gangrene is due to *C. novyi* type A (*C. novyi* types B, C, and D are differentiated by toxin permutation and soluble antigen production, and do not cause human disease). Compared to *C. perfringens*, *C. novyi* bacilli are larger and more pleomorphic. It is a stricter anaerobe and has peritrichous flagella, but its motility is inhibited in the presence of oxygen. The oval spores are central or subterminal. There are at least four toxins, which possess haemolytic, necrotizing, lethal, lipase, and phospholipase activities. There have been outbreaks amongst PWID.
- *Clostridium sporogenes* is probably not pathogenic in its own right. It is usually encountered in a mixed wound culture containing accepted pathogens, and may have a role in enhancing local conditions and accelerating an established anaerobic infection.
- *Clostridium septicum* usually lives in the soil, human, or animal gut, and can cause gas gangrene in humans and animals. *C. septicum* bacteraemia is seen with breakdown of gut integrity (e.g. in leukaemia). Gram stain appearance of the organism may be variable, with long, short, and filamentous GPRs, together with some older Gram-negative cells. Spores start off as swollen Gram-positive 'citron bodies', then tend to be oval, bulging, and either central or subterminal. *C. septicum* grows well on ordinary media at 37°C and has numerous peritrichous flagella; hence, it is actively motile. Colonies are often initially transparent and 'droplet-like', with projecting radiations, then become grey and opaque with time. The α exotoxin has lethal, haemolytic, and necrotizing properties, and can be demonstrated in cultures.
- *C. difficile* (➲ see *Clostridioides difficile* infection, pp. 196–200) is a healthcare-associated infection (HCAI), subject to mandatory reporting. It can cause *C. difficile* infection (CDI) and colitis. Clinical features vary, and diagnosis is usually by toxin tests, rather than by culture. Infection control measures are paramount to control spread.

Actinomyces

Actinomyces spp. are mouth, gut, and vaginal commensals that may cause the chronic granulomatous infection actinomycosis. The main species of human importance are *Actinomyces israelii* and *Actinomyces gerencseriae*. Others include *Actinomyces meyeri* (isolated from brain abscesses), *Actinomyces viscosus* (found in dental caries), and also *Actinomyces naeslundii* and *Actinomyces odontolyticus*.

Pathogenesis

Actinomycosis is endogenously acquired, and those with dental caries and intrauterine contraceptive devices (IUCDs) are at increased risk. Historically, rural farm workers were affected more than those living in towns, purportedly because of poor dental hygiene. Chronic abscesses, tissue destruction, fibrosis, and sinus formation are typical findings. The masses of mycelia in relatively young lesions may be visible as yellow sulfur granules; later on, they form dark brown, hard granules due to calcium phosphate deposition.

Clinical features

Most human cases of actinomycosis are in the cervicofacial area, especially around the jaw. Infection may follow dental procedures. Haematogenous spread to the liver, brain, and other organs is well recognized. In addition to facial disease, clinical presentations include thoracic actinomycosis (due to aspiration of oral *Actinomyces*; characterized by chest wall sinuses and bony erosion of the ribs and spine), appendix or colonic diverticular actinomycosis, pelvic actinomycosis (linked with IUCDs), cerebral actinomycosis, and 'punch actinomycosis' (knuckle infection due to human bite).

Diagnosis

- **Histology**—tissue biopsies of suspect lesions are stained with fluorescein-labelled antisera, to demonstrate characteristic sulfur granules and mycelia. Any sulfur granules available should be crushed and Gram-stained—organisms appear as branching GPRs. *Nocardia* spp. are morphologically indistinguishable. However, *Actinomyces* are NOT acid-fast, and *Nocardia* are weakly acid-fast.
- **Culture**—*Actinomyces* often fail to grow aerobically. Growth requires enriched culture (e.g. brain–heart infusion medium or selective media) incubated under micro-aerophilic conditions (i.e. 5–10% CO_2). Colonies may appear after 3–7 days but may take up to 14 days. *A. israelii* and *A. gerencseriae* colonies have a 'molar teeth' shape on agar. Further identification can be confirmed by MALDI-TOF or at a reference laboratory usually by molecular methods. Note that sputum often contains oral *Actinomyces*.

Treatment

Surgical involvement is vital, and debridement reduces scarring, deformity, and recurrence rate. Removal of an IUCD is the primary treatment for pelvic disease. Actinomycosis is usually treated with penicillin or ampicillin, for up to 6 months. Broad-spectrum antibiotics (e.g. co-amoxiclav, or ceftriaxone and metronidazole) may be needed if there are concomitant pathogens. Despite large doses of antibiotics given for long periods, recurrence is common. The issue seems to be one of tissue penetration, rather than drug resistance.

Nocardia

Nocardia spp. are environmental saprophytes that occasionally cause chronic granulomatous infections Thirty-three species of *Nocardia* have been shown to cause disease in humans, with members of the *Nocardia asteroides* complex (*Nocardia asteroides sensu stricto*, *Nocardia farcinica*, and *Nocardia nova*) being the commonest worldwide.

Pathogenesis

Nocardiosis is acquired through inhalation (pulmonary) or direct inoculation (cutaneous). Subsequent haematogenous dissemination, typically to the CNS, results in abscess formation.

Clinical features

Pulmonary nocardiosis is commoner in the immunosuppressed (prophylaxis against *Pneumocystis jirovecii* with co-trimoxazole may be protective against nocardiosis, but not when alternative agents are used) and those with pre-existing lung disease. Presentation and clinical/radiological findings are variable, making the diagnosis difficult. Secondary abscesses, mainly in the brain, occur in approximately one-third of patients with pulmonary nocardiosis, and can be misdiagnosed as malignant lesions due to an indolent presentation. Other clinical presentations include cutaneous disease (e.g. post-trauma) with lymphatic involvement (sporotrichoid), which may progress to a fungating mycetoma.

Diagnosis

- Branching, aerobic GPRs, weakly acid-fast when decolorized with 1% sulfuric acid (modified ZN stain). Other specialist stains that aid in the diagnosis of *Nocardia* include the Gomori methenamine silver method.
- Colonies of *Nocardia* may be coloured (orange/cream/pink), and the surface may be dry or chalky. *Nocardia* can take up to a month to grow on standard media (e.g. Lowenstein–Jensen media, brain–heart infusion agar, and trypticase–soy agar with blood enrichment).
- *Nocardia* organisms can be differentiated from *Actinomyces*, because they are strict aerobes (whereas *Actinomyces* organisms are facultative anaerobes), and *Nocardia* grow over a wide range of temperatures (whereas *Actinomyces* only grow at 35–37°C). *Actinomyces* are not acid-fast.

Treatment

Seek expert advice. Sensitivity testing should be performed. Usually a long course with combination therapy (e.g. >3 months in normal hosts, 6 months if immunocompromised) is required. Antibiotic sensitivity varies with the species; co-trimoxazole is the most widely used empirical drug (most species are sensitive). Alternatives include a carbapenem or amikacin. Ceftriaxone is often used and PO agents, such as minocycline, moxifloxacin, and linezolid, have a role, but long-term use may be limited by side effects.

Actinomadura and *Streptomyces*

Actinomadura and *Streptomyces* spp. are aerobic filamentous actinomycetes implicated in mycetoma, also known as Madura foot. Mycetoma can be divided into actinomycetoma (bacterial) or eumycetoma (fungal), which has important treatment implications. This is a chronic granulomatous condition that mainly occurs in Africa, Asia, and Central America. The important subspecies are *Actinomadura madurae*, *Actinomadura pelletieri*, and *Streptomyces somaliensis*. Other actinomycetes are implicated in Madura foot (e.g. *Nocardia*), along with a wide variety of mould species such as *Madurella* and *Exophilia*.

Diagnosis

Clinically, grains seen within host tissues or in the discharge from sinus tracts are diagnostic of mycetoma. These grains are colonies of the organism, and should be crushed in potassium hydroxide (KOH) and Gram-stained to distinguish between actinomycetoma (Gram-positive filaments) and eumycetoma (septate fungi). These grains should be rinsed in 70% alcohol before culture, to try to eliminate any surface contaminants, and appropriate plates set up at 26°C and 37°C. Macroscopically, grains are often red. *Actinomadura* spp. show many similar properties to *Actinomyces* spp. but are not acid-fast when decolorized with 1% sulfuric acid.

Clinical features

Mycetomas usually involve the hand or foot, and arise from traumatic inoculation from soil or plants, usually via thorns or splinters. Chronic granulomata of the skin, subcutaneous tissue, and bone may progress to sinus formation.

Treatment

Seek expert advice. *Actinomadura* and *Streptomyces* are usually penicillin-resistant. Prolonged antimicrobials are required; actinomycetoma tend to respond to therapy better than eumycetoma. The role of surgery is limited but may be required in select cases. Co-trimoxazole, aminoglycosides, macrolides, carbapenems, and tetracyclines are commonly used, often in combination.

Gram-negative cocci—overview

Gram-negative cocci include a variety of pathogenic and non-pathogenic species (see Table 7.6 and Figure 7.4).
- Also ⤳ see Overview of fastidious Gram-negative rods), p. 338.

Table 7.6 Gram-negative cocci

Organism	Microbiology	Syndrome
Neisseria meningitidis	Aerobic, Gram-negative diplococci, oxidase-positive, grow at 37°C on blood and chocolate agar, glucose- and maltose-positive	Meningitis Septicaemia Others
Neisseria gonorrhoeae	Aerobic, Gram-negative diplococci, oxidase-positive, grow at 37°C on blood and chocolate agar, glucose-positive	Gonorrhoea Septic arthritis Ophthalmia neonatorum
Non-pathogenic *Neisseria* spp.	Aerobic, Gram-negative diplococci, oxidase-positive, grow at 22°C on nutrient agar	Oral commensals—rarely cause invasive infections
Moraxella catarrhalis	Aerobic, Gram-negative cocci, oxidase-positive, grow at 37°C on blood and chocolate agar	Respiratory pathogen
Anaerobic Gram-negative cocci (e.g. *Veillonella* spp.)	Anaerobic, Gram-negative cocci	Unclear Dental caries?

NB *Acinetobacter* spp. are Gram-negative rods that may appear coccoid or bacillary. Unlike *Neisseria* spp., they are oxidase-negative. They are discussed further in ⤳ *Acinetobacter*, pp. 332–4.

Neisseria meningitidis

Vieusseaux first described epidemic cerebrospinal fever in 1805. In 1887, Weichselbaum isolated *N. meningitidis* from the CSF. In the late nineteenth century, meningococcal carriage was described. In 1909, different serotypes of *N. meningitidis* were recognized.

Epidemiology

Humans are the only known reservoir of *N. meningitidis*, and ~20% of the population carry the organism in their throat. However, half of these carriage strains are non-capsulated, and thus non-pathogenic. During outbreaks, the carrier rate of an epidemic strain may reach 90%. Risk factors for meningococcal disease include:

- lack of bactericidal antibody;
- age—bimodal distribution: 3 months to 3 years and 18–23 years;
- travel to endemic areas (e.g. Africa, Mecca);
- complement deficiencies;
- splenectomy;
- host genetic polymorphisms (e.g. *MBL, TNFA Fc/RIIa, PAI-1*).

Pathogenesis

To cause infection, the organism must cross the nasopharyngeal mucosa and enter the circulation. The type IV pilus (encoded by *pilC*) is involved in mucosal colonization. The polysaccharide capsule is important in avoiding host immunity (and defines the serogroup of the isolate; see Table 7.7). Various secretion systems help deliver toxins, and IgA protease enhances survival within epithelial cells.

Clinical features

- Acute—meningitis and septicaemia, purulent conjunctivitis (occasionally becomes systemic), monoarthritis, endocarditis, pericarditis, pneumonia.
- Chronic septicaemia with joint and skin involvement is less common.

Table 7.7 Major serogroups of *Neisseria meningitidis*

Serogroup	Pattern of disease	Vaccines
A	Epidemic meningitis, associated with different clones	Yes
B	Epidemic strains (and outbreaks). Main serotype in the UK	Yes. Introduced into routine UK schedule in 2015
C	Local outbreaks	MenC vaccine introduced into routine schedule in 1999
W-135	Pilgrims returning from the Hajj	Yes—in high-risk groups
X, Y, Z, 29E, Z'	Rare	

Diagnosis

- *N. meningitidis* is hazard group 2. Suspected and known isolates of *N. meningitidis* should always be handled in a safety cabinet.
- **CSF examination**—in meningitis, the CSF pressure is elevated and the CSF appears turbid. CSF polymorphs and protein are normally raised, and CSF glucose level is low (normal is >60% of serum level). In very early infection, CSF results may be normal, as the meningeal reaction has not had time to take place.
- **Microscopy**—Gram-negative intracellular diplococci. Note that, in meningococcal meningitis, the CSF usually has a higher yield than BCs. If Gram staining is negative, methylene blue staining may pick up scanty meningococci.
- **Culture**—fastidious, transparent, non-pigmented, non-haemolytic colonies. May be mucoid if capsule production. Oxidase-positive. Identified by API NH, MALDI-TOF, and molecular methods.
- **Meningococcal PCR (send to the meningococcal reference laboratory)**—can be performed on CSF, serum, plasma, EDTA blood, or joint fluids. ➲ See meningitis flow chart (back inside cover of second edition). Serogrouping—capsular polysaccharide antigens are identified by slide agglutination test with using polyclonal antibodies. There are at least 13 serogroups, the commonest of which are summarized in Table 7.7.
- **Serotyping**—identification of (PorB) class 2/3 outer membrane protein (OMP) by a dot-blot EIA with using monoclonal antibodies.
- **Serosubtyping**—identification of (PorA) class 1 OMP by a dot-blot EIA using monoclonal antibodies.
- MLST and WGS can identify genetic relationships between organisms during outbreaks as they evolve over time, but are of limited use in outbreak management.
- MenB characterization with use of the Meningococcal Antigen Typing System (MATS) would be ideal for identification of vaccine-preventable strains but is yet to be implemented on a real-time basis.
- *N. meningitidis* produces a capsule which forms the basis of the serogroup typing system. There are now at least 13 serogroups, but the commonest ones are summarized in Table 7.7.

Treatment

- See management of acute bacterial meningitis (➲ see Acute meningitis, p. 764) and septicaemia. Reduced susceptibility to penicillin has resulted in empirical therapy for meningitis being a third-generation cephalosporin (usually ceftriaxone in the UK).
- After treatment, antibiotics—usually ciprofloxacin—should be given for nasopharyngeal eradication, unless ceftriaxone was used for treatment.

Infection control issues

This is a notifiable condition. Droplet infection control precautions are recommended, particularly before the patient has completed 24h of appropriate antibiotic therapy. Public health will arrange chemoprophylaxis—indicated for those who had prolonged close contact in a household-type setting during the 7 days before illness, or transient close contact if exposed to respiratory droplets or secretions at around the time of admission.

Ciprofloxacin is recommended for all ages and in pregnancy. The advantages of ciprofloxacin over rifampicin (previous choice) are single dose, no interaction with the oral contraceptive pill (OCP), and availability in community pharmacies. The risk of complications is negligible from a single dose. The alternatives (e.g. if ciprofloxacin-allergic) include ceftriaxone. Vaccination may also be offered. For complete guidelines, web search 'PHE meningococcal public health 2012' and see *Meningococcal: the green book* (available at: 🔗 https://www.gov.uk/government/publications/mening ococcal-the-green-book-chapter-22).

Vaccination

- Group C conjugate vaccine—capsular polysaccharides linked to a carrier protein. Part of the routine UK schedule since 1999. Reported cases fell by 90% in all age groups that were immunized, and by 66% in other age groups as a result of herd immunity. A booster dose was introduced in 2006, as a result of studies demonstrating waning protection during the second year of life. Similarly, an adolescent booster dose was started in 2013 (for further details, see the UKHSA website and *Meningococcal: the green book* (available at: 🔗 https:// www.gov.uk/government/publications/meningococcal-the-green-book-chapter-22). Given at 3 months 12 months, and 14 years of age. Also available combined with *H. influenzae* type b (Hib) vaccine.
- Quadrivalent ACWY vaccine—conjugate and polysaccharide versions available. Conjugate is preferred. Recommended for those travelling to areas of risk, including Hajj pilgrimage parts of Africa, and Asia (see 🔗 http://nathnac.net).
- Group B protein vaccine—three *N. meningitidis* proteins produced by recombinant technology and a preparation of Group B-derived outer membrane vesicles. Shown to be immunogenic and may protect against 88% of MenB strains in the UK. Effectiveness has been shown through an observed reduction in infections,[4] though it does not appear to reduce the rates of carriage.[5] Initially restricted to risk groups (asplenic children, laboratory workers, etc.) due to issues of cost; entered the routine UK vaccination schedule in 2015. Doses at 2, 4, and 12 months.

References

4 Ladhani SN, Andrews N, Parikh SR, *et al*. Vaccination of infants with meningococcal group B vaccine (4CMenB) in England. *N Engl J Med*. 2020;**382**:309–17
5 Marshall HS, McMillan M, Koehler AP, *et al*. Meningococcal B vaccine and meningococcal carriage in adolescents in Australia. *N Engl J Med*. 2020;**382**:318–27.

Neisseria gonorrhoeae

N. gonorrhoeae only infects humans and causes the sexually transmitted infection (STI) gonorrhoea (➔ see Gonorrhoea pp. 755–7). This is the second commonest bacterial STI in the UK. Increasing rates of antimicrobial resistance, together with its persistence and association with poor reproductive health outcomes, have made it a major public health concern.

Pathogenicity

Gonococci are divided into four Kellogg types, according to colonial appearance, ability to auto-agglutinate, and virulence. Kellogg types T1 and T2 are more virulent and possess many fimbriae, whereas types T3 and T4 are non-fimbriate and avirulent. In gonococci, the fimbriae are associated with attachment to mucosal surfaces and resistance to killing by phagocytes. Traditional typing methods are being replaced by molecular techniques.

Clinical features

Gonorrhoea commonly presents as a purulent disease of the urethral mucous membrane, or of the cervix in ♀. Secondary local complications (e.g. epididymitis, salpingitis, pelvic inflammatory disease (PID; ➔ see Pelvic inflammatory disease, pp. 750–2)) and metastatic complications (e.g. arthritis) may occur if the primary infection is inadequately treated. Other manifestations of disease include disseminated gonococcal infection (skin lesions, painful joints, and fever), ophthalmia neonatorum (purulent conjunctivitis of the newborn—a notifiable condition), perihepatic inflammation (Fitz-Hugh–Curtis), and rarely endocarditis or meningitis. Rectal or pharyngeal infection is often asymptomatic and identified through contact tracing. If cultured, gonococcus should always be treated, as it is never a commensal.

Diagnosis

- **Microscopy**—Gram-negative intracellular diplococci. This can be done within the GU medicine (GUM) clinic, ensuring prompt treatment of patients.
- **Culture**—culture remains essential where infection persists after treatment and treatment failure is suspected. Culture is specific, sensitive, and cheap. Urethral swabs from ♂ and endocervical swabs from ♀ should be Gram-stained, and then immediately inoculated onto selective media and placed in enriched CO_2 conditions. Typical Gram staining appearance of *N. gonorrhoeae* (Gram-negative diplococci in association with neutrophils) from urethral/endocervical swabs, together with a consistent clinical presentation, is regarded as adequate for treatment in many cases. However, culture is critical for legal cases and for antimicrobial sensitivity testing. After 24–48h, oxidase-positive colonies appear, and identification can be confirmed by testing for acid production from sugars (API® NH) or MALDI. Identification must be confirmed by two different methods. Selective agars (e.g. NYC or VCAT—containing vancomycin, colistimethate sodium, amphotericin, and trimethoprim) are used. Most laboratories no longer test for β-lactamase production with use of the nitrocefin strip method, as patients are likely to be treated with a third-generation cephalosporin according to current guidelines.
- Nucleic acid amplification tests (NAATs) are generally more sensitive (96% in both symptomatic and asymptomatic infections), compared to culture. ♂ should send first-pass urine, and ♀ a vaginal or an endocervical swab. Other specimen types can be tested—NAATs are recommended for asymptomatic individuals (urethral/endocervical) and

MSM (rectal/pharyngeal). Positive NAATs from extragenital sites and low-prevalence populations must be confirmed.

- If gonococcus is isolated from a prepubertal girl with vulvovaginitis, it may indicate sexual abuse. A paediatrician should deal with the case sensitively, and senior laboratory staff should be involved. 'Chain of evidence' documentation is required, since evidence may be needed in court.
- Testing for co-infection with *Chlamydia* is recommended, as *Chlamydia trachomatis* commonly accompanies genital gonorrhoea (35% of heterosexual men and 41% of women with gonorrhoea).
- For further details, see assets.publishing.service.gov.uk/government/uploads/system/uploads/attachment_data/file/972388/Guidance_for_the_detection_of_gonorrhoea_in_England_2021.pdf

Treatment

The *UK national guideline for the management of gonorrhoea in adults, 2018* (available at: 🔗 https://www.bashh.org/guidelines) recommends IM ceftriaxone 1g monotherapy (the dose has increased over time due to concerns over rising MICs) for uncomplicated infection. Dual therapy is no longer recommended. A quinolone is preferred when sensitivity has been proven by testing prior to therapy being initiated. Ciprofloxacin resistance rates in the UKHSA sentinel surveillance were 36.4% in 2017, with limited alternatives: in 2017, resistance to penicillin (10.8%), tetracyclines (48.5%), and azithromycin (9.2%), and reduced susceptibility to cefixime. Infection with a resistant organism results in an adverse clinical outcome for the patient and in transmission to other contacts. The 2018 guidelines recommend a test of cure for all cases. A screen for further STIs and contact tracing are indicated in all cases.

Non-pathogenic *Neisseria*

Non-pathogenic *Neisseria* spp. are upper respiratory tract commensals and include: *Neisseria lactamica*, *Neisseria polysaccharea*, *Neisseria subflava*, *Neisseria sicca*, *Neisseria mucosa*, *Neisseria flavescens*, *Neisseria elongata*, *Neisseria cinerea*, and *Neisseria weaveri*.

Microbiology

N. lactamica and *N. polysaccharea* are the species most commonly isolated from nasopharyngeal swabs during meningococcal surveys. Colonies appear similar to *N. meningitidis* and also grow on selective media, unlike nasopharyngeal commensals. *N. lactamica* is easy to distinguish, as it produces acid from glucose, maltose, and lactose, and gives a positive ONPG test result for β-galactosidase. MALDI identification is also useful. It is thought that non-pathogenic species have contributed to the acquisition of resistance mechanisms by pathogenic organisms. *Neisseria* spp. are naturally competent for DNA uptake; thus, *N. meningitidis* and *N. gonorrhoeae* have acquired penicillin resistance by picking up the genes from other 'neisserial' flora.

Clinical features

Can occasionally cause invasive diseases such as meningitis, endocarditis, bacteraemia, ocular infections, pericarditis, osteomyelitis, and empyema—in such cases, full susceptibility testing should be performed, as penicillin resistance is increasing.

Moraxella

For decades, *Moraxella catarrhalis* was regarded as an upper respiratory tract commensal. However, since the 1970s, it has been recognized as an important and common respiratory tract pathogen.

Microbiology

M. catarrhalis grows well on many media, including blood and chocolate agar. It shows the 'hockey-stick' sign, in that it slides across the agar surface when pushed and can be difficult to pick up onto a loop. *M. catarrhalis* is oxidase-positive, catalase-positive, and DNase-positive, and produces butyrate esterase.

Clinical features

M. catarrhalis causes otitis media, lower respiratory tract infections (LRTI) in COPD patients, pneumonia (particularly in the elderly), nosocomial respiratory tract infections, sinusitis, and occasionally bacteraemia. OMPs, lipo-oligosaccharide (LOS), and pili are probably important in pathogenesis.

Treatment

Almost all strains of *M. catarrhalis* produce an inducible β-lactamase. Regardless of the results of ampicillin susceptibility testing, ampicillin should not be used. Suitable agents include co-amoxiclav, cephalosporins, fluoroquinolones, or tetracyclines.

Anaerobic Gram-negative cocci

- *Veillonella* spp. are part of the normal flora of the GI tract of humans and animals. *Veillonella* may be isolated from a variety of clinical conditions, though their role in causing infection is unclear. The commonest species is *Veillonella parvula*, which fluoresces red under ultraviolet (UV) light. *Veillonella* are able to use some of the lactic acid produced by streptococci, lactobacilli, and other bacteria that may induce dental caries. They are associated with supragingival dental plaque and are also found as part of the tongue microflora. They are generally regarded as minor components of mixed anaerobic infections.
- *Acidaminococcus* spp. and *Megosphora* spp. are other anaerobic Gram-negative cocci found in the human gut. They are considered non-pathogenic.

Escherichia coli

E. coli is the type species of the genus *Escherichia* n the order *Enterobacterales*. It contains a variety of strains, ranging from commensal organisms to highly pathogenic variants. Infections tend to involve the gut and urinary tract, but almost any extraintestinal site may be involved. *E. coli* may be a marker of faecal contamination (e.g. in food and water testing), as it does not otherwise exist outside the animal body.

Pathogenesis

- O and K polysaccharide antigens protect *E. coli* from complement and phagocytic killing, unless antibodies are present. Phagocytosis is usually successful if there are antibodies to K antigens present alone, or to both O and K antigens.
- Haemolysin is more commonly produced by strains causing extraintestinal infections, and is thought to increase virulence.
- The ColV plasmid, harboured by some *E. coli*, encodes an aerobactin-mediated iron uptake system. This is commoner in strains isolated from cases of septicaemia, pyelonephritis, and lower UTIs than in commensal faecal strains.
- Fimbriae—type 1 fimbriae adhere to cells containing mannose residues, possibly contributing to pathogenicity, but their role in UTIs is debated. Other filamentous proteins may cause mannose-resistant haemagglutination (e.g. colonization factor antigens (CFAs) in human enterotoxigenic *E. coli* (ETEC), K88 in pigs). F fimbriae bind specifically to receptors on P blood group antigens of human erythrocytes and uroepithelial cells.
- Other—enteric strains demonstrate specific interactions with the GI mucosa, release toxins, and may harbour plasmid-encoded virulence factors.

Epidemiology

Serotyping of *E. coli* is based on O (somatic), H (flagellar), and K (surface/capsular) antigens, as detected in agglutination reactions.

- There are >160 O antigens, and cross-reactions occur between *E. coli* O antigens and O antigens of other species (e.g. *Citrobacter*, *Salmonella*).
- H antigens are usually monophasic and are determined from cultures on semi-solid agar.
- Heat labile K antigens traditionally prevented O antigen (heat stable) agglutination thus agglutination tests are done on boiled samples. K antigens are acidic polysaccharide capsular antigens and divided into groups I and II.

Clinical features

Urinary tract infections

E. coli is the commonest cause of community-acquired, uncomplicated UTIs (➔ see Chapter 17, Introduction, pp. 724–5), and also causes nosocomial UTIs. Clinical manifestations range from urethritis and cystitis to pyelonephritis and sepsis. Many uropathogenic strains originate in the patient's own gut and cause infection by the ascending route. Specific P fimbriae, or 'pili associated with pyelonephritis' (known as the PAP pilus), which attach to uroepithelial cells, are important in pathogenesis. These uropathogenic strains may contain additional virulence factors such as haemolysin, ColV plasmids, and resistance to complement-dependent bactericidal effect of serum.

Enteric infections

E. coli is responsible for many cases of diarrhoeal disease, ranging from acute gastroenteritis, particularly in the tropics ('traveller's diarrhoea'; ➜ see Infectious diarrhoea, pp. 691–3), to life-threatening haemorrhagic colitis. The strains involved fall into 4–5 groups, with different pathogenic mechanisms (see Table 7.8).

Bacteraemia

Usual sources of nosocomial *E. coli* bacteraemia are the urogenital, GI, and respiratory tracts, and foreign bodies such as IV lines and endotracheal tubes. The hallmark of cases of Gram-negative bacteraemia is the systemic reaction to LPS or endotoxin, which may be fatal. Many health systems require reporting of nosocomial cases.

Neonatal sepsis

E. coli may cause neonatal meningitis and septicaemia, especially in premature babies. The strains responsible may express the K1 or K5 surface/capsular antigens, which have enhanced virulence.

Table 7.8 Clinical features and pathogenic mechanisms of different *Escherichia coli*

Abbreviation	Full name	Clinical features	Pathogenesis
EHEC VTEC STEC	Enterohaemorrhagic *E. coli* Verotoxin-producing *E. coli* Shiga toxin-producing *E. coli*	Haemorrhagic colitis/HUS	**Verotoxins** (VT1 and 2), also called shiga-like toxins (SLT1 and 2), are phage-encoded toxins thought to target vascular endothelial cells. The A subunit mediates biological activity, whereas the B subunit is responsible for binding and toxin uptake. The risk of developing HUS depends on the type of shiga toxin plus on host and environmental factors

Table 7.8   (Contd.)

Abbreviation	Full name	Clinical features	Pathogenesis
ETEC	Enterotoxigenic *E. coli*	Traveller's diarrhoea	**ST (heat-stable enterotoxin)** causes increased GMP, thus altering ion transport, and increased fluid secretion by mucosal cells of the small intestine
			LT (heat-labile enterotoxin)— B polypeptide binds to the mucosal surface of the small intestine, allowing the A polypeptide to enter the cell and catalyse adenosine diphosphate ribosylation of the guanine nucleotide component of adenylyl cyclase, thus causing increased AMP and increased fluid secretion (as with *Vibrio cholerae*)
			Colonization/adherence factors—see text
EIEC	Enteroinvasive *E. coli*	Disease similar to shigella-like dysentery	
EPEC	Enteropathogenic *E. coli*	Childhood diarrhoea	
EAEC	Enteroaggregative *E. coli*	Traveller's diarrhoea, especially in Mexico and North Africa	

NB a novel strain of *E. coli* O104:H4 caused a serious outbreak of bloody diarrhoea/HUS in Germany in 2011. This was an EAEC strain which had acquired the shiga toxin Stx2.

AMP, adenosine monophosphate; GMP, guanosine monophosphate; HUS, haemolytic uraemic syndrome.

Other non-enteric infections
E. coli may cause post-operative wound infections and deep abscesses. Respiratory tract infection is usually opportunistic, often in debilitated patients such as diabetics or alcoholics. Nosocomial pneumonia (±empyema) is usually due to aspiration, rather than haematogenous spread.

Diagnosis

E. coli usually form smooth, colourless colonies on non-selective media and may appear haemolytic on BA. Most ferment lactose, appearing yellow on CLED agar (and produce acid and gas in 24–48h), but ~5% are non-lactose fermenters. Usually motile, and those responsible for extraintestinal infections often have a polysaccharide capsule. Usually positive for indole production, ornithine decarboxylase, lysine decarboxylase, and methyl red, and negative for urease, citrate utilization, H_2S production, and Voges–Proskauer test. *E. coli* O157 are usually non-sorbitol fermenters (appear colourless/white on CT-SMAC agar). However, some do ferment sorbitol, so if high clinical suspicion (e.g. haemolytic uraemic syndrome (HUS)), send to the reference laboratory for PCR testing. Remember *E. coli* O157 is an ACDP category 3 organism.

Treatment

Management of *E. coli* infection depends on the site and severity of the infection. Simple *E. coli* UTIs may respond to nitrofurantoin, trimethoprim, or ampicillin. Some hospital-acquired *E. coli* infections are due to multiresistant organisms and may require treatment with other agents. Susceptibility data vary geographically (due to prior antibiotic usage), so follow your hospital antibiotic policy. Be guided by antibiotic susceptibility results, and use the narrowest possible targeted therapy. Antibiotics may be harmful in cases of *E. coli* O157.

Klebsiella

Klebsiella spp. are usually harmless colonizers of the human gut. The classification can be confusing, but the main species defined by DNA hybridization studies are *Klebsiella pneumoniae* subspecies *aerogenes* (formerly *Klebsiella aerogenes*), *K. pneumoniae* subspecies *pneumoniae* (formerly *Klebsiella pneumoniae*), and *Klebsiella oxytoca*. Other rare respiratory subspecies include *K. pneumoniae* subspecies *ozaenae* and *K. pneumoniae* subspecies *rhinoscleromatis*. Note that some *Klebsiella* have recently been reclassified as *Raoultella* (e.g. *Raoultella ornithinolytica* and *Raoultella terrigena*; ➔ see Other *Enterobacterales*, pp. 327–8), and also *Enterobacter aerogenes* has been reclassified as *K. pneumoniae* subspecies *aerogenes*.

Pathogenesis

Klebsiella that express capsular K antigens are resistant to complement-mediated serum killing. Those with O antigens are resistant to phagocytosis. *Klebsiella* spp. have two iron uptake systems—one uses aerobactin (related to virulence), and the other uses enterochelin (plasmid-encoded).

Epidemiology

There are about 80 K (capsular) antigens recognized overall, and K2, K3, and K21 are common in the UK. There are also five different somatic O antigen types, but these are rarely used for typing. There is an association between the antigenic structure, habitat, and biochemical reactivity—for example, capsular types 1–6 are commonest in the human respiratory tract). Capsular serotyping, bacteriocin typing, and phage typing, in addition to molecular methods and WGS, are used for epidemiological studies.

Clinical features

Klebsiella infections are rare in the immunocompetent host. They tend to cause nosocomial and opportunistic infections (UTIs, pneumonia, other respiratory infections, surgical wound infections, bacteraemia) in those with risk factors (diabetes, COPD, alcoholism). Severe pneumonia with 'redcurrant jelly' sputum and multiple lung abscesses is called Friedlander's pneumonia and has high mortality. A 'hypervirulent' strain of often very mucoid *K. pneumoniae* (hvKp) has been recognized over the last decade as a cause of unusually severe infections (classically liver abscesses, but numerous syndromes are described) in immunocompetent hosts, with a higher incidence in the Asia Pacific region. The ability to cause metastatic disease is unusual.

Diagnosis

Klebsiella spp. are facultatively anaerobic, catalase-positive, and oxidase-negative, and ferment glucose. Organisms are capsular, which may give colonies a mucoid appearance. The capsule is made of glucuronic acid and pyruvic acid. On Gram staining, organisms may look fat and chunky. They are lactose fermenters and are usually fimbriate, but non-motile. They are H_2S- and indole-negative (except *K. oxytoca* which is indole-positive), are Voges–Proskauer-positive, grow in KCN, and can use citrate as a sole carbon source. Different species of *Klebsiella* are usually recognized by different biochemical tests. They can be identified biochemically (API® 20E), via MALDI-TOF, or by using automated systems.

Treatment

Most *Klebsiella* spp. are inherently resistant to ampicillin and other penicillins. Many are now multiresistant due to extended-spectrum β-lactamases (ESBLs), depressed ampCs, and *K. pneumoniae* carbapenemase (KPCs). Aminoglycoside susceptibility varies across regions. Treat according to local hospital policy and sensitivity data.

Proteus

Proteus mirabilis is most commonly isolated from community UTIs, whereas *Proteus vulgaris* and *Proteus myxofaciens* tend to cause nosocomial infections. *Proteus* belongs to the tribe *Proteae*.

Pathogenesis

Factors that contribute to the ability of *Proteus* to colonize and infect the urinary tract include:

- production of the enzyme urease, which splits urea into ammonium hydroxide. This increases urinary pH and encourages struvite stone formation. These stones act as a nidus for persistent infection and also obstruct urinary flow;
- fimbriae help uroepithelial colonization;
- flagella-dependent motility helps spread in the urinary tract;
- uropathogenic *Proteus* synthesizes several haemolysins.

Clinical features

In addition to urine infections, *Proteus* also causes bacteraemia, wound infections, and respiratory infections in debilitated hospital patients. The human GI tract is the main reservoir of infection for patients who subsequently become infected.

Diagnosis

Proteus organisms rapidly hydrolyse urea. The presence of hundreds of flagellae on each organism makes them extraordinarily motile, appearing as 'swarming' on agar plates, and can produce the Dienes phenomenon (a line of inhibited growth where two strains meet). *Proteus* organisms give positive methyl red reactions, are usually Voges–Proskauer-negative (except some strains of *P. mirabilis*), and can grow in the presence of KCN. Most *P. mirabilis* strains are indole-negative, whereas the other subspecies are indole-positive. *Providencia* and *Morganella* have many similarities to *Proteus*, but can be differentiated by biochemical tests and MALDI.

Phage typing, bacteriocin typing, and serotyping schemes have been developed. The Dienes phenomenon may be exploited for typing—two test organisms are viewed as identical if they show no line of demarcation where the swarming growths meet (after inoculation onto the surface of an agar plate).

Treatment

Antibiotic resistance is increasing, but the indole-negative *P. mirabilis* is generally more sensitive than the indole-positive species (e.g. *P. vulgaris*), which may carry inducible AmpC β-lactamase. Amikacin and carbapenems may be the only options. Note that *Proteus* is inherently resistant to colistimethate sodium, tetracyclines, and nitrofurantoin.

Enterobacter

The genus *Enterobacter* includes *Enterobacter cloacae*, *Enterobacter sakazakii*, *Enterobacter taylorae*, *Enterobacter gergoviae*, *Enterobacter asburiae*, *Enterobacter hormaechei*, *Enterobacter cancerogenus*, *Enterobacter agglomerans*, and the recently described *Enterobacter bugandensis*. The genus was previously known as *Aerobacter* spp. and belongs to the tribe *Klebsielleae*. *E. aerogenes* has been reclassified as *K. pneumoniae* subspecies *aerogenes* (formerly *K. aerogenes*).

Epidemiology

Enterobacter organisms are common human gut commensals, which rarely cause infection in the immunocompetent host.

Clinical features

Enterobacter spp., most commonly members of the 'E. cloacae complex', can colonize hospital inpatients and cause nosocomial opportunistic infections such as wound infections, burn infections, pneumonia, and UTIs. Risk factors for infection include indwelling lines, frequent courses of antibiotics, a recent invasive procedure, diabetes, and neutropenia. They can often be isolated from diabetic ulcers. *Enterobacter* infections have been associated with IV fluid contamination. *E. sakazakii* has been implicated in severe neonatal meningitis (mortality rate of 40–80%), and there have been outbreaks associated with dried infant formula. *E. bugandensis* emerged as a highly pathogenic species, following a neonatal outbreak in Tanzania and isolation from environmental sampling on the International Space Station.

Diagnosis

In common with the other *Enterobacterales*, *Enterobacter* spp. are facultative anaerobes that give a positive catalase result and a negative oxidase result. They ferment glucose (with the production of acid and gas) and also lactose. They do not produce H_2S on triple sugar iron media; they are indole-negative and methyl red-negative; they are Voges–Proskauer-positive and can grow in the presence of KCN. They use citrate as a sole carbon source and are ONPG-positive. Unlike *Klebsiella*, they are usually motile and are less likely to be heavily capsulated. *Enterobacter* can be identified by biochemical properties (API® 20E), MALDI-TOF, or automated methods.

Treatment

Enterobacter organisms (except *E. sakazakii*) are usually resistant to first-generation cephalosporins, and readily develop resistance to second- and third-generation cephalosporins due to inducible β-lactamases such as AmpC. Carbapenems are the mainstay of treatment; alternatives include ciprofloxacin and aminoglycosides. *E. sakazakii* tends to be more sensitive to antibiotics overall, and ampicillin and gentamicin in combination are the usual treatment of *E. sakazakii* neonatal meningitis.

Further reading

Mshana S. Outbreak of a novel *Enterobacter* sp. carrying blaCTX-M-15 in a neonatal unit of a tertiary care hospital in Tanzania. *Int J Antimicrob Agents*. 2011;**38**:265–9.

Singh NK. Multi-drug resistant *Enterobacter bugandensis* species isolated from the International Space Station and comparative genomic analyses with human pathogenic strains. *BMC Microbiol*. 2018;**18**:175.

Citrobacter

Citrobacter koseri (formerly *Citrobacter diversus*), *Citrobacter freundii*, and occasionally *Citrobacter amalonaticus* are associated with nosocomial respiratory tract infections and UTIs. Their role as primary pathogens or secondary infections/colonizers is debated. *C. koseri* has also been associated with outbreaks of neonatal meningitis.

Pathogenesis

Animal studies on neonatal meningitis showed that pathogenic strains of *C. koseri* were more virulent and had an extra OMP, compared to non-pathogenic strains.

Clinical features

The clinical significance of isolation of *Citrobacter* spp. from the urinary and respiratory tracts in debilitated hospital patients is often unclear. When isolated from BCs, it is usually one of a number of species present, and such polymicrobial infections are often associated with a poor clinical outcome (probably due to the patient's general debilitated state, rather than the organism's virulence). However, *Citrobacter* is a recognized cause of endocarditis, and in neonates, *Citrobacter* organisms (particularly *C. koseri*) can cause severe meningitis and brain abscesses.

Diagnosis

Citrobacter is so named because the organisms can grow on Simmons citrate media. They are usually motile and methyl red-positive and Voges–Proskauer-negative, and slowly hydrolyse urea. They are usually non-lactose fermenters but may appear as late lactose fermenters. *C. freundii* may be mistaken for *Salmonella*, as it produces H_2S. Note there is considerable cross-reactivity with the O antigens of other *Enterobacterales*.

Treatment

Like many of the other *Enterobacterales* that cause nosocomial infections, *Citrobacter* tend to be multiresistant, so reliance on laboratory antimicrobial susceptibility testing is paramount. *C. freundii* has the inducible AmpC β-lactamase. Plasmid-mediated ESBLs are becoming commoner. Treatment options may include aminoglycosides, antipseudomonal penicillins, carbapenems, and quinolones.

Serratia

There are many named species of *Serratia*, which belong to the tribe *Klebsielleae*. *S. marcescens* is the main species that causes human disease. Infections with *Serratia liquefaciens*, *Serratia rubidaea*, and *Serratia odorifera* are very uncommon.

Epidemiology

Unlike the other *Enterobacterales*, *Serratia* is more likely to colonize the respiratory and urinary tracts of hospital patients (rather than the gut). However, in neonates, the GI tract may be the reservoir for cross-contamination. There have been reports of outbreaks in the USA due to contaminated syringes.

Clinical features

Serratia spp. are opportunistic pathogens, particularly in the healthcare setting, and cause respiratory tract infections and UTIs, bacteraemias, and skin and wound infections. Patients with IVCs and urinary catheters are at increased risk. *Serratia* infections have been associated with contaminated

IV therapy and septic arthritis in patients who have had intra-articular injections. *Serratia* also causes endocarditis and osteomyelitis in PWID, and cellulitis in patients on haemodialysis.

Diagnosis

Serratia can be recognized by the production of a characteristic red/deep pink pigment. They are slow or non-lactose fermenters, and usually motile. Like *Enterobacter*, most *Serratia* do not produce H_2S or lactose on triple sugar iron media, are Voges–Proskauer-positive, grow in the presence of KCN, and use citrate as a sole carbon source. *Serratia* can be differentiated from the other *Enterobacterales* by the production of an extracellular DNase, or by MALDI or automated methods.

Treatment

Serratia are often multiresistant to antibiotics. Treat according to local epidemiology, until sensitivity results are available. Options are often limited to amikacin, piperacillin–tazobactam, and carbapenems. Efforts focused on good infection control practice, especially handwashing, are vital in reducing horizontal transmission between patients. Note that *Serratia* organisms are inherently resistant to colistimethate sodium.

Salmonella

Salmonellae belong to the family *Enterobacterales*. There are seven subspecies and over 2400 serovars. The correct nomenclature is *Salmonella enterica*, followed by the serotype (e.g. *Salmonella enterica* serotype Typhimurium). This is commonly abbreviated to *S.* Typhimurium (serotype not italicized).

Epidemiology

Salmonellae are commensals and pathogens of a wide range of domesticated and wild animals. Some species (e.g. *S.* Typhi and S. Paratyphi) are well adapted to humans and have no other host. Others are more adapted to animals and rarely affect humans (e.g. *S.* Arizonae and reptiles). In humans, salmonellae can be divided into those that cause enteric fever (*S.* Typhi and S. Paratyphi) and the non-typhoidal *Salmonella* spp. (NTS). Salmonellae are usually transmitted by the faeco-oral route.

Pathogenesis

- Infection begins with ingestion of organisms in contaminated food and water.
- Salmonellae express an array of distinct fimbriae that help them to adhere to the intestinal wall.
- They also encode a type III secretion system (T3SS) within *Salmonella* pathogenicity island 1 (SPI-1) that is needed for bacteria-mediated endocytosis and intestinal epithelial evasion.
- A number of SPI-1 translocated proteins (SipA, SipC, SopE, and SopE2) promote membrane ruffling and *Salmonella* invasion.
- Salmonellae are also adapted to survival and replication in the intracellular environment.

Clinical features

- Gastroenteritis (➜ see Infectious diarrhoea, pp. 691–3), enteric fever (➜ see Enteric fever, pp. 693–5), bacteraemia and endovascular infection, localized infections, chronic carrier state.
- *Salmonella* bone and joint infections are seen in patients with underlying haemoglobinopathies.
- Salmonellosis in uncontrolled HIV—20- to 100-fold increased risk. More likely to have severe invasive disease (enterocolitis, bacteraemia, meningitis).

Diagnosis

- *S. typhi* and *S. paratyphi* are ACDP category 3 organisms.
- Salmonellae are facultative anaerobic GNRs, which grow readily on routine media. Their growth in specialized media is summarized in Table 7.9. They are motile, oxidase-negative, urease-negative, non-lactose fermenters.
- Salmonellae possess LPS somatic (O) heat-stable antigens, and flagellar (H) heat-labile antigens. Usually, the H antigens exhibit diphasic variation, so they can exist in phases 1 and 2 (see Table 7.10).
- *S.* Typhi, *S.* Paratyphi C, and some strains of *S.* Dublin and *Citrobacter* produce the Vi ('virulence') polysaccharide capsule, which may mask the O antigens. If only the Vi antiserum is positive, heat the bacterial suspension in boiling water to remove the capsule and test it again using the same antisera. Rough strains, in which the O antigens are absent, tend to cross-agglutinate with different antisera.
- Most diagnostic laboratories identify the organism as *Salmonella* by biochemical tests (e.g. API® 20E or shorter panel) or MALDI-TOF, and partially determine the antigenic structure with different Poly-O and

Table 7.9 Appearance of *Salmonella* spp. in different media

Agar	*Salmonella* spp.
MacConkey agar	Non-lactose fermenters appear white
CLED (cysteine, lactose, electrolyte-deficient)	Non-lactose fermenters appear blue
DCA (deoxycholate citrate)	Yellow or colourless, often with a dark centre
XLD agar (xylose–lysine–deoxycholate)	*Salmonella* appear red, some with black centres
SSA (*Salmonella, Shigella*)	Non-lactose fermenters appear colourless, some with black centres
Hektoen agar	*Salmonella* are blue-green. *S.* Typhimurium and others that reduce sulfur produce a black precipitate
Brilliant green agar	Red-pink colonies surrounded by brilliant red zones
Selenite broth	Growth of *Salmonella* results in a cloudy tube
Tetrathionate broth	Tetrathionate-reducing bacteria (*Salmonella* and *Proteus*) can grow

Table 7.10 Antigenic structure of some *Salmonella* spp

Serotype	O antigen	H (phase 1)	H (phase 2)
Typhi	9, 12 (Vi)	d	–
Paratyphi A	1, 2, 12	a	–
Paratyphi B	1, 4, 5, 12	b	1, 2
Paratyphi C	6, 7 (Vi)	c	1, 5
Typhimurium	1, 4, 5, 12	i	1, 2
Enteritidis	1, 9, 12	g, m	1, 7
Virchow	6, 7	r	1, 2
Hadar	6, 8	z10	e, n, x
Heidelberg	1, 4, 5, 12	r	1, 2
Dublin	1, 9, 12 (Vi)	g, p	–

Box 7.7 Resistance

S. typhi resistant to third-generation cephalosporins (due to CTX-M-15) was first isolated from a traveller returning to the UK from Pakistan in 2017. Consider empirical therapy with ceftriaxone plus azithromycin until AST results are available (➜ see Enteric fever, pp. 693–5).

Poly-H antisera (see Table 7.10). This identifies the causes of enteric fever or invasive serotypes.

- All *Salmonella* should be submitted to a reference laboratory for confirmation of the serotype by WGS and further epidemiological investigations, as necessary.
- *Salmonella* isolates are notifiable.

Treatment

- Enteric fever—the first-line treatment for imported cases of typhoid fever in the UK is ceftriaxone. When susceptibility results are available, options may include ciprofloxacin, azithromycin, ampicillin, or co-trimoxazole (see Box 7.7). Notifiable disease.
- NTS—gastroenteritis does not usually require treatment, except in the immunosuppressed, neonates, the elderly, and those at risk of bacteraemia. Suitable antibiotics may include ampicillin, ciprofloxacin, trimethoprim, or chloramphenicol, depending on *in vitro* susceptibility.
- Invasive disease due to NTS (e.g. bacteraemia, meningitis)—always requires therapy. Ceftriaxone penetrates the CSF well, so it may be used for *Salmonella* meningitis. Source of infection should be investigated.
- Chronic asymptomatic carriers (e.g. Typhoid Mary)—management of chronic carriers is debated. Good personal hygiene should prevent spread of disease. In the absence of biliary disease, prolonged

antibiotics (e.g. ampicillin, ciprofloxacin) may cure 80% of carriers. Cholecystectomy may be considered for patients with gallstones or chronic cholecystitis, but there is a risk of contiguous spread during surgery.

Shigella

The genus *Shigella* is divided into four species: *Shigella dysenteriae*, *Shigella flexneri*, *Shigella boydii*, and *Shigella sonnei*, based on serology and biochemical reactions (see Table 7.11). The organisms cause bacillary dysentery via an invasive mechanism identical to enteroinvasive *E. coli* (EIEC). *Shigella* belongs to the tribe *Escherichiaeae*. DNA hybridization studies show that *E. coli* and *Shigella* are a single genetic species, hence they cannot be distinguished from each other by MALDI.

Epidemiology

There are 10 serotypes of *S. dysenteriae* and 15 serotypes of *S. boydii*. *S. flexneri* can be divided into six serotypes by group- and type-specific antigens, and each serotype can be further subdivided. *S. sonnei* must be typed by other means, such as colicine production or plasmids, as they are serologically homogeneous. Most cases of shigellosis in the UK occur in young children, though infection occurs at any age after travel to areas where hygiene is poor. *S. sonnei* is endemic in the UK, whereas *S. boydii* and *S. dysenteriae*, and most *S. flexneri*, infections originate outside the UK.

Pathogenesis

The infecting dose of *Shigella* is only 10–100 organisms—when one member of a family has acquired the disease, the secondary attack rate is high. Infection can spread rapidly in institutions, especially amongst young

Table 7.11 Biochemical reactions of *Shigella*

Shigella spp.	Gas from glucose	ONPG	Indole	Catalase	Acid from		
					Lactose	Mannitol	Dulcitol
Shigella dysenteriae 1	–	+	–	–	–	–	–
Shigella dysenteriae 2–10	–	V	V	+	–	–	–
Shigella flexneri 1–5	–	–	V	+	–	+	–
Shigella flexneri 6	V	–	–	+	–	V	V
Shigella boydii	–	–	V	+	–	+	V
Shigella sonnei	–	+	–	+	(+)	+	–

(+), positive after incubation for ≥48h; ONPG, ortho-nitrophenyl-β-D-galactopyranoside; V, variable.

children. It is commonly spread by food and water. Laboratory-acquired infection has been reported.

Dysentery results from invasion of the wall of the large bowel, with accompanying inflammation and capillary thrombosis. As the organisms invade and multiply within epithelial cells, cell death results in ulcer formation. Shiga toxin (Stx) inhibits protein synthesis within target cells via a mechanism similar to ricin toxin production. Some strains also produce an exotoxin, which results in water and electrolyte secretion from the small bowel (similar to cholera toxin), which may result in watery diarrhoea preceding bloody diarrhoea.

Clinical features

- *S. dysenteriae* usually causes a more severe illness, possibly with marked prostration, paediatric febrile convulsions, toxic megacolon, and HUS.
- *S. flexneri* and *S. boydii* may also cause severe disease, whereas *S. sonnei* usually causes mild symptoms (**➲** see Gastroenteritis, pp. 691–3).
- *Shigella* rarely invades elsewhere; metastatic infection is unusual.

Diagnosis

Shigella organisms are non-motile, non-capsulated GNRs. Most appear as non-lactose fermenters after 18–24h of incubatior on MacConkey or DCA (deoxycholate citrate) agar, but *S. sonnei* is a late lactose fermenter. *Shigella* is urease-, citrate-, and H_2S-negative. *S. dysenteriae* is the only species that cannot ferment mannitol. Suspicious colonies should be confirmed with species-specific antisera, followed by type-specific antisera for all, except *S. sonnei*. *S. dysenteriae* type 1 is an ACDP category 3 organism.

Note that MALDI cannot reliably differentiate *Shigella* from *E. coli* due to their close relatedness, so any non-lactose-fermenting coliform with risk factors or clinical suspicion should be tested with *Shigella* antisera.

Shigella isolates are notified to the UKHSA automatically via the CoSurv system.

Treatment

Most cases of *Shigella* infection are mild and self-limiting, so they are treated with oral rehydration therapy, rather than with antibiotics. Antibiotics may be indicated in severe infections, patients at extremes of age, or the immunocompromised. Options include ciprofloxacin, azithromycin, ampicillin, co-trimoxazole, tetracycline, or cephalosporins according to *in vitro* susceptibility testing. Antibiotics are unlikely to reduce the period of excretion, so strict infection control measures are paramount.

Other *Enterobacterales*

- *Elizabethkingia meningoseptica* or *meningosepticum*—colonies grow slowly and are very pale yellow. Found in fresh and salt water, plants, and soil. Initially recognized as a cause of outbreaks of neonatal meningitis. Linked to nosocomial pneumonia, endocarditis, postoperative bacteraemia, and meningitis in immunocompromised adults. Associated with sepsis and soft tissue infection in the immunocompetent. Isolates are usually multi resistant to antibiotics, and co-trimoxazole/fluoroquinolones may be beneficial. Colistimethate sodium resistance and vancomycin sensitivity/intermediate growth are paradoxical for a Gram-negative bacterium.

- *Edwardsiella tarda*—infections in humans probably originate from contact with cold-blooded animals. Non-lactose fermenters, so may be mistaken for *Salmonella* spp. on enteric media. *Edwardsiella* spp. rarely cause disease but are occasionally associated with gastroenteritis, which usually resolves without antibiotics. Reports of bacteraemia, liver abscess, soft tissue infection, and meningitis.
- *Hafnia alvei* (formerly an *Enterobacter*)—belongs to the tribe *Klebsielleae*. Found in human and animal faeces, sewage, soil, water, and dairy products. Produces greyish colonies on BA and ferments fewer sugars than *Enterobacter*. All *H. alvei* are lysed by a single phage, which does not act on any other *Enterobacterales*. *H. alvei* occasionally causes opportunistic/nosocomial infections, and antibiotic sensitivities are usually similar to those of the *Enterobacter* group.
- *Kluyvera*—*Kluyvera ascorbata* is a potentially virulent pathogen, isolated from various clinical specimens; reports of UTIs, GI infections, soft tissue infections, and bacteraemia. *Kluyvera cryocrescens* is an environmental organism. Usually resistant to penicillins and cephalosporins.
- *Morganella morganii*—member of tribe *Proteeae*. Most hydrolyse urea rapidly (see Table 7.8). *Morganella* organisms cause hospital-acquired infections (HAIs), which are often multiresistant, carrying inducible AmpC, so treatment is usually with carbapenems.
- *Pantoea agglomerans* (previously known as *E. agglomerans*)—occasionally causes opportunistic infections in humans (UTIs, bacteraemia, and chest infections) and has contaminated IV fluids in the past. May be isolated from superficial skin swabs and respiratory specimens.
- *Providencia alcalifaciens*, *Providencia stuartii*, and *Providencia rettgeri*—also tribe *Proteeae*. *Providencia* causes nosocomial infections in debilitated patients, and treatment is often with carbapenems.
- *Raoultella*—oxidase-negative, capsulated GNRs (formerly designated *Klebsiella*), named after the French bacteriologist Didier Raoult. Unlike most *Klebsiella*, they grow at 10°C, consistent with their recovery from plants, soil, and water. Human infections are rare.

Overview of GNR non-fermenters

These organisms derive energy from carbohydrates by oxidative (rather than fermentative) metabolism.

Pseudomonads

Pseudomonads are a large and diverse group of aerobic, oxidative GNRs. Most are saprophytes found in soil, water, and moist environments. *P. aeruginosa* is the species most commonly associated with human disease, particularly nosocomial infections. Other opportunistic species of *Pseudomonas* include *Pseudomonas putida*, *Pseudomonas fluorescens* (which has been associated with blood transfusions), and *Pseudomonas stutzeri*. Organisms recently allocated to new genera include *Burkholderia*

(*Burkholderia cepacia* and *Burkholderia pseudomallei*), *Stenotrophomonas* (*Stenotrophomonas maltophilia*), *Comamonas* (➔ see *Delftia acidovorans* below), and *Brevundimonas* (➔ see *Brevundimonas* below).

Delftia acidovorans

Formerly known as *Comamonas acidovorans* or *Pseudomonas acidovorans*, this rare organism may cause endocarditis in drug users. Confusion arises, as it may grow on *B. cepacia*-selective media and may be resistant to colistimethate sodium and gentamicin.

Brevundimonas

Brevundimonas diminuta and *Brevundimonas vesicularis* are rare and of uncertain clinical significance. There are recent reports of bacteraemia in immunocompromised hosts, treated with piperacillin–tazobactam, amikacin, carbapenems, and tigecycline.

Glucose non-fermenters

This diverse group is taxonomically distinct from the oxidative pseudomonads and the carbohydrate-fermenting *Enterobacterales*. They are mainly opportunistic pathogens and often multiresistant to antibiotics. Identification difficulties arise because they tend to be biochemically inert.

- *Agrobacterium*—plant pathogens, usually non-pathogenic to humans, with <50 case reports of human disease in the literature.
- *Alcaligenes*—three clinically relevant species: *Alcaligenes xylosoxidans*, *Alcaligenes faecalis*, and *Alcaligenes piecnaudii*. Found in soil and water, and in the GI and respiratory tracts of hospital patients. Nosocomial outbreaks have occurred (generally in immunocompromised patients) with a wide range of clinical manifestations. *A. xylosoxidans* is often multiresistant; carbapenems or co-trimoxazole may be required.
- *Chryseobacterium*—other than *Chryseobacterium meningosepticum* (➔ see Other *Enterobacterales*, pp. 327–8), isolation of these organisms from clinical samples usually reflects colonization.
- *Chryseomonas*—infection with the rare *Chryseomonas luteola* is usually associated with peritoneal dialysis catheters or indwelling lines, and may result in peritonitis, endocarditis, bacteraemia, or meningitis.
- *Eikenella corrodens*—oral commensal and cause of endocarditis ('E' in HACEK; ➔ see HACEK organisms, pp. 342–4), meningitis, skin and soft tissue infections (particularly human bites), and pneumonia. Facultative anaerobe, requiring incubation in CO_2. The colonies pit ('corrode') the surface of the agar.
- *Flavimonas oryzihabitans*—found in soil, water, and damp environments, and may cause line-associated bacteraemias in the immunocompromised.
- *Flavobacterium*—this group of yellow-pigmented organisms is so genetically diverse that many have been reclassified. *Flavobacterium meningosepticum* is now *Elizabethkingia meningoseptica* (➔ see Other *Enterobacterales*, pp. 327–8). Other flavobacteria now belong to the genus *Sphingobacterium* (➔ see *Sphingobacterium* below).

- *Ochrobactrum*—previously called *Achromobacter*, *Ochrobactrum anthropi* causes nosocomial opportunistic infections, particularly catheter-related bacteraemia.
- *Oligella*—*Oligella urethralis* (formerly *Moraxella urethralis*) is a GU tract commensal, whereas *Oligella ureolytica* is usually found in patients with long-term indwelling urinary catheters. They are of low pathogenicity.
- *Roseomonas*—known as the 'pink-pigmented coccoid' group. *Roseomonas gilardii* is the commonest species isolated from humans and has been reported to cause community-acquired bacteraemia.
- *Shewanella*—*Shewanella putrefaciens* (formerly *Pseudomonas putrefaciens*) is commonly isolated from water and the environment, but rarely causes human disease. It is usually found as part of a polymicrobial infection, typically from cellulitis complicating a leg ulcer or burn.
- *Sphingobacterium*—contains high amounts of sphingophospholipid compounds in the cell membrane. Most human isolates of this genus are *Sphingobacterium multivorum* and *Sphingobacterium spiritivorum*, which can cause nosocomial infections in various sites. Isolation from respiratory samples from CF patients are of uncertain significance.
- *Sphingomonas paucimobilis*—implicated in nosocomial outbreaks associated with contaminated water. It may be confused with flavobacteria, as it produces a non-diffusible yellow pigment.

Pseudomonas aeruginosa

P. aeruginosa is widespread in soil, water, and moist environments. Hospitalized patients may be colonized with *P. aeruginosa* at moist sites such as the perineum, ear, and axilla. It is a highly successful opportunistic pathogen, largely due to its resistance to many antibiotics, its ability to adapt to a wide range of physical conditions, and minimal nutritional requirements.

Epidemiology

P. aeruginosa is found almost anywhere in the environment, including surface waters, vegetation, and soil. It usually colonizes hospital and domestic sink traps, taps, and drains. It also colonizes moist areas of human skin, leading to 'toe web rot' in soldiers stationed in swampy areas, and otitis externa in divers in saturation chambers.

Pathogenesis

The broad range of conditions caused by *P. aeruginosa* may be explained by the fact that the pathogen is both invasive and toxigenic. *P. aeruginosa* has low intrinsic virulence in man and animals. Infection occurs when host defences are compromised or the skin/mucous membranes are breached (e.g. neutropenia, burns patients, intensive care patients, indwelling devices), or when a relatively large inoculum is introduced directly into the tissues. The process can be divided into three stages: bacterial attachment/colonization, local invasion, and dissemination/systemic disease. Different virulence factors are produced, depending on the site and nature of the infections, and include:

- exotoxins (exotoxin A and exo-enzyme S) and endotoxins (LPS);

- cytotoxic substances—proteases (elastase and alkaline phosphatase (ALP)), cytotoxin (previously called leucocidin), haemolysins, phospholipases, rhamnolipids, pyocyanin;
- porins;
- pili and fimbriae (important in epithelial adherence, e.g respiratory).

Clinical features

P. aeruginosa causes a wide spectrum of conditions.

- Community-acquired infections are rare, and tend to be mild and superficial. Examples include otitis externa, varicose ulcers, and folliculitis associated with jacuzzis.
- Nosocomial infections with *P. aeruginosa* tend to be more severe and more varied than community infections. *P. aeruginosa* may account for ~10% of all HAIs. Examples include pneumonia, UTIs, surgical wound infections, bloodstream infections (BSIs), and respiratory infections.
- CF patients (see Box 7.8), burns patients, and mechanically ventilated patients are at particular risk.
- Other conditions associated with *P. aeruginosa* include endocarditis (PWID and prosthetic valves), eye infections, bone and joint infections, post-operative neurosurgical infections, and ear infections.

Box 7.8 *Pseudomonas aeruginosa* in patients with cystic fibrosis

P. aeruginosa colonizes up to 80% of CF patients and causes chronic lung infection. Once established, it is refractory to treatment, partly due to the formation of biofilms. Many isolates appear mucoid due to the production of an alginate-like exopolysaccharide capsule (glycocalyx) that resists phagocytosis and contributes to biofilm formation. Isolates may have atypical growth requirements such as appearing auxotrophic for specific amino acids and non-motile. Primary culture plates often show mixed colonial forms that are usually genetically identical. Results for susceptibility testing often vary, and CF clinicians may base their choice on multiple factors, including prior response to treatment. Some strains, such as the Liverpool epidemic strain (LES), are transmissible and may be more aggressive. Typing is available, and CF patients colonized with LES may be segregated to prevent transmission.

Diagnosis

Non-sporing, non-capsulate, motile GNR. Strict aerobe (hence often used in testing anaerobic cabinets) but can grow anaerobically in the presence of nitrate. It grows in many different culture media and produces a characteristic 'freshly cut grass' odour. The typical green-blue colour is due to the diffusible pigments pyocyanin (blue phenazine pigment) and pyoverdin (yellow-green fluorescent pigment; principal siderophore). Other pigments include pyorubrin (red) and pyomelanin (brown). Note that ~10% do not produce detectable pigments, even in pigment-enhancing media. *P. aeruginosa* is oxidase-positive (usually within 10s) and appears relatively inactive in carbohydrate fermentation tests (only glucose is used). It grows best at 37°C and also at 42°C, but not at 4°C. Confusion occasionally arises in differentiating *P. aeruginosa* from other *Pseudomonas* spp. with use of commercial kits—growth at 42°C; flagella stains and differential sugar fermentation tests may prove useful.

For epidemiological studies, serotyping may be useful; four 'O serotypes' account for ~50% of clinical and environmental isolates. PFGE may help to discriminate between serotypes. Molecular typing (e.g. VNTR or WGS) is useful for cross-infection and outbreak investigations, and for surveillance amongst CF patients.

Treatment

Antipseudomonal agents include ciprofloxacin (quinolones provide the only PO option), ceftazidime, ticarcillin, piperacillin, carbapenems, aminoglycosides (gentamicin, tobramycin, amikacin), polymyxins (colistimethate sodium), and aztreonam. Newer agents include ceftolozane–tazobactam, ceftazidime–avibactam, and cefiderocol. Theoretically, the use of dual therapy should reduce the development of antibiotic resistance and may also have the potential for bacterial synergy, but there is little clinical evidence for this.

Acinetobacter

Historically, a pathogen of tropical climates, *Acinetobacter* spp. are an important cause of nosocomial infections. They accumulate multiple antibiotic resistance mechanisms. Increasing antibiotic-selective pressure and the ability to survive well in the environment (including on curtains and in dust) have contributed to its success as an opportunistic pathogen. There are ~19 genospecies, based on DNA–DNA hybridization studies; seven of these have species names (see Table 7.12).

Table 7.12 Genomic species of *Acinetobacter*

Genospecies	Species name
1	*Acinetobacter calcoaceticus*
2	*Acinetobacter baumannii*
4	*Acinetobacter haemolyticus*
5	*Acinetobacter junii*
7	*Acinetobacter johnsonii*
8	*Acinetobacter lwoffi*
12	*Acinetobacter radioresistens*
Other	*Acinetobacter* spp. unnamed (>14)

Epidemiology

Acinetobacter has been an increasingly common nosocomial pathogen since the 1970s, affecting debilitated patients. Infections tend to peak in summer, and are associated with wars and natural disasters. Nosocomial spread in ICUs is common, and may occur via fomites, the environment, and colonized HCWs. Dramatic multi-hospital outbreaks have occurred. Colonization of British military casualties repatriated to the UK from Iraq and Afghanistan has caused infections and onward transmission to other hospitalized patients. In the UK, there have been outbreaks of two multiresistant clones carrying carbapenem-hydrolysing class D β-lactamases (OXA-23 and OXA-51). These are now widespread.

Risk factors

Risk factors include:
- community-acquired infections—alcoholics, smokers, chronic lung disease, diabetes, and living in a tropical developing country;
- HAIs—ICU, ventilation, urinary catheter, IV lines, length of stay, treatment with broad-spectrum antibiotics, total parenteral nutrition (TPN), surgery, wounds.

Pathogenesis

This organism has very few virulence factors, which explains why it only causes opportunistic infections. It occurs naturally as a saprophyte in soil and water, and occasionally colonizes moist human skin. The ability to survive in the environment is probably related to the capsule, the production of bacteriocin, and prolonged viability under dry conditions.

Clinical features

Acinetobacter spp. are able to infect almost every organ system, though it is vital to distinguish true infection from pseudo-infection (e.g. pseudo-bacteraemia due to skin colonization). The commonest site of infection is the respiratory tract where it causes nosocomial pneumonia, particularly ventilator-associated pneumonia (VAP), adult community-acquired pneumonia (CAP), and community-acquired tracheobronchitis and bronchiolitis in children. Other sites include the urinary tract, intracranial (usually postneurosurgery), soft tissue (burns, wounds, and device-associated cellulitis), the eye, heart (endocarditis), and bone. Nosocomial bacteraemia is usually associated with the respiratory tract or IV catheters, and has a reported mortality rate of 17–46%. *Acinetobacter baumannii* bacteraemia tends to be more severe.

Diagnosis

Acinetobacter spp. classically appear as Gram-negative coccobacilli, though they may retain crystal violet, so they appear Gram-positive. They are generally encapsulated, non-motile organisms, which readily grow in routine media as white, mucoid, oxidase-negative, catalase-positive colonies. Misidentification may arise using API® profiles, as they are biochemically relatively unreactive, but acidification of glucose, haemolysis of RBCs, and the ability to grow at 44°C are more reliable characteristics. They are readily identified on MALDI.

Treatment

- International surveillance systems have observed increasing resistance in *Acinetobacter* spp. In 2009, 61% of isolates were resistant to ceftazidime, and 86% to carbapenems. Carbapenem susceptibility may be discordant (e.g. imipenem-susceptible, meropenem-resistant). Polymyxins (e.g. colistimethate sodium) usually have activity, but resistance may occur. Susceptibility testing should include carbapenems, aminoglycosides (including amikacin), sulbactam, and polymyxins (e.g. colistimethate sodium, tigecycline). There is some evidence to support combination therapy with rifampicin and colistimethate sodium ± carbapenem. Cefiderocol is an emerging option.
- Empirical treatment might include a combination of a cephalosporin or carbapenem with a fluoroquinolone, aminoglycoside, or colistimethate sodium if local resistance rates are high.
- Once susceptibility is known, the usual rules of antibiotic stewardship should apply (i.e. the narrowest-spectrum effective agent)—there are no data to demonstrate that combination therapy reduces the emergence of resistance.
- Inhaled/nebulized colistimethate sodium may be useful in pneumonia, and intrathecal or intraventricular administration in meningitis caused by highly resistant strains. IV colistimethate sodium achieves low lung and CSF concentrations.
- Involve the reference laboratory and infection prevention control team as appropriate.

Stenotrophomonas maltophilia

Previously called *Pseudomonas maltophilia* or *Xanthomonas maltophilia*, this opportunistic pathogen of relatively low virulence has an amazing ability to survive in a wide range of environments, especially in hospitals. It is inherently resistant to most antibiotics, including carbapenems.

Epidemiology

Ubiquitous in the environment, *S. maltophilia* has been isolated from multiple sources in hospitals, including water (tap and distilled), nebulizers, dialysis machines, solutions, IV fluids, thermometers, etc. Transmission of nosocomial infections has been associated with hospital water or contaminated disinfectant solutions. Studies have shown that most outbreaks result from antibiotic-selective pressure (especially extensive use of carbapenems, to which *S. maltophilia* is intrinsically resistant), rather than from cross-infection.

Risk factors

Risk factors for nosocomial infections include: ICU stay, increased length of stay, treatment with broad-spectrum antibiotics, malignancy (especially if immunosuppressed), instrumentation (e.g. urinary catheter, IV lines, intubation, TPN, CAPD), patients with COPD, and neutropenia.

Pathogenesis

Potential virulence factors include those involved in adherence to plastics, and production of exo-enzymes such as elastase and gelatinase.

Clinical features

S. maltophilia can cause a variety of infections, ranging from superficial to deep tissue to disseminated disease. It is most commonly isolated from the respiratory tract, and distinguishing true infection from colonization can be difficult. *S. maltophilia* pneumonia has a high mortality rate. Other common sites of *S. maltophilia* infection include skin and soft tissues, intra-abdominal, the urinary tract, the eyes (especially in contact lens wearers), and device-related.

Diagnosis

A motile, non-lactose-fermenting GNR that grows readily on standard media. It is a strict aerobe. It is often pale yellow on BA, with an ammonia-like smell. Most are oxidase-negative and catalase-positive. Resistance to a carbapenem may be a useful marker. Note that *S. maltophilia* is increasingly isolated from sputum in patients with CF. It grows well on colistimethate sodium-containing media, so it may be misidentified as *B. cepacia*.

Treatment

Unfortunately, results of antibiotic susceptibility testing correlate poorly with treatment outcome. The drug of choice is co-trimoxazole. Other options to consider include ticarcillin–clavulanic acid, doxycycline, minocycline, newer-generation quinolones, and third-generation cephalosporins. There is clinical evidence that co-trimoxazole and moxifloxacin may be synergistic. Most strains are resistant to aminoglycosides.

Burkholderia cepacia complex

Previously classified as *Pseudomonas cepacia*, these opportunistic pathogens are a particular problem in CF patients. Other risk factors for infection include chronic granulomatous disease and sickle-cell haemoglobinopathies. There are at least 18 different phylogenetically similar, but genomically distinct, species (termed genomovars) in the *B. cepacia* complex. Most important are *B. cepacia*, *Burkholderia multivorans*, and *Burkholderia cenocepacia* (genomovars I, II, and III, respectively). The prevalence of each varies with geographical region.

Epidemiology

Members of the complex are found in the natural environment and have been isolated from multiple sources in hospitals. Environmental transmission may occur via contact with respiratory equipment, water supplies, or disinfectants. However, transmission between colonized patients to other CF patients is more significant, and patients should be segregated into separate groups (e.g. for outpatient clinics and summer camps). This can be a highly emotive issue. Patient-to-patient transmission is commonest with *B. cenocepacia* but has also been reported for *B. multivorans* and *Burkholderia dolosa*. The epidemiology within CF units has changed as a result of segregation—B. *cenocepacia* has declined in many European units, and *B. multivorans* (now commonest) strains acquired by patients are genotypically unrelated, suggesting an environmental source, rather than patient-to-patient transmission.

Pathogenesis

These organisms can survive in a wide range of environments. Virulence factors include adherence to plastics, production of elastase, gelatinase, adhesin (a mucin-binding protein), siderophores, flagella, efflux pumps, haemolysin, exopolysaccharide, quorum-sensing systems, and metalloproteases. Resistance to non-oxidative neutrophil killing may be important.

Clinical features

Genomovars II and III are the commonest causes of *B. cepacia* colonization in CF patients. The three main patterns of infection are:
- chronic asymptomatic carriage;
- progressive deterioration over months, with frequent hospital admissions, recurrent fevers, and weight loss (similar to *P. aeruginosa*);
- necrotizing pneumonia and bacteraemia, associated with rapid deterioration, which is nearly always fatal. Risk factors for this pattern include ♀ with poor lung function and severe CXR changes ('cepacia syndrome')—particularly associated with *B. dolosa*, *B. multivorans*, and *B. cenocepacia*;
- pre-lung transplant colonization is associated with high post-transplant mortality. This effect is most pronounced with *B. cenocepacia*. Death in the early post-transplant period may be characterized by cepacia syndrome. Abscess and empyema are later complications.

In other patients, *Burkholderia* spp. can cause a range of other infections, from superficial to deep tissue to dissemination disease, but these are rare.

Diagnosis

Burkholderia spp. are motile, non-lactose fermenting aerobic GNRs. Selective media are necessary for culture. Colistimethate sodium resistance may be a useful indicator. Identification can be difficult—MALDI and commercial systems or kits have significant limitations in identifying members of the *B. cepacia* complex, so they should be confirmed by molecular (genotypic) methods at a reference laboratory because of implications for the patient and infection control. Full details of the lab processing are in the UK SMI document "Investigation of bronchoalveolar lavage, sputum and associated specimens" available at: www.gov.uk/government/publications/smi-b-57-investigation-of-bronchoalveolar-lavage-sputum-and-associated-specimens

Treatment

B. cepacia complex members show high rates of resistance to antipseudomonal antibiotics, including colistimethate sodium. Agents, such as co-trimoxazole, chloramphenicol, minocycline, and carbapenems, show good *in vitro* activity against *Burkholderia* spp. However, there are limited clinical data on the best approach to treatment. Clearance of some drugs is increased in the CF population, which may make dosing difficult. Use of combination therapy is debated, but in general, two or more drugs with *in vitro* activity are used. Synergy has not been consistently demonstrated clinically or *in vitro*—the aim is to reduce the development of resistance. Note that all *Burkholderia* spp. are constitutively resistant to colistin, and many become multiresistant on treatment. Commonly used combinations include meropenem with ceftazidime or tobramycin.

Burkholderia gladioli

Formerly known as *Pseudomonas marginata* and closely related to *B. cepacia* complex. Can be distinguished from the other *Burkholderia* microbiologically, because it is oxidase-negative. An opportunistic pathogen in CF and associated with a poor outcome.

Burkholderia pseudomallei

B. pseudomallei (formerly known as *Pseudomonas pseudomallei*) causes melioidosis, which is endemic in parts of South East Asia, Northern Australia, and the Caribbean. It is a major cause of community-onset septicaemia in North East Thailand.

Epidemiology

In endemic areas, *B. pseudomallei* can be cultured from moist soil, surface water (rice paddies), and the surface of many fruits and vegetables. Rodents carry it.

Pathogenesis

B. pseudomallei can survive and multiply within phagocytes; hence, a long course of antibiotics is recommended and antibiotics active *in vitro* do not always lead to clinical cure.

Clinical features

B. pseudomallei is usually acquired through inhaling contaminated particles or cutaneously through skin abrasions. It can infect almost any organ. Manifestations range from subclinical infection to pneumonia (may cavitate with profound weight loss, resembling TB), skin ulcers/abscesses, genital infection and prostatitis, bone and joint infection, encephalomyelitis, or overwhelming septicaemia. Parotid infection occurs in children. May present years after exposure, due to the intracellular nature of the organism.

Diagnosis

- *B. pseudomallei* is a hazard group 3 organism. All specimens should be handled in containment level (CL) 3 if melioidosis is suspected clinically.
- **Samples**—if case is suspected, culture blood, sputum, urine, throat, and rectal swabs, as well as any lesion/pus
- **Gram staining**—may show small bipolar GNRs.
- **Culture**—grows well on blood or Ashdown medium nutrient agar, after 1–2 days. They appear either wrinkled and dry, or mucoid and, after prolonged incubation, may turn orange. A strict aerobe, and oxidizes glucose and breaks down arginine. The API® 20NE reliably identifies most isolates, as does MALDI. Characteristically resistant to gentamicin and colistimethate sodium.

- Early involvement of the reference laboratory is recommended for confirmatory tests (e.g. PCR, IgM- and IgG-specific EIAs, serology, but note there are problems with sensitivity and specificity).

Treatment

Even mild disease should be treated intensively. The first 14 days should be with an IV agent (ceftazidime or a carbapenem) or longer if clinical improvement is slow. This should be followed by at least 3 months' PO therapy to prevent relapse (6 months for bone or neurological infection). Co-trimoxazole is preferred. Co-amoxiclav is an alternative—but less effective. Note that resistance to these PO agents may develop during treatment; seek expert advice.

Overview of fastidious Gram-negative rods

These organisms often require specialist supplementation or media for culture. They can be divided by appearance on Gram staining as follows:
- coccobacilli:
  - *Haemophilus*;
  - HACEK organisms;
  - *Gardnerella*;
  - *Bordetella*;
  - *Brucella*;
  - *Yersinia*;
  - *Pasteurella*;
  - *Francisella*.
- rods with pointed ends:
  - *Legionella*;
  - *Capnocytophaga*.
- curved rods:
  - *Vibrio*;
  - *Aeromonas*, *Plesiomonas*;
  - *Campylobacter*;
  - *Helicobacter*.

Streptobacillus moniliformis causes rat bite fever, as does *Spirillium minor*.

B. mallei causes glanders, which is a rare disease of horses in Asia, Africa, and the Middle East. It is a hazard group 3 organism but has not been isolated in the UK since the 1940s. In humans, it causes symptoms similar to melioidosis.

Haemophilus influenzae

H. influenzae is a small, fastidious Gram-negative coccobacillus, belonging to the family *Pasteurellaceae*. It is highly adapted to humans and found in the nasopharynx of 75% of healthy children and adults.

Epidemiology

Polysaccharide encapsulated (serotypes a–f) and non-encapsulated 'non-typeable' strains. Droplet transmission. *H. influenzae* serotype b (Hib) used to be a common cause of invasive infections in children, including meningitis, septic arthritis, and epiglottitis. The annual incidence of invasive Hib disease dropped dramatically after the introduction of the Hib conjugate vaccine in 1993. The lack of a toddler booster saw the incidence rising due to waning immunity and rising cases from 1999. Booster vaccination to those under 4 years old from 2004 onwards saw a reduction in invasive disease across all age groups, as carriage fell.

Pathogenesis

H. influenzae inhabits the upper respiratory tract of humans; 25–80% of healthy people carry non-capsulated organisms, whereas 5–10% carry capsulated strains (~50% of which are capsular type b). In addition to the polysaccharide capsule that facilitates invasion, virulence factors of capsular type b include fimbriae (involved in attaching to epithelial cells), IgA proteases (aid in colonization), and OMPs (involved in invasion). There is evidence that simultaneous viral infection may initiate invasion. Other serotypes and unencapsulated strains are rarely invasive but can cause pneumonia or severe disease in high-risk groups.

Clinical features

- Invasive infections (e.g. meningitis, epiglottitis, bacteraemia with no clear focus, septic arthritis, pneumonia, cellulitis). Mostly caused by capsular type b. Types e and f and non-capsulated strains may also cause serious disease. Infections generally occur between 2 months and 2 years of age, as babies aged <2 months are protected by maternal antibody.
- Non-invasive infections (e.g. otitis media, sinusitis, endometritis, purulent exacerbations of COPD). These local infections are usually associated with non-capsulated organisms. There may be an underlying abnormality (anatomical or physiological). Intercurrent viral infection may precipitate an infection.

Diagnosis

- **Culture**—growth in the presence of X (haemin) and V (nicotinamide adenine dinucleotide (phosphate), NAD(P)) factors. X is needed to synthesize certain respiratory enzymes that contain iron (e.g. cytochrome c, cytochrome oxidase catalase, peroxidase). V is required for oxidation–reduction processes in metabolism. BA contains both X and V, but *H. influenzae* grows poorly. NAD supplementation improves growth on BA, as will streaking an organism that excretes NAD (e.g. *S. aureus*)—this phenomenon is called **satellitism**. *H. influenzae* grows well on chocolate agar, which is made by heating BA at 70–80°C for a few minutes to inactivate the NADase, which normally limits

utilization of V factor. Growth is also better in CO_2-enriched conditions. Oxidase-positive.
- Antibiotic susceptibility testing with discs may be unreliable. Nitrocefin strips are recommended to test for β-lactamases. MIC is needed for invasive infections.
- Antigen detection (e.g. latex agglutination) is rarely used now. Molecular tests (e.g. PCR) are available.
- **Capsule detection**—encapsulated strains of *H. influenzae* are responsible for most invasive infections (e.g. meningitis, epiglottitis), whereas respiratory infections and otitis media are usually associated with non-encapsulated strains. The polysaccharide capsule can be demonstrated by the Quellung reaction with type-specific antisera at a reference laboratory.
- **Antigenic type**—there are six antigenic types (a–f). Hib causes the most severe invasive infections.
- **Biotypes**—there are eight biotypes of *H. influenzae* (I–VIII), based on indole, ornithine decarboxylase, and urease reactions.

Treatment
- Severe infection—first line: third-generation cephalosporins (e.g. ceftriaxone). Bactericidal, penetrates the CSF and clinically effective. Alternatives include co-trimoxazole, ampicillin (but ~20% of UK type b strains produce β-lactamase), or chloramphenicol.
- Non-invasive infection—PO ampicillin (~20% of UK non-capsulated strains are β-lactamase-positive), co-amoxiclav, or azithromycin. Note there are reports of increasing resistance to macrolides and quinolones.
- β-lactamase-negative, ampicillin-resistant (BLNAR) *H. influenzae* are becoming increasingly recognized worldwide. The mechanism of resistance is altered PBPs. β-lactamase is absent phenotypically, but the ampicillin MIC is ≥4mg/L. They are usually sensitive to ceftriaxone.

Prevention
- Vaccine—the Hib conjugate vaccine (capsular polysaccharide and protein) was introduced in the UK in 1992. Now given at 2, 3, 4, and 12 months. The impact of vaccination far exceeded that predicted, due to the added benefit of herd immunity. Give to unimmunized contacts of index cases. For detailed information about the use of the Hib vaccine, web search 'UK Green Book Hib'.
- Chemoprophylaxis—only required if the index case is confirmed or probable and under 10 years of age, or if there is a vulnerable individual in the household (ideally within 48h, but up to 4 weeks after index diagnosis). The preferred agent is rifampicin. Reduces carriage and onward transmission. May be considered for close contacts in school outbreaks. For full details, see Public Health England 2013 guidance '*Revised recommendations for the prevention of secondary Haemophilus influenzae type b (Hib) disease*' (available at: ℘ www.gov.uk/governm ent/publications/haemophilus-influenzae-type-b-hib-revised-recommen dations-for-the-prevention-of-secondary-cases).

Other *Haemophilus* species

Haemophilus spp., other than *H. influenzae*, are usually considered rare causes of human disease. Most are normal flora of the human mouth and upper respiratory tract. However, they may be associated with infections such as endocarditis, respiratory tract infections, septicaemia, brain abscess, meningitis, and soft tissue infections.

Haemophilus parainfluenzae

H. parainfluenzae is increasingly recognized as a cause of human infection. Clinical infections are similar to those caused by *H. influenzae*, but *H. parainfluenzae* tends to be less virulent. *H. parainfluenzae* has been reported as a cause of pharyngitis, epiglottitis, otitis media, conjunctivitis, dental abscess, pneumonia, empyema, septicaemia, endocarditis, septic arthritis, osteomyelitis, meningitis, abscesses, and urinary and genital tract infections. *H. parainfluenzae* differs from *H. influenzae* in that it is V factor-dependent only.

Haemophilus haemolyticus and *Haemophilus parahaemolyticus*

These species rarely cause human disease, but *H. haemolyticus* may be difficult to distinguish from *H. influenzae*, so it may be commoner than previously considered.

Aggregatibacter aphrophilus

Haemophilus aphrophilus and *Haemophilus paraphrophilus* have been reclassified as a single species on the basis of multiple locus sequence analysis—*Aggregatibacter aphrophilus*, which includes V-factor-dependent and V-factor-independent isolates. *Actinobacillus actinomycetemcomitans* has also been renamed *Aggregatibacter aphrophilus*.

Haemophilus segnis has been reclassified as *Aggregatibacter segnis*.

Organisms require CO_2 for growth and are independent of the X factor. They cause a variety of infections, including sinusitis, otitis media, pneumonia, empyema, bacteraemia, endocarditis, septic arthritis, osteomyelitis, meningitis, abscesses, and wound infections

Haemophilus ducreyi

This causes chancroid, an STI, common in Africa and South East Asia. It presents as a painful penile ulcer associated with inguinal lymphadenopathy. Microbiological diagnosis may be made when Gram-negative coccobacilli are isolated from a lymph node aspirate or from ulcer swabs. Microscopy is classically described as a 'shoal of fish' appearance. Treatment options include tetracyclines, erythromycin, and co-amoxiclav.

Haemophilus influenzae biogroup *aegyptius*

H. influenzae biogroup *aegyptius* was previously known as *Haemophilus aegyptius* or the Koch–Weeks bacillus. It is very similar biochemically to *H. influenzae* biotype III but can be differentiated by PCR. It causes Brazilian purpuric fever (conjunctivitis leading to fulminant septicaemia, with high mortality) and epidemic purulent conjunctivitis. Combination therapy with ampicillin and chloramphenicol is usually recommended.

HACEK organisms

The HACEK organisms (see Box 7.9) are rare causes of endocarditis (➔ see Infective endocarditis, pp. 672–4), which tends to be insidious in onset (mean time to diagnosis ~3 months). Most are part of normal human mouth flora and are occasionally associated with periodontitis and infections elsewhere (e.g. joints). They grow slowly and may need prolonged incubation (14 days) in CO_2 supplementation. High index of suspicion and close liaison with the laboratory are crucial.

> ## Box 7.9 The HACEK organisms
> * *Haemophilus influenzae*
> * *Haemophilus parainfluenzae*
> * *Haemophilus parahaemolyticus*
> * *Aggregatibacter aphrophilus*
> * *Aggregatibacter segnis*
> * *Aggregatibacter actinomycetemcomitans*
> * *Cardiobacterium hominis*
> * *Eikenella corrodens*
> * *Kingella kingae*

Aggregatibacter actinomycetemcomitans

A mouth commensal and major pathogen of the genus *Aggregatibacter*. There are two other *Aggregatibacter* spp.: *A. aphrophilus* (includes *H. aphrophilus* and *H. paraphrophilus*) and *A. segnis* (formerly *H. segnis*).

* Diagnosis—difficult to culture. Fastidious and grows slowly, so BCs should be incubated for at least 14 days. Growth is enhanced by CO_2 supplementation (5–10%). *Aggregatibacter* may form 'granules' in BCs or broth (the media remains clear). On Gram staining, often looks coccoid or coccobacillary, resembling *Haemophilus*. Catalase-positive. Does not grow on MacConkey and is biochemically similar to *Pasteurella* spp.
* Pathogenesis—periodontal disease is associated with the ability to invade and multiply within gingival epithelial cells, and with the production of a leucotoxin that lyses neutrophils. Other potential virulence factors include bacteriocin, endotoxin, chemotaxis-inhibiting factor, and fibroblast-inhibiting factor.
* Clinical—can cause endocarditis, joint infections, and severe periodontal disease. Has been found (together with some *Haemophilus* spp., fusiforms, and anaerobic streptococci) in actinomycotic lesions.
* Treatment—usually susceptible to third-generation cephalosporins (4 weeks for native, and 6 weeks for prosthetic, valve endocarditis). Periodontitis requires debridement plus antibiotic treatment (e.g. tetracyclines).

Cardiobacterium hominis

C. hominis is the only species in the genus. It is normal flora in the human mouth, nose, and throat, and occasionally other mucous membranes and the GI tract. Unlike the other HACEK organisms, it rarely causes diseases other than endocarditis.

- Diagnosis—GNR with a pleomorphic appearance and may be difficult to decolorize during Gram staining. Culture is enhanced in 5–10% CO_2 and high humidity. It grows well on BA and chocolate agar, with slight β-haemolysis, but poorly on MacConkey agar. It is catalase-negative and oxidase-positive.
- Treatment—sensitivity testing is difficult, because of slow growth, but usually susceptible to β-lactams, tetracycline, and chloramphenicol. Cephalosporin resistance has been reported, so MICs are critical. Hence, the current first-line recommendation of ceftriaxone for HACEK organisms may not be optimal for *C. hominis* endocarditis—an alternative regimen to consider is co-amoxiclav and gentamicin.

Eikenella corrodens

E. corrodens exists as normal mouth and upper respiratory tract flora.
- Diagnosis—facultative anaerobic GNR. Oxidase-positive and catalase-negative. About 50% of strains create a depression in the agar ('corroding bacillus'). As with the other HACEK organisms, culture is slow and enhanced in 5–10% CO_2.
- Clinical features—subacute endocarditis, but is more commonly found as part of mixed infections (e.g. human bite wounds, head and neck infections, respiratory tract infections). It often coexists with *Streptococcus* spp. Infections are usually indolent, taking >1 week from time of injury to clinical symptoms of disease. Suppuration is common and may smell like an anaerobic infection.
- Treatment—usually susceptible to β-lactams, tetracyclines, and fluoroquinolones. It is uniformly resistant to clindamycin, erythromycin, and metronidazole, and often resistant to aminoglycosides.

Kingella kingae

There are four species of *Kingella*, all of which colonize the respiratory tract and rarely cause human disease: *K. kingae* (previously known as *Moraxella kingae*), *Kingella indologenes* (now known as *Suttonella indologenes*), *Kingella denitrificans*, and *Kingella oralis*. *K. kingae* is the commonest, and a recent increase in cases is likely to be due to increased awareness of the organism and improved diagnostics.
- Diagnosis—they are short GNRs with tapered ends, which sometimes appear coccoid. They tend to resist decolorization, so they may look Gram-positive. *Kingella* is catalase-negative and oxidase-positive. *K. kingae* grows on BA and chocolate agar, but not on MacConkey agar. To increase the chance of recovering *K. kingae* from joint fluid, the fluid should be inoculated into BC bottles, rather than just plated out directly onto agar plates.
- Clinical features—most cases of invasive disease occur in children aged between 6 months and 4 years. *K. kingae* most commonly causes bacteraemia, endocarditis (of native and prosthetic valves), and septic

arthritis. *K. indologenes* and *K. denitrificans* also cause endocarditis. *K. oralis* is found in dental plaque, but its relationship with periodontal disease is unknown.
- Treatment—most *Kingella* spp. appear susceptible to penicillins and cephalosporins; however, β-lactamase producers have been reported. Alternatives include aminoglycosides, co-trimoxazole, tetracyclines, erythromycin, and quinolones.

Gardnerella

Gardnerella vaginalis is found in the ♀ genital tract and is associated with bacterial vaginosis (BV)/non-specific vaginitis (➔ see Bacterial vaginosis, pp. 741–3). It is usually classified with GNRs, though it is normally susceptible to vancomycin. Of interest, electron microscopy (EM) studies have noted the cell wall to be either Gram-negative or Gram-positive, or to show an atypical laminated appearance.

Epidemiology
There is debate on whether specific biotypes have been associated with BV. Newly acquired strains of *G. vaginalis* may precipitate BV, rather than overgrowth of previously colonizing biotypes.

Pathogenesis
Adherence of *G. vaginalis* to vaginal and urinary epithelial cells may play a role in the pathogenesis of BV and UTIs. Pili have been seen on *G. vaginalis*, and *G. vaginalis* also produces a cytolytic toxin (haemolysin). It is serum-resistant, which may aid survival during bloodstream invasion at childbirth.

Clinical features
- BV—*G. vaginalis* is almost universally present in women with BV along with mixed anaerobic flora.
- UTI—*G. vaginalis* is isolated from <1% of UTIs and, because of its presence in the ♀ genital tract, could represent vaginal contamination. However, it has been found from suprapubic aspirates, and also in association with renal disease and interstitial cystitis.
- Bacteraemia—this rare event is associated with ♀ genital tract conditions such as chorioamnionitis, post-partum endometritis, and septic abortion. Neonatal infection has also been reported.

Diagnosis
Gardnerella is a facultative anaerobe, which appears as a pleomorphic Gram-variable rod. It is oxidase- and catalase-negative, non-encapsulated, and non-motile. It needs enriched media for growth. Note that *G. vaginalis* is susceptible to sodium polyanetholesulfonate (SPS), which is found in most BC bottles, so bacteraemia figures may be underestimated. In clinical practice, BV is diagnosed using the Amsel criteria.

Treatment
G. vaginalis is usually susceptible to penicillin, clindamycin, and vancomycin, and resistant to colistimethate sodium, cefalexin, and tetracyclines. Metronidazole is usually the preferred treatment for BV. See 'UK National

Guideline for the management of bacterial vaginosis 2012' (available at: ✆ https://www.bashh.org/documents/4413.pdf).

Bordetella

Bordetella pertussis and *Bordetella parapertussis* cause whooping cough, which is a notifiable disease in England and Wales. The other species only cause human infections under special circumstances—these are *Bordetella bronchiseptica* (causes kennel cough in dogs and snuffles in rabbits), *Bordetella avium* (bird pathogen), *Bordetella hinzii*, *Bordetella holmesii*, and *Bordetella trematum*.

Epidemiology

The organism is spread by droplets and is highly infectious. Pertussis has the highest incidence in infants but also occurs in adolescents and adults. Morbidity and mortality are higher in ♀ than in ♂, and in those <6 months old. In the UK, pertussis displays 3- to 4-yearly peaks in activity.

Pathogenesis

B. pertussis produces a number of biologically active substances that are thought to play a role in disease:
- surface components (e.g. filamentous haemagglutinin (FHA), pertactin, and fimbriae);
- toxins such as pertussis toxin (PT), adenylyl cyclase toxin (ACT), tracheal cytotoxin (TCT), and dermonecrotic toxin (DNT);
- other products (e.g. tracheal colonization factor and BrKA (*Bordetella* resistance to killing)).

Clinical features

- Incubation of 7–10 days is followed by a 'catarrhal stage' similar to a viral upper respiratory tract infection (URTI). Fever is unusual. Cough gradually worsens over 1–2 weeks.
- A 'paroxysmal stage' follows. In children, there may be distinctive whoops, gagging, cyanosis, conjunctival haemorrhage, and vomiting. These are most bothersome at night. Lasts for 2–8 weeks. Symptoms are less severe in vaccinated children and adults, in whom prolonged cough may be the only symptom.

Diagnosis

- **Microscopy**—tiny coccobacilli, occur singly or in pairs. *B. pertussis* and *B. parapertussis* are non-motile.
- **Culture**—on Bordet–Gengou agar, pearly colonies on days 3–4; CCBA agar (charcoal cephalexin): *B. pertussis* produces glistening greyish-white colonies, whereas *B. parapertussis* colonies are larger and duller and become visible sooner. Do not grow on nutrient agar and grow poorly on BA. Culture lacks sensitivity.
- **Molecular**—PCR for toxin promoter or insertion sequence IS481 (occurs in *B. pertussis*, *B. holmesii*, and some *B. bronchiseptica*). Consider reference laboratory confirmation (per nasal swab or NPA) in cases

of compatible respiratory illness in a child <12 months on paediatric intensive care unit (PICU) or paediatric ward.
- **Serology**—anti-PT IgG antibody levels are determined using an EIA, on paired sera or single samples taken >2 weeks after onset for any individuals with prolonged cough.

Treatment

- Whooping cough is a notifiable condition.
- Antibiotics are recommended for children with clinical pertussis (even in the absence of laboratory diagnosis) or asymptomatic with a positive PCR for the purposes of reducing transmission. Treatment has to be early (within 7 days of symptoms) to decrease severity; thus, it is of limited help in the paroxysmal phase—it does, however, eliminate carriage. Patients are most contagious in the catarrhal phase and first 2 weeks of cough.
- Adults can be considered for treatment if symptoms are under 2 weeks or if cough persists after 4 weeks, particularly if they are in one of the priority groups mentioned under the point 'Antibiotic prophylaxis' below.
- Usual agents are clarithromycin or azithromycin for 7 days. Co-trimoxazole for 14 days is an alternative.
- Antibiotic prophylaxis—a 2007 Cochrane review concluded there was insufficient evidence to determine the benefit of prophylactic treatment of pertussis contacts. UK guidelines recommend offering prophylaxis to close contacts of an index case if disease onset was within 21 days AND one of the contacts belongs to a priority group—in which case, all close contacts should be offered treatment. Priority groups include those aged under 1 year who have received <3 doses of pertussis vaccine, pregnant women, HCWs working with infants and pregnant women, and those who work, or share a house, with an infant under 4 months of age (and thus not fully vaccinated). See 'Guidelines for the public health management of pertussis' (2018; available at: ℘ www.gov.uk/government/publications/pertussis-guidelines-for-public-health-management).

Vaccine

- Acellular pertussis (aP) vaccine is given in the primary immunization course as DTaP/IPV/Hib, at ages 2, 3, and 4 months. A further booster as dTaP–IPV is given with preschool boosters, as vaccine immunity wanes over time. There were major epidemics of whooping cough in 1977/9 and 1981/3, after immunization coverage dropped from >80% to 30%, following a report linking the vaccine to brain damage.
- A national outbreak in the UK in 2011/12 affected all age groups, including infants <3 months of age. An enhanced surveillance scheme was set up, and pertussis immunization offered to pregnant women to protect infants from birth (see Pertussis: the green book, available at: ℘ https://www.gov.uk/government/publications/pertussis-the-green-book-chapter-24).

Brucella

Brucella spp. (see Table 7.13) cause brucellosis (undulant fever, Mediterranean fever, Malta fever) and contagious/infectious abortion in cattle. This zoonosis is transmitted via contaminated or untreated milk and milk derivatives, or by direct contact with infected animals or their carcasses. *Brucella* spp. survive well in aerosols and resist drying, so they are candidates for agents of bioterrorism (➔ see Bioterrorism, pp. 882–3).

Table 7.13 Main species of *Brucella*

Brucella spp.	Animal infected	Human manifestations
B. *abortus*	Cattle; bison and elk in North America	Brucellosis
B. *suis*	Pigs (swine brucellosis)	Brucellosis
B. *melitensis*	Goats/sheep	Brucellosis
B. *canis*	Dogs (mainly beagles in the USA)	Mild disease only
B. *ovis*	Sheep (Australia and New Zealand)	No evidence this species infects man

NB the host relationship is not absolute, and man and domestic animals may be susceptible to infections by different species.

Epidemiology

Virtually eliminated from most developed countries, including the UK (animal vaccination, pasteurization, screen/slaughter of infected herds). It remains endemic in Africa, the Middle East, central and South East Asia, South America, and some Mediterranean countries (including Greece, Turkey, Portugal, Spain, Italy, and Southern France). Human–human transmission has been documented but is rare—methods include breast milk, sexual transmission, and congenital disease. Around 10 cases occur in the UK annually—almost always acquired abroad. Brucellosis also occurs through occupational exposure of laboratory workers, vets, and slaughterhouse workers. A careful epidemiological patient history is crucial, regarding travel, diet (e.g. unpasteurized dairy produce), and possible exposure.

Pathogenesis

After ingestion (or entry via skin abrasions or inhaling infected dust), the bacteria live in the regional lymph nodes during the incubation period (usually 2–8 weeks). They then enter the circulation and subsequently localize in different parts of the reticuloendothelial system, forming granulomatous lesions that may result in complications in many organs. *Brucella* organisms surviving within granulomas may cause relapses of acute disease or result in chronic brucellosis.

Clinical features

Brucellosis has a wide variety of clinical presentations. The 'undulant' or wave-like fever rises and falls over weeks in ~90% of untreated patients. Malodorous perspiration is said to be pathognomonic. Localized infection occurs in 30%, osteoarticular most commonly, with epididymo-orchitis in ~6%. Other symptoms include weakness, headaches, depression, myalgia, and body pain. Hepatomegaly and splenomegaly may occur. Sequelae are also variable, and include granulomatous hepatitis, anaemia, leucopenia, thrombocytopenia, meningitis, uveitis, and optic neuritis. Infection in pregnancy is associated with abortion, premature delivery, and intrauterine infection with fetal death.

Diagnosis

- *Brucella* is a hazard group 3 organism. Laboratory exposure is a Health and Safety Executive (HSE)-reportable clinical incident, requiring RIDDOR (Reporting of Injuries, Diseases and Dangerous Occurrences Regulations) reporting and thorough risk assessment of laboratory staff. Guidance on prophylaxis and follow-up of staff can be found via the brucellosis reference laboratory (available at: ℘ https://www.gov.uk/guidance/bru-reference-services).
- **Culture from blood or bone marrow**—marrow culture is the gold standard, most sensitive, especially in chronic disease, and less affected by prior use of antibiotics. Growth can take up to 8 weeks. Coccobacilli or short bacilli. May occur singly, in chains, or in groups. Non-motile, non-sporing, and non-capsulated. Aerobic, and *B. abortus* requires 5–10% CO_2 to grow. The three main species (*Brucella melitensis*, *B. abortus*, *Brucella suis*) can be differentiated biochemically and by antigenic structure. Each species can be further divided into biotypes—there are >9 biotypes of *B. abortus*, >3 of *B. melitensis*, and >5 of *B. suis*.
- **Serology**—raised (1:160) or a 4-fold rise in antibody titre over 2 weeks in symptomatic patients suggests the diagnosis of active *Brucella*. Difficult to interpret in those from endemic areas or with relapsed infection. Demonstration of antibodies: standard agglutination, mercaptoethanol test, rose Bengal reactions, EIA. At the reference laboratory, all sera are screened with a *Brucella* antibody assay and specific IgG/IgM EIA. Positive samples then undergo further testing with in-house micro-agglutination and complement fixation.
- **Other**—histology (e.g. granulomatous hepatitis), radiology (e.g. the 'pedro-pons sign', preferential erosion of the antero-superior corner of lumbar vertebrae), PCR (usually positive within 10 days of infection).

Treatment

Drugs must enter macrophages and be active in an acidic environment.
- Uncomplicated—doxycycline 6 weeks, with either 14–21 days of streptomycin OR 6 weeks of rifampicin. Fluoroquinolones (also in combination) have a role in relapsed or resistant disease.
- Focal infection, including articular and neurological—at least 12 weeks' treatment and three-drug regimens may be required for neurological disease or endocarditis (which also needs surgery).
- Antibody levels may be measured to monitor response to therapy.

Prevention

Good standards of hygiene in the production of raw milk and its products, or pasteurization of all milk, will prevent brucellosis acquired from ingestion of milk. Also avoid contact with infected animals. Vaccination of young cattle helps to protect animals against *B abortus* but is not completely effective. However, it helps to limit the spread of disease and thus aids in eradication. Only by testing all animals, and slaughtering those with positive results, can the disease be truly eradicated.

Yersinia pestis

Y. pestis causes plague. There are three clinical syndromes: bubonic, pneumonic, and septicaemic (see Table 7.14). Found worldwide, but most cases are reported from developing countries of Africa and Asia. There are ~10 cases annually from rural areas of the USA. The last case acquired in the UK was in 1918.

Pathogenesis

The somatic (heat-stable) and capsular (heat-labile) antigens are important in virulence and immunogenicity. Somatic antigens V and W help to resist phagocytosis, and the capsular antigen containing the immunogenic fraction (F1) is antiphagocytic also. Other virulence factors include an LPS endotoxin,

Table 7.14 Features of the main clinical forms of plague

	Bubonic	Pneumonic	Septicaemic
Transmission	Rat flea bites *Xenopsylla cheopis*	Respiratory aerosols from rat fleas. Person-to-person spread in crowded, unhygienic conditions, during epidemics. May arise as a complication of bubonic or septicaemic plague	Primary infection. Complication of bubonic or pneumonic plague
Diagnostic specimen	Fluid from buboes	Sputum	BCs/blood films
Clinical symptoms	Fever, painful buboes, inguinal lymphadenopathy	Cough or haemoptysis ± bubo	Fever, hypotension, no buboes
Incubation period	2–8 days	1–4 days (maximum 6 days)	2–8 days
Mortality if untreated	~60%	High mortality (approaching 100%)	High mortality (approaching 100%)

the ability to absorb iron as haemin, and temperature-dependent coagulase and fibrinolysin.

Diagnosis

- **Culture**—short Gram-negative coccobacillus, occurs singly or in pairs (or as chains in fluid culture). Old cultures are pleomorphic and may resemble yeast cells. Non-sporing, non-motile, and often capsulated at 37°C. Methylene blue shows bipolar staining. *Yersinia* spp. grow between 14°C and 37°C, with optimal growth at 27°C. Small, non-haemolytic colonies are seen on BA at 24h. Catalase-positive and oxidase-negative. Although *Y. pestis* grows on MacConkey agar, it tends to autolyse after 2–3 days. Usually cultured from a bubo aspirate, but may also grow from blood, CSF, or sputum. Cefsulodin–Irgasan–Novobiocin (CIN) agar is selective for *Yersinia* and *Aeromonas* spp. ('bullseye' appearance).
- Direct immunofluorescence is a more rapid diagnostic method.
- Serological tests for yersiniosis (acute and convalescent) include the complement fixation test and haemagglutination of tanned sheep red cells onto which F1 capsular antigen has been adsorbed.

Treatment

Early antibiotic therapy for suspected cases (e.g. streptomycin, gentamicin, or doxycycline) reduces the otherwise high mortality to ~10%. Contacts may also be given antibiotic prophylaxis. Patients with pneumonic plague should be isolated until they are sputum smear-negative (usually ~3 days since starting treatment). There is no vaccine currently available. It is a notifiable disease.

Yersinia enterocolitica

Epidemiology and clinical features

- *Y. enterocolitica* resembles *Y. pestis* and *Yersinia pseudotuberculosis* on culture and morphologically, but differs antigenically and biochemically. The commonest serotypes causing human infection in Europe are 3 and 9. Acquired from eating infected meat or milk. Patients with conditions associated with iron overload (e.g. haemochromatosis) and the immunosuppressed are at increased risk of *Yersinia* infections.
- Usually presents as a febrile illness associated with bloody diarrhoea, and may mimic salmonellosis, shigellosis, or appendicitis. Other presentations include mesenteric lymphadenitis and septicaemia, which may be fatal in the elderly. Secondary complications include erythema nodosum, polyarthritis, peritonitis, reactive arthritis (previously known as Reiter's syndrome), meningitis, osteomyelitis, and hepatic, renal, and splenic abscesses. *Y. enterocolitica* has been cultured from pseudotuberculous lesions in animals.

Treatment

- Gastroenteritis usually resolves without antibiotics. In severe infection, the recommended regimen is doxycycline plus an aminoglycoside.

Alternatives—ceftriaxone, co-trimoxazole, and fluoroquinolones. Note resistance to penicillin.
- If the patient is on desferrioxamine, this should be stopped, as it may increase the severity of infection.

Yersinia pseudotuberculosis

Epidemiology and clinical features
- Strains can be differentiated by somatic and flagellar antigens, some of which are shared with *Y. pestis*. Most human infections are due to serotype 1.
- Causes fatal septicaemia in animals and birds. Humans usually acquire the infection from contact with water polluted by infected animals or from eating contaminated vegetables—infection due to direct contact with animals is rare. In humans, yersiniosis ranges from asymptomatic to a fatal typhoid-like illness with fever, purpura, and hepatosplenomegaly. Mesenteric adenitis ± erythema nodosum may mimic appendicitis.

Diagnosis and treatment
- GNR, slightly acid-fast, grows poorly on MacConkey agar (like *Y. pestis*). Can produce urease and motile at 22°C, unlike *Y. pestis*.
- Shows *in vitro* susceptibility to ciprofloxacin, tetracyclines, aminoglycosides, sulfonamides, and penicillin. Mesenteric adenitis is usually self-limiting.

Pasteurella

The genus *Pasteurella* includes the species *Pasteurella multocida*, *Pasteurella haemolytica* (now known as *Mannheimia haemolytica*), *Pasteurella canis*, *Pasteurella stomatis*, and *Pasteurella pneumotropica*. *Pasteurella* live in the mouth, and GI and respiratory tracts of many animals (especially dogs and cats) ± humans. *P. multocida*, the most frequent human isolate, usually causes skin and soft tissue infections.

Epidemiology
Fifteen serotypes of *P. multocida* have been identified, based on four capsular antigens and 11 somatic antigens. PFGE can be used to compare strains. Humans acquire infection from animal bites or inhaling air contaminated by infected animals' coughing.

Pathogenesis
In animals, *P. multocida* causes haemorrhagic septicaemia, which is usually fatal. Most virulent *Pasteurella* strains have a polysaccharide capsule, which is antiphagocytic and protects against intracellular killing by neutrophils. Also, some strains produce a leucotoxin, and some bind transferrin.

Clinical features
- *P. multocida* causes skin and soft tissue infections after animal bites, most commonly a localized abscess, with cellulitis and lymphadenitis. *P. multocida* has also been associated with URTIs and LRTIs. Other sites

of infection are uncommon—these include meningitis post-head injury, bone and joint infections, septicaemia, endocarditis, and intra-abdominal infections.

- *P. haemolytica* is not thought to be pathogenic for humans. It causes pneumonia in sheep and cattle, and septicaemia in lambs, and also infects poultry and domestic animals.
- *P. pneumotropica* may be isolated from the respiratory tract of laboratory animals. There are reports of it causing human infections (e.g. animal bite wound infections, septicaemia, URTIs).

Diagnosis

P. multocida is a facultatively anaerobic Gram-negative coccobacillus, which appears pleomorphic in culture and does not grow on MacConkey agar. At 37°C, organisms are capsulated, non-sporing, and non-motile. They show bipolar staining with methylene blue. Most are fermentative, and oxidase-positive and catalase-positive.

Treatment

Penicillin is the mainstay of treatment, and there is a wealth of clinical experience to support this. It is resistant to PO first-generation cephalosporins, flucloxacillin, clindamycin, and erythromycin. It is sensitive *in vitro* to fluoroquinolones, which may be considered in penicillin-allergic patients.

Francisella

Francisella tularensis is primarily an animal pathogen (rabbits and hares), which occasionally infects humans as accidental hosts, as a result of contact with infected animals or invertebrate vectors (especially in summer months). Only two of the five subspecies are clinically important: type A (*F. tularensis* subspecies *tularensis*) is highly virulent, and type B (*F. tularensis* subspecies *holarctica*) less virulent. It is a potential agent of bioterrorism (➔ see Bioterrorism, pp. 882–3).

Epidemiology and pathology

Tularaemia is endemic in North America and parts of Europe, Asia, northern Australia, and Japan. Most cases in man are sporadic, though outbreaks have been reported. It may survive for days in moist soil and in water polluted by infected animals, and for years in culture at 10°C. Organisms are killed in 10min after exposure to moist heat at 55°C. There is evidence from animal experiments of intracellular multiplication of *F. tularensis*. The capsule and citrulline ureidase activity contribute to virulence.

Clinical features

Infection (tularaemia) ranges from asymptomatic to septic shock, depending on the virulence of the particular strain, host immune response, route of entry, and degree of systemic involvement. A history with relevant epidemiology is vital. There are two main forms:

- **ulceroglandular**—commonest, patients usually report animal contact; acute-onset fever, headache, and rigors, usually followed by glandular lesions, and skin ulceration may occur (hands/arms after animal exposure, head/neck, trunk, or perineum after tick exposure, e.g. eschar);

- **typhoidal/pulmonary**—follows insect exposure or inhaling infected dust, or eating contaminated food or water Acute-onset fever, headache, and rigors, followed by respiratory or typhoid-like symptoms.

Diagnosis

F. tularensis is a hazard group 3 organism. It is a small, non-motile, non-sporulating, capsulated Gram-negative coccobacillus, which shows characteristic bipolar staining with carbol fuchsin (10%). It stains poorly with methylene blue. It is a strict aerobe, and culture requires the addition of egg yolk or rabbit spleen to agar. Traditional microbiological methods are being replaced by immunological and molecular tests, including EIA and immunoblots for antibodies (but tests relying on antibody detection are limited in early clinical stages of disease). If a case is suspected, involve the UKHSA Reference Unit at Portor Down promptly. It is a notifiable organism.

Treatment

Seek expert advice. Streptomycin or gentam cin are antibiotics of choice, with the addition of chloramphenicol for meringitis. Ciprofloxacin is a PO option for those with mild illness. A 10- to 14-day course is required. Relapse is commoner with tetracycline or chloramphenicol, as they are bacteriostatic for *F. tularensis*. The live vaccine is based on an attenuated strain of *F. tularensis*. PEP with doxycycline or ciprofloxacin may be considered after potential inhalation.

Legionella

This organism is named after the outbreak of pneumonia affecting >180 members of the American Legion at a convention in Philadelphia in 1976. *Legionellaceae* naturally live in water and only incidentally infect humans. This may result in either legionnaire's disease or Pontiac fever. There are 52 different genetically defined species of *Legionella*, of which ~50% infect humans. *L. pneumophila* serogroup 1 is the most pathogenic and accounts for ~95% of human cases.

Epidemiology

Legionella is acquired via inhalation of contaminated aerosolized water (e.g. from spas, showers, air conditioning systems, water storage tanks, nebulizers) or environmental sources (e.g. potting soil can contain *Legionella longbeachae*). Water systems are more likely to be contaminated with *Legionella* if the temperature is outside the recommended range (it should be <20°C or >55°C), if the flow is obstructed, or if biofilms have formed. It is an intracellular organism and can survive in amoebae, within the environment. The incubation period is 2–10 days, and occasionally symptoms may develop up to 3 weeks post-exposure. It is not transmitted from person to person. Most cases are isolated, but clusters and outbreaks occur.

Pathogenesis

After the infection is established, pneumonic consolidation develops, characterized by proteinaceous fibrinous exudates pouring into the alveoli. The mechanism of distant toxic changes (e.g. confusion, hallucinations, focal neurology) is poorly understood. *Legionella* organisms are engulfed by monocytes and may survive intracellularly for prolonged periods of time.

Clinical features

In addition to the two main clinical syndromes, rare conditions (e.g. prosthetic valve endocarditis, wound infections) have been reported:

- **legionnaire's disease**—rapidly progressive pneumonia, characterized by fever, respiratory distress, and confusion. Mortality of >10% in healthy people. May be associated with hyponatraemia. Risk factors include age >50 years, hospital admission, immunosuppression, and smoking. Men are affected more than women;
- **Pontiac fever**—a brief flu-like illness, with a high attack rate, but low mortality.

Diagnosis

- **Microscopy/culture**—short rods/coccobacilli may be difficult to see on Gram staining, so fluorescent antibody staining or silver impregnation may help. Grows best on media such as BCYE agar, which contains iron plus cysteine as an essential growth factor. Some strains prefer 2.5–5% CO_2 at 35–36°C. *L. pneumophila* colonies usually appear by day 5, but other species may require 10 days. Colonies may autofluoresce under UV light. Serogroups can be differentiated by slide agglutination or fluorescent antibody tests (FATs), which are available at reference laboratories.
- **Antigen detection**—*Legionella* urinary antigen test (EIA) only detects serogroup 1 of *L. pneumophila*; thus, it will be negative in outbreaks caused by other serogroups.
- **Molecular methods**—*Legionella* PCR is available at some reference centres.
- **Antibody detection**—FAT, rapid micro-agglutination test (RMAT), or EIA. A >4-fold rise or titre 1:256 is usually diagnostic. Remember that antibodies may take >8 days to develop after onset of infection and may persist for months/years post-infection. Some cross-reactivity with *Campylobacter*.

Treatment

- Conventional susceptibility tests in broth and agar are unreliable. Many antibiotics with *in vitro* activity (e.g. β-lactams, aminoglycosides) are ineffective.
- Macrolides (azithromycin, clarithromycin), quinolones, tetracyclines, and rifampicin are effective, as they have good intracellular penetration.
- Levofloxacin may bring about more rapid defervescence, but outcomes are similar. Duration of 7–10 days.
- Combination therapy may have a role for the treatment of endocarditis.

Control and prevention

Legionnaire's disease is a notifiable condition. Control relies on good design and maintenance of water systems to prevent growth of *Legionella* organisms, and on subsequent treatment of the source (e.g. contaminated water systems) if a case occurs (see Box 7.10). The main approaches to control are **physical** (heat, UV light, sonication), **chemical** (inhibiting scale

Box 7.10 Legio\nella guidance

A full list of UK guidance, including water system maintenance, case investigation, and prevention, is available at: ℗ https://www.gov.uk/government/collections/legionnaires-disease-guidance-data-and-analysis.

formation, use of biocides to kill amoebae, use of charcoal filters), and attention to **plumbing** (maintenance, no dead legs in the system, pumps in series (not in parallel), no dead spaces in heaters, regular flushing of the system).

Capnocytophaga

Genus *Capnocytophaga* in the family *Flavobacteriaceae*. Two groups:
- species associated with dog bite infections (and occasionally bites from other animals such as rabbits or cats)—*Capnocytophaga canimorsus* and *Capnocytophaga cynodegmi*;
- species found in the human mouth—*Capnocytophaga ochracea*, *Capnocytophaga gingivalis*, *Capnocytophaga sputigena*, *Capnocytophaga haemolytica*, and *Capnocytophaga granulosa*.

Epidemiology

While *C. canimorsus* and *C. cynodegmi* are most commonly associated with bites, occasionally infections occur merely after exposure to dogs. Species found in the human mouth produce a variety of enzymes that help invasion of periodontal tissue (e.g. acid and alkaline phosphotases, aminopeptidases, IgA, proteases, trypsin-like enzymes).

Clinical features

Amongst animal bite infections, those caused by *C. canimorsus* are commoner and more severe than those by *C. cynodegmi*, with a mortality rate approaching 30%. Risk factors—asplenic patients (it is encapsulated), alcoholics, and those on steroids. Asplenic patients with *C. canimorsus* infection may present with shock, disseminated purpuric lesions, and DIC. Fulminant infections may also occur in healthy people, though infections tend to be milder. Meningitis, endocarditis, pneumonia, corneal ulcer, cellulitis, and septic arthritis due to *C. canimorsus* have also been reported.

Species found in the human mouth may be important in localized juvenile periodontitis. May colonize the ♀ genital tract, and is associated with intra-uterine infection, amnionitis, and neonatal infections in premature babies. Rare presentations—endocarditis, eye infections, and peritonitis.

Diagnosis

- Long, thin, delicate GNRs, typically fusiform, but older cultures often show pleomorphic sizes and shapes. Facultative anaerobes, grow best with CO_2 enrichment. On BA or chocolate agar, may appear yellowish, with a spreading edge with finger-like projections due to typical gliding motility. No growth on MacConkey agar.
- Differentiation of individual species usually requires reference laboratory assistance. In general, species from the human mouth are

oxidase-negative and catalase-negative, whereas those from animals' mouths are oxidase-positive and catalase-positive.
- *C. canimorsus* is more fastidious than the others and may be difficult to grow from BCs—culture on enriched agar (e.g. heart infusion agar with rabbit or sheep blood) for 14 days in 10% CO_2 may help.

Treatment

Co-amoxiclav is usually recommended. Asplenic patients should be given prophylaxis after a dog bite, pending culture, as the organism may take a while to grow, and mortality is high. Resistance to β-lactams has been reported in the human mouth species—for example, *C. haemolytica* and *C. granulosa* are often resistant to β-lactams and aminoglycosides. All species are usually sensitive to clindamycin, erythromycin, tetracyclines, and quinolones.

Vibrios

The genus *Vibrio* (family *Vibrionaceae*) includes over 30 species. The most important ones that result in human infections are *Vibrio cholerae*, *Vibrio parahaemolyticus*, and *Vibrio vulnificus*. Other species, such as *Vibrio alginolyticus*, *Vibrio damsela* (now known as *Listonella damsela*), *Vibrio fluvialis*, *Vibrio hollisae* (now known as *Grimontia hollisae*), and *Vibrio mimicus*, occasionally cause opportunistic infections.

Vibrio cholerae

There are ~20 cases of cholera (➲ see Cholera, pp. 696–8) imported into the UK every year. These are most commonly O1-El Tor. In the mid 1990s, a new serogroup (O139) appeared in the Bay of Bengal—this was the first time a non-O1 serogroup had resulted in epidemic cholera.

Epidemiology

Cholera is prevalent in Central and South America, Africa, and Asia. There are >130 different O (somatic antigen) serogroups of *V. cholerae*. Serogroup O1 (the 'cholera vibrio') causes epidemic cholera, and some strains of non-O1 (the 'non-cholera or non-agglutinable vibrios) can also cause diarrhoea. Serogroup O1 is usually acquired by the faecal–oral route, whereas non-O1 *V. cholerae* may be associated with consumption of seafood or exposure to saline environments. The two biotypes of serogroup O1 (**El Tor**, which is the commonest, and **classical**) can be distinguished by susceptibility to phage and the fact that El Tor is haemolytic and resistant to polymyxin B. The subtypes of serogroup O1 are Ogawa (commonest), Inaba, and Hikojima (which possesses determinants of both other subtypes).

Pathogenesis

The potent cholera enterotoxin, produced by serogroup O1 and some non-O1 strains, comprises five B (binding) subunits and one A (active) subunit. Insertion of the B subunits into the host cell membrane forms a channel for subunit A to enter the cell. By causing the transfer of adenosine diphosphate (ADP) ribose from nicotinamide adenine dinucleotide (NAD) to another protein, adenylyl cyclase is irreversibly activated and cAMP is overproduced. The resulting hypersecretion of chloride ion (Cl^-) and bi-carbonate ion (HCO_3^-) causes massive loss of water and electrolytes (rice-water stool). Other features important in the pathogenesis of serogroup O1 include production of mucinase and other proteolytic enzymes (which help the organism reach the enterocytes), the motility of the organism, and adhesive haemagglutinins (aid in close adherence to the enterocyte surface). Non-O1 strains may produce other enterotoxins, cytotoxins, haemolysins, and colonizing factors.

Cholera is transmitted by contaminated food or water, and requires a large infective dose. Humans are the only host. Only a handful of those infected are symptomatic (ratios quoted are 40 asymptomatic carriers to one symptomatic individual for El Tor, and 5:1 for classical), which underscores the need for good hygiene.

Clinical features

V. cholerae usually causes the typical profuse watery diarrhoea of cholera, which may rapidly lead to hypovolaemic shock and death from dehydra-tion. Milder cases are similar to other causes of secretory diarrhoea, and asymptomatic infections also occur. Non-O1 *V. cholerae* usually causes mild, sometimes bloody, diarrhoea but may occasionally be severe and resemble cholera. Patients exposed to aquatic environments may suffer from wound infections, and bacteraemia and meningitis have been reported.

Diagnosis

During an epidemic, cholera is a clinical diagnosis. Otherwise, diagnosis is based on high clinical suspicion, together with culture or dark-field mi-croscopy of faecal samples (comma-shaped organisms are seen moving around, which ceases when diluted O1 antisera is added). Vibrios are short, curved, or 'comma-shaped' aerobic GNRs, which are motile by a single polar flagellum. They ferment both sucrose and glucose, but not lactose. Most are oxidase-positive (the test must be performed from non-selective media). The growth characteristics of vibrios are summarized in Table 7.15.

Table 7.15 Growth characteristics of *Vibrio* spp.

Species	TCBS agar	Biochemistry	Salt requirement	Growth at 42°C
Vibrio cholerae	Yellow	Oxidase-positive	Not halophilic (0–3% NaCl)	Yes
Vibrio parahaemolyticus	Green		Halophilic (3–6% NaCl)	Yes
Vibrio vulnificus	Green (85%), yellow (15%)	Lactose-negative	Halophilic (3–5% NaCl)	No
Vibrio alginolyticus	Yellow		Halophilic (3–10% NaCl)	Yes

NaCl, sodium chloride.

V. cholerae is non-halophilic (i.e. it can grow on media without added salt), provided the necessary electrolytes are present. *V. cholerae* can grow at 42°C (along with *V. parahaemolyticus* and *V. alginolyticus*). Vibrios are tolerant of alkali but have a low tolerance to acid. Vibrios accumulate on the surface of alkaline peptone water. If a loopful is inoculated onto TCBS agar, *V. cholerae* appears as a yellow sucrose fermenter. *V. cholerae* is killed by most detergents and by heating at 55°C for 15min. However, it can survive for up to 2 weeks in salt water at ambient temperatures, and also on chitinous shellfish for 2 weeks, even if refrigerated.

Treatment

Cholera is a notifiable condition. Rehydration is key. Antibiotics (e.g. azithromycin, ciprofloxacin) reduce the duration of disease and the period of excretion of *V. cholerae* in faeces of infected patients. Antibiotic treatment is not routinely required but should be considered in those with severe illness or during an outbreak. In the UK, a killed oral vaccine is licensed for relief workers and travellers to remote endemic areas. However, the most important preventative strategies are improvement of sanitation and food and water standards.

Vibrio parahaemolyticus

V. parahaemolyticus is ubiquitous in fish and shellfish, and in the waters they inhabit. Outbreaks of diarrhoea occur infrequently in the UK.

Epidemiology

V. parahaemolyticus infection is common in South East Asia, particularly Singapore and Japan. However, it also occurs in the UK and USA, particularly during summer months.

Pathogenesis

Kanagawa-positive strains (➔ see Diagnosis below) of *V. parahaemolyticus* adhere to human enterocytes and produce a heat-stable cytotoxin.

Clinical features

V. parahaemolyticus is usually acquired through ingesting seafood and causes acute explosive diarrhoea. Extraintestinal infections arise from handling contaminated seafood or exposure to the aquatic environment, the commonest being wound infections.

Diagnosis

This organism is halophilic (salt-loving); hence, it will not grow on CLED agar. Clinical strains of *V. parahaemolyticus* usually appear as green, non-sucrose-fermenting colonies on TCBS agar, but isolates from estuary and coastal waters may ferment sucrose. Faecal samples should be enriched in alkaline peptone water containing 1% NaCl. The Kanagawa phenomenon refers to haemolysis of human erythrocytes on Wagatsuma's agar by strains of *V. parahaemolyticus* which cause gastroenteritis.

Treatment

Rehydration is the main intervention for patients with diarrhoea. Severe infections require treatment with fluoroquinolones, doxycycline, or third-generation cephalosporins. Antibiotics do not shorten the duration of symptoms. Prevention strategies involve good food hygiene standards.

Vibrio vulnificus

V. vulnificus has been called the 'terror of the ceep' due to the severe fulminant infection it can cause.

Epidemiology

Infections are commonest in areas with higher water temperatures such as the mid-Atlantic and Gulf Coast states of the USA. Septicaemia arises from eating contaminated raw shellfish, whereas wound infections are due to injuries sustained in aquatic environments.

Pathogenesis

The polysaccharide capsule helps to resist phagocytosis and bactericidal effects of human serum. The association with liver disease (with increased serum iron levels) may be explained by the ability of virulent strains to use transferrin-bound iron. Toxin production is also important.

Clinical features

There are three main infections associated with *V. vulnificus*:
- fulminant septicaemia, followed by cutaneous lesions—this is associated with high mortality (50%). Immunosuppressed patients are at increased risk, particularly elderly ♂ alcoholics with liver dysfunction;
- wound infection, rapidly progressing to cellulitis, oedema, erythema, and necrosis—patients may develop septicaemia and it may be fatal;
- acute mild diarrhoea—usually in those with mild underlying conditions.

Diagnosis

This organism is halophilic. For further growth characteristics, see Table 7.15.

Treatment

Early treatment with ceftazidime and doxycycline is key.

Other *Vibrio* species

- *V. alginolyticus* is the commonest *Vibrio* organism found in seafood and seawater in the UK. It is a halophilic organism, which does not grow on CLED but grows in 10% NaCl. Colonies are large and yellow (sucrose-fermenting) on TCBS agar, and there is swarming on non-selective media. Causes opportunistic wound infections associated with exposure to seawater, usually self-limiting.
- *V. fluvialis* is phenotypically similar to *Aeromonas hydrophila* (➔ see *Aeromonas*, pp. 360–1). Implicated in outbreaks of diarrhoea; acquired from seafood.

- *V. damsela* (now known as *Listonella damsela*) is a halophilic organism acquired in warm coastal areas. Cause of wound infection.
- *V. hollisae* (now known as *Grimontia hollisae*) has been associated with diarrhoea and bacteraemia in areas of warm seawater in the USA. It is acquired from raw seafood.
- *V. mimicus* is associated with gastroenteritis from eating raw oysters. There are also reports of ear infections. It occurs in environments similar to *V. cholerae*.

Aeromonas

Aeromonas spp. are aquatic organisms. *A. hydrophila*, *Aeromonas sobria*, and *Aeromonas caviae* are the main species, and *Aeromonas salmonicida* is an economically important fish pathogen. The genus *Aeromonas* has undergone a number of taxonomic and nomenclature revisions recently, and has been moved from the family *Vibrionaceae* to the new family *Aeromonadaceae*.

Epidemiology

A cause of diarrhoea and soft tissue infections. Diarrhoea is commoner in summer months when water concentrations of aeromonads are higher. Outbreaks may occur.

Pathogenesis

Gastroenteritis is the commonest disease associated with *Aeromonas*, but its role is debated. It is capable of producing an enterotoxin, and antibiotics active against *Aeromonas* may improve patient symptoms. It may be that only specific subsets of *Aeromonas* are pathogenic.

Clinical features

Diarrhoea tends to be watery and self-limiting, but is occasionally more severe. Chronic colitis following diarrhoea has been reported. In addition to gastroenteritis, there are reports of *Aeromonas* septicaemia in the immunocompromised, and wound infections in healthy people and those undergoing leech therapy. It should be considered as a cause of soft tissue infection in those with water exposure. There are rare reports of nosocomial bacteraemia, peritonitis, meningitis, and eye and bone and joint infections.

Diagnosis

This facultatively anaerobic GNR is usually β-haemolytic on BA and ferments carbohydrates to produce acid and gas. It grows readily on MacConkey agar, and lactose fermentation is variable. Growth on TCBS agar is also variable. It is oxidase-positive, so it can be distinguished from oxidase-negative *Enterobacterales*. Suitable plates for detection of *Aeromonas* from faeces samples include CIN agar or BA containing ampicillin. Note that not all laboratories routinely culture faeces for *Aeromonas*, and some enteric media actually inhibit its growth.

Treatment

There are no controlled trials, but clinical improvement has been seen with antibiotics that are active *in vitro* such as fluoroquinolones, co-trimoxazole, and aminoglycosides (except streptomycin). Resistance to carbapenems has been reported due to chromosomal carbapenemases.

Plesiomonas

Plesiomonas shigelloides, the only species in the genus, is associated with outbreaks of gastroenteritis in warm climates. In the literature, it has been known as *Pseudomonas shigelloides*, C27, *Aeromonas shigelloides*, and *Vibrio shigelloides*. The taxonomic status has varied—it is related to *Proteus* but is currently placed in the family *Enterobacterales*.

Epidemiology

P. shigelloides is found in soil and water (mainly fresh water, but also salt water in warm weather). It is usually transmitted to humans via water or food (e.g. shrimp, chicken, oysters), and also co on zes many animals. Most patients recently travelled abroad.

Pathogenesis

There is no animal model, and no pathogenic mechanism has been identified. Volunteer studies have been largely unsuccessful in causing disease. Hence, it has been difficult to prove a causal relationship.

Clinical features

Symptoms vary from mild, self-limiting diarrhoea to mucoid bloody diarrhoea, with features of entero-invasive disease. It has occasionally resulted in serious extraintestinal infection such as osteomyelitis, septic arthritis, endophthalmitis, SBP, pancreatic abscess cellulitis, cholecystitis, and neonatal sepsis with meningitis. Bacteraemia is rare and usually in the immunocompromised.

Diagnosis

This motile, facultatively anaerobic GNR does not ferment lactose. It grows readily at 35°C on most enteric agars, such as MacConkey agar, but does not grow on TCBS agar. It appears non-haemolytic and is oxidase-positive. Selective techniques are needed to isolate it from a mixed culture.

Treatment

The role of antibiotics is unclear, and results of studies conflicting. *In vitro*, it is usually sensitive to quinolones, cephalosporins, and carbapenems.

Campylobacter

Campylobacter organisms are spiral-shaped flagellate bacteria belonging to the rRNA superfamily VI. *Campylobacter jejuni* is the commonest cause of diarrhoea in most developed countries. *Campylobacter coli* also causes diarrhoea. *Campylobacter fetus* is the type species of the genus and causes abortion in sheep and cows. It occasionally causes septic abortions in humans and bacteraemia/soft tissue infections in the immunocompromised. Some species, including *Campylobacter lari* and *Campylobacter upsaliensis*, cause diarrhoea in children in developing countries, whereas species such as *Campylobacter concisus* and *Campylobacter rectus* are associated with periodontal disease.

Pathogenesis

Campylobacter organisms are ingested (faeco-oral transmission), and they then colonize the jejunum, ileum, and terminal ileum, occasionally extending to the colon and rectum. Mesenteric lymph node involvement and transient bacteraemia may occur. Histological findings of acute inflammation ± superficial ulceration are the same as in *Salmonella*, *Shigella*, or *Yersinia* infections.

Clinical features

Campylobacter gastroenteritis is variable in terms of symptoms and severity. In severe cases, GI haemorrhage, toxic megacolon, and HUS have been reported. Other complications include meningitis, deep abscesses, cholecystitis, and reactive arthritis; ~25% of cases of Guillain–Barré syndrome (GBS) have documented *Campylobacter* gastroenteritis as a precedent—the lipo-oligosaccharide cell surface structures act as critical factors in triggering GBS through ganglioside mimicry.

Diagnosis

This small, spiral GNR has a single, unsheathed flagellum at one or both poles and is extremely motile. Staining with carbol fuchsin reveals a characteristic 'seagull' appearance. Selective blood-free agar is used (e.g. charcoal–cefoperazone–deoxycholate agar (CCDA) containing charcoal, sodium pyruvate, and ferrous sulfate). It is micro-aerophilic and grows best at 42°C. Like *Helicobacter*, *Campylobacter* organisms undergo coccal transformation under adverse conditions and are biochemically inactive. However, they are oxidase-positive. Typing methods include serotyping, biotyping, phage typing, and molecular methods.

Treatment

Rehydration and symptom relief are usually adequate, as *Campylobacter* infection is usually self-limiting in 5–7 days. However, in severe dysenteric disease, macrolides or ciprofloxacin may be prescribed. Resistant strains, especially *C. coli*, may respond to trimethoprim or co-trimoxazole. Bacteraemia associated with severe disease should be treated with aminoglycosides or carbapenems until sensitivity testing is performed. Good hygiene standards are important in prevention. Infective organisms may be excreted in the faeces for ~3 weeks after resolution of diarrhoea. There is no vaccine.

Helicobacter

The genus *Helicobacter* contains up to 17 species, which colonize the stomach of different animals. *Helicobacter pylori* is a spiral-shaped flagellate bacteria belonging to the rRNA superfamily VI, which colonizes humans (it is found in ~50% of the world population). *H. pylori* was discovered in 1983 in Australia by Warren and Marshall, who went on to receive the Nobel Prize for Medicine in 2005. Its importance in the pathogenesis of peptic ulcer disease and malignancy soon became clear. *Helicobacter cinaedi* and *Helicobacter fennelliae* are associated with proctitis in homosexual men.

Pathogenesis

As with other bacteria in the rRNA superfamily VI, *H. pylori* is adapted to colonizing mucous membranes (in this case, the gastric mucosa only) by penetrating mucus. The cagA protein is important in virulence. After phosphorylation by tyrosine kinase, cagA is injected into epithelial cells by a type IV secretion system. This alters signal transduction and gene expression in host epithelial cells.

Clinical features

H. pylori is associated with 95% of duodenal, and 70% of gastric, ulcers. Epidemiological studies have highlighted the association of *H. pylori* and gastric cancer, and the World Health Organization (WHO) classifies *H. pylori* as a group 1 carcinogen.

Diagnosis

This GNR is shaped like a helix and has a tuft of sheathed unipolar flagella. It is strictly micro-aerophilic and requires CO_2 for growth. It is relatively inactive biochemically, except for strong urease production. Under adverse conditions, it undergoes coccal transformation. The UKHSA/British Infection Association (BIA) have produced guidelines on testing and management of *H. pylori*. Options for testing patients are as follows:

- serology—if positive, this indicates the patient has been infected but does not differentiate between active and past infection. Not advised for use in the elderly. High negative predictive value in low-prevalence countries;
- biopsy of the stomach or duodenum—histology ± urease test ± culture;
- urea breath tests—the patient drinks ^{14}C- or ^{13}C-labelled urea, which is metabolized by *H. pylori*, producing labelled CO_2 that can be detected in the breath. This test is also used to assess effectiveness of treatment but is affected by proton pump inhibitor (PPI) use;
- rapid urease test (the enzyme urease produced by *H. pylori* catalyses the conversion of urea to ammonia and HCO_3^-, which is reflected by a rise in pH)—this is usually performed on a biopsy sample;
- faecal antigen tests—affected by PPI use.

The urea breath test and faecal antigen test have greater sensitivity and specificity than serology for diagnosis, and can also be used to confirm eradication. The patient should receive no antibiotics for 4 weeks before the tests, and no PPI for 2 weeks before the tests. Molecular typing of *H. pylori* is more useful than serotyping.

Treatment

NICE has issued clinical guidelines on the investigation and management of dyspepsia (web search 'NICE guidance CG184').[3] Eradication of *H. pylori* in patients testing positive is beneficial in duodenal/gastric ulcers and low-grade MALToma (mucosa-associated lymphoid tissue), but **not** in gastro-oesophageal reflux disease (these patients should be offered a PPI). Triple therapy consists of a PPI (e.g. omeprazole) and two antibiotics (e.g. amoxicillin, clarithromycin, or metronidazole), and achieves >85% eradication. Clarithromycin or metronidazole should not be given if they have been used for any infection in the previous year; ~10% of patients fail treatment, possibly due to antibiotic resistance (see Box 7.11).

Box 7.11 Antibiotic resistance in *Helicobacter pylori*

Antibiotic resistance varies geographically; the rise in resistance in *H. pylori* is recognized by the World Health Organization as a global threat of high priority since 2017. Metronidazole resistance varies from ~50% in Europe to 90% in developing countries. Clarithromycin resistance is usually <10% in Europe but may be rising. A meta-analysis has shown that pre-treatment clarithromycin resistance may reduce the effectiveness of therapy by 55%. Resistance correlates with prior use of the antibiotic in question; clarithromycin resistance rates are higher in regions with higher macrolide consumption. Second- and third-line options include quadruple therapy, bismuth-based regimens, or use of levofloxacin or rifabutin. Earlier sensitivity testing is advocated but requires invasive sampling and technically difficult laboratory methods. Consult recent guidelines, and seek expert help.

A Cochrane review (2006) of eradication therapy for peptic ulcer disease in *H. pylori*-positive patients found that treatment had a small benefit in initial healing of duodenal ulcers, and a significant benefit in preventing the recurrence of both gastric and duodenal ulcers, once healing had been achieved.[7] Other treatment includes probiotics (which improved eradication rates and reduced adverse events in a recent meta-analysis) and bismuth compounds.

References

6 National Institute for Health and Care Excellence (2014, updated in 2019). *Gastro-oesophageal reflux disease and dyspepsia in adults: investigation and management*. NICE clinical guideline [CG184]. Available at: ℬ https://www.nice.org.uk/guidance/cg184

7 Moayyedi P, Soo S, Deeks J, et al. Eradication of *Helicobacter pylori* for non-ulcer dyspepsia. *Cochrane Database Syst Rev*. 2006;**2**:CD002096.

Bacteroides

More than 30 genera of anaerobic GNRs are recognized, but human infections are largely restricted to four of these: *Bacteroides*, *Prevotella*, *Porphyromonas*, and *Fusobacterium* (see Table 7.16). These organisms are found in the mouth, GI tract, and vagina, and are amongst the most important constituents of 'normal flora'. They may cause a variety of infections in humans, particularly polymicrobial infections and abscesses. *Bacteroides fragilis* is the most important species; it is found in the GI tract and is associated with a wide variety of infections.

Pathogenesis

Virulence factors of *Bacteroides* spp. include:
- capsular polysaccharide—inhibits opsonization/phagocytosis, and promotes abscess formation and adherence to epithelial cells;
- pili and fimbriae—promote adherence to epithelial cells and mucus;
- succinic acid—inhibits phagocytosis and intracellular killing;
- enzyme production—contributes to tissue damage and/or promotes invasion and spread (e.g. heparinase, fibrinolysin, hyaluronidase, neuraminidase);

Table 7.16 Characteristics of anaerobic Gram-negative rods

Organism	Pigmented	Fluorescence	Usually resistant to	Usually sensitive to
Bacteroides fragilis	No	No	Penicillin Vancomycin Kanamycin Colistimethate sodium	Erythromycin Rifampicin
Fusobacterium	No	No	Erythromycin Vancomycin	Colistimethate sodium Penicillin Kanamycin
Prevotella	Brown/black	Brick red	Vancomycin	Rifampicin Colistimethate sodium Penicillin
Porphyromonas	Brown/black	Brick-red		Rifampicin Penicillin Vancomycin

- synergy between anaerobic and facultative bacteria (see Box 7.12).

Clinical features

- Intra-abdominal infections—*B. fragilis* is the commonest anaerobic isolate in intra-abdominal abscesses, often polymicrobial infections.
- Diarrhoea—enterotoxin-producing strains have been implicated in diarrhoea in children.
- Bacteraemia—*B. fragilis* is the commonest isolate in anaerobic bacteraemias. The source is usually intra-abdominal and associated with abscesses, malignancy, bowel perforation, or surgery. Septic shock is less common in *B. fragilis* bacteraemia than in bacteraemia caused by aerobic Gram-negative bacilli; this is presumably related to the absence of lipid A in the endotoxin of *B. fragilis*.
- Endocarditis—associated with large vegetations and a high frequency of thromboembolic complications.
- Skin and soft tissue infections—often found as part of mixed flora in diabetic and decubitus ulcers. *B. fragilis* has also been isolated from cutaneous abscesses of the lower limbs.
- Bone and joint infections—*B. fragilis* may rarely cause osteomyelitis and septic arthritis.
- CNS infections—anaerobic meningitis is rare, and most laboratories do not culture CSF anaerobically. In cases of anaerobic meningitis that have been described, *B. fragilis* is the commonest isolate. In contrast, anaerobes are frequently implicated in brain abscesses.

Diagnosis

- *Bacteroides* are non-spore-forming, non-motile anaerobic GNRs.
- On BA, *Bacteroides* appear as glistening, non-haemolytic colonies, which are aerotolerant.
- Gram staining may reveal pale pink, pleomorphic coccobacilli, with irregular or bipolar staining.
- Commercial identification kits (e.g. API® 20A, MASTRING ID, Rapid ID 32A) identify *B. fragilis* through biochemical properties and/or susceptibility pattern (usually sensitive to erythromycin and rifampicin, but resistant to penicillin, vancomycin, kanamycin, and colistimethate sodium). Molecular identification and MALDI can also be used.

Box 7.12 Synergy in anaerobic infections

- Infections involving anaerobes usually contain multiple obligate anaerobic bacteria, as well as facultative anaerobic bacteria.
- Evidence suggests true synergy between anaerobic and facultative bacteria, with formation of abscesses occurring more readily with infections involving both groups of bacteria than involving either alone.
- Facultative organisms may lower the oxidation–reduction potential in the microenvironment, promoting more favourable conditions for anaerobes.
- Anaerobic bacteria may inhibit phagocytosis of facultative bacteria.
- *Bacteroides fragilis* produces β-lactamases in abscess fluid that may protect other normally susceptible bacteria from antimicrobials.

Treatment

- Drainage of abscesses and debridement of necrotic tissue are the mainstay of treatment for anaerobic infections. However, some abscesses (e.g. brain, liver, tubo-ovarian) have been managed with antimicrobial therapy alone.
- The choice of antibiotics to treat anaerobic infections is usually empirical, as most of the infections are polymicrobial and require broad-spectrum therapy.
- *Bacteroides* is usually sensitive to antimicrobials such as metronidazole, clindamycin, chloramphenicol, carbapenems, cefoxitin, and β-lactam/β-lactamase inhibitor combinations (e.g. co-amoxiclav, piperacillin–tazobactam).

Prevotella and *Porphyromonas*

Prevotella and *Porphyromonas* formerly belonged to the genus *Bacteroides* (⊃ see *Bacteroides*, pp. 364–7).
- The genus *Prevotella* includes *Prevotella melaninogenica*, *Prevotella bivia*, *Prevotella oralis*, and *Prevotella buccalis*.
- The genus *Porphyromonas* includes *Porphyromonas gingivalis*, *Porphyromonas endodontalis*, and *Porphyromonas asaccharolytica*.

Pathogenesis

- Virulence in *P. melaninogenica* is associated with the capsular polysaccharide, which inhibits opsonophagocytosis, and promotes abscess formation and adherence to epithelial cells.
- In *P. gingivalis*, pili and fimbriae aid adherence to epithelial cells and mucus.
- Production of various enzymes may also aid evasion of the host immune response or promote tissue destruction.

Clinical features

Prevotella and *Porphyromonas* contribute to the formation of abscesses and soft tissue infections in various parts of the body. They also cause infections of the oral cavity (such as periodontal and endodontal disease), ♀ genital tract infections, osteomyelitis of the facial bones, and human bite infections.

Diagnosis

- These are non-spore-forming, non-motile, anaerobic Gram-negative bacilli.
- They are usually isolated (along with other anaerobes) from abscesses and soft tissue infections.
- *Prevotella* and *Porphyromonas* may both appear pigmented—usually brown/black.
- Young, unpigmented colonies can show brick-red fluorescence under UV light.
- Gram staining reveals small, pale pink coccobacilli.

Treatment

- The mainstay of treatment for anaerobic infections is surgical drainage of abscesses and debridement of necrotic tissue.
- *Prevotella* and *Porphyromonas* are usually sensitive to agents such as metronidazole, clindamycin, chloramphenicol, and cefoxitin. Penicillin resistance is common, but isolates are usually susceptible to co-amoxiclav and other β-lactam/β-lactamase inhibitor combinations.

Fusobacterium

Fusobacterium spp. colonize the mucous membranes of animals and humans, and occasionally cause infections of the oral cavity and head and neck. Clinically, the most important species are:

- *Fusobacterium nucleatum* (subspecies *nucleatum*, *polymorphum*, and *fusiforme*);
- *Fusobacterium necrophorum* (subspecies *necrophorum* and *fundiliforme*).

Epidemiology

Fusobacteria are commensals of the oral cavity. As with other obligate anaerobes, the significance of these organisms is being increasingly recognized.

Pathogenesis

Fusobacterium spp. produce LPS endotoxin which is biologically active. They also produce metabolites that are important to oral spirochaetes.

Clinical features

- *F. necrophorum* causes severe systemic infections such as Lemierre's disease, post-anginal sepsis, and necrobacillosis.
- Lemierre's disease is a severe systemic disease which occurs in previously healthy young adults, and usually presents initially as severe sore throat, followed by fever, cervical lymphadenopathy, and unilateral thrombophlebitis of the internal jugular vein. Metastatic infection with spread to the lungs, pleural cavity, bones, or brain may occur. If untreated, the condition leads to death in 7–15 days.
- Other species commonly isolated from oral infections include *Fusobacterium periodonticum*, *Fusobacterium alocis*, *Fusobacterium sulci*, and *Fusobacterium naviforme*.
- Species found in the GI or GU tracts (e.g. *Fusobacterium mortiferum*, *Fusobacterium necrogenes*, *Fusobacterium varium*, and *Fusobacterium gonidiaformans*) may cause intra-abdominal infections, osteomyelitis, ulcers, and skin/soft tissue infections.
- *Fusobacterium ulcerans* was originally isolated from tropical ulcers but may be found in other sites.

Diagnosis

- *Fusobacterium* are long, thin GNRs with pointed ends ('fusiform') that are often arranged in pairs. They are non-spore-forming and non-motile.
- They may be haemolytic on BA but are often difficult to grow.

- They can be identified by using commercial tests (e.g. MASTRING™ ID (Mast Diagnostics) and API® 20A or Rapid D® 32A (bioMérieux) or MALDI.
- Molecular techniques (e.g. PCR) have been developed.

Treatment

- The mainstay of treatment for anaerobic infections is surgical drainage of abscesses and debridement of necrotic tissue.
- Lemierre's syndrome and other severe invasive disease is usually treated with a combination of penicillin and metronidazole, for 2–6 weeks.
- Alternatives include clindamycin monotherapy, co-amoxiclav, piperacillin–tazobactam, or chloramphenicol.

Spirochaetes—an overview

Spirochaetes are a group of helical organisms sharing many properties with Gram-negative bacteria. The vast majority are non-pathogenic, but a few are important causes of disease in humans (see Table 7.17). There are aerobic and anaerobic species, both free-living and parasitic. Axial filaments, fixed at each end of the organism, run along the outside of the protoplasm within the outer sheath and give the characteristic coiled appearance. These are similar to bacterial flagella and are capable of constricting, warping the cell body, and enabling the bacterium to move by rotating it in space.

Treponema species

Four members of the genus *Treponema* cause human disease: *Treponema pallidum* subspecies *pallidum* (syphilis) and three 'non-venereal' treponematoses.

Microbiology

Morphologically identical, *Treponema* spp. appear as motile, helical rods on dark-field microscopy. They are thin, around 10 micrometres long and 0.15 micrometres wide. They cannot be cultured *in vitro* (unlike the non-pathogenic treponemes) but remain motile in specific enriched media for several days at 35°C. Organisms remain viable after freezing. The organisms all share a significant degree of DNA homology and are very similar antigenically; thus, all cause positive serological tests for syphilis.

Epidemiology and clinical features

- *T. pallidum* subspecies *pallidum*—the causative agent of syphilis. An increasing incidence in the UK, beginning in the 1960s, plateaued in the mid 90s, but several large outbreaks between 1998 and 2003 saw diagnoses of infectious syphilis in men rise 15-fold. Transmission—sexual contact, direct vascular inoculation (PWID, transfusions), direct cutaneous contact with infectious lesions, or transplacental infection (congenital syphilis; ➔ see Syphilis, pp. 760–2). Interacts

Table 7.17 Overview of spirochaetes of clinical significance

Genus	Species	Clinical disease	Morphology	Culture	Diagnosis
Treponema	T. pallidum subsp. pallidum	Syphilis	Appear identical. Thin helical cells 10×0.15 micrometres. Visible on dark-field microscopy	Cannot be cultured in vitro; remain motile in specific enriched media at 35°C for several days	Direct detection methods in primary syphilis; mainstay is serology; cross-reactivity between species
	T. pallidum subsp. pertenue	Yaws			
	T. pallidum subsp. endemicum	Endemic syphilis			
	T. carateum	Pinta			
Borrelia	B. recurrentis	Louse-borne relapsing fever	Helical; $3–20 \times 0.25$ micrometres. Can be stained with aniline dyes	Can be cultured, but not practical	Demonstration of spirochaetes in peripheral blood smears; immunological and PCR-based tests available
	B. hermsii and others	Tick-borne relapsing fever			
	B. burgdorferi	Lyme disease		Culture possible from biopsy of rash	Serology; can remain positive for years
Leptospira	L. interrogans	Leptospirosis	Motile, 10×0.1 micrometres. Stain poorly—visible on dark-field or phase contrast	Specialized media. Allow minimum of 6 weeks	Serology; molecular techniques available

with HIV in both acquisition and diagnosis. For clinical features, ➔ see Syphilis, pp. 760–2. For details of treatment, ➔ see Syphilis, Management, p. 762.

- *T. pallidum* subspecies *pertenue*—the causative agent of yaws, a chronic non-venereal disease endemic in the humid tropics (Central Africa, South America, South East Asia, and parts of the Indian subcontinent). Acquired in childhood through contact with infectious skin lesions. Incubation of 3 weeks. Affects the skin (papular skin lesions which may ulcerate) and bones (periosteitis, dactylitis):
  - primary stage—lesion at inoculation site; secondary stage— dissemination of treponemes, causing multiple skin lesions;
  - latent stage—usually asymptomatic (most patients remain non-infectiously latent for their lifetime);
  - tertiary stage (<10% of patients 5–10 years later)—bone, joint, soft tissue deformities.
- *T. pallidum* subspecies *endemicum*—the causative agent of non-venereal endemic syphilis or 'bejel'. Endemic in dry subtropical or temperate areas of the Middle East, India, Asia, and parts of Africa. Infection occurs in childhood and is associated with poor standards of hygiene. Transmission: contact with mucosal lesions or contaminated eating utensils/water. Incubation of 10–90 days. Primary lesions (1–6 weeks): patches in the mouth, followed by skin lesions resembling the chancres of venereal syphilis; secondary stage (6–9 months): macerated patches on the lips and tongue, anogenital hypertrophic condyloma lata, painful osteoperiostitis of long bones; tertiary stage: destruction of cartilage and bone, gummata of skin, bones, and nasopharynx. CNS/cardiovascular system (CVS) disease is very rare.
- *Treponema carateum*—the causative agent of pinta, the most benign of the endemic treponematoses, affecting only the skin. Endemic to South/Central America. Spread by contact with infected skin. Incubation: 2–3 weeks. Primary lesion: papule or erythematous plaque on exposed surfaces of the legs, foot, forearm, or hands, which slowly enlarges, becoming pigmented and hyperkeratotic. May be associated with regional lymphadenopathy. Secondary lesions: disseminated lesions of similar appearance, appearing 3–9 months later. Late/tertiary pinta: disfiguring pigmentary changes and atrophic lesions.

General diagnosis

- Direct detection—culture (the gold standard) is expensive and time-consuming, and is used primarily in research. Direct detection of organisms by microscopy (dark-field or immunofluorescence) of material scraped from a lesion is the usual means of diagnosis in primary infection. PCR of such material, CSF, or vitreous fluid may be helpful in some circumstances.
- Serological diagnosis—the mainstay. Serological tests fall into two groups. Both show cross-reactivity amongst the four *Treponema* spp.:
  - non-treponemal tests (e.g. Venereal Disease Research Laboratory (VDRL), rapid plasma reagin (RPR))—detect antibodies (both IgG and IgM) to cardiolipin produced as a response to treponemal infection, and are not specific but are very sensitive. Samples with very high antibody titres may give false-negative results (the 'prozone'

phenomenon) in early infection or HIV. Poor sensitivity in late-stage infection. Quantitative, with antibody titres tending to decline with time—a phenomenon accelerated by therapy. False positives occur in pregnancy, TB, and endocarditis, amongst others;
* treponemal tests—use specific treponemal antigens and are consequently more specific. Qualitative. They can detect late-stage infection and remain positive after successful therapy (e.g. *T. pallidum* haemagglutination assay (TPHA), EIA, fluorescent treponemal antibody absorption (FTA-ABS) test).

Diagnosis of syphilis

Traditionally, diagnosis was made by a sensitive non-treponemal screening test, with positive samples followed up by using a more specific treponemal assay. Recent guidelines reverse this.[8]
* Specific tests should be performed first line, including EIA IgM if primary syphilis is suspected (detected by the end of week 2 after infection).
* Perform quantitative non-treponemal tests when treponemal tests are positive—this helps to stage disease and indicates the need for treatment. A VDRL/RPR titre >16 and/or positive IgM indicate active disease within the appropriate clinical context. Yaws/pinta may give identical results—it may be appropriate to manage as if they had latent syphilis.
* Tests are often negative in late syphilis, but this does not exclude the need for treatment. Repeat positive tests on a second specimen for confirmation. Discrepant results are repeated by using an immunoblot. FTA-ABS is no longer recommended for this purpose.
* Repeat screening in seronegative patients at recent risk of acquiring disease—there is a seronegative window in early primary syphilis (➔ see Syphilis, pp. 760–2).

Treatment

Early syphilis and pinta/yaws/bejel—prolonged antibiotic therapy is required due to the slow dividing rate of *T. pallidum* (averages one doubling *in vivo* per day). Highly sensitive to penicillin and a long-acting depot injection of benzathine benzylpenicillin is the standard therapy. A single dose is sufficient for early infection. Alternative: 10-day course of azithromycin (increasing reports of resistance) or 14 days of doxycycline. For further management advice, ➔ see Syphilis, pp. 760–2.

References

8 Kingston M, French P, Goh B, *et al*.; Syphilis Guidelines Revision Group 2008, Clinical Effectiveness Group. UK national guidelines on the management of syphilis 2008. *Int J STD AIDS*. **19**:729–40.

Borrelia species

Relapsing fever

Relapsing fever is caused by several *Borrelia* spp. transmitted by arthropods, characterized by recurring episodes of fever. Two distinct clinical forms were recognized as far back as ancient Greece: epidemic louse-borne and endemic tick-borne relapsing fever. The presentation of abrupt fever, muscle aches, and joint pains with crisis, remission, and then relapse are similar for both, but the periodicity tends to be characteristic (e.g. 5.5 days for louse-borne versus 3.1 days for tick-borne). The recurrent nature is thought to be due to antigenic variation of the spirochaetal OMPs.

Epidemiology

- Tick-borne relapsing fever is worldwide and transmitted by soft-bodied *Ornithodoros* ticks. Most tick species carry distinctive borreliae. Epidemiology depends on the local vector—for example, *Ornithodoros hermsi* is the commonest vector in California and Canada, and lives in dead trees and on rodents and transmits *Borrelia hermsii*. Infection is passed down the tick generations; thus, disease tends to be endemic.
- Louse-borne relapsing fever has occurred in Africa, the Middle East, and Asia. Human body louse inhabits only humans, and *Borrelia recurrentis* is not transmitted vertically within lice; thus, it is maintained by passage from louse to human and then back to another louse, which remains infective for its entire life. Therefore, infection is associated with poverty and overcrowding, and disease tends to be epidemic.

Clinical features

Incubation and symptoms are similar in both conditions. Three to 8 days after exposure, there is abrupt-onset fever, headache, myalgia, arthralgia, chills, weakness, anorexia, epistaxis, cough/haemoptysis, and weight loss. Examination findings include hypotension, hepatosplenomegaly, lymphadenopathy, nuchal rigidity, jaundice, photophobia, injected conjunctiva, and iritis.

- Tick-borne disease—the primary episode lasts 3–6 days and is followed by a critical episode that may cause fatal shock. The first relapse occurs 7–10 days later. Subsequent relapses are less severe. The average number of relapses experienced is three but can be as many as 10.
- Louse-borne disease—there are fewer relapses than with tick-borne infection, and hepatic or splenic involvement is commoner, as are neurological manifestations (coma, hemiplegia, meningitis, seizures).

Diagnosis

Culture is possible, but not practical, and serology is not diagnostically helpful. Five per cent of patients have a positive VDRL. Most useful is demonstration of spirochaetes in peripheral blood smears (and other body fluids—marrow aspirates, CSF). Unlike the other spirochaetes, borreliae stain well with acid aniline dyes such as Giemsa. They are most likely to be found during febrile episodes when the sensitivity of blood smears is around 70% for louse-borne fever (lower for tick). Multiple thick and thin smears may need to be examined. Immunological and PCR-based tests are available. Other laboratory findings include deranged clotting tests and elevated LFTs.

Treatment

- Tick-borne relapsing fever—tetracycline is the drug of choice, given for 7–14 days. Other: doxycycline 7 days, erythromycin 10 days.
- Louse-borne relapsing fever—a single dose of doxycycline (preferred), tetracycline, erythromycin, or benzy penicillin.
- Jarisch–Herxheimer reactions can occur (usually within the first 2h after antibiotic administration), particularly in louse-borne relapsing fever. Features: sweating, tachycardia, hypertension, followed by profound

hypotension. It can be fatal and appears to be mediated partly by tumour necrosis factor (TNF)-α. Pre-administration of steroids does not appear to limit the reaction significantly. Anti-TNF-α antibodies may help.

Lyme disease

Caused by infection with, and the host immune response to, *B. burgdorferi*. Acquired by the bite of *Ixodes* (hard) ticks, and co-infection with other tick-borne organisms can occur (e.g. babesiosis).

Epidemiology

Ticks acquire and spread infection through feeding on infected animals (particularly deer). A tick must be attached for 2–3 days to pass on infection. Only small numbers of bacteria are present in the tick until it feeds. Eighty-five per cent of human infections occur while the tick is in the nymph stage (spring to summer), and 15% in the adult stage (autumn). Cases are commonest in children aged 5–9 years and in adults aged 60–69 years. Only 40% give a definite history of tick bite. Cases occur across Europe, China, Japan, Australia, and parts of the USA. It is relatively rare in the UK, with most cases occurring in the south (New Forest and Salisbury Plain), East Anglia, Cumbria, and the Scottish Highlands.

Clinical manifestations

Clinical features may be a result of direct bacterial infection (particularly in the early stages of disease) or a consequence of an immune response leading to symptoms in many organs (e.g. arthritis). They differ with the strain of *Borrelia* involved. Less than 10% of those in endemic areas with no history of symptoms are seropositive. Features may be seen in three overlapping stages:

- **early localized**—around 7 days after a tick bite, patients may develop erythema chronicum migrans (EM), an expanding painless annular skin lesion centred on the bite, with or without local lymphadenopathy. It is probably a result of the inflammatory response to the organism in the skin. Multiple lesions can occur, following a single bite. Lasts 2–3 weeks if untreated. Lymphocytoma is a rare local blue/red nodule or plaque on the ear, nipple, or scrotum. It may be mistaken for cutaneous lymphoma;
- **early disseminated**—weeks/months after the bite, patients develop constitutional symptoms, malaise, generalized lymphadenopathy, hepatitis, arthritis (50%—initially intermittent and migratory, it may evolve into chronic monoarticular arthritis in 10% of cases), neurological features (15%—meningitis, meningoencephalitis, cranial nerve lesions, and neuropathy), and cardiac features (10%—atrioventricular (AV) block, pericarditis, congestive cardiac failure (CCF));
- **late persistent** (but can occur within the first year)—arthritis (usually of the knee with synovitis/effusion), neurological (including focal deficits, fatigue, and neuropsychiatric problems). Acrodermatitis chronica atrophicans (ACA) is decoloration of the skin on the extremities (similar in appearance to peripheral vascular disease), mostly associated with *Borrelia afzelii*.

Microbiology

Three members of the B. burgdorferi sensu lato complex cause Lyme disease: *Borrelia garinii* and *B. afzelii* in Asia, and *B. burgdorferi sensu stricto* in North America. *B. garinii* and *B. afzelii* are the commonest European clinical isolates. These differences account for the variation in clinical manifestations across the world (*B. garinii* associated with neurological disease, *B. afzelii* with ACA, and *B. burgdorferi sensu stricto* with joint symptoms).

Diagnosis

Laboratory support is not required for a clear clinical diagnosis of EM but should be sought for all later manifestations. Treat unvalidated investigations offered by commercial 'Lyme specialty' laboratories with caution.

- **Direct detection**—culture is possible from EM biopsy, but requires specialist media and takes 2–6 weeks. PCR may be useful on CSF in acute neuroborreliosis (10–30% sensitivity), tissue from ACA (>90% sensitivity) or lymphocytoma (80% sensitivity), and synovial fluid in refractory arthritis.
- **Serology**—most patients are seropositive within 2–4 weeks. Guidelines recommend a 2-stage approach: a sensitive EIA, followed by immunoblot (western) of those with reactive or equivocal results. EIA may give false positives in the presence of other spirochaetes (syphilis), glandular fever, and autoimmune disease. IgM immunoblots are also prone to false positives—reserve for those with acute presentations and a high probability of disease. Specific response is sensitive but develops late (30% positive in the acute phase, 70% at 2–4 weeks, 90% at 4–6 weeks). Prompt antibiotic therapy may prevent a good antibody response. Some patients remain positive for years; thus, active and inactive infection cannot be distinguished. Interpret tests with caution in those without a travel history or a presentation consistent with Lyme disease. Do not test those with no symptoms, even with a history of tick bite. Serology is nearly always positive in late neuroborreliosis, ACA, and arthritis.
- **Lumbar puncture**—for cell count and serology in those patients with neurology if the diagnosis is not obvious.

Treatment

- Early-stage skin manifestations, arthritis, or Bell's palsy—doxycycline or amoxicillin PO for 14–21 days. If arthritis persists, repeat the course or consider IV ceftriaxone for 14–21 days. Azithromycin is a third-line agent and associated with treatment failures.
- Late or neurological disease—ACA, 21–28 days of doxycycline; isolated meningitis, 14–21 days of doxycycline; encephalitis/myelitis, 14 days of IV ceftriaxone; third-degree heart block, 14–21 days of IV ceftriaxone; late neuroborreliosis, 14–28 days of IV ceftriaxone.

Prevention

- Patients probably remain at risk of reinfection after treatment.
- Practice tick avoidance, and promptly remove any attached ticks.
- Doxycycline prophylaxis (single dose) is practised in the USA for those within 3 days of a bite from a tick that has been attached for >36h in an endemic area. European guidance is less categorical, as tick infection

rates are lower, *Borrelia* spp. less pathogenic, and the window for treatment less reliable.

'Seronegative chronic Lyme disease' should be considered rare, with only two case reports of seronegative ACA and no reliable reports of seronegative late-stage neuroborreliosis. 'Post-Lyme syndrome' refers to non-specific symptoms for >6 months after effective treatment. Physicians should ensure alternative diagnoses have not been missed (e.g. multiple sclerosis, malignancy, etc.). Prolonged antibiotic courses have not been shown to be effective.

Further reading

British Infection Association. The epidemiology, prevention, investigation and treatment of Lyme borreliosis in United Kingdom patients: a position statement by the British Infection Association. *J Infect.* 2011;**62**:329–38.

Leptospira species

Leptospira are motile, obligately aerobic spirochaetes. They stain poorly but can be visualized on dark-field or phase contrast microscopy. Two species are identified: *Leptospira interrogans* (includes all human pathogens) and *Leptospira biflexa* (a saprophytic species). *L. interrogans* has >200 serotypes, and antigenically related organisms are grouped into serovars (a synonym for serotype) for classification. Recent DNA analysis does not correlate well with serological classification. The 'type' strain is *L. interrogans* serovar *icterohaemorrhagiae*, and the type disease leptospirosis.

Leptospirosis

A biphasic disease with initial septicaemia and a secondary phase characterized by immune phenomena (vasculitis, aseptic meningitis). Weil's disease is a severe form characterized by jaundice and acute renal failure.

Epidemiology

Leptospira are found worldwide. The primary reservoirs of most leptospiral serovars are wild mammals. These continually reinfect domestic populations, and at least 160 mammalian species are affected. The organism has been recovered from rats, pigs, dogs, cats, and cattle, amongst others, but rarely causes disease in these hosts. Rodents are the most important reservoir, and rats the commonest worldwide source. There are associations between particular animals and serovars (e.g. *L. interrogans* serovar *icterohaemorrhagiae* and rats). Humans are incidental hosts, and onward transmission is rare. Transmission occurs when people come into contact with infected animal urine (e.g. canoeing, swimming in lakes and rivers, farming). It is primarily a disease of tropical and subtropical regions, and infection in temperate regions is uncommon.

Pathogenesis

After gaining entry via the skin or mucous membranes, the organism replicates in blood and tissue. Leptospiraemia particularly affects the liver and kidney, causing centrilobular necrosis and jaundice, or interstitial nephritis and tubular necrosis, respectively. Renal failure may occur, exacerbated by hypovolaemia. Other organs affected include muscle (oedema and focal necrosis), capillaries (vasculitis), and the eye (chronic uveitis).

Clinical features

- Incubation 7–12 days. The majority of patients (90%) develop mild disease without jaundice; 5–10% develop the severe form (Weil's).
- First phase ('septicaemic')—organism can be cultured from blood, CSF, and most tissues. Lasts 4–7 days. Characterized by a flu-like illness, cough, haemoptysis, rash, meningism, and headache. One to 3 days of improvement follows. Patients may become afebrile.
- Second stage ('immune' or 'leptospiruric phase')—antibodies may be detected, and the organism isolated from urine. Features are due to the immunological response to infection and may last up to a month. Disease may be anicteric (in which death is rare) or icteric. Aseptic meningitis is the most important feature of anicteric disease and is seen in 50% of cases. Icteric disease is characterized by jaundice, hepatosplenomegaly, nausea/vomiting, anorexia, and diarrhoea/constipation. Organisms can be isolated from blood <48h after jaundice onset. Weil's disease is characterized by jaundice, renal failure, hepatic necrosis, lung disease, and bleeding. It starts at the end of stage one.
- Other features—uveitis (<10%—can occur <1 year after initial illness), subconjunctival haemorrhage (92% of patients), renal impairment (uraemia, haematuria, oliguria), and pulmonary (haemorrhage, acute respiratory distress syndrome (ARDS)).
- Overall mortality is 10%; up to 40% in those with hepatorenal involvement.

Diagnosis

- **Direct examination**—dark-field examination of blood, CSF, or urine may demonstrate *Leptospira*. High false-positive rate (misinterpretation of fibrils, red cell fragments), so not recommended.
- **Culture**—there has been little change in culture techniques over the years. It is difficult and insensitive, and requires several weeks of incubation. Specialized culture media should be inoculated within 24h of specimen collection (either blood or CSF in heparin or sodium oxalate). Organisms can be isolated from blood and CSF in the first week of illness in 50% of cases. In the second phase of illness, they can be found only in the urine where they may be isolated for up to 1 month. Cultures can be reported as negative after 6–12 weeks.
- **Molecular techniques**—PCR assays to detect leptospiral DNA can distinguish different species, and allow early diagnosis before antibodies develop. Usually performed on urine and serum in the first week of infection, nucleic acid can be detected after antibiotic therapy has been initiated.
- **Serology**—the mainstay of diagnosis. Commercial tests with genus-specific antigens are used to screen sera, and positive reactions confirmed in a reference laboratory using the micro-agglutination test (MAT) with live *Leptospira* (killed have lower sensitivity). The MAT detects agglutinating antibodies in patient serum and is relatively serovar-specific, so a large number of antigens must be tested. Interlaboratory variation is high. A positive MAT is considered to be a 4-fold increase in antibody titre, or a switch from seronegative to a

titre of 1/100 or over. Early samples tend to cross-react; convalescent samples are more specific and diagnostic. EIA for IgM is useful for diagnosing current infection, but cross-reactions occur.

Treatment
- Mild disease—doxycycline (preferred as also effective for rickettsial disease which may be confused with leptospirosis) or amoxicillin PO for 5–7 days.
- Severe disease—penicillin G, ceftriaxone IV for 5–7 days.
- Children or pregnant women can be treated with amoxicillin or ceftriaxone. Azithromycin is an alternative in severe allergy.
- Prophylaxis—doxycycline reduces morbidity and mortality in endemic areas, but has no impact on infection rates, as measured by seroconversion. It is likely to be useful in cases of accidental laboratory exposure or military and adventure travel. Animal vaccines are available against specific serovars.

Overview of *Rickettsia*

Microbiology

Rickettsiae are fastidious, obligate intracellular Gram-negative coccobacilli (0.3 micrometres by 1–2 micrometres). They survive only briefly outside a host (unlike *Coxiella*, with which they were previously classified) and are maintained in a cycle involving mammal reservoirs and arthropod vectors. Isolation is usually only performed in reference laboratories.

Epidemiology

Zoonotic reservoirs are varied and include wild rodents, dogs, and live-stock. Humans are incidental hosts, with the exception of louse-borne ty-phus, for which humans are the main reservoir. *Rickettsia rickettsii*, *Rickettsia typhi*, *Rickettsia tsutsugamushi*, and *Rickettsia akari* can exist as vector com-mensals. *Rickettsia prowazekii*, however, kills its human body louse vector within 3 weeks. For geographical distribution, see Table 7.18.

Diagnosis

- Usually based upon clinical features and epidemiological history. The presence of a typical rash or eschar suggests the diagnosis.
- **Culture**—usually only performed in reference laboratories. Blood or biopsy tissue from skin lesions should be frozen at −70°C. Organisms may be isolated in small laboratory animals or in embryonated eggs. Highly infectious if aerosolized—fatal laboratory-acquired infections have occurred.
- **Detection of antigen**—direct immunofluorescence of skin lesions in spotted fevers (rash or eschar) can identify organisms. Sensitivity is around 70%, with specificity approaching 100%. Organisms are most likely to be in a blood vessel near the centre of the lesion—the biopsy should include this to increase chance of successful culture. Availability is limited.
- PCR assays are available for various specimens (e.g. blood, biopsy tissue, CSF), usually at reference laboratories such as Rare and Imported Pathogens Laboratory (RIPL) (available at: ℘ www.gov.uk/government/collections/rare-and-imported-pathogens-laboratory-ripl).

Table 7.18 Overview of rickettsial disease

	Species	Syndrome	Vector (geography)	Clinical features
Spotted fever group	*Rickettsia rickettsii*	Rocky Mountain spotted fever	Ixodid ticks (Western hemisphere)	Incubation ~7 days. Fever, headache, myalgia, eschar, rash. Multisystem involvement; untreated, 20% mortality
	Rickettsia conorii	Mediterranean spotted fever	Ixodid ticks (Mediterranean, Africa, and India)	Incubation ~5 days. Eschar and local lymphadenopathy. Rash. Mild
	Rickettsia africae	African tick bite fever	Tick (sub-Saharan Africa, East Caribbean)	5–7 days. Mild illness, minimal rash, eschar with lymphadenopathy
	Rickettsia akari	Rickettsial pox	Mite (USA, Africa, Korea, and Russian Federation)	Incubation ~7 days. As for *R. conorii* plus vesicular rash resembling chickenpox
Typhus group	*Rickettsia prowazekii*	Epidemic typhus	Body louse (South America, Africa, Asia)	Incubation ~10 days. Fever, headache, neurological, and GI symptoms. Rash. Untreated, 20–50% mortality
		Brill–Zinsser disease	Nil—recurrence years after primary attack	Similar, milder illness than epidemic typhus, developing years after recovery—in the West, was seen in East European immigrants after World War II. Lasts around 2 weeks
	Rickettsia typhi	Murine (endemic) typhus	Flea (worldwide where human/rat coexist)	Similar to epidemic typhus, but much milder
	Rickettsia tsutsugamushi	Scrub typhus*	Mite (South Pacific, Asia, Australia)	Eschar common. Similar to epidemic typhus

* So-called 'scrub' typhus, as the vector is harboured in scrub vegetation. The chigger mites stay within several metres of where they hatch and are transovarially infected. Infection therefore occurs in very focused rural 'mite islands'.

- **Serology**—not useful acutely, but the main means of confirming diagnosis. Antibodies first appear at around days 7–10 after infection. A 4-fold rise on a convalescent sample is required for diagnosis, but a single titre of over 1:64 is very suggestive of infection (sensitivity 95%). Most tests cannot distinguish between spotted fever group species.
  - Micro-immunofluorescence is the most sensitive/specific test—it requires trained personnel and a fluorescence microscope.
  - Latex agglutination tests are available for Rocky Mountain spotted fever (RMSF). A single positive test is considered diagnostic. Rarely produce positive reactions in convalescence.
  - Complement fixation and the Weil–Felix* tests are neither sufficiently sensitive nor specific.

Rickettsial diseases

Rickettsiae replicate within the cytoplasm of infected endothelial and smooth muscle cells of capillaries and small arteries. They cause necrotizing vasculitis, with consequent protean manifestations. The classic triad of fever, headache, and rash, with appropriate travel and exposure history, should alert to a possible diagnosis. An eschar (black, ulcerated lesion) may develop at the bite site. Severity varies greatly with species—any organ can be involved.

Spotted fevers

Rocky Mountain spotted fever

- Clinical features—the most virulent spotted fever, with 20% mortality if untreated. Fever, myalgia, and headache follow a 2- to 14-day incubation. GI involvement may suggest an acute surgical abdomen. Maculopapular rash (90% of cases, more likely to be spotless in the elderly or black) appears at around days 3–5, often starting on the hands, and may become petechial or necrotic. Gangrene in 4% of cases. Severe multisystem involvement is common, including lung (pneumonia, effusion, oedema), nervous system (meningitis, focal deficits, e.g. deafness), and renal impairment. Thrombocytopenia and DIC can occur. Death at around 10 days, sooner in fulminant cases (more frequently in black ♂ with glucose-6-phosphate dehydrogenase (G6PD) deficiency).
- Treatment—tetracycline, chloramphenicol (preferred in pregnancy), or doxycycline for 7 days, continuing for 2 days after the patient becomes afebrile. It is recommended that doxycycline is used, even in children with suspected RMSF, given the life-threatening nature of the disease. No demonstrated benefit from steroid therapy.

Other spotted fevers

- Mediterranean spotted fever (boutonneuse fever) is a much milder disease; 5–7 days after inoculation, patients develop an eschar, with local tender lymphadenopathy and a generalized maculopapular rash, with abrupt onset of fever and headache. Mortality is rare, but disease severity varies with the specific strain. Severe disease is more likely in those with diabetes, cardiac disease, and G6PD deficiency, and in the elderly.

---

* In 1915, in Poland, Weil and Felix found that serum from patients with typhus agglutinated certain strains of *Proteus vulgaris*. It was the mainstay of diagnosis for many years.

- African tick bite fever (*R. africae*) causes mild clinical illness (fever, headache, myalgia), eschars, and regional lymphadenopathy, with scant or absent rash. May be a common cause of fever in returning travellers.
- Rickettsial pox (*R. akari*, transmitted by house mouse mite) outbreaks typically occur after mouse extermination programmes result in starving mites that seek an alternative source of blood. Presentation is similar to Mediterranean spotted fever, with the addition of a vesicular rash that resembles chickenpox.

Treatment of all these fevers is with doxycycline for 5–7 days.

Typhus group

Epidemic typhus

- In recent decades, epidemic typhus has been reported in Burundi, Rwanda, Ethiopia, the highlands of Algeria, and a few remote regions of mountainous South and Central America.
- Clinical features—unusual in that humans are the reservoir,* and outbreaks are thus commonest in conditions of crowding, especially in winter and war. The louse feeds on an infected person, and bites and defecates on the next, and infected faeces (which may remain infectious for as long as 100 days) are scratched into the bite.
  - Acute disease—after 1-week incubation, abrupt onset of headache and fever is followed by maculopapular rash at day 5. This involves the entire body within days. Neurological features (confusion, drowsiness, coma) are common, as is multisystem involvement (DIC, jaundice, myocarditis, pulmonary infiltrates). Mortality is 20–50% if untreated—low in children, high in the elderly.
  - Brill–Zinsser disease—a recudescence years after the initial episode. Usually a mild illness. Abrupt onset with fever, headache, malaise, and often rash. Patients are often elderly, and symptoms may be attributed to pre-exisiting ailments.
- Prevention—delousing, doxycycline prophylaxis for HCWs in affected areas.
- Treatment—as for RMSF. Early therapy nearly eliminates fatal illness.

Murine typhus

- Clinical features—longer incubation (up to 2 weeks), and patients rarely recall flea exposure. Fever, headache, and myalgia are followed by rash in 50%. Some may develop multisystem features, but this is less common than with epidemic louse-borne typhus. Mortality is <1%, higher in the elderly and those with G6PD deficiency.
- Treatment—spontaneous recovery usually occurs within 2 weeks if untreated. Antibiotic treatment is as for RMSF.

Scrub typhus

- Clinical features—not as severe as epidemic typhus. An individual is inoculated by the bite of the chigger mite, and develops abrupt fever and headache 6–18 days later. Usually tender lymph nodes and an eschar at the inoculation point. Severity varies widely—neurological features can occur. Untreated, mortality varies—up to 30%. Many serotypes (unlike the other organisms), so people may become infected again.

---

* However, *R. prowazekii* infection has been demonstrated amongst flying squirrels in the USA, with the squirrel flea and louse as vectors.

- Treatment—as for RMSF, but resistance to doxycycline and chloramphenicol has been seen in Northern Thailand. Treatment may need to be prolonged to avoid relapse (2 weeks). Azithromycin may be an alternative.

Coxiella burnetii

Q fever (as in 'Query') is the name coined by the medical officer in Queensland, Australia, who first investigated the outbreak of febrile illness that hit 20 employees of a Brisbane meat works.

Microbiology

C. burnetii is morphologically similar to rickettsiae but, with a variety of genetic and physiological differences, is now classified separately (more closely related to *Legionella*). It is a significantly hardier organism and may be transmitted by aerosol or infected milk. It can form spores and is able to survive outside a host for some time—over 40 months in skimmed milk at room temperature. It grows in the phagosomes of infected cells, rather than in the cytoplasm (as other *Rickettsia*)—appreciating the more acidic environment the phagosome affords. A characteristic feature is its antigenic 'phase' variation. If isolated from humans/animals, it is highly infectious and expresses phase I antigens. However, once subcultured within cells, its capsule LPS antigens change (phase II) and it is not infectious. This shift allows differentiation between acute and chronic Q fever.

Epidemiology

Found around the world, and a zoonosis, the organism is usually acquired from occupational exposure to cattle or sheep but can be caught from many different animals—exposure to parturient cats is an important risk factor. Acquisition from unpasteurized dairy products has occurred, and person-to-person spread is possible, but unusual. It exists in a tick reservoir, but this is thought to be an insignificant route of direct human infection—it is likely they infect those animals from which it may be acquired by humans. Infected ungulates are usually asymptomatic, though abortion/stillbirth may result. Organisms from a heavily infected placenta may be found in the soil for 6 months, and the air for 2 weeks after parturition. The largest outbreak yet described took place in the Netherlands in 2009 where it was previously unknown. It is a common cause of fever in armed forces personnel returning from Iraq and Afghanistan. Other risk factors—those living downwind from farms or contaminated manure, abattoir workers, vets.

Clinical features

- Incubation—humans are infected by inhalation (occasionally ingestion). Rare cases have occurred by transplacental transmission, intradermally, and via blood transfusions. Organisms proliferate in the lungs, and bacteraemia follows. Up to 50% of cases may be asymptomatic. Presentation is 2–5 weeks after infection.

- Acute Q fever—ranges from a self-limiting febrile illness (commonest), to prolonged pyrexia of unknown origin (PUO) with granulomatous hepatitis, to pneumonia. Pneumonia may be an incidental finding, as part of PUO, or a severe atypical pneumonia with dry cough, fever, fatigue, pleuritic chest pain, pleural effusion, and diarrhoea. It may be rapidly progressive, resembling legionnaire's disease. Hepatomegaly and rashes are common. Acute Q fever can be complicated by behavioural disturbances, GBS, myo-/pericarditis, arthritis, glomerulonephritis, severe headache, and aseptic meningitis, amongst others. Autoantibodies are often found (anti-mitochondria, anti-smooth muscle). Mortality is around 1% and is associated with myocarditis. Acquisition during pregnancy increases the risk of obstetric complications.

- Chronic Q fever—defined as infection lasting >6 months. Occurs in 1–5% of cases and may present years later. The commonest manifestation is culture-negative endocarditis. It usually occurs in those with pre-existing valve damage (<40% of such patients with acute Q fever develop endocarditis, unless treated promptly). Thus, patients diagnosed with Q fever should have valvular disease excluded. Hepatitis, osteomyelitis, vascular graft infection, and neurological infection are also recognized. Immunocompromised and pregnant hosts are at higher risk of chronic disease.

Diagnosis

- **Culture**—difficult and hazardous for laboratory staff; a category 3 organism.
- **Serology**—the organism has two biological phases. Antibodies to phase II are produced first. Phase I antibodies appear weeks later. If antibodies to both phases are present simultaneously, chronic infection (specifically endocarditis) should be considered. Cross-reactions occur with *Bartonella* infection. Immunofluorescence is the most widely used test. Seroconversion may be detected 7–15 days after symptom onset, and 90% have detectable antibodies by day 21. A high phase II titre indicates acute infection, whereas a high phase I titre suggests chronic infection—notably, it remains high 6 months after treatment completion. Those at high risk of chronic disease (valve abnormalities, immunodeficiency, pregnancy) should undergo serial serological testing for at least 6 months.
- **Molecular**—PCR tests exist but are not in widespread use outside of specialist reference laboratories.

Treatment

- Pneumonia—infection is nearly always self-limiting. Even without therapy, people begin to recover at around 2 weeks. However, treatment is indicated in all cases to reduce the chance of chronic disease—doxycycline, or chloramphenicol for 2–3 weeks. Long-term co-trimoxazole is an alternative during pregnancy. Patients should have echocardiography to exclude valve abnormalities. If normal, they should have serological follow-up testing at 3 and 6 months to ensure resolution.

- Valve abnormalities—those with acute Q fever who are found to have an underlying valve disease should be considered for prophylaxis (12 months of hydroxychloroquine with doxycycline), even in the absence of endocarditis, given the high risk of its development.
- Endocarditis—combination antibiotic therapy for a prolonged period (minimum 18 months; lifelong has been noted in some cases) (e.g. tetracycline with rifampicin, doxycycline with hydroxychloroquine). Valve replacement may be required.
- Consider Q fever in the diagnosis of culture-negative endocarditis.

Bartonella species

Microbiology

Bartonellae are Gram-negative intracellular organisms belonging to the genus *Bartonella*, closely related to *Brucella*, based on 16S rRNA analysis. Most species causing human infection are associated with mammalian reservoirs that may experience chronic asymptomatic infection.

Clinical syndromes

- Bartonellosis (*Bartonella bacilliformis*)—a biphasic disease transmitted by *Phlebotomus* sandflies. Endemic to Andean regions (Peru, Colombia, Ecuador).
  - Oroya fever—3–12 weeks after inoculation. Mild or severe (fever, headache, confusion, acute anaemia due to erythrocyte invasion). Complications: abdominal pain, thrombocytopenia, seizures, dyspnoea, hepatic/GI dysfunction, angina; untreated, 40% mortality. Treatment: chloramphenicol plus a beta-lactam for 14 days. Risk of opportunistic infections in survivors (e.g. *Salmonella*, toxoplasmosis). Asymptomatic bacteraemia with *B. bacilliformis* occurs in 15% of survivors.
  - Verruga peruana is a late-stage manifestation, usually experienced by populations native to the Andes. Crops of skin lesions appear weeks to months after an untreated acute infection. Initially miliary, they become nodular, then 'mulaire' (red, round lesions, 5mm in diameter). Occur on mucosal surfaces and internally. Histology demonstrates neovascular proliferation with occasional organisms.
- Cat-scratch disease (*Bartonella henselae*)—commonest cause of lymphadenopathy in children/young adolescents; 3–10 days after inoculation, a papule or pustule may be visible at the site. Most present at 2–3 weeks with the onset of regional lymphadenopathy and fever. Rarely, headache, sore throat, and skin rash. Lymph nodes settle over 2–4 months, even without treatment. Complications (commoner in the immunocompromised): encephalopathy, retinitis, bone/skin involvement, granulomatous hepatitis. Conjunctival exposure may present as Parinaud's oculoglandular syndrome (ocular granuloma/ conjunctivitis, preauricular lymphadenopathy). Other atypical presentations: PUO, osteomyelitis, hepatic/splenic granulomas. Diagnosis is based on history. Biopsy may be necessary to exclude lymphoma. Blood or tissue culture should be attempted in cases of PUO, neuroretinitis, or encephalitis after cat exposure, especially

if immunocompromised. Treatment: mild, 5 days of azithromycin; disseminated, 14 days of rifampicin plus azithromycin; neuroretinitis, 4–6 weeks of doxycycline or azithromycin plus rifampicin.

- **Bacillary angiomatosis** (BA)—unusual vascular proliferation caused by *B. henselae* or *Bartonella quintana* infection. Usually occurs in the immunocompromised, mostly HIV patients with CD4 count of <100/mm^3, but also in transplant patients and those on chemotherapy. Lesions begin as small papules that grow into round, red/purple nodules that ulcerate. May also appear as flat, hyperpigmented plaques. Occur in the skin, liver, spleen, bone, mucosal surfaces, heart, CNS, and bone marrow. Pathogenesis: the organism's outer membrane adhesin binds to endothelial cells, and induces endothelial proliferation and new vessel formation. Numerous organisms are visible in lesions stained with Warthin–Starry silver stain. Diagnosis: lesion biopsy. All patients should be treated—6–8 weeks of erythromycin or doxycycline for cutaneous disease, longer if recurrence occurs. Skin lesions may be excised. Without therapy, systemic infection (fever, abdominal pain, anorexia) can occur.

- **Bacterial peliosis** (BP)—characterized by blood-filled cystic lesions scattered throughout a visceral organ. Cases involving the liver (peliosis hepatis) and spleen present with weight loss, diarrhoea, abdominal pain, nausea, fever, hepatosplenomegaly, and elevated liver enzymes. Caused by *B. henselae* or *B. quintana* (less common, affecting bone). Most patients also have BA and previous cat exposure.

- **Fever, bacteraemia, endocarditis** (*B. quintana*)—acquired by scratching infected louse faeces into skin lesions. Epidemics occur in conditions of overcrowding and poor sanitation (e.g. soldiers in World War I—'trench fever'). Bacteraemia has been described in homeless alcoholics. Incubation is 3–40 days, followed by relapsing fever with headache, rash, and splenomegaly. Recognized cause of culture-negative endocarditis in those with uncontrolled HIV and immunocompetent alcoholics. *B. henselae* bacteraemia occurs in the immunocompetent, as well as in those with HIV. Diagnosis is by culture, or PCR/serology if culture-negative. Treatment: 4–6 weeks of macrolides and tetracyclines. Endocarditis may need surgery and very prolonged antibiotic courses.

Diagnosis

- **Direct examination**—Giemsa-stained blood films may detect *B. bacilliformis* in areas of endemic Oroya fever (large number of organisms). Not useful in detection of *B. henselae* or *B. quintana*, due to low levels of blood-borne organisms. May be visible by silver staining of lesions in BA or BP and in lymph nodes in early cat-scratch disease.

- **Culture**—may fail to trigger CO_2 detection systems; *B. henselae* grows on chocolate agar, with characteristic white, dry, cauliflower-like colonies. These become visible 5–14 days after incubation at 37°C in 5% CO_2. On Gram staining, they are small, curved bacilli, 2 micrometres by 0.5 micrometres, and display twitching motility when mounted in a saline drop. They are non-reactive in many standard biochemical tests. Colonies with appropriate morphological characteristics can have their identity confirmed by cellular fatty acid analysis, immunofluorescence antibody, or commercial enzyme substrate kits.

- **Molecular**—PCR or DNA hybridization techniques can be used to speciate isolates. Direct detection of *Bartonella* organisms in pus or tissue is possible by using PCR, with wide-ranging sensitivity depending on the technique and sample.
- **Serology**—EIA or immunofluorescence kits may be used to demonstrate anti-*Bartonella* antibodies in culture-negative endocarditis, those with cat-scratch disease, or HIV-associated aseptic meningitis, etc. There is substantial cross-reactivity between *B. henselae* and *B. quintana*, as well as with certain *Chlamydia* spp.

Mycoplasma

Microbiology

Amongst the smallest free-living organisms (0.2 micrometres in diameter) and lack a cell wall (bound only by a trilaminar membrane). Possess a small genome, with limited biosynthetic capabilities. Require enriched media for growth. The term '*Mycoplasma*' refers to a member of the class *Mollicutes*, thus encompassing the genera *Mycoplasma* and *Ureaplasma*. Many species have been isolated, but only four are significant human pathogens, a property attributed to tip organelles that interact with host cells.

Mycoplasma pneumoniae

Common cause of respiratory tract infection all year round (peaking in winter), affecting all ages, but with most disease from the age of 5 years to young adulthood. Droplet transmission. The organism attaches to respiratory epithelial cells and multiplies locally, producing H_2O_2, which results in epithelial damage. Incubation is for 2–3 weeks, and presentation is usually insidious (e.g. flu-like, wheeze, especially in children, intractable cough). Fewer than 10% of patients develop pneumonia (commonest cause of 'atypical'). Multiple lobes may be involved, but without consolidation; effusions in 20%. Disease is usually self-limited, resolving over 3–10 days without antibiotics. CXR abnormalities may take 6 weeks to clear. Antibiotic therapy (e.g. erythromycin) speeds resolution but rarely eradicates the organisms—recurrences can occur. Antibodies produced against *M. pneumoniae* cross-react with brain cells and erythrocytes (cold agglutinins). Immunity is not long-lasting. Complications (many immune-mediated): pleuritis, pneumothorax, lung abscess, haemolytic anaemia (cold agglutinins), thrombocytopenia, arthritis, rashes (e.g. erythema nodosum and multiforme), myocarditis, GBS, transverse myelitis, acute disseminated encephalomyelitis. Meningoencephalitis is thought to be due to direct invasion. Immunodeficiency predisposes to severe disease.

Ureaplasma urealyticum and Mycoplasma hominis

Part of the commensal flora in ♂ and ♀ urogenital tracts. Sexually transmitted, the rate of transmission is related to sexual activity and is much lower amongst women using barrier contraception. They are associated with GU infections, including non-gonococcal urethritis (NGU), epididymitis (rare), endometritis, chorioamnionitis, PID, pyelonephritis, and neonatal bacteraemia/abscesses. Additionally, they are statistically linked with prematurity, low birthweight, and infertility, and—in the case of *U. urealyticum*—colonization of the respiratory tract is linked to the development of chronic lung disease of the newborn. Both may be isolated from BCs in women with post-partum fever (10% of cases), and may cause septic arthritis and s/c abscesses in those with immunodeficiency. Sternal wound infections with *M. hominis* have occurred in heart and lung transplant patients.

Mycoplasma genitalium

Mycoplasma genitalium is an increasingly recognized sexually transmitted cause of NGU, cervicitis, and PID. Urethral discharge is the commonest reported symptom; most cases are asymptomatic. Screening is not currently recommended. Men with NGU (and partners) and women with PID (and partners) should be tested and treated in a GUM setting. Macrolide resistance is high, probably due to overuse of single-dose azithromycin, which should no longer be used for any STI. ➜ See Treatment below.

Other *Mycoplasma* organisms

Mycoplasma fermentans, *Mycoplasma penetrans* and *Mycoplasma pirum* have been isolated in those with HIV and are unusual in their ability to actively invade cells. Certain organisms found in animal hosts have caused human disease if sufficient exposure and predisposing comorbidity (e.g. *Mycoplasma arginini*, *Mycoplasma canis*—in dogs).

Diagnosis

- **Direct detection**—indirect fluorescent antibody tests to detect *M. hominis* in genital samples have been developed (not widely used).
- **Culture**—specimens should be inoculated to culture media as soon as possible. Several media are used—most are diphasic (media with agar overlayed by media without agar). All species grow at 35–37°C but differ in their optimal pH, atmospheric conditions, and substrate utilization.
  - **M. pneumoniae**—rarely attempted, as requires up to 4 weeks. Growth is indicated by pH change. Positives are subcultured to agar, and colonies should then be visible after a week. Identity is confirmed by serological methods or enzyme substrate tests.
  - Genital *Mycoplasma* samples are inoculated into broth and onto agar, and should be kept for 8 days (although *M. genitalium* and *M. fermentans* can take longer and are not routinely looked for). Broths that exhibit a change in colour are plated to the appropriate agar. Plates are examined by microscope each day for colonies. Selective plates and colonial morphology are usually sufficient to allow identification. Antisera are available to confirm *M. hominis*.
- **Molecular**—PCR techniques are available and are perhaps most useful in acute respiratory illness. Not yet in widespread use.
- **Serology**—*M. pneumoniae* complement fixation tests detect early IgM, and IgG to a lesser extent. EIAs are supplanting them, being more sensitive than culture in detecting acute infection (sensitivity 97.8%). A 4-fold rise between acute and convalescent (14 days) samples is diagnostic of recent infection.

Treatment

- *M. pneumoniae* is sensitive to a wide range of agents—tetracyclines, quinolones, or macrolides (resistance emerging, e.g. in Japan and China) (e.g. azithromycin for 5 days, doxycycline for 7–14 days).
- *M. hominis* is usually resistant to macrolides. Some genital *Mycoplasma* isolates have been found to be tetracycline-resistant and carry the *tetM* resistance determinant (also found in other genital tract organisms, e.g. GBS). Doxycycline considered first line. Fluoroquinolones usually active. Clindamycin may be appropriate in neonates.
- *U. urealyticum*—usually resistant to clindamycin and less susceptible to quinolones. Doxycycline first line. Erythromycin or azithromycin is effective.
- *M. genitalium*—macrolide resistance has increased to high levels along with usage. A combination of 7 days' doxycycline therapy, followed sequentially by 3 days of azithromycin, is recommended for uncomplicated cases. Quinolones (e.g. moxifloxacin) are preferred in macrolide-resistant or complicated infections (see British Association for Sexual Health and HIV (BASHH) guidelines, available at: ✆ www. bashhguidelines.org/current-guidelines/urethritis-and-cervicitis/myc oplasma-genitalium-2018/).

Chlamydia

Small obligate, intracellular (unable to produce ATP) Gram-negative organisms. Outside a host cell, they are tiny (300nm in diameter), inactive 'elementary' bodies. They infect cells by receptor-mediated endocytosis, inhibit lysosome fusion, and reside in a membrane-protected 'inclusion' body where they grow (800nm in diameter). Three species produce human disease. The family *Chlamydiaceae* was reorganized in 1999 on the basis of genetic similarities. *Chlamydia trachomatis* remains in the genus *Chlamydia*, but *psittaci* and *pneumoniae* were moved to a new genus *Chlamydophila*. They differ antigenically in host preference and antibiotic susceptibility.

Chlamydia trachomatis

Clinical features

There are 15 different serovars causing distinctive clinical syndromes. Natural infection confers only short-lived protection against reinfection.

- **Lymphogranuloma venereum** (LGV) (serovars L1, L2, L3)—endemic in Africa, India, South East Asia, South America, and the Caribbean. Sexually transmitted. The organism enters through skin abrasions and causes a small papule or ulcer (primary lesion) on the genital mucosa or nearby skin 3–30 days after infection. It heals rapidly, and weeks later, the patient develops secondary symptoms: lymphadenopathy (usually inguinal/femoral), fever, headache, myalgias, proctitis (particularly in MSM, and may resemble inflammatory bowel disease (IBD)), and occasionally meningitis. Nodes may coalesce, forming abscesses and buboes.

- **Trachoma** (serovars A, B1, B2, C)—chronic follicular keratoconjunctivitis that leads to corneal scarring and is the commonest cause of preventable blindness in the developing world (500 million affected, around 9 million blind). First infection acquired in childhood. Resolves, but multiple reinfections, and the consequent host response results in conjunctival scarring and corneal damage. The inner surface of the eyelid scars, and inturning eyelashes further abrade the cornea (see Box 7.13).
- **Inclusion conjunctivitis** (serovars D to K)—sexually transmitted eye infection in adults (of whom slightly over half have concurrent genital tract infection) and a cause of neonatal conjunctivitis (probably from the mother's genital tract, but can occur even if delivered by caesarean section—5 days to 6 weeks after delivery). No corneal scarring.
- **Neonatal pneumonia** (serovars D to K)—most acquired from the mother's genital tract. Seen in 10–20% of infants born to infected mothers. Usually symptomatic by 8 weeks, with nasal congestion, cough, etc., and only moderate illness.
- **STIs** (serovars D to K)—epididymitis (along with *N. gonorrhoeae*, the common cause in the under 35s) urethritis, proctitis (usually asymptomatic), salpingitis, cervicitis with consequent PID and infertility. Reactive arthritis/Reiter's syndrome may follow. Perihepatitis (Fitz-Hugh–Curtis syndrome) is an inflammation of the liver capsule and adjacent peritoneum seen in the setting of PID, presenting with right upper quadrant pain.

Box 7.13 WHO grading of trachoma
- Trachomatous inflammation follicular—5+ follicles in upper tarsal conjunctiva
- Trachomatous inflammation intense—pronounced tarsal conjunctival inflammation obscuring at least half of deep tarsal vessels
- Trachomatous conjunctival scarring—scars on tarsal conjunctiva
- Trachomatous trichiasis—1+ eyelash rubs on eyeball
- Corneal opacity—opacity obscuring part of pupil margin

Diagnosis
Trachoma may be diagnosed on clinical grounds. Other clinical presentations require laboratory identification for a definitive diagnosis. The majority of genital STIs are asymptomatic.
- **NAAT**—the test of choice, performed on vaginal swabs (best), ♂ first-catch urine, rectal or conjunctival swabs. PCR, transcription-mediated amplification (TMA), and strand displacement amplification techniques are all sensitive (80–99%, depending on assay and sample) and specific (>98%).
- **Immunoassay rapid testing**—rapid tests based on monoclonal antibody binding of chlamydial antigens from patient-collected samples have been developed, allowing same-day results.

- **Direct detection**—microscopy of certain Giemsa-stained clinical specimens (particularly neonatal conjunctivitis) may allow direct visualization if there are sufficient bacterial inclusion bodies in the cytoplasm. Monoclonal antibodies and immunofluorescence increase sensitivity.
- **Culture**—research tool only, as being obligate intracellular organisms, the techniques for culturing are similar to those used in virus culture.
- **Serology**—most useful for epidemiological studies.

Treatment

- Trachoma—transmission is by flies or eye-to-hand in endemic areas; thus, hygiene is important for control (rates fall quickly with socio-economic improvement). Systemic therapy (erythromycin or doxycycline) is effective in areas of low transmission (where reinfection is less frequent). Eyelid surgery can prevent further mechanical damage. In endemic areas, treatment is best delivered over an entire region (reduces reinfection). WHO guidelines recommend mass treatment if the prevalence of active trachoma amongst 1- to 9-year olds in a region is over 10%.
- LGV—aspirate buboes. Doxycycline for 3 weeks.
- Genital and ocular infections in adults—single-dose azithromycin, or doxyciline for 7 days. Longer courses of amoxicillin may be effective in pregnant women. Remember that gonococcal infection may coexist.
- Neonatal infections—erythromycin PO for 14 days for conjunctivitis (TOP therapy will not eliminate carriage) and pneumonia. Prenatal screening of mothers and treating those infected with *Chlamydia* infection are 90% effective in preventing infants from acquiring infection.

Chlamydophila psittaci

C. psittaci infects many kinds of birds; thus, the classic term for infection caused by this bacterium 'psittacosis' (derived from the Greek word for parrot) is not so accurate a description as 'ornithosis'. It is an occupational disease of zoo workers, pet shop workers, and poultry farmers. Human-to-human transmission occurs but is very rare. Infection is primarily acquired by inhalation of organisms from aerosolized avian excreta or respiratory secretions from sick birds (mouth-to-beak resuscitation has been implicated in acquisition). Transient exposure is sufficient (e.g. pet shop customers, gardening), and cases have occurred following exposure to other infected animals (e.g. dogs, sheep). The disease is found worldwide. Incubation is 5–14 days, and the presentation is with fever, chills, malaise, cough, headache, breathlessness, mild pharyngitis, and epistaxis. Less commonly, nausea, vomiting, and jaundice may be seen. Examination may demonstrate the features of an atypical pneumonia. Other features: bradycardia, peri-/myocarditis, culture-negative endocarditis, splenomegaly, meningitis, encephalitis, GBS, rashes, acute glomerulonephritis, severe respiratory failure, sepsis, shock. Relapses can occur. Infection in pregnancy may be life-threatening. Diagnosis: serology, micro-immunofluorescent antibody (MIF) test is sensitive and specific for *C. psittaci*. A 4-fold rise in titre or a high IgM titre is considered diagnostic. Complement fixation tests are more widely available but cannot differentiate between chlamydial species. Culture is avoided due to risks to laboratory staff. PCR-based tests are available. Treatment: tetracycline or doxycycline for 2–3 weeks (reduces the risk of relapse). Erythromycin may be used in children and pregnant women.

Chlamydophila pneumoniae

The cause of 3–10% of CAP cases amongst adults. Adolescents tend to experience mild pneumonia/bronchitis. Older adults can experience more severe disease. Fifty per cent of young adults have serological evidence of previous infection. Unlike *C. psittaci* human-to-human transmission by respiratory secretions is the norm. In most populations, infection is commoner in ♂ (may reflect cigarette use). Incubation is 3–4 weeks, and URTI symptoms are followed by bronchitis or pneumonia 1–4 weeks later. Most infections are mild or asymptomatic. Other features: hoarse voice, non-productive cough, headache. Fever is often absent. Extrapulmonary features: meningoencephalitis, GBS, myocarditis, reactive arthritis. Symptoms can be very prolonged, even with treatment. Diagnosis: serology, preferably MIF test. A definite case requires a 4-fold rise in titre—single elevated IgG titres may be seen in the uninfected elderly as a consequence of repeated infections. Antibody tests may be negative in the early weeks after infection—it can take as long as 8 weeks for a significant IgG response to develop after primary infection. Other tests: PCR, direct immunofluorescence, and immunoassay cell culture tests. Treatment: doxycycline or erythromycin for 10–14 days. Response is often slow.

Mycobacterium tuberculosis

The *Mycobacterium tuberculosis* (MTB) complex comprises several species, including *M. tuberculosis*, *Mycobacterium bovis*, *Mycobacterium africanum*, *Mycobacterium microti*, and *Mycobacterium caprae*. The term tuberculosis (TB) describes a broad range of clinical diseases caused by MTB (and less commonly by *M. bovis*). For treatment of TB disease, ➔ see Antituberculous agents, pp. 75–9.

Epidemiology

MTB is estimated to infect one-third of the world population and is the second most frequent infectious cause of death worldwide after HIV. There are around 10 million new cases of active TB every year, causing around 1.2 million deaths. Most cases occur in the developing world. In the developed world, despite a general downward trend, there has been an increase in incidence in certain groups (e.g. immigrants from high-prevalence countries, HIV-infected patients). Infection is acquired by inhalation of infectious droplet nuclei or occasionally skin inoculation. The resurgence of TB in Africa has been fuelled by HIV, which increases the risk of developing all forms of TB. The emergence of MDR- (resistance to at least isoniazid and rifampicin) and XDR- (resistance to rifampicin, isoniazid, a quinolone, and an injectable agent) TB has further complicated management and is discussed further elsewhere (➔ see Antituberculous agents, pp. 75–9).

Microbiology

Mycobacteria are aerobic, non-sporing, non-motile, weakly Gram-positive bacilli, characterized by their cell envelope, of which mycolic acid is a key component. It is this that enables them to resist destaining with acid–alcohol after staining with aniline dyes—hence acid-fast bacilli (AFB). MTB is slow-growing, with a generation time of >24h in laboratory media. At least 3–4 weeks are needed to grow the organism on solid media in most cases. Liquid culture systems are faster, with BACTEC™ detecting the growth of MTB in as little as 8 days with smear-positive specimens. Once grown, identification is by morphology/biochemical properties or nucleic acid detection.

Immunology and pathogenesis

Inhaled infectious droplets lodge in the alveoli. They may either be cleared by the innate immune system or establish infection. Such infection may be immediately active (primary disease) or latent, and/or activate many years later, determined by the interplay between the organism and the host cell-mediated immune response. Disease occurs in 10% of otherwise healthy infected people, half of whom within the first 3 years after infection.

- Primary infection—inhaled TB bacilli multiply in alveolar macrophages that, in turn, produce cytokines (TNF-α, platelet-derived growth factor, transforming growth factor-β, fibroblast growth factor), attracting neutrophils and other phagocytic cells. These form a nodule or 'tubercle' (granulomatous in histology). This will enlarge if infection is progressive, and bacilli may reach regional lymph nodes. A tubercle plus regional lymphadenopathy is termed the Ghon complex. Bacilli proliferate until an effective cell-mediated immune response is mounted. If this is ineffective, progressive lung disease and dissemination may occur.
- Reactivation—otherwise healthy individuals with latent TB infection have a 5–10% chance of reactivating and developing active disease over their lifetime. The chance is much higher in those with comorbidities associated with immunosuppression (e.g. diabetes, malignancy), and rates with advanced HIV are ~10% a year. Disease is more likely to be localized than that seen with primary infection.

Clinical features

Pulmonary TB is the commonest presentation. TB may also disseminate (miliary TB) or affect almost any other organ (extrapulmonary TB): pleural cavity, pericardium, lymph nodes, GI tract and peritoneum, GU tract, skin, bones and joints, and CNS (➔ see Tuberculous meningitis, pp. 772–3).

Diagnosis

- Diagnosis is based on a combination of compatible clinical syndrome, supportive radiological investigations, and detection of AFB or culture of MTB from clinical specimens. The gold standard for diagnosis is culture.
- Samples of sputum or tissue are liquefied, decontaminated (to prevent overgrowth of media by bacteria), neutralized, and centrifuged, and the deposit inoculated into solid or liquid media. Sterile site samples (e.g. CSF) do not need decontamination, and loss of viability may occur.
- Acid-fast stains:

- ZN stain (carbol fuchsin stain, decolorizes with acid-alcohol, counterstain with methylene blue)—a sputum specimen needs at least 10 000cfu/mL to give a positive smear. The Kinyoun stain is similar, but modified to make heating unnecessary;
- auramine stain (fluorochrome phenolic auramine or auramine–rhodamine stain, acid–alcohol decolorization, potassium permanganate counterstain). Up to 10 times more sensitive than ZN, and advances in fluoroscopic lighting (e.g. long-life LEDs) are making the technology more suitable for resource-poor settings.

- Nucleic acid detection tests allow rapid diagnosis of MTB infection in clinical specimens, detecting as few as 1–10 organisms/mL. They are usually used as an adjunct to smear, culture, and full drug sensitivity testing. The Cepheid Xpert® MTB/RIF (Ultra) assay is a widely used automated PCR system that can identify TB and rifampicin resistance (and others) from clinical specimens (including sputum, pus, and CSF). Sensitivity for detecting TB is >98% on smear-positive sputa, and 75–90% if smear-negative. Detection of rifampicin resistance (*rpoB* gene) is >97% sensitive and >98% specific. Results can be available within 2h. The WHO has recommended the system, in place of smear microscopy, for the diagnosis of drug-resistant TB or TB in HIV-infected patients. Other nucleic acid detection methods are available (e.g. TB-LAMP).
- Culture methods can detect as few as 10 organisms/mL. Media are classically egg- (Lowenstein–Jensen, better growth), agar- (Middlebrook 7H10, better speed and allows colony morphology examination), or liquid- (Middlebrook 7H12) based. Growth in liquid media is faster (<8 days for smear-positive sputum) than in solid (3–8 weeks). Specimens are generally inoculated into both solid (e.g. an LJ slope) and liquid media systems. This provides a backup, should liquid culture fail. Commercial liquid culture systems include BACTEC™ and MGIT™.
- Identification is usually done at reference laboratory level, once a mycobacterium has been isolated. Techniques include high-pressure liquid chromatography (HPLC) of mycolic acids, DNA sequencing of 16S rRNA, PCR restriction enzyme assay, and DNA probe hybridization (INNO-LiPA® MYCOBACTERIA). Typing can be performed for epidemiological purposes (e.g. mycobacterial interspersed repetitive unit VNTRs (MIRU-VNTRs)).
- Drug susceptibility testing—phenotypic testing takes >3 weeks, depending on growth speed. Rapid tests include:
  - microscopic observation drug susceptibility—media with and without antibiotics are inoculated with the patient specimen and examined for growth. Concerns regarding biosafety;
  - nucleic acid amplification to identify known drug resistance mutations. Line probe assays (e.g. Hain Genotype MTBDRplus) are recommended by the WHO for rapid screening for MDR-TB in low- or middle-income settings. They can be performed on positive cultures or smear-positive sputum. DNA is extracted from the specimen, multiplex PCR used to amplify those regions of the genome associated with known resistance mutations, and reverse hybridization performed in which single-stranded amplicons bind to specific probes attached to test strips which can be read visually.

- WGS—the introduction of WGS as a method for complete identification, prediction of drug susceptibility, and epidemiological analysis occurred in the UK in 2017. Accurate prediction is possible for the majority of first-line drugs, but phenotypic results are still required for detection of many resistance patterns. The method has greatly improved the time to results and provides detailed information on relatedness for outbreak management.
- Tuberculin skin test (TST)—purified protein derivative (PPD) is a standardized protein precipitate of tuberculin. The Mantoux test is performed by intracutaneous injection of five tuberculin units of PPD in 0.1mL of solution. The reaction diameter is read after 48–72h (induration, NOT erythema which may be larger). Specifics of interpretation vary with guidelines. In the UK, <6mm is negative; 6–14mm is positive but could be due to bacille Calmette–Guérin (BCG) vaccination or exposure to non-tuberculous mycobacteria (NTM); 15mm or greater is strongly positive and suggestive of TB infection or disease. False-negative reactions occur in up to 20% of patients with TB and in HIV-infected patients. Delayed reactivity (>10mm induration after 6 days) may occur in certain populations (e.g. Indo-Chinese immigrants). Sensitivity and specificity vary with the specific cut-offs chosen, but overall 97% specific for latent TB amongst non-BCG-vaccinated (around 60% in vaccinated) populations and 80% sensitive.
- Interferon-γ release assays ('IGRAs') (T-SPOT®, QuantiFERON®-TB Gold) detect T cells responsive to antigens specific to MTB (e.g. ESAT-6, CFP-10), thus avoiding issues of BCG cross-reactivity. They are used for the diagnosis of latent TB and cannot distinguish this from active infection. A negative result does not rule out active TB. Specificity is >95% for the diagnosis of latent TB; sensitivity is around 90%. Sensitivity remains high in children aged <3 years and in HIV co-infection. In the UK, TST is first line for screening, with follow-up IGRA if necessary, unless HIV-positive or immunocompromised when IGRA (alone or with TST) is recommended.

Prevention

- Vaccination—BCG is a live attenuated vaccine derived from *M. bovis*. It is given to infants and children in high-prevalence areas and results in a 60–80% reduction in the incidence of TB. It should only be given to infants aged <12 weeks or children who are TST-negative. Although it does not prevent infection, BCG vaccination reduces the risk of disseminated disease in children. BCG is contraindicated in HIV-infected individuals. Vaccination can occasionally cause disseminated BCG infection, usually in immunosuppressed patients. Intravesical BCG (used to treat bladder cancer) can cause liver or lung granulomas, psoas abscess, or osteomyelitis. Trials of novel vaccine candidates are ongoing.
- Treatment of latent disease—the aim of testing people for latent TB is to find those at higher risk of developing active disease who would therefore benefit from preventative therapy. There is no point in testing those in whom treatment would not be considered. Risk groups include those likely to have recently acquired infection (e.g. tested as part of contact tracing; the risk of TB disease is highest in the first 2–3 years), HCWs, and the immunosuppressed (e.g. in anti-TNF therapy). For

detailed indications, see the 2016 UK NICE guidance (available at: ✍ www.nice.org.uk/guidance/ng33). The usual regimen is isoniazid for 6 months, or rifampicin and isoniazid for 3 months. The risk of isoniazid hepatotoxicity increases with age (<1% in those aged <35 years, >5% in the over 65s); thus, testing is not indicated in older people with a moderate/slightly increased risk of reactivation.

Mycobacterium leprae

Leprosy, or Hansen's disease, is caused by infection with *M. leprae*, an obligate intracellular parasite, the only natural hosts of which are humans and armadillos. Experimental infections can be induced in the mouse footpad. Clinical manifestations of leprosy include skin lesions, deformities, and peripheral neuropathy, making it one of the most socially stigmatizing diseases. Leprosy exhibits a spectrum of clinical features, ranging from lepromatous (multibacillary) to tuberculoid (paucibacillary) forms.

Epidemiology

The WHO began an ambitious leprosy elimination programme (defined as <1 case per 10 000 in endemic countries) in the 1990s. Multidrug treatment was made available free to all patients, and the number of new cases has fallen from 763 000 in 2001 to 202 185 in 2019. Only a couple of endemic countries still have to achieve the 'elimination threshold. The greatest number of new cases in 2019 occurred in India, Brazil, and Indonesia. Leprosy is associated with poverty and rural residence, but not with HIV infection. Distribution in endemic countries is non-homogeneous, suggesting that genetic factors may play a role in disease expression. The mode of transmission is unclear but thought to be human-to-human, or via nasal droplet infection or direct inoculation into the skin. Incubation is long, with an average of 5–7 years (range of 2–40 years), and peak onset is in young adulthood.

Microbiology

M. leprae is an AFB with a dense lipid capsule outside the cell wall, best visualized by a modified Fite stain (it may be decolorized by the ZN stain). It grows best at temperatures of 27–33°C, consistent with its preference for cooler areas of the body. It multiplies very slowly (doubling time of 12–13 days) and, as an obligate intracellular organism, cannot be cultured in artificial media. Experimental infection of the mouse footpad can be used to assess antimicrobial susceptibility.

Clinical features

Disease ranges from 'tuberculoid' (or paucibacillary), with few organisms and a robust cell-mediated immune response, to 'lepromatous' (or multibacillary) with a weaker immune response, a higher number of organisms, and greater infectivity. Clinical manifestations are largely confined to the skin, upper respiratory tract, and peripheral nerves. Most serious sequelae are a result of peripheral nerve damage, resulting in deformities (e.g. ulnar, median, peroneal nerve palsies), loss of peripheral parts of the digits, and plantar ulceration.

- **Lepromatous leprosy**—characterized by numerous skin nodules, plaques, and a thickened dermis that typically occur in cool areas of the body (e.g. earlobes, feet). No apparent resistance, with poor cell-mediated immune response. Involvement of the nasal mucosa results in congestion, epistaxis, and rarely septal collapse ('saddle nose'). May also cause loss of eyebrows and eyelashes, trichiasis, corneal scarring, uveitis, lagophthalmos, testicular dysfunction, and amyloidosis.
- **Tuberculoid leprosy**—characterized by hypopigmented, anaesthetic skin plaques, and asymmetrical peripheral nerve involvement. It is typically paucibacillary (non-infectious) and associated with a good cell-mediated immune response.
- **Borderline leprosy**—the majority of patients, with manifestations intermediate between the two polar forms.
- **Reversal reactions ('type 1 reaction')**—an abrupt increase in inflammation within previously quiescent skin lesions, new skin lesions, neuritis, and fever in borderline leprosy patients either before (downgrading reaction) or after (reversal reaction) starting therapy. If the neuritis is not treated promptly, irreversible nerve damage may occur.
- **Erythema nodosum leprosum ('type 2 reaction')**—affects >50% of lepromatous and borderline leprosy patients after initiation of therapy. Clinical features include painful nodules (usually on extensor surfaces, may pustulate or ulcerate), neuritis, fever, malaise, anorexia, uveitis, lymphadenitis, orchitis, anaemia, leucocytosis, and glomerulonephritis.

Diagnosis

- **Biopsy**—full-thickness skin biopsies should be taken from skin plaques or nodules in lepromatous patients and from the periphery of lesions in tuberculoid patients. Nerve biopsies may result in loss of function and should only be performed if diagnostic uncertainty justifies the risk.
- **Mycobacterial cultures**—should be performed on biopsy material to exclude cutaneous TB.
- **PCR**—assays are available and, when performed on biopsies, have a sensitivity of >90% in lepromatous, and 34% in tuberculoid, disease.
- A firm diagnosis of leprosy requires the presence of a characteristic peripheral nerve abnormality or the demonstration of AFB in skin biopsies or split skin smears. In atypical cases, two of the following three criteria are required: a clinically compatible skin lesion, dermal granuloma on skin biopsy, hypoaesthesia within the lesion.

Treatment

Treatment requires combination therapy with two or more agents (e.g. dapsone, clofazimine, rifampicin). Ethionamide, prothionamide, and certain aminoglycosides have also been used. Newer agents, such as minocycline, clarithromycin, fluoroquinolones, look promising. For treatment regimens, ➔ see Antileprotics, pp. 79–81. Drug resistance is uncommon. Relapses occur (usually within 5–10 years), but are rare (around 1%) and more likely if treatment is not completed.

Prevention

Household contacts of cases should be monitored annually for evidence of disease, but drug prophylaxis is not justified. BCG vaccination offers some protection (single dose is around 50% protective).

Non-tuberculous mycobacteria

This group of organisms comprises about 50 species of mycobacteria, excluding those in the MTB complex and *M. leprae*. Other names for NTM include atypical mycobacteria, opportunistic mycobacteria, or mycobacteria other than tuberculosis (MOTT).

Classification

NTM were previously classified according to growth rate, colonial morphology, and pigmentation (Runyon classification). This has been superseded by molecular methods but nonetheless remains useful to separate NTM into three groups:

- **rapidly growing mycobacteria** (≤7 days' incubation) (e.g. *Mycobacterium fortuitum* complex, *Mycobacterium chelonae/abscessus* group, *Mycobacterium mucogenicum*, *Mycobacterium smegmatis*);
- **slow-growing mycobacteria** (>7 days' incubation) (e.g. *Mycobacterium avium* complex (MAC), *Mycobacterium kansasii*, *Mycobacterium xenopi*, *Mycobacterium simiae*, *Mycobacterium szulgai*, *Mycobacterium scrofulaceum*, *Mycobacterium malmoense*, *Mycobacterium terrae/nonchromogenicum* complex, *Mycobacterium haemophilum*, *Mycobacterium genavense*);
- **intermediate-growing mycobacteria** (7–10 days) (e.g. *Mycobacterium marinum* (fish tank granuloma), *Mycobacterium gordonae*).

Clinical features

The NTM can cause a wide spectrum of diseases (see Table 7.19).

Diagnosis

Because the signs and symptoms of NTM lung disease are often variable and non-specific, diagnosis requires multiple positive respiratory cultures. Diagnosis of NTM infections at other sites requires positive cultures from pus, tissue biopsies, or BCs.

- **Microscopy**—the acid-fast stains used for identifying MTB (→ see Diagnosis, p. 392) also work well for identifying NTM.
- **Culture**—appropriate culture media include Middlebrook 7H10 or 7H11 agar or BACTEC™ broth. Samples from skin and soft tissue infections need to be plated at 28–30°C, as well as at 35–37°C, as some species only grow at low temperatures (e.g. *M. chelonae*, *M. haemophilum*, *M. marinum*). *M. xenopi* grows best at 42°C. Other species have special growth requirements (e.g. *M. genavense*, BACTEC™ broth for 6–8 weeks; *M. haemophilum*, iron supplementation).
- **Identification**—although traditional biochemical and other standard tests may be performed, identification of NTM increasingly uses rapid molecular methods such as HPLC of mycolic acids, PCR–restriction fragment length polymorphism (RFLP) analysis of the heat-shock

Table 7.19 Clinical syndromes caused by non-tuberculous mycobacteria

Syndrome	Commonest causes
Chronic bronchopulmonary disease (adults, cystic fibrosis patients)	*Mycobacterium avium* complex (MAC), *Mycobacterium kansasii*, *Mycobacterium abscessus*
Cervical lymphadenitis (children)	MAC
Skin and soft tissue infections	*Mycobacterium fortuitum* group, *Mycobacterium chelonae*, *Mycobacterium abscessus*, *Mycobacterium marinum*, *Mycobacterium ulcerans*
Bone and joint infections	*M. marinum*, MAC, *M. kansasii*, *M. fortuitum* group, *M. abscessus*, *M. chelonae*
Disseminated infection (HIV-positive)	*Mycobacterium avium*, *M. kansasii*
Disseminated infection (HIV-negative)	*M. abscessus*, *M. chelonae*
Catheter-related infections	*M. fortuitum*, *M. abscessus*, *M. chelonae*

protein gene, genetic probes for mycobacterial RNA, 16S ribosomal RNA sequencing, and WGS.
- **Drug susceptibility testing**—various methods are used, including agar disc elution, broth microdilution, E-test, and BACTEC™ radiometric detection. However, the clinical utility for susceptibility results is not as well established for many NTM as it is for TB. Rapid growers, in particular, tend to be resistant to classic TB medications.
  - **MAC**—clinical breakpoints exist for clarithromycin (from which azithromycin sensitivity can be inferred), which correlate with outcome. No clear link between *in vitro* susceptibility and clinical response for other drugs.
  - *M. malmoense*, *M. xenopi*—there is no correlation between *in vitro* susceptibility and *in vivo* response.
  - *M. kansasii*—rifampicin susceptibility testing is recommended, but evidence of correlation to outcomes is limited.
- **Strain comparison**—for epidemiological studies, standard biochemical identification and susceptibility testing have been superseded by molecular methods.

Treatment

Treatment may be medical, surgical, or a combination of the two. The choice of drugs and duration of treatment depend on the causative organism, site of infection, and patient's HIV status. Treatment is summarized in Table 7.20.

Table 7.20 Treatment of atypical mycobacterial infections

Causative organism	British Thoracic Society (BTS) guidelines*	American Thoracic Society (ATS) guidelines**	Comments
Mycobacterium avium complex (MAC), normal host	Pulmonary: rifampicin + ethambutol + isoniazid for 24 months	Clarithromycin (or azithromycin) + rifabutin (or rifampicin) + ethambutol (until culture negative for 1 year)	May add streptomycin for initial 2–3 months for severe disease; extrapulmonary disease: surgical excision
MAC, immunocompromised	Rifabutin + ethambutol + clarithromycin (or azithromycin)	Clarithromycin (or azithromycin) + ethambutol + rifabutin. Amikacin or streptomycin initially for severe disease	Primary prophylaxis if CD4 count <50/mm³. Lifelong treatment required
Mycobacterium abscessus	Rifampicin + ethambutol ± clarithromycin	Amikacin + cefoxitin for severe disease. Newer macrolides	Surgical excision
Mycobacterium chelonae	Pulmonary: rifampicin + ethambutol + clarithromycin; extrapulmonary: ciprofloxacin + aminoglycoside or imipenem ± clarithromycin	Tobramycin + cefoxitin or imipenem for severe disease. Clarithromycin or clofazimine PO	Surgical excision
Mycobacterium fortuitum	Pulmonary: rifampicin + ethambutol + clarithromycin; extrapulmonary: ciprofloxacin + aminoglycoside or imipenem ± clarithromycin	Pulmonary: two agents (macrolides, quinolones, doxycycline, minocycline); extrapulmonary: amikacin + cefoxitin or imipenem	Optimal regimen not defined; surgical excision
Mycobacterium haemophilum	Pulmonary: rifampicin + ethambutol + clarithromycin	Ciprofloxacin + rifabutin + clarithromycin	Optimal regimen not defined; surgical excision

(Continued)

Table 7.20 (Contd.)

Causative organism	British Thoracic Society (BTS) guidelines[*]	American Thoracic Society (ATS) guidelines[**]	Comments
Mycobacterium kansasii	Pulmonary: rifampicin + ethambutol (9 months)	Isoniazid + rifabutin + ethambutol (18 months, with 12 months smear-negative)	
Mycobacterium malmoense	Pulmonary: rifampicin + ethambutol ± isoniazid (24 months)	Rifampicin + isoniazid + ethambutol ± quinolones and macrolides	Extrapulmonary: excision
Mycobacterium marinum	Rifampicin + ethambutol or co-trimoxazole or tetracycline	Clarithromycin or minocycline or doxycycline or co-trimoxazole or rifampicin + ethambutol (± 3 months)	Surgical excision
Mycobacterium scrofulaceum		Clarithromycin + clofazimine ± ethambutol	Chemotherapy rarely indicated; surgical excision
Mycobacterium ulcerans	Rifampicin + ethambutol + clarithromycin	Rifampicin + amikacin or ethambutol ± co-trimoxazole (4–6 weeks)	Surgical excision and skin grafting
Mycobacterium xenopi	Pulmonary: rifampicin + ethambutol ± isoniazid for 24 months	Macrolide + rifamycin + ethambutol ± streptomycin	Extrapulmonary: excision

[*] British Thoracic Society (BTS) guidelines. *Thorax*. 2000;**55**:210–18.

[**] American Thoracic Society (ATS) guidelines. *Am J Respir Crit Care Med*. 2007;**175**:367–416.

Mycobacterium chimaera

A global outbreak of this slow-growing NTM (a subspecies of *M. avium*) was identified in 2015. Invasive infections, including endocarditis, surgical site infections, and metastatic infections, have all been described. Genomic analysis has proposed contamination of heater–cooler units used in open cardiac surgery as the likely source, with patients undergoing valve surgery most at risk.[9] Infection can be insidious and may present many years after the initial surgery; a high index of suspicion is required, including in patients presenting with PUO or unexplained granulomatous inflammation. Diagnosis is confirmed by positive cultures of clinical specimens, including blood, and multiple samples should be sent. Antimicrobial therapy is broadly similar to treatment for MAC infection, with clarithromycin and amikacin used in combination with rifampicin, ethambutol, linezolid, or quinolones, depending on the context and sensitivity testing (proven breakpoints only exist for macrolides). Removal of infected prosthetic material is almost always required.[10] Seek expert help.

References

9 Chand M, Lamagni T, Kranzer K, *et al.* Insidious risk of severe *Mycobacterium chimaera* infection in cardiac surgery patients. *Clin Infect Dis.* 2017;**64**:335–342.

10 Hasse B, Hannan MM, Keller PM, *et al.* International Society of Cardiovascular Infectious Diseases guidelines for the diagnosis, treatment and prevention of disseminated *Mycobacterium chimaera* infection following cardiac surgery with cardiopulmonary bypass. *J Hosp Infect.* **104**:214–53.

Viruses

Introduction to virology

At first, clinical virology can be an intimidating topic. Admittedly, there is a critical threshold of terminology, along with an understanding of molecular cell biology that needs to be crossed to yield the fullest dividend. However, the reader is highly encouraged to make these initial investments as the comprehension gained will provide an invaluable and transferrable foundation. This will serve to enhance bedside clinical virology practice, as well as critical appraisal of new diagnostics/therapeutics for inevitable future epidemics. As bacteriology/parasitology become more molecular in their diagnostics, these skills are immediately transferable.

It can be useful to approach this in two distinct, but complementary, ways:
- virus classification;
- viral replication.

Virus classification

Viruses can be classified by a number of methods (e.g. structure, genome composition, or concordant clinical syndrome). An awareness of each is helpful towards a foundation in clinical virology.

Properties and structure

Viruses are obligate intracellular parasites, dependent on living cells for the replication of their genome in order to reproduce. They have colonized all life forms, including bacteria, plants, insects, animals, and even other viruses.

Viruses are very small (20–150nm in diameter) protein packages that contain genetic material (DNA or RNA)—the viral genome. This contains all the information needed to make new virus. The viral particle is composed of structural proteins. A capsid (protein coat) protects the nucleic acid contents. It is composed of many capsomeres (protein subunits). The term nucleocapsid refers to the capsid and viral genome. Nucleocapsids may take several geometric forms:
- helical (spiral staircase)—nucleic acid forms the central core, with the nucleocapsid proteins forming the steps. It is made of a single protein, which requires less coding capacity on the genome and is easier to assemble. Most human helical nucleocapsid viruses have RNA genomes and are enveloped (e.g. Ebola, influenza, measles, rabies);
- icosahedral (spherical)—the commonest structure, with all animal DNA viruses (except *Poxviridae*) and some RNA (e.g. enterovirus, hepatitis C virus (HCV)) viruses taking this shape. Unit architecture varies in the number of proteins used to make the subunits and overall structural composition;
- complex (look like a space rocket)—these viruses do not fall into neat structural categories and are of a rare conformation (e.g. pox viruses, bacteriophages).

Some viral capsids have an outer envelope (derived from the plasma membrane of the infected cell from which it was released). Amongst human DNA viruses, only *Herpesviridae*, *Poxviridae*, and *Hepadnaviridae* are enveloped. Most human RNA viruses are enveloped, except *Picornaviridae*, *Caliciviridae*, and *Reoviridae*.

Protein spikes (crucial for mediating attachment) can be embedded directly from the nucleocapsid or envelope. Beneath the envelope, some viruses may have a stabilizing membrane protein. The entire particle is referred to as a virion. Certain viruses also contain enzymes.

Viral genomes and the Baltimore classification

The viral genome provides numerous ways for viral classification, based on size, composition, and conformation. It may be DNA or RNA, and encodes both structural and non-structural (NS) proteins (proteins required for viral expression, replication, or immune evasion). Genome size is expressed in base pairs (bp). The base refers to one of the four components that make up either DNA (guanine, cytosine, adenine, or thymine) or RNA (thymine is substituted for uracil in RNA). They join like the rungs of a ladder to make base pairs. When these bases form bonds with five-ring sugar structures, they become nucleosides. Many antiviral drugs are nucleoside analogues (e.g. aciclovir, remdesivir, entecavir, emtricitabine).

Viral genomes are generally smaller than their bacterial counterparts; for example, *Escherichia coli* has a genome of 4.6 million bp and the human genome has 6 billion bp (accounting for diploidy) Bacteria may have several thousands of genes, but even the largest viruses have <200 genes, and the smallest perhaps only four (many viruses may produce >1 protein from the same gene by means of RNA splicing or frameshifting to conserve genomic space). Amongst viruses, RNA viruses tend to have smaller genomes that their DNA counterparts; for example, cytomegalovirus (CMV) has a genome of 236 000 bp. Accordingly, DNA viruses have proofreading mechanisms built into their polymerases to ensure fidelity when replicating their larger genomes. Conversely, RNA viruses have higher error rates. Many mutations are detrimental or neutral to viral replication, but some will allow the virus to evade host immune responses and medical therapies. This is more likely to occur in environments that promote favourable mutations arising (e.g. suboptimal antiviral drug concentrations or weakened host immune systems where replication continues to occur under a selection pressure). Viruses evolve rapidly due to the high number of genome duplications undergone in short spaces of time.

Genome composition can take many forms: single-stranded (ss), double-stranded (ds), segmented, or circular. Broadly, all DNA viruses are ds, except for *Parvoviridae*, whereas all RNA viruses are ss, except for *Reoviridae*. Some ssRNA virus genomes exist in a positive sense and can be translated directly into protein by host ribosomes. All other viral genome conformations must produce positive messenger RNA (mRNA) from their genomes for this purpose. The Baltimore classification uses these features to produce seven groups:

- dsDNA viruses (e.g. herpes simplex type 1);
- ssDNA viruses (e.g. parvovirus);
- dsRNA viruses (e.g. rotavirus);
- positive sense (+) ssRNA viruses (e.g. hepatitis C virus);
- negative sense (−) ssRNA viruses (e.g. influenza virus);
- ssRNA with a DNA intermediate (e.g. HIV);
- dsDNA with an RNA intermediate (e.g. hepatitis B).

Taxonomy

Viral taxonomy is a dynamic field that is reviewed constantly. The International Committee on Taxonomy of Viruses (ICTV) represents a fantastic online resource (available at: ℅ https://ictv.global/). There are no consistent rules governing the naming of individual viruses. Some are named according to the disease they produce (poxvirus), others by acronyms (papovavirus—papilloma polyma vacuolating virus), some by appearance (coronavirus (CoV)), and still others after the location in which they were first identified (Marburg). They may rarely be called after their discoverers (Epstein–Barr). It is recommended that the species name is written in italics, with the letter of the first word given a capital, whereas an individual virus name is usually neither italicized nor given a capital.

Viral replication

All viral replication cycles will vary according to their Baltimore classification and individual properties, but many trends are generalizable.

Entry

Viral entry is the pivotal initial step and generally involves the interaction of a viral surface protein and a host cell receptor (originally intended for other functions and simply exploited by the virus). The cellular receptor used contributes towards viral tropism. After successful attachment, internalization follows. Once in the cell, the virus uncoats (sheds its protein shell) and frees its genome.

Transcription

Viral infection hijacks cellular ribosomes to translate the viral mRNAs to make proteins. Protein transcription is a heavily regulated process and may be separated into phases—'early' proteins may be involved in DNA synthesis or act as transcriptional activators to speed viral expression over host proteins; 'late' proteins are produced from mRNA transcribed from newly synthesized viral nucleic acid and tend to be structural. After translation, a wealth of biochemical post-translational modifications may occur to ensure correct protein formation.

Viral genome replication

The genome of a positive-sense RNA virus can immediately act as mRNA and be translated from directly. A negative-sense RNA virus must carry an RNA polymerase within the virion to turn the negative-sense RNA genome into positive-sense mRNA (antigenome) for translation. DNA viruses usually exploit host cell polymerases to make mRNA. RNA retroviruses use an exceptional polymerase called reverse transcriptase (RT) to turn RNA into DNA, which is then turned into mRNA by host polymerases. Most DNA viruses replicate in the nucleus, except *Poxviridae*, whereas most RNA viruses replicate in the cytoplasm, except the influenza virus.

The fidelity of genome replication is not guaranteed, and genetic variation may arise by three main mechanisms:

- errors in replication and absence of proofreading activity in enzymes such as RNA polymerase and RT (misreading of bases)—give rise to point mutations;
- recombination of genetic material—can occur either within a genome or between two viruses of the same kind if the host cell is co-infected with both viruses;
- reassortment—can occur in segmented RNA viruses (e.g. influenza virus or rotavirus) whereby whole segments are swapped. This can give rise to progeny virus with very different characteristics from either parent (➋ see Influenza, pp. 407–11).

Viral assembly

This may occur predominantly in the nucleus (e.g. adenovirus) or in the cytoplasm (e.g. poliovirus (PV)). Viral release then occurs by budding from the cell surface (e.g. measles), lysis of the cell (e.g. polio), or even cell-to-cell spread, thereby avoiding extracellular immune defences. Some, such as HIV, may require a phase of post-release maturation. Overall a complete viral life cycle typically takes 6–8h, with the potential to produce thousands of viruses from each infected cell.

Influenza

Virology

Influenza viruses are enveloped negative-sense ssRNA viruses, with a genome that is broken up into eight different segments (about 1300bp in total). This segmented genome is unusual and key to their pandemic potential. There are four influenza viruses, named influenza A (IAV) to D, and each is the sole member of its own genus (*alpha, beta, gamma, delta-influenzavirus*). All belong to the family *Orthomyxoviridae*. Influenza C virus and the recently discovered influenza D virus are far more antigenically stable than IAV, and the burden of disease they cause in humans is considered minimal. Only IAV/IBV are considered significant human pathogens, with IAV alone capable of causing pandemics.

The viral envelope is spiked with two glycoproteins that are important to viral entry and exit; the majority comprises haemagglutinin (HA) (80%), followed by neuraminidase (NA) (20%). AV is further divided into subtypes, based on the antigenic differences of HA and NA. At least 18 HA and 10 NA variants have been identified in IAV (although not all cause human infection). It is against these specific subtypes that immunity is based and consequently fails, such that immunity against H1N1 will likely not protect against H7N9. Viruses are named in a formula that follows: type/place of initial isolation/strain number/year of isolation/antigenic subtype (e.g. A/Victoria/3/75 (H3N2)). IBV are classified into two lineages B/Yamagata and B/Victoria.

Replication occurs in respiratory epithelial cells following binding of HA to sialic acid receptors on the cell surface. The virion is internalized by endosome-mediated transport where acidification (aided by the M2 ion channel protein) fuses the viral envelope and endosome membrane to release the ribonucleoprotein (RNP), which is composed of viral RNA and RNA-associated protein (polymerase and regulatory functions), into the cytosol. Notably, despite being an RNA virus, replication takes place in the nucleus and so the RNP is transported to the nucleus for replication. Transcription takes place by using a process called cap-snatching (whereby a short piece of host mRNA is cleaved and used to initiate viral RNA transcription). Newly synthesized immature virions are transported to the cell membrane and released by budding (thereby gaining their host-derived envelope).

The concept of antigenic variation is of critical importance for influenza. It involves the alteration of key viral protein structures (surface glycoproteins) to produce variants to which there may be little or no pre-existing immunity. This variation involves changes in the HA and NA glycoproteins, and takes place via two mechanisms: drift and shift:

- antigenic drift—gradual accumulation of multiple genetic point mutations that occur through a lack of proofreading mechanism of RNA polymerase. There is a selective pressure imposed by the host immune response for changes that are less well recognized to predominate. This accounts for the annual seasonal influenza epidemic;
- antigenic shift—occurs through genetic reassortment. This occurs when a cell infected with two different 'parent' influenza viruses produces a new virus by swapping genetic material (called reassortment). The progeny virus will contain one or more RNA genome segments from both parents. While viral reassortment is not uncommon, it usually does not result in a virus that is capable of replicating or being readily transmissible in humans. If it does, it can cause an influenza pandemic. A flu pandemic is a global outbreak of a new IAV that is very different from recently circulating strains, with little to no existing population immunity. During pandemics, the mortality burden is usually shared across all age groups (even shifted towards the young). This is in contrast to the annual seasonal epidemic where the burden of morbidity is primarily linked to age/comorbidities.

Numerous strains will be circulating in the human population at any time, and IAV can move between humans and animals (particularly birds/avian, pigs/swine, and bats), increasing potential genetic diversity exponentially. As the global population, human–animal interactions, and healthcare inequality increase, influenza pandemics represents a clear threat to global public health.

Epidemiology

The epidemiology of seasonal influenza is complex.

- The influenza season in temperate climates last for a few months after reaching a sudden 2- to 3-week peak (usually in late December/January in the northern hemisphere). It occurs in reverse in the southern hemisphere. Tropical climates experience influenza year-round.
- Infection rates are underestimated due to a large spectrum of illness (asymptomatic to subclinical infection is common). Estimates of mortality that are attributed to influenza (rather than to complications) are difficult to make, as not all influenza-related deaths present as pneumonia. The economic loss due to missed work attendance is significant.

- Attack rates (estimated at up to 20% of the population) are highest in the young, but mortality is highest in the elderly who are at greatest risk of complicated influenza. Children are significant vectors.

Historical influenza pandemics include the following.
- The first well-documented pandemic was in 1918 (Spanish influenza; H1N1 and almost 50 million people died—more than in the First World War). Contemporary genetic analysis has revealed the presence of exceptional virulence factors and it was primarily avian in origin.
- A shift to H2N2 prompted a pandemic in 1957, followed by a less severe pandemic in 1968 caused by H2N3.
- In 1977, a shift to H1N1 disproportionately affected the young, who lacked immunity by virtue of not experiencing the previous H1N1 pandemic.
- In 2009, a H1N1 strain called (H1N1)pdm09 emerged (composed of mostly swine, but also human/avian, reassortment). Again, the young were disproportionally affected. Unlike the seasonal H1N1 circulating previously, (H1N1)pdm09 was almost completely sensitive to oseltamivir. This has since become the dominant seasonal H1N1 strain.

Clinical features

- Influenza is a respiratory virus, and transmission is through droplets and fomites. In closed environments (schools, hospitals, workplaces), person-to-person transmission is enhanced. Incubation period of 1–4 days. Spectrum of disease ranges from asymptomatic to minor subclinical infection, to progressive hypoxia and development of complications that can be fatal.
- Uncomplicated disease, defined as not needing hospital admission—fever, chills, headache, malaise, myalgia, eye pain, anorexia, dry cough, sore throat, and nasal discharge. After around day 3, respiratory features predominate, as fever and other systemic features settle. Elderly patients may present with fever and confusion and few respiratory features. Convalescence may take two or more weeks.
- Complicated influenza, defined as illness requiring hospital admission due to signs of a lower respiratory tract infection (LRTI; hypoxia/ abnormal CXR) or deterioration of an underlying medical comorbidity.
  - Risk factors include pregnancy (including 2 weeks post-partum), age >65 years, chronic cardiac/lung/renal/liver disease, diabetes, immunosuppression, and morbid obesity.
  - In a pandemic, the traditional population 'risk groups' are less applicable.
- The main complication of influenza infection is primary viral pneumonia. This presents with rapidly worsening cough, breathlessness, and hypoxia (resembles acute respiratory distress syndrome (ARDS)). Mortality is high. Secondary bacterial pneumonia may occur, developing shortly after an initial period of improvement. Synergism between viral and respiratory bacterial pathogens is increasingly recognized. Expectant causative organisms include: *Streptococcus pneumoniae*, *Haemophilus influenzae*, *Klebsiella pneumoniae*, and *Staphylococcus aureus*. Fungal disease in the form of invasive aspergillosis is increasingly recognized,

and clinicians should be mindful of its development. Screening strategies are an area of intense research. Other respiratory complications, including croup, chronic obstructive pulmonary disease (COPD), and cystic fibrosis (CF) exacerbations, in addition to extra-respiratory complications of IAV (myositis, myo-/pericarditis, encephalitis, and Guillain–Barré syndrome (GBS)), are recognized.

Diagnosis

The diagnosis of influenza can be made, with some confidence, based on clinical/syndromic criteria alone during an outbreak—with 85% accuracy in some studies. Treatment and, in particular, infection prevention control (IPC) measures should not be delayed, pending test results.

- In general, the performance of rapid antigen detection or point-of-care assays is considered inferior (due to sensitivity) compared to clinical laboratory-performed molecular techniques. They can provide a role in some specific settings.
- Molecular techniques (PCR) are considered gold standard. They can be performed on throat swabs (most commonly), but also on bronchoalveolar lavage (BAL) and nasopharyngeal aspirate (NPA) specimens. Allows typing and sequencing.
- Viral culture—almost never performed for routine clinical samples.
- Serology—almost never performed in routing clinical service due to the need for paired samples (10–20 days apart).

Treatment

- The true efficacy of influenza antivirals is debated but are recommended by most guidelines in certain settings.
- Uncomplicated infection can be managed in the community by self-administered supportive care. The use of antivirals is advocated in certain groups once circulating influenza crosses a defined threshold each year. It is aimed at preventing progression to complicated disease in those deemed at risk. The use of antivirals in complicated infection is usually clearly mandated.
- Their choice and use are discussed in ⟳ Antivirals for influenza, pp. 98–9).

Prevention

- Good IPC practice, a successful vaccination programme (note that uptake amongst healthcare staff averages 50%), and use of antivirals as post-exposure prophylaxis (PEP) (limited efficacy) together form the basis of influenza prevention.
- The aim of vaccination is to attenuate disease while reducing transmission, thereby providing a bidirectional approach to protecting those most likely to suffer serious morbidity or mortality. It also aims to provide an 'immunity ring' surrounding the precise groups most likely to mount a suboptimal vaccine response.
- There is an increasing array of influenza vaccines available. All but one are inactivated, administered IM, and so cannot cause influenza. Quadrivalent vaccines contain two IAV and two IBV strains, whereas trivalent vaccines contain only a single IBV strain. A live vaccine containing attenuated virus, modified to replicate at lower body

temperatures (limited to the nose) and administered intranasally, is used in children. Most of these vaccines were made by using virus derived from culture in chicken eggs. Some are produced by using virus from cell culture, and a recombinant protein-derived one exists. The development of a highly effective pan-influenza vaccine remains one of virology's most highly desirable, but elusive, goals.

- Immunity is usually achieved 14 days post-administration and lasts a year. The magnitude of vaccine-derived immunity declines steadily with age (and immunosuppression). In terms of efficacy, every year, there is a prediction (educated guesswork) as to which strains will predominate the upcoming season. It takes around 6 months to manufacture these vaccines, and changes cannot be made in a timely fashion. Usually a good match is achieved, with 2014/15 a notable exception due to significant drift occurring. Efficacy is strain-, host-, and end point-dependent (prevent mortality or hospitalization)—crude rates of 10–90% are documented, depending on the variables used.
- Vaccines should be offered to:
  - everyone aged >65 years;
  - people aged 6 months or older in a clinical risk group (chronic respiratory/heart/kidney/liver disease, diabetes, immunosuppression, asplenia, pregnancy (any stage), morbid obesity);
  - children aged between 2 and 17 years not in clinical risk groups;
  - household contacts of immunocompromised people and healthcare workers (HCWs);
  - others as clinical judgement suggests.
- There are very few contraindications to the influenza vaccine. Full indications and administration schedules are available at: ℘ https://www.gov.uk/government/publications/influenza-the-green-book-chapter-19.
- PEP using antiviral agents:
  - is likely to be of modest benefit in a specific subpopulation and specific circumstances;
  - should be offered to the contact if deemed at risk of development of complicated disease and if unvaccinated or the vaccine was not well matched that year or if vaccinated <14 days previously;
  - comprises oseltamivir (within 48h of exposure) od for 10 days, or zanamivir (within 36h of exposure) inhaled (INH) od for 10 days.
- Influenza activity is under surveillance by numerous bodies that regularly publish contemporary guidance—UK Health Security Agency (UKHSA, available at: ℘ https://ukhsa-dashboard.data.gov.uk/topics/influenza), European Centre for Disease Prevention and Control (ECDC, available at: ℘ https://www.ecdc.europa.eu/en/seasonal-influenza), World Health Organization (WHO, available at: ℘ https://www.who.int/tools/flunet), and Centers for Disease Control and Prevention (CDC, available at: ℘ https://www.cdc.gov/flu/about/keyfacts.htm)).

Parainfluenza

Virology

Parainfluenza viruses (PIVs) (family *Paramyxoviridae*) are enveloped negative-sense ssRNA viruses (linear genome ~15 500bp) that circulate as four genetically and antigenically distinct species (PIV-1 to 4). They are further placed into two genera: PIV-1 and 3 in *Respirovirus*, and PIV-2 and 4 in *Rubulavirus*. Two surface glycoproteins—haemagglutinin–neuraminidase (HA) (more genetically stable than in influenza virus) and fusion (F)—mediate attachment and entry. Transmission is by respiratory droplet spread. Replication occurs in respiratory epithelial cells, peaking 2–5 days after infection. Types 1 and 2 usually infect the larynx and upper trachea (croup), and type 3 the distal airway (bronchiolitis, pneumonia). Reinfection is both possible and common.

Epidemiology

- Globally, PIVs are amongst the commonest cause of respiratory infections, with infection almost ubiquitous by adulthood.
- PIV-3 is endemic and the most frequently isolated member, followed by PIV-1 (epidemics in alternate years) and PIV-2 (annual epidemics). Type 4 is rarely isolated.

Clinical features

- Generally difficult to differentiate, based on clinical features alone, from other respiratory viruses without molecular testing.
- Spectrum of disease is dependent on age and host immune status, ranging from asymptomatic to mild coryzal illness to fatal pneumonia. Bacterial and fungal (less frequent) co-infection is not uncommon and should be actively excluded.
- Healthy individuals:
  - children—otitis media, croup, bronchiolitis (<6 months) progressing to upper respiratory tract illness (<5 years);
  - adults—asymptomatic to usually mild upper respiratory tract infection (URTI). Known to provoke exacerbations of asthma and COPD.
- Immunocompromised:
  - severe disease in bone marrow transplant (BMT) or lung transplant patients in all age groups. Typically causes pneumonia. Patients with immunodeficiencies are expectantly associated with prolonged viral shedding.

Diagnosis

- Diagnosed by PCR on respiratory sample (e.g. throat swab).
- Serology requires paired samples, therefore rarely performed.

Treatment

- No specific antiviral therapy. Supportive care. No proven benefit with immunoglobulin. Reduce immunosuppression where relevant. Treat bacterial/fungal co-infection.
- No vaccine is currently available.

Respiratory syncytial virus

Virology

Respiratory syncytial virus (RSV) is an enveloped negative-sense ssRNA virus (linear genome ~15000bp) that contains 10 genes producing 11 proteins. It is a member of the *Pneumoviridae* family (along with human metapneumovirus (HMPV); ➔ see Human Metapneumovirus, pp. 414–15) in the genus *Orthopneumovirus*. Two virulence proteins—non-structural protein 1 (NS1) and NS2—enhance viral replication by inhibiting apoptosis and interferon responses. RSV enters cells via two surface glycoproteins—attachment (G) and fusion (F). Two RSV subtypes A and B (differentiated on G protein sequence) co-circulate with subtype A, causing more severe disease. The F glycoprotein causes infected cells to merge (fuse), forming the eponymous large multinucleated cells (syncytia). After replicating in the upper respiratory tract, RSV can spread lower down to the bronchioles and alveoli. Spread by direct contact (via fomites) and likely droplets. Although primary infection is ubiquitous by the age of 2, immunity is incomplete and reinfection occurs.

Epidemiology

- RSV causes annual worldwide seasonal outbreaks. In the northern hemisphere, these occur in the winter months and usually precede the influenza season. In more tropical climates, RSV outbreaks do not reach the same peaks but circulate for a large proportion of the year.
- RSV is the commonest cause of LRTI in children aged <1 year, with mortality of 2–7%. Increasingly recognized cause of adult illness.

Clinical features

- Lymphocytic infiltration of the areas around the bronchioles, with wall and tissue oedema, is observed, followed by proliferation and necrosis of the bronchiolar epithelium, causing bronchiolitis. This leads to sloughed epithelium and mucus blocking small airway lumens, resulting in air trapping and hyperinflation. Air absorbed distally to obstructed airways leads to areas of atelectasis.
- Clinical disease is attributed to mechanical vulnerability of the small airways in young children to inflammation and obstruction due to their diameter (resistance to airflow being inversely related to the cube of the radius).

Clinical features

- Clinical consequences of infection depend on age and comorbidities, and range from a trivial URTI to life-threatening pneumonia.
- Young children—bronchiolitis, bronchospasm, pneumonia, and acute respiratory failure.
- Older children and adults—repeat RSV infections tend to cause an URTI picture, in addition to LRTI features seen in younger children. RSV is more likely to cause ear, nose, and throat (ENT) infections, compared to other viruses. Secondary bacterial infections may occur.
- Immunocompromised—extremes of age, particularly the young (premature <35 weeks' gestation or age <6 months), concomitant cardiac/respiratory disease (congenital cardiopulmonary disease,

CF), and haematopoietic stem cell transplantation (HSCT) or organ recipients are at risk of severe RSV pneumonia and mortality.

Diagnosis

- Diagnosis by PCR on a respiratory sample (throat swab, NPA in neonates).
- Clinical diagnosis can be made, with some confidence, in children during an outbreak. Serology is only useful epidemiologically.

Treatment

- An effective antiviral agent or a vaccine remains a desirable, yet elusive, goal. A disastrous vaccine was trialled in the 60s and changed the landscape of vaccinology for years to come. Vaccinated children tragically showed enhanced respiratory disease post-vaccination. This was attributed to vaccine-induced low-avidity, poorly neutralizing antibody response, which paradoxically enhanced infection.
- Basic IPC practice (handwashing, environmental cleaning, and cohorting patients) can decrease nosocomial transmission, and is cheap and underappreciated.
- Supportive care is the mainstay—oxygen, fluids, respiratory support. Bronchodilators may help wheeze in some children but are not routinely recommended. No proven benefit from steroids.
- The use and efficacy of ribavirin are debated in the management of RSV infection (➜ see Antivirals for respiratory syncytial virus, p. 100). Not routinely used, but occasionally given with multidisciplinary team (MDT) support in cases of refractory RSV in those severely immunocompromised.
- Immunoprophylaxis of high-risk infants with a humanized monoclonal antibody directed against the F glycoprotein (palivizumab) is recommended in certain high-risk groups (➜ see Antivirals for respiratory syncytial virus, pp. 100–1; see also *Respiratory syncytial virus: the green book*, available at: ⌗ https://www.gov.uk/government/publications/respiratory-syncytial-virus-the-green-book-chapter-27a):
  - age <2 years and treated for bronchopulmonary dysplasia (BPD) in the last 6 months;
  - age <2 years with congenital heart disease;
  - age <2 years with primary severe combined immunodeficiency disease (SCID);
  - born under 35 weeks' gestation and aged under 6 months at the onset of the RSV season.

Human Metapneumovirus

Virology, epidemiology, and clinical features

HMPV is an enveloped negative-sense ssRNA virus (linear genome ~13 300bp) in the genus *Metapneumovirus* in the family *Pneumoviridae* (along with RSV; ➜ see respiratory syncytial virus, pp. 413–14). There are two subgroups A and B, and two clades within each group termed 1 and 2 (A1–2 and B1–2). It is a seasonal respiratory virus that, from a clinical viewpoint, is very similar to RSV and parainfluenza infections (➜ see respiratory syncytial virus, pp. 413–14). It is spread by droplets, with almost ubiquitous exposure occurring by the age of 5. It predominantly presents as a mild, self-limiting URTI, but more severe disease is possible at extremes of age or in the immunosuppressed.

Diagnosis and treatment

Diagnosis is via molecular testing on a respiratory sample (commonly a throat swab). Treatment is supportive. No proven effective antiviral therapy exists.

Rhinovirus

Virology, epidemiology, and clinical features

Rhinovirus is a member of the family Picornaviridae (genus Enterovirus) and is a positive-sense ssRNA virus (genome ~8000bp). Like all Picornaviridae, it is non-enveloped, unusual amongst respiratory viruses. Consequently, enhanced robustness in the environment may contribute to fomite spread as a particular route of transmission. The genome carries a single gene, with its translated precursor polyprotein cleaved by proteases into 11 viral proteins. There are three species described A–C, with >100 serotypes. Most serotypes use intercellular adhesion molecule 1 (ICAM-1) as an entry receptor.

Rhinovirus is the aetiological agent causing the 'common cold'—a mild URTI. One of the commonest respiratory viruses, it can cause year-round infection and the global burden of disease (economic and morbidity) is difficult to overestimate. Although it predominantly presents as a mild, self-limiting URTI, there is increasing recognition of more severe disease at extremes of age or in the immunosuppressed.

Diagnosis and treatment

Diagnosis is via molecular testing on a respiratory sample (commonly a throat swab). Treatment is supportive. No effective antiviral therapy exists.

Coronaviruses

Enveloped viruses of the family Nidovirus. Large positive-sense ssRNA genome that replicates by using a set of nested mRNAs ('nido' for 'nest'). The name derives from Latin 'corona' (crown), reflecting the electron microscopy (EM) appearance of the viral spike protein that populates the surface of the virus and determines its host tropism.

Classic community-acquired coronavirus

Found worldwide. In temperate climates, human coronavirus (HcoV) respiratory infections tend to occur in winter. Spread is by aerosol or contact with infected secretions. Immunity is acquired, but reinfection is common (by either waning immunity or antigenic variation). Outbreaks occur in hospitals and residential care homes. Presentations may be:
- respiratory—HcoV account for <20% of all adult acute URTIs and may cause acute otitis media in children. They have been isolated from infants with pneumonia and associated with wheeze in children, and may trigger asthma attacks in adults and children. In the elderly,

they cause flu-like illnesses, pneumonia, and acute exacerbations of bronchitis;
- enteric—there is an association between the presence of CoV particles on EM of faecal samples and diarrhoea in infants or necrotizing enterocolitis in neonates;
- diagnosis is rarely helpful, as treatment is supportive. RT-PCR tests are available.

Severe acute respiratory syndrome coronavirus

Severe acute respiratory syndrome coronavirus (SARS) was recognized in China in November 2002 and had spread to affect 29 countries across the world by February 2003. The epidemic had died out by July 2003; 8096 cases were reported, with a fatality rate of 11% (43% in those over 60 years of age). Between July 2003 and May 2004, there were four small and rapidly contained outbreaks of SARS, three of which were associated with laboratory releases and the fourth thought to be due to an animal source. The cause was a novel CoV. Animals are thought to be the main reservoir. Transmission is by droplets and contact with contaminated surfaces—nosocomial transmission was common in the early stages of the outbreak. The virus is present in the faeces and may cause diarrhoea.

- Clinical features—incubation is 2–10 days. A 3- to 7-day febrile prodrome follows, notable for the absence of upper respiratory symptoms. The respiratory phase typically starts with a dry cough, progressing to breathlessness and progressive pulmonary infiltrates on CXR.
- Diagnosis—during the outbreak, RT-PCR was performed, but sensitivity appeared limited (<70% positive on NPAs in week 2 of illness). No systematic study was performed to validate tests. Serological testing by enzyme-linked immunoassay (EIA) at 3 weeks appeared most sensitive.
- Treatment—no specific therapy. Care is supportive. Patient isolation and infection control precautions were key to the control of the 2002/3 outbreak. This was greatly facilitated by the relatively long prodrome that enabled patients to be identified and isolated before they became infectious.

Middle East respiratory syndrome (MERS) coronavirus

This betacoronavirus, closely related to several bat CoVs, was identified in 2012 from a man admitted to hospital in Saudi Arabia with pneumonia and renal failure. Shortly after his admission, an identical virus was identified in Qatar in a patient with similar features who had travelled to Saudi Arabia. Cases followed across the Middle East and were reported in five other countries amongst patients returning from the Middle East. The UK, France, Italy, and Tunisia reported limited human-to-human transmission to close contacts of the index cases. The case fatality rate was reported as 60%.

- Clinical features—incubation around 5 days (but <10 days). Symptoms range from none (positive RT-PCR tests were found in several asymptomatic close contacts) to mild respiratory illness to severe pneumonia requiring ventilation or extracorporeal membrane oxygenation. Other symptoms: pericarditis, renal failure, disseminated intravascular coagulopathy (DIC), diarrhoea. Those with underlying medical problems seem at greater risk of severe disease.

- Diagnosis—RT-PCR testing of lower respiratory tract specimens is most sensitive. Testing multiple specimens taken at different times from different sites increases the likelihood of detecting virus. Guidance should be sought from national public health authorities regarding who to test, based upon contemporary epidemiology.
- Treatment is supportive, and infection control paramount.

SARS-CoV-2

Virology

An entirely novel CoV (➜ see Coronaviruses, pp. 415–17) was first recognized in late 2019 in the city of Wuhan in the Hubei province of China as the aetiology of a series of pneumonia cases. This virus would eventually be named severe acute respiratory syndrome coronavirus 2 (SARS-CoV-2). It is the causative pathogen of the coronavirus disease 2019 (Covid-19) pandemic. The pandemic is ongoing, and any printed nformation will be quickly outdated—see the excellent online resources signposted by WHO (available at: ✍ https://covid19.who.int), CDC (available at: ✍ https://www.cdc.gov/coronavirus/2019-ncov/index.html), and ECDC (available at: ✍ https://www.ecdc.europa.eu/en/covid-19).

SARS-CoV-2, like SARS-CoV-1 (the viral aetiology in the 2002 SARS pandemic), are in the genus *betacoronavirus*, along with numerous other mammalian and bat CoVs. It is generally accepted (though not definitively proven) that SARS-CoV-2 originated through a zoonotic spillover event (potentially numerous) from a bat CoV. It may have involved an intermediate host, before human-to-human transmission became the mainstay. Numerous alternate origin theories have been postulated, with little scientific evidence of merit to support them.

It is a respiratory virus, and transmission is primarily through inhalation of respiratory droplets through close contact. Fomites and overt airborne transmission likely represent incidental routes of unknown significance.

It is an enveloped positive-sense ssRNA virus, with a large genome (30 000kilobase pair). The CoV polymerase is thought to have proofreading ability, unusual for an RNA polymerase, but unsurprising, given its large genome. Unique to CoV replication is the process of discontinuous transcription to produce 'nested mRNA'. This involves producing different-length subgenomic mRNA strands coding for differing structural proteins, but each with a common 5′ end (nested), thereby enhancing the repertoire of viral protein-coding capability. Attachment is mediated via the viral surface glycoprotein (S, spike) binding to the host cellular angiotensin-converting enzyme 2 (ACE2) receptor (TMPRSS2 is a host co-receptor protease integral to subsequent virion–cellular fusion). SARS-CoV-1 and HCoV-NL63 also utilize ACE2.

S protein is composed of two subunits: S1 and S2. The outermost S1 component contains a region called the receptor binding domain (RBD) that most intimately engages with the host receptor. It is this region that defines tropism and contributes heavily to pathogenicity. It is in the S gene that mutations are of the most consequence. While most mutations will have either neutral or deleterious effects on viral replication, advantageous mutations in the S gene can pose problems:

- Enhanced viral binding to the receptor can result in increased replication, transmission, and potentially disease severity.
- Laboratory molecular assays designed to detect existing S gene regions can fail to detect new mutant S gene mutants (this happened at the onset of Omicron). This has been referred to as S gene target failure.
- Immune escape can arise whereby existing immunity (derived naturally or through vaccine) is less effective towards this new S protein. This has been amply demonstrated by the numerous waves of reinfection following the emergence of viral variants and is a source of much concern.

The immune response to SARS-CoV-2 is incompletely understood, but it is likely that both humoral and cellular components are necessary for viral elimination. The neutralizing antibody response is directed primarily against the S protein. There is variation in zenith titres achieved following natural infection, uncertainty about what constitutes a protective threshold, and concerns regarding decreased neutralization with new variants and the waning of immunity with time. A cell-mediated immune response is crucial to viral clearance. For an ill-described cohort of patients, infection triggers a highly inflammatory state and is associated with a poorer prognosis, hence the use of immunomodulators as treatment.

The nomenclature surrounding Covid variants has evolved—in 2021, the WHO brought together groups with established naming systems (GISAID, available at: ℘ https://gisaid.org; Nextstrain, available at: ℘ https://nextstrain.org; Pango, available at: ℘ cov-lineages.org/) and concluded future strains would be primarily labelled after letters of the Greek alphabet (available at: ℘ https://www.who.int/activities/tracking-SARS-CoV-2-variants). Variants fall into two categories:

- variants of interest (VOIs)—contain mutations predicted or known to affect viral characteristics (transmission, disease severity, diagnostics, treatment escape, or decreased response to vaccine or public health interventions) and have epidemiological evidence of increasing or multifocal transmission;
- variants of concern (VOCs)—as per VOIs and through further assessment, have been deemed to be significant at a global public health level.

Alpha was the first variant identified in 2020 and displaced globally the 'index virus' (first identified in December 2019). Large Beta and Gamma outbreaks would follow, but only Delta would become a dominant global strain itself, until its own displacement by Omicron. The onset of each variant was associated with uncertainty over the potential for changes in morbidity (Delta), immune escape (Beta/Omicron), or transmission (Alpha/Delta/Omicron).

Epidemiology

See the Johns Hopkins University resource centre for up-to-date information on cases and spread (available at: ℘ https://coronavirus.jhu.edu/map.html).

Diagnosis

- Molecular testing of the upper airway is the gold standard. RNA detection alone is not synonymous with a replicative competent or infectious virus, leading to confusion in public health/IPC policy in the early years of the pandemic.
- Antigen testing is the technology behind portable 'lateral flow tests'. Advantages include ease of use by the general public and specificity; however, sensitivity was lower than that of molecular testing.
- Serology for respiratory viruses is fraught with difficulty and is of almost no real use in acute diagnostics. Use of serology to demonstrate Covid immunity is an admirable, but unachievable, goal due to evolving variants, no agreed standardized quantitative threshold of immunity, and variable antibody responses.

Clinical features

- Typically, there is an incubation period of 5–10 days, during which the patient will be asymptomatic and highly infectious for the latter 3–5 days. Once symptoms arise, infectivity falls, with transmission rare beyond 8–10 days in otherwise immunocompetent populations.
- Consequences of infection range from asymptomatic (30% of cases prior to vaccination deployment, higher in a seropositive population) to mild URTI to life-threatening pneumonia and ARDS.
- Clinical severity has changed over the course of the pandemic as immunity is acquired (either through vaccination or natural infection) and new viral strains emerge. Amongst those with symptomatic infection in the early waves, 80% were mild (typical URTI symptoms—cough, malaise, and coryzal symptoms); about 15% had more severe symptoms requiring hospital admission, and 5% needing higher-level support. Case fatality rate <3%, varying greatly with age and comorbidities. Omicron's emergence saw significant reductions in hospital admissions and mortality.
- Extrapulmonary manifestations—confusion, diarrhoea, increased incidence of thromboembolic events, a hyperinflammatory state, secondary infections (particularly fungal), and neurological sequelae.
- In children, an inflammatory syndrome similar to Kawasaki disease has been observed—paediatric inflammatory multisystem syndrome (PIMS), also called multisystem inflammatory syndrome in children associated with Covid (MISC-C). Fever, rash, GI symptoms, and conjunctivitis predominate, with cardiac abnormalities described. Treatment is typically with intravenous immunoglobulin (IVIG) and steroids (see ♒ https://www.rcpch.ac.uk/resources/paediatric-multisystem-inflammat ory-syndrome-temporally-associated-covid-19-pims-guidance).
- Long Covid syndrome represents a significant diagnostic and management challenge. It is a focus of intense research.

Treatment

- Treatments change regularly and vary by patient cohort. Check local policy and review the WHO-managed Covid-19 *Living guideline*' (available at: ♒ https://www.bmj.com/content/370/bmj.m3379).
- For the majority of infections, supportive care is the mainstay.

- For non-hospitalized high risk cohorts, antiviral therapy has been shown to reduce progression to severe disease and is recommended. Risk groups are given here www.nice.org.uk/guidance/ta878/chap ter/5-Supporting-information-on-risk-factors-for-progression-to-sev ere-COVID-19.
- Molnupiravir is a mutagenic nucleotide analogue that mimics cytidine. Once incorporated into the RNA chain, it is misread, causing a cascade of detrimental mutations that will eventually cause 'error catastrophe'.
- Paxlovid PO (combination of the protease inhibitors nirmatrelvir and ritonavir).
- Remdesivir IV for 3 days
- For hospitalized patients, non-specific therapy consists of respiratory support, nutritional adjuncts, screening for secondary infection (serum procalcitonin), and prevention of venous thromboembolism. Treatment shown to be of benefit include:
  - glucocorticoids—clear mortality benefit in those with an oxygen requirement (usual agent used is dexamethasone);
  - immunomodulatory agents—interleukin-6 (IL-6) antagonists (tocilizumab, sarilumab) and JAK inhibitor (baricitinib) for those with viral penumonitis
  - monoclonal antibodies targeting the S protein—had benefit in seronegative patients early in the pandemic, but efficacy against new variants was greatly reduced. Both casirivimab/imdevimab and sotrovimab were initially included in international guidelines and later removed;
  - direct antiviral agents—remdesivir is an adenosine analogue that acts as a delayed chain terminator in viral polymerase. Its true efficacy is debated, but it remains in widespread use.
- Numerous agents have been investigated and found to have been of no benefit (e.g. hydroxychloroquine, vitamin D, ivermectin). Some of these agents with purported activity never had any credible scientific merit to begin with and misinformation became an additional threat of the pandemic.

Prevention

- IPC is a key part of the pandemic response and has been employed amongst the general public, as well as in healthcare settings. Face masks, handwashing, and behavioural interventions (social distancing, limiting contacts) became the mainstay.
- It is accepted that such measures reduce transmission, but to what extent is unclear, as are the wider societal costs of implementation.
- Deployment of Covid vaccines was a fundamental part of reducing disease severity and spread, saving numerous lives and facilitating a return to more normal daily life. Inactivated, viral vector, and mRNA-based vaccines were all approved and deployed. All currently use elements derived from the spike protein and are thus vulnerable to mutations/variant changes. A multivalent vaccine is extremely desirable.

Measles

Virology

The measles virus (MeV) is an enveloped negative-sense ssRNA virus (linear genome ~15 800bp) in the family *Paramyxoviridae*, genus *Morbillivirus*. Crucially, despite >20 genotypes across eight clades, there is a single sero-type; thus, antibodies directed against one genotype (e.g. vaccine-derived) demonstrate cross-protection. The virion is composed of two glycopro-teins on its envelope surface: haemagglutinin (H) and fusion (F), which me-diate attachment and entry. This surrounds the helical RNP complex, which is composed of the viral genome that is associated with three structural proteins: nucleoprotein (N), phosphoprotein (P), and large protein (L). The membrane protein (M) sits below the envelope and interacts with both sur-face glycoproteins and the RNP. The non-structural proteins C and V are notable virulence factors involved in evasion of the host immune response. A well-recognized post-infection period of immunosuppression with in-creased susceptibility to opportunistic/secondary bacterial infections can persist for weeks to months. Destruction of memory cells towards pre-viously encountered pathogens is described. Replication follows a typical format for a negative-sense RNA virus—initially focusing on transcription of mRNA to form protein, before switching to genome replication. An air-borne pathogen that utilizes numerous host cellular receptors at different stages—initially infecting the epithelial cells of the respiratory tract before being amplified in regional (primary viraemia) and peripheral lymphoid tissue, which leads to disseminated systemic infection (subsequent sec-ondary viraemia). One of the most transmissible infections, with an R_0 (basic reproduction number R nought; average number of cases caused by a single case in a susceptible population) of 12–18. The incubation period is 7–18 days, and patients are infectious from first symptom development (prodrome) to ~4 days post-appearance of rash.

Epidemiology

- Notifiable illness. Despite favourable biology and a highly effective vaccine, measles remains a leading cause of mortality in children. Largely due to decreases in vaccination rates, driven by misinformation and the disproven link between the measles, mumps, and rubella (MMR) vaccine and autism.
- Outbreaks primarily occur in two scenarios—low-resource settings with limited access to vaccines and pockets of low vaccine uptake (hesitancy, incomplete vaccination course) within high-resource settings.
- In the UK, pre-introduction of the measles vaccine in 1968, there were up to 800 000 cases, with ~100 fatalities annually, with biannual peaks. The combined MMR vaccine was introduced in 1988, and incidence plummeted. Multiple catch-up campaigns were implemented to target partially or non-immunized children and teenagers.

Clinical features

- Following the incubation period, a prodromal phase (coinciding with secondary viraemia) of malaise, fever, anorexia, and the 3Cs (conjunctivitis, coryza, and cough) is seen. About 48h before the exanthem on the body, Koplik's spots (blue-grey spots with a red base,

classically found on the buccal mucosa opposite the second molars) can appear. Although not sensitive, it is a specific sign.
- The exanthem of measles is erythematous and maculopapular, and may become confluent. Initially blanching but can progress to petechiae or haemorrhagic. Rash begins on the face and proceeds down and out, involving the palms and soles last. Resolves in the same pattern. Lasts around 5 days, may desquamate as it heals. Clinical improvement normally observed within 2 days after appearance of the rash.
- Complications are reported in 30% of MeV cases and are commonest in patients aged <5 or >20 years and those who are immunocompromised or pregnant. Although the commonest complications are diarrhoea (8%) and otitis media (7%), it is respiratory (6%) (pneumonia, bronchiolitis) or neurological complications (encephalitis, acute disseminated encephalomyelitis (ADEM), and subacute sclerosing panencephalitis (SSPE)) that carry the greatest mortality. Encephalitis (0.1%) and ADEM (0.1%) present a few days and ~2 weeks after the viral exanthem, respectively. ADEM is thought to represent a triggered post-infectious autoimmune process rather than direct viral infection per se. SSPE is a rare progressive, devastating, and usually fatal complication that occurs many years after the primary infection. The exact pathogenesis is unknown, but persistent neuronal MeV with a defective M gene is thought contributory.
- Pregnant women have increased rates of MeV complications. Although MeV is not thought to cause congenital infection to the developing fetus, rates of pregnancy complications (intrauterine death and preterm delivery) are increased.

Diagnosis

Both the immunization history and the age of the patient are critical pieces of the history. Do not wait for laboratory confirmation before implementing infection control procedures and public health notification.
- Oral swab—for serology (IgM/IgG), and PCR is optimal. Oral sampling is the preferred specimen, as a multitude of serological and molecular tests can be performed. In the UK, testing is arranged via public health laboratories (web search: UK Gov Measles test).
- Blood—IgM is usually detectable by day 3 post-appearance of exanthem, with IgG appearing later (should be present by day 14). Paired serology (showing >4-fold increase in antibody titre) may be necessary. Viral RNA is present up to day 3 post-exanthem.

Treatment

- Supportive therapy and treatment of bacterial superinfection.
- Use of vitamin A in hospitalized children with measles is recommended by WHO, but benefits in adults are less clear.
- Ribavirin has been used in severe cases but lacks robust evidence.

Prevention/vaccine

- Measles vaccine is available as part of the MMR formulation. It is a live vaccine containing attenuated strains of each virus. It is highly effective, resulting in >95% efficacy at preventing clinical MeV infection. The normal schedule is two doses at least 3 months apart, from the age of

12 months. For full details, see *Measles: the green book* (available at: ℘ https://www.gov.uk/government/publications/measles-the-green-book-chapter-21).
- MMR vaccination is part of the routine national vaccination programme, and most people are eligible (as it is a live vaccine, some exclusions do exist).
- PEP with immunoglobulin (and occasionally the MMR vaccine) is recommended for those exposed and susceptible people considered at risk of severe or fatal measles (neonates, pregnancy, immunosuppression). It should be administered as soon as possible, ideally within 72h, but up to 6 days post-exposure. Full guideline is available at: ℘ https://assets.publishing.service.gov.uk/media/653b8 80ae6c9680014aa9c1f/national-measles-guidelines-october-2023.pdf

Mumps

Virology
Mumps virus (MuV) is an enveloped negative-sense ssRNA virus (linear genome ~15 000bp) in the genus *Orthorubulavirus*, family *Paramyxoviridae*. Although there are 12 genotypes, there is only a single serotype. Seven genes code for nine proteins. Two surface glycoproteins—haemagglutinin–neuraminidase (HN) and fusion (F)—mediate cellular attachment and entry. This surrounds an M protein, which interacts with the ribonucleoprotein complex (RNP) composed of the genome, viral polymerase, and associated proteins. Viral replication is typical for a negative-sense RNA virus, occurring in the cytoplasm. Spread is by droplets and/or direct contact.

Epidemiology
- Endemic globally. Prior to widespread vaccination, MuV was the commonest cause of viral meningitis, occurring in epidemics every 2–5 years, mainly infecting children aged 2–7 years. Consequently, >85% of adults showed signs of previous infection.
- Passive immunity due to transmitted maternal antibody makes infection uncommon in children aged under 1 year.
- Today the incidence of MuV outbreaks is increasing. These are mainly amongst young adults aged 15–34 in colleges/universities where most (64%) are unvaccinated. While MuV infection can occur in those who are fully vaccinated (secondary vaccine failure), this is unusual and does not account for most cases.
- In the UK, vaccine-derived immunity to MuV is intrinsically linked to age, as pre-1988, there was no routine immunization against MuV (see *Mumps: the green book*, available at: ℘ https://www.gov.uk/government/publications/mumps-the-green-book-chapter-23).

Clinical features
- Incubation period is between 14 and 25 days. Cases are infectious for 1 week before and after the onset of parotiditis, mirroring the presence of the virus in saliva.

- A prodrome of fever, myalgia, malaise, headache, and anorexia precedes parotiditis. Between a third to a half of cases either are asymptomatic or show mild respiratory symptoms with(out) a fever.
- The hallmark of clinical MuV is salivary gland swelling, typically the parotids. The gland swells (usually bilateral in 75%) over 2–3 days, typically resolves in a week, and is associated with severe pain.
- CNS involvement—is extremely common (based on CSF pleocytosis), with <50% of MuV meningitis showing no glandular involvement). Symptomatic infection is unusual: meningitis (5–10%) and encephalitis (<0.5%). Encephalitis is seen in 1 in 6000 and takes two forms: an early onset which represents direct neuronal damage due to viral invasion, and a larger late-onset (7–10 days) group representing a post-infectious demyelinating process. Recovery takes around 2 weeks, and sequelae (e.g. psychomotor retardation) and death (1.4% of cases) may be seen. Unilateral deafness occurs in 4% and is not associated with CNS involvement.
- Epididymo-orchitis; the commonest extra-glandular manifestation in post-pubertal ♂ (20–30%). Abrupt onset (5–10 days post-parotiditis), with fever and a warm, swollen (up to four times normal), tender testicle (unilateral in 60–80%), with erythema of the overlying skin. Fever resolves at 5 days, with gonadal symptoms following. Some degree of atrophy may be seen in 50%, once recovered. Hypofertility is uncommon, whereas infertility is very rare. No association with the development of testicular cancer has been identified.
- Oophoritis (5% of post-pubertal women with mumps—impaired fertility and premature menopause have been reported but are rare).
- Pancreatitis is rare (4%), along with arthritis and myocardial involvement.
- Mumps infection during pregnancy does not appear to be more severe nor increase complications of pregnancy. Does not appear to cause congenital disease. No specific PEP is recommended.

Diagnosis

- Diagnosis is usually clinical in the context of an unvaccinated individual with parotiditis. Laboratory confirmation is required for epidemiological purposes or when the disease is atypical.
- An oral swab for viral RNA detection (PCR) and IgM (antibody detection/serology) is the specimen of choice. These are available from local public health services. It should be taken as quickly as possible after the onset of parotitis. IgM can be detected from about 1 week post-symptom onset and is detectable for a few weeks.
- Blood for serum—IgM (acute infection) and IgG (past infection/vaccination) can be tested. IgM may not appear until day 5 post-symptom onset. Demonstrating infection in those with previous vaccination is difficult, as viral loads may not reach the same zenith and an IgM response will not always be mounted. These individuals will likely have some IgG.
- Notably, many other viruses are capable of causing parotiditis and a broad differential should be borne in mind (PIV, Epstein–Barr virus (EBV), enterovirus, and influenza).

Treatment
- Supportive care is the mainstay.
- No benefit of steroid use has been demonstrated.

Prevention
The 2-dose schedule MMR vaccine is ~88% effective. Occasionally, a third dose is administered in some outbreaks. For full details, see *Mumps: the green book* (available at: ✆ https://www.gov.uk/government/publications/mumps-the-green-book-chapter-23).

Rubella

Virology
Rubella virus (RuV) is an enveloped positive-sense ssRNA virus (linear genome ~10 000bp) in the genus *Rubivirus*, family *Matonaviridae* (previously in the family *Togavirus*). The genome contains two non-overlapping reading frames. The first codes for two non-structural proteins: p90 and p150. The second codes for three structural proteins: the two surface glycoproteins E1 and E2 (mediate attachment and entry), and C protein (the nucleocapsid). After entry, the virion is transported to the cytoplasm via acidic endosomes, losing its capsid in the process, at which point replication and assembly can take place at the endoplasmic reticulum and Golgi apparatus. There is only one serotype, but almost 13 genotypes based on the E1 sequence. An airborne pathogen spread by inhalational of contaminated droplets, enhanced by close contact.

Epidemiology
- Before the introduction of the vaccine RuV was a common childhood exanthem, with >80% of adults showing serological evidence of past infection. Now infection is very rare.
- Almost all UK cases of congenital rubella syndrome (CRS) now occur in women born overseas.
- After infection or vaccination, most people develop lifelong protection against the disease. Reinfection is possible, but with considerably diminished viraemia and an attenuated clinical course (the majority asymptomatic). CRS described in this cohort, but rare (<5–10%).

Clinical features
- The incubation period is 14–21 days. Individuals with rubella are infectious from one week before symptoms appear to 4 days after the onset of the rash.
- Postnatal rubella is a mild infection. Many cases are subclinical. Adults may experience a prodrome of malaise, fever, and anorexia. The main symptoms are lymphadenopathy (cervical and posterior auricular) and a maculopapular rash (starting on the face and moving down) that may be accompanied by coryza and conjunctivitis and last 3–5 days. Splenomegaly can occur.
- Complications are uncommon; arthritis affecting the wrists, fingers, and knees and resolving over a month may be seen, as the rash appears (women > men); haemorrhagic manifestations occur in 1 in 3000 (children > adults) and may be due to thrombocytopenia, as well as

vascular damage; encephalitis occurs in 1 in 5000 (adults > children), with mortality of up to 50%.

- CRS is the most feared complication; it is catastrophic in early pregnancy, leading to fetal death, premature delivery, and a multitude of congenital defects. Maternal–fetal infection occurs through haematogenous spread. The risk of CRS is inversely related to gestation: <10 weeks (80–90%), 11–20 weeks (10–20%), and >20 weeks (<1%). In the first 2 months of gestation, there is an up to 85% chance the fetus will develop multiple defects or spontaneous abortion. The constellation of CRS findings includes cataracts/congenital glaucoma, cardiac abnormalities, hearing impairment, purpura, hepatosplenomegaly, jaundice, microcephaly, low birthweight, developmental delay, meningoencephalitis, and radiolucent bone disease.
- Developmental defects may become apparent as the infant grows (e.g. hearing loss, myopia, mental retardation, diabetes, behavioural and language disorders).
- Infection in the mother is mild and self-limiting. Infected neonates may excrete infectious RuV for months, and IPC measures must be taken.

Diagnosis

- Its mild nature makes clinical diagnosis difficult. All results must be taken in the context of whether a clinically compatible syndrome exists. If a case of rubella is being investigated, close liaison with local virology/public health departments is critical.
- Serology—seroconversion with detection of viral RNA by PCR is gold standard. IgM should be detectable a few days after the appearance of rash and persist for a few weeks.
- A positive IgM on a single sample should be taken with extreme caution, and a diagnosis of rubella should not be made (cross-reactive IgM positivity can occur with other acute viral infections (e.g. CMV/EBV).
- The evolution in antibody response over time is critical to making a diagnosis. A seroconversion in IgG/IgM, rising IgM, or a 4-fold rise in IgG in paired sera is suggestive. IgG antibody avidity can play a role in determining the timing of infection; low IgG avidity implies a recent infection. IgM may be positive in cases of reinfection (albeit weakly reactive).
- Diagnosis of congenital rubella in neonates may necessitate the analysis of several samples over time to determine whether antibody titres are falling (maternal antibody) or rising (recent infection). Detection of rubella IgM in a newborn's serum suggests infection.
- PCR to look for viral RNA can be performed on a variety of samples and can complement serological testing; negative PCR does not exclude infection. Intrauterine diagnosis has been made by placental biopsy and by cordocentesis with detection by PCR.

Treatment/prevention

- No specific treatment for rubella, regardless of whether the patient is pregnant or not. There is no PEP (use of immunoglobulin is not recommended).

- MMR is a live vaccine, and a single vaccination achieves a seroconversion rate of 95%. Women should not become pregnant for 1 month following vaccination. For full details, see *Mumps: the green book* (available at: ⅍ https://www.gov.uk/government/publications/mumps-the-green-book-chapter-23).

Parvovirus

Virology

Parvovirus B19 is a non-enveloped ssDNA virus (linear genome 5600bp) and a notable exception to the consensus that most human DNA viruses are double-stranded. It is in the genus *Erythroparvovirus*, family *Parvoviridae*. The family is unusual, as they can only replicate in the presence of a rapidly dividing cell (parvovirus B19) or a helper virus (other genera). Although there are three genotypes (showing geographical distribution), there is only a single serotype (infection usually confers lifelong immunity). The icosahedral capsid is composed of the structural proteins VP1 and VP2 (majority). Three non-structural proteins are coded for, with NS1 deemed responsible for stimulating cellular apoptosis of infected cells. The virus binds to a receptor called globoside, or P antigen which is present in high concentrations in rapidly proliferating CD36+ erythroid progenitor cells. These are the only cells capable of sustaining the complete viral replication cycle. Those who lack P antigen on their erythrocytes are resistant to infection. Following entry, the rest of the viral replication cycle takes place in the nucleus before cell lysis occurs. The virus was found in 1974, while evaluating assays for HBsAg—sample 19 in panel B of a microtiter plate gave a 'false positive', and EM revealed the newly discovered virus. It is primarily an airborne pathogen spread by inhalation of contaminated droplets; however, vertical (to the developing fetus) and blood product transmissions are reported. Due its lack of an envelope, it is difficult to inactivate/decontaminate surfaces/blood products.

Epidemiology

- Infection common in childhood; 50% are IgG-positive by 15 years, and 90% antibody-positive by 90 years. About 30–40% of pregnant woman are seronegative (i.e. susceptible to infection).

Clinical features

- Cases are infectious for 7–10 days before the viral prodrome. By the time a rash appears, the viraemia is usually gone.
- In immunocompetent hosts—~25% are asymptomatic, 50% will have non-specific viral illness, and 25% will develop classical rash or arthralgia (both thought to be immune complex-mediated).
- Erythema infectiosum, or fifth disease, is the classic childhood exanthem: 5–7 days of fever, coryza, and mild nausea/diarrhoea, followed by the classic 'slapped cheek' rash (fiery, red eruption with surrounding pallor). A second erythematous maculopapular rash may follow on the trunk and limbs 1–2 days later, fading to produce a lacy appearance. Adults have milder manifestations. Pruritus (especially on the soles of the feet) can occur.

- Arthralgia: women > men, 75% will have concurrent rash. Symmetrical, mainly small joints of the hands/feet. Lasts 1–3 weeks and is non-destructive.
- Transient aplastic crisis (TAC)—causes a temporary (4–8 days) pause in erythropoiesis (as infected cells are destroyed), leading to severe anaemia (leucopenia and thrombocytopenia are also described). This is usually clinically silent in those with normal erythroid turnover. Described in a wide range of haemolytic conditions: sickle-cell (nearly 90% of TAC episodes), thalassaemia, pyruvate kinase deficiency, glucose-6-phosphate dehydrogenase (G6PD) deficiency, autoimmune haemolytic anaemia.
- Pure red cell aplasia (PRCA)—chronic infection is possible in immunocompromised hosts (haematological malignancies, advanced HIV, congenital immunodeficiency, patients undergoing transplantation), causing severe long-lasting anaemia. Administration of immunoglobulin may be beneficial.
- Congenital infection—infection in first 20 weeks' gestation can lead to intrauterine death due to hydrops fetalis (incidence ~3–11%, with 40–50% mortality). Hydrops fetalis refers to the accumulation of fluid in fetal soft tissues and serous cavities. The infected fetus may have severe manifestations (anaemia, myocarditis, heart failure) due to high red cell turnover and an immature immune response. Fetal complications after 20 weeks' gestation is very rare (<1%). Children who survive hydrops fetalis are not considered to have increased rates of neurological sequelae, although large cohort studies are lacking.

Diagnosis

- Serology—IgM normally detectable by the time symptoms develop and lasts for up to 3 months. IgG is detectable by day 7 of illness and remains detectable for life. It is not useful in diagnosing acute infection or in attributing manifestations such as chronic arthropathy to parvovirus B19. Seroconversion (IgG) in pregnancy is diagnostic.
- PCR—can be performed on blood or amniotic fluid. Note viraemia is usually gone by the time symptoms develop in immunocompetent hosts. Mainly of use for diagnosis of chronic infection in immunocompromised hosts.

Treatment/prevention

- Supportive care is mainstay for immunocompetent hosts. No effective antiviral therapy is currently available.
- For patients with transient aplastic anaemia or those with chronic infection, a reduction in immunosuppression and/or IVIG is recommended. If disease recurs, they may require repeated courses. In some HIV-infected patients, chronic B19 infection will resolve with the initiation of antiretroviral therapy (ART).
- Suspected cases of fetal infection should be referred to fetal medicine to determine whether intrauterine blood transfusion is necessary. For details of management of parvovirus B19 in pregnancy, see ℘ https://www.gov.uk/government/publications/viral-rash-in-pregnancy
- From an infection control viewpoint, cases of TAC and PRCA require basic personal protective equipment (PPE) and ideally isolation (glove and gown, own room, mask, etc.). Pregnant HCWs should not care for such patients.

Adenovirus

Virology

The genus *Mastadenovirus* in the family *Adenoviridae* contains seven species of human adenovirus (HadV) A–G (based on haemagglutination characteristics) that comprise >80 viral types (numbered) capable of causing morbidity. HadV are non-enveloped, icosahedral-shaped dsDNA viruses (linear 35 000bp genome). Surrounding the genome is the viral capsid that is composed of three proteins termed hexons, pentons, and fibres—that project outwards to form a trimeric surface glycoprotein. Organ tropism can be predicted by species and likely reflects differences in fibre–host cell interactions: respiratory tract (B, C, and E), GI tract (A, F, and G), and GI/ocular (D). Cellular infection is classically cytopathic due to induced lysis. HadV are important research tools where they are used as vectors for genes that can form the basis of immunotherapy and in some vaccines due to a wide variety of cells being susceptible to infection.

Epidemiology

- Primary infection is worldwide and ubiquitous by age 10, with reinfection likely. Outbreaks in crowded settings are common.
- Up to 10% of childhood febrile illness cases may be attributable to HadV.
- Transmission is widespread through inhalation of droplets via the respiratory route, faecal–oral route, or contact through fomites.
- As HadV are non-enveloped, they can persist for long periods on surfaces and are resistant to some disinfectants, but are sensitive to bleach, formaldehyde, and heat.

Clinical features

- Clinical manifestations vary widely according to age, host immunocompetence, and HadV type (listed as numbers henceforth). Most infections are mild and self-limiting, but serious morbidly is possible (7, 14, 21, 5).
- Respiratory infection (1, 2, 5, 6, 7)—incubation is around 4–5 days, and illness takes the form of mild pharyngitis/tracheitis (cough, fever, sore throat, and rhinorrhoea) or, less commonly in infants, bronchiolitis and atypical pneumonia (7). Bacteria superinfection is possible. Viral pneumonia is recognized, but differentiation from other causes is paramount. Commoner in young children with underlying comorbidities.
- Pharyngoconjunctival fever (3, 7)—a syndrome of conjunctivitis (usually bilateral), pharyngitis, fever, and cervical adenitis. Symptoms last 3–5 days (self-limiting); bacterial superinfection is uncommon, and there is no permanent eye damage. Respiratory involvement rarely progresses to the lungs. Contaminated swimming areas have been implicated in some outbreaks.
- Epidemic keratoconjunctivitis (EKC) (8, 19, 37, 53)—similar to pharyngoconjunctival fever, but follows a far more protracted clinical course. Consists of (usually bilateral) conjunctivitis, with preauricular lymphadenopathy. Painful corneal infiltrates can last for a month, causing significant blurring of vision. Although self-limiting, it causes significant

distress. Highly contagious, and secondary spread to household contacts occurs in 10% of cases.

- GI tract—HadV is the primary aetiology behind 5–10% of infantile diarrhoea (40, 41), which presents with watery diarrhoea and fever that can last for up to 2 weeks. However, due to protracted viral secretion after infection and asymptomatic infection, possible detection of HadV in faecal samples requires close clinical correlation before attributing causality. Intussusception and mesenteric adenitis are reported.
- Haemorrhagic cystitis (7, 11, 21)—benign, self-limiting (3 days) macroscopic haematuria in children, more commonly ♂. No fever is observed, and renal function remains normal.
- Encephalitis/meningoencephalitis (7, 1, 6, 12)—rare, usually in the context of severe systemic/respiratory infection.
- Myocarditis, pancreatitis and myositis and arthritis are reported.
- Immunocompromised—HadV is an increasingly recognized opportunistic pathogen in this cohort. Differentiation between non-pathogenic carriage/detection and causative pathogen can be difficult.
  - HSCT—causes more morbidity in children (3%) than in adults (1%), which is attributed to infection being primary. Commonest manifestation is GI, although expectant pneumonia, cystitis, and encephalitis are described. Akin to monitoring for CMV disease, pre-emptive monitoring for HadV appears to be able to predict invasive disease.
  - Solid organ transplant (SOT)—incidence rates low overall (<5%). Highest in the liver, followed by cardiac and renal transplants. In contrast to HSCT, however, disease is more likely to occur in the transplanted organ rather than be systemic (although this is described). It is associated with increased rates of organ rejection and, to a lesser extent, disseminated severe HadV disease.

Diagnosis

- Antigen detection and culture are almost never undertaken in a clinical setting, although they remain in use in academic centres. Serology is also rarely undertaken.
- PCR for HadV is the mainstay. It is sensitive/specific and quantitative, and can be performed on a variety of specimens (CSF, fixed tissues, blood). Typing is possible in some reference centres.

Treatment

- There is no generally accepted effective antiviral agent against HadV. Most infections in immunocompetent hosts are self-limiting.
- Only in immunocompromised cohorts is treatment with cidofovir (limited by nephrotoxicity) or brincidofovir even considered (➔ see Antivirals for cytomegalovirus, pp. 95–8). Their proven efficacy is debated. IVIG is of no proven benefit. Consideration towards lowering iatrogenic immunosuppression should be made.

Human papillomavirus

Virology

The family *Papillomaviridae* contains over 100 species that can infect a wide range of hosts: reptiles, fish, birds, and various mammals (e.g. human papillomavirus (HPV)). They are non-enveloped, isohedral-shaped dsDNA viruses (circular genome ~7500bp). The genome typically codes for 6–9 proteins designated early (E) and late (L), based on their expression. The viral capsid is composed of two viral proteins called L1 (the majority), which mediates cell attachment, and L2 (these are antigenic and serve as components for the HPV subunit vaccine). The ability of HPV to establish latency is debated. The genus *Alphapapillomavirus* contains several HPV species of particular interest, mainly due to their oncogenic ability (associated with cancers of the head and neck, along with the anogenital tract), although they cause a range of other benign clinical manifestations. Different types show different tissue tropism. They are risk-categorized, based on their association with cervical cancer, into low- (HPV-6, 11) and high- (HPV-16, 18) risk types.

Following a micro-abrasion, HPV gains access to, and almost exclusively infects, epithelial cells (starting in the basal layer called stratum germinativum). HPV classically generates little to no viraemia, thus efficiently evading host immunity, which contributes to its ability to persist and establish long-lived infection. Stages of the viral replication cycle are closely linked to cellular differentiation to maximize efficiency and transmission. Two viral proteins called E1 (a helicase) and E2 (a crucial viral regulator controlling transcription) act to ensure both the transfer and amplification of viral genomes to daughter cells as cellular differentiation progresses. Consequently, the top layer (which will be profusely shed) of HPV-infected skin cells contains a high burden of infectious HPV virions. The viral proteins E6 and E7 are particularly notable oncogenes, which transform host cells through their antagonistic interactions on the tumour suppressor proteins p53 (negative regulator of cell growth and division) and retinoblastoma (stops cell division in the presence of DNA damage).

Transmission is through close contact with infected skin cells. Vertical transmission during vaginal delivery is recognized. Fomite transmission is debated.

Epidemiology

- Global prevalence with almost ubiquitous human infection.

Clinical features

- Most HPV infections are asymptomatic and self-resolve within 12 months (70%) to 24 months (90%). Persistent infection from a high-risk type is a risk factor for malignancy. HPV (type number) and their associations are listed.
- Cutaneous HPV episodes are extremely common, aesthetically unpleasant, and occasionally painful. Close personal contact important in their transmission. The majority of cases resolve (90%) within 5 years. Very rarely progress to verrucous carcinoma. Young children may develop genital warts from hand contact with non-genital lesions; their presence should, however, prompt the consideration of abuse.

- Common warts/verruca vulgaris (71%) (1, 2, 4)—occur frequently amongst school-aged children, with a well-defined, exophytic appearance. Commonly found on the back of the hands, between fingers, and on the palms and soles. May coalesce.
- Plantar warts/verruca plantaris (34%) (3, 10)—commonest amongst adolescents/young adults. Appear as raised bundles of fibres and are often painful.
- Planar warts/verruca plana (4%)—irregular, slightly elevated papules. Seen in childhood.

- Recurrent respiratory papillomatosis (6, 11)—commonest paediatric benign laryngeal tumour (median age of 3). Infection is probably acquired intrapartum. Patients presenting with hoarseness or an altered cry. Disease may spread to the trachea and lungs, resulting in obstruction, stridor, infection, and respiratory compromise. May require surgical excision. Adult disease is associated with a high number of sexual partners and oral–genital contact. Presentation is less aggressive, with rare malignant transformation.
- Anogenital warts/condylomata acuminata (6, 11, although co-infection with high-risk types is common)—represents the commonest sexually transmitted infection (STI) in the UK, although this is trending down following the introduction of HPV vaccination. Transmitted by close skin-to-skin contact; therefore, barrier contraception reduces, but does not eliminate, risk. Incubation period is 3–34 weeks. Clinically apparent disease occurs in 50–60% of cases following exposure; 30% of cases resolve spontaneously within 4 months, although resolution of lesion does not correlate with resolution of HPV carriage. Immunosuppression and smoking are associated with worse disease. Lesions are typically found on the vulva, penile shaft and glans, and perineal skin. Lesion appearance is highly variable. Lesions can be singular/multiple and look flat/dome-like/verruca-like. They can be sessile or pedunculated, and small (<1mm) or coalesce into larger plaques. Lesion colour is also heterogeneous, with white, erythematous, violaceous, or brown manifestations all described. Although typically benign, the potential for anogenital warts to induce significant psychological stress should not be underestimated. Additionally, those with a large burden of disease or with lesions involving the anogenital area/urethra may experience issues with micturition/defecation/bleeding.
- Malignancy—HIV infection, if present, plays an additive role in genital tract malignancy:
  - cervical—fourth commonest cancer in women; 90% can be attributed to HPV infection (16, 18 responsible alone for 70%);
  - anal—80–90% of anal canal malignancies are associated with HPV infection (16, 18, 32);
  - penile—30–50% attributable to HPV infection (16, 18, 6);
  - oropharyngeal—50–80% attributable to HPV infection (16, 18, 31), typically at tongue base and tonsil area.

Diagnosis

- Cutaneous HPV manifestations are usually made on clinical examination by an experienced practitioner. Biopsy may be indicated to confirm the diagnosis (➔ see Genital warts, pp. 745–7).
- Molecular detection of HPV DNA from tissue samples (cervical swabs, tissue biopsies) is highly sensitive and allows typing. More detailed testing is not usually undertaken.

Treatment

- Cutaneous/anogenital warts—most cutaneous warts undergo spontaneous resolution. Treatment strategies vary considerably and should be tailored to the patient/site.
  - Chemical destruction is first line; daily salicylic acid-based preparations or cryotherapy 3-weekly (both achieve cure in up to 70% of cases). Salicylic acid cures around 80% of deep plantar warts, but only 50% of mosaic plantar warts. This can be enhanced by curettage, cryotherapy, and electrosurgery.
  - Enhancing the local immune response can be achieved by using either TOP imiquimod (a Toll-like receptor 7 agonist) or interferon (IFN).
  - Antiproliferative therapy (TOP pocophyllotoxin). If no response seen by 3–4 weeks, consider switching therapy
  - Treatment options are more limited in pregnancy; salicylate and cryotherapy are the mainstay.
- There are no effective HPV antiviral therapies available to supplement the treatment of HPV-associated cancer.

For guidelines, see ℘ https://www.bashhguidelines.org/current-guidelines/skin-conditions/anogenital-warts-2015/

Prevention

- Barrier contraception reduces, but does not eliminate, HPV transmission.
- HPV vaccination is preventative only and does not act as a therapeutic vaccine. It is unknown what effect (if any) it has on HPV infection at the time of receipt. It does not replace the need for cervical screening, which should occur in tandem to vaccination schedules.
- The HPV vaccine was introduced into routine immunization of girls aged 12–18 in 2008, and extended to boys in 2019. It was expanded to include men who have sex with men (MSM) aged <45 years in 2018. The full extent of these measures will be seen in the coming years, but international experience shows vaccination is highly effective in preventing both benign and malignant HPV disease.
- Vaccinations—three subunit vaccines are available, made from the L1 protein of the capsid that forms a virus-like particle devoid of DNA, which is therefore neither infectious nor live. The vaccines differ by the number of types they cover with a 2, 4 and 9 HPV type composition available. It is a highly effective vaccine, with seroconversion rates of >95% and disease prevention rates of >99%. For administration schedules and more detailed information, see *Human papillomavirus (HPV): the green book* (available at: ℘ https://www.gov.uk/government/publications/human-papillomavirus-hpv-the-green-book-chapter-18a).

Human polyomaviruses

Virology

The family *Polyomaviridae* contains over 100 species across six genera that infects a range of hosts; fish, birds, and mammals. They are non-enveloped, icosahedral dsDNA viruses (circular genomes ~5,000bp). There are ~14 species of human polyomavirus (HpyV). A capsid composed of viral proteins (VP) 1–3 surrounds the genome; the majority is VP-1, which is used as an antigenic target to differentiate amongst species. A region of the genome, called the non-coding control region (NCCR), regulates the expression of viral genes to enhance replication. When NCCRs were compared between immunocompromised and immunocompetent hosts, NCCRs from immunocompromised hosts had more mutations (were less conserved). Purportedly, as a consequence, viral replication and cytopathic damage are enhanced. Two viral proteins, called small and large tumour (T) protein, manipulate the progression of cell cycle phase towards maximal enhanced viral replication. HpyV is generally not considered an oncogenic virus *in vivo* (a notable exception is HpyV-5). Following primary infection, latency is established (multi-site, but mainly in the kidney). Precise routes of transmission are not proven, but respiratory and faecal–oral routes seem likely. HpyV are important opportunistic causes of disease in the immunosuppressed.

Notable HpyV (BK and JC refer to initials of the index patient case) include:
- HpyV-1 (BKV)—four serotypes, largely reflecting geographical variation;
- HpyV-2 (JCV)—single serotype;
- HpyV-5—called Merkel cell polyomavirus and is highly associated with Merkel cell carcinoma (an aggressive skin malignancy);
- Simian virus 40—is a virus of unknown, yet fiercely debated, pathogenicity following the inadvertent exposure of people receiving polio vaccination in the 1950s.

Epidemiology

- Infection is almost ubiquitous, with varying reported seroprevalence rates—these approach 50–90% to JCv, BKv, or both.

Clinical features

Primary infection is usually asymptomatic, but children may experience mild upper respiratory tract symptoms. Viruria alone (presence of virus in the urine) requires particular clinical correlation (10–30% of immunocompetent hosts, rising to 50% in immunocompromised).
- BKv:
  - BKv-associated renal nephropathy—occurs in renal transplant recipients (rare in other transplants), mainly in the first year post-grafting (10%). Linked with iatrogenic immunosuppression. This can present as an acute or a progressive decline in renal function that, if replication goes unchecked, is associated with graft loss. Viraemia heralds frank disease and is therefore a useful screening marker;
  - ureteric stenosis (due to obstruction secondary to infection of the epithelium). Notably, pain is absent, as this graft is not innervated. Decoy cells may be seen (virally infected epithelial cells, with enlarged

nuclei and large inclusion bodies reflecting viral replication) in the urine;
- haemorrhagic cystitis—mainly seen in the HSCT population, particularly in the first 2 months post-grafting.
- JCv:
  - progressive multifocal leukoencephalopathy (PML) is the most feared manifestation of JCv infection. Almost exclusively seen in immunocompromised cohorts (HIV, HSCT) and those receiving immunomodulatory agents (notably natalizumab for multiple sclerosis). Uncontrolled viral replication promotes spread to the CNS where destruction of various glial cells ensues, especially myelin-producing oligodendrocytes. Patients present with a spectrum of neurological symptoms (hemiparesis, visual field defects, aphasia, ataxia, and cognitive impairment), and a few PML subtypes exist. Abnormalities best seen on magnetic resonance imaging (MRI) (non-enhancing foci not aligning to vascular territories) occur predominantly in the cerebral white matter, sparing the cord.

Diagnosis

- Serology use is limited, given seroprevalence. JCv serology is sometimes used in a screening capacity pre-immunosuppression.
- Viral culture remains the remit of academia. Urine cytology is of limited utility. Molecular analysis of blood/CSF/urine is the mainstay.
- BKv-associated nephropathy—screening of appropriate patient cohorts with blood/urine quantitative PCR monitoring is usual practice. Histology is possible.
- JCv-associated PML—based on clinically compatible syndrome with concordant MRI findings. Molecular analysis of CSF is possible (negative result does not exclude diagnosis due to sensitivity issues). Brain biopsy is gold standard.

Treatment

- The majority of patients with BKv and JCv infection are asymptomatic and do not require treatment. There is no broadly accepted effective antiviral therapy. New therapies are highly desirable.
- BKv-associated nephropathy may respond to reduction of immunosuppression. IVIG is only of use in certain cases (concurrent hypogammaglobulinaemia). The use of cidofovir is generally considered to be of extremely limited use. The use of leflunomide or quinolone antibiotics is not recommended.
- PML—almost uniformly fatal (<1 year). No effective antiviral treatment exists and centres around decreasing host immunosuppression.

Poxviruses

Virology

The family *Poxviridae* contains >80 viral species across >20 genera, but only a handful cause notable human infections. Poxviruses are large enveloped, pleomorphic-shaped dsDNA viruses (linear genome ~130 000–350 000bp). Despite being a DNA virus, replication takes place in the cytoplasm. Two antigenically distinct forms of poxvirus virions are made during replication due to the presence/absence of a second membrane envelope gained during assembly at the Golgi apparatus. The cross-neutralizing ability amongst viral species within the genus *Orthopoxvirus* is the biological foundation that made variola (smallpox) eradication possible (i.e. immunity towards one conferred immunity to all). Transmission is through close contact with broken skin and via the respiratory route.

Genus Orthopoxvirus
- Vaccinia:
  - Vaccinia virus infections are not thought to occur naturally.
  - Most notable for its widespread use in research and as the component of the live smallpox vaccine.
  - Jenner observed in 1798 that inoculating people with pustular material from presumed cowpox gave protection from smallpox, inventing 'vaccination'. Crucially, cowpox is a different virus to vaccinia (frequently mistaken as the same entity), but both members of the same genus. It is unclear when vaccinia replaced cowpox virus (if it ever even was) as the component of the smallpox vaccine. The reader is encouraged to read further into this fascinating origin.
  - Routine vaccination for smallpox has been discontinued.
  - Vaccinia vaccination against smallpox carries one of the highest rates of complications: fever, regional lymphadenopathy, post-infectious encephalitis (1–2 weeks later), and skin eruptions.
- Variola (smallpox):
  - In 1980, the WHO declared smallpox was eradicated, although interest remains due to bioterrorism. The last natural case was in Somalia in 1977 and an occupational case occurred following a laboratory accident in Birmingham, UK in 1978.
  - Most clinicians will never have seen a case, but it should be in the differential (albeit at the bottom) for any fever and vesicular/pustular rash. Early infectious diseases consultation is crucial.
  - Two (clinically similar) viral strains—the particularly virulent variola major (mortality 20–50%) and the milder variola minor (mortality <1%). Different clinical subtypes exist, which affect mortality.
  - Incubation is <12 days; then a 2-day prodrome is followed by a rash. Classically, in contrast to varicella-zoster virus (VZV) infection, variola lesions are all in the same stage of development (VZV lesions are clustered in different stages). Also, variola lesions have a centrifugal distribution, concentrating more at the peripheries, including the hands and soles (VZV lesions have a centripetal distribution and rarely involve the hands/soles).
  - Viraemia precedes the rash; thus, PCR analysis of swab/throat/urine is necessary. IPC is paramount.
  - Treatment experience is limited and composed of supportive care, the antivirals tecovirimat and brincidofovir, and immunoglobulin (robust evidence obviously lacking). A vaccine is available for those deemed at risk of contracting illness.
- Monkeypox:
  - Cause of a vesicular illness ("mpox") in humans similar in appearance to smallpox. There are 2 distinct strains—clade I in the Congo region (reported case fatality rate 10% and classified as an HCID

in the UK), and the less virulent clade II in West Africa (CFR 3–4% and not considered HCID in the UK since January 2023). The classic illness of fever, myalgia, lymphadenopathy and rash occurs in these regions or sporadically elsewhere associated with travel. Rates here increased following the end of routine smallpox vaccination in the 1980s. Transmission is through contact with an infected animal/human—likely with a rodent reservoir. Monkeys and humans are incidental hosts. In 2022 there was a global outbreak caused by clade IIb. The majority of cases had no relevant travel history and the burden of disease was experienced by MSM. Many patients presented with genital and anal lesions without systemic illness. Transmission was by close contact with data suggesting infectivity up to 4 days before symptoms onset. By April 2023 there had been almost 3800 cases reported in the UK and no deaths. Treatment is supportive—antivirals (e.g. tecovirimat) may have a role in those at risk of, or with, severe disease.

Genus Parapoxvirus
- Orf virus:
  - Zoonotic infection usually acquired from sheep and goats. Causes skin lesions at the site of inoculation. No specific therapy needed.
- Pseudocowpox virus:
  - Zoonotic agent acquired from cows, causing 'milkers nodule'.

Genus Molluscipoxvirus
- Molluscum contagiosum:
  - The only poxvirus specific for humans in the post-smallpox era. Found worldwide (10–20% seroprevalence) and spread by close human contact.
  - A common disease of childhood and adolescents as a result of sexual transmission or contact sports.
  - Causes small, firm, umbilicated papules on exposed epithelial (children) or genital areas (adults). Usually resolve spontaneously (6–12 months) but can persist in immunosuppressed hosts.
  - Diagnosis is clinical but may be confirmed, if necessary, by histology, as lesions can resemble those of other conditions, including cryptococcosis and histoplasmosis.
  - Management is by local therapy (cryotherapy, excision, podophyllotoxin, etc.) and improving immunological function. Severe cases associated with immunocompromise are treated with IFN alfa or cidofovir (disappointing efficacy).

Herpesviridae

A large and important family of human viral infections that occupy significant resources in terms of clinical and laboratory time Almost every human being is infected with at least one herpesvirus. They cause a wide spectrum of morbidity, ranging from asymptomatic (primary EBV) to mild illness (childhood VZV) to life-threatening (HSV-associated neonatal infection or encephalitis). They play an increasingly recognized role in immune modulation, as well as possessing oncogenic potential (the *Gammaherpesvirinae*; human herpesvirus (HHV)-4 and 8). Large enveloped csDNA viruses (linear genome ranges from 120000 to 230000bp), grouped into three subfamilies, based on genetic sequencing and cell tropism. Between the icosahedral nucleocapsid and the viral envelope lies the tegument—a matrix of proteins that enhance replication and assist in immune evasion and direct intracellular trafficking. Although the genome organization can vary dramatically amongst herpesviruses, numerous genes are conserved, with members of individual subfamilies showing most similarities. Following viral attachment and entry, the viral capsid and tegument proteins are released into the cytoplasm, with subsequent transport of the genome containing the capsid to the nucleus where replication takes place. From here, either a lytic (active viral gene expression with genome replication and particle assembly that results in eventual cell death) or a latent (maintenance of the viral genome without active gene expression) pathway follows. This requires controlled division of viral replication by early and late gene expression.

A key property of all herpesviruses is that of latency, the ability to establish a persistent lifelong infection from which periodic reactivation can occur. This requires a degree of immune evasion (partially achieved through downregulation of cell surface major histocompatibility complex (MHC)), coupled with maintaining integrity of the genome. The precise mechanisms underpinning latency are unknown and vary amongst individual herpesviruses.

In addition to the eight numerical HHV nomenclature, some herpesviruses have a more colloquial terminology. A ninth herpesvirus (B-virus) is listed for completion. B-virus infects macaques and can rarely infect humans, causing fatal encephalitis unless PEP is started.

- *Alphaherpesvirinae*—HHV-1, 2 (herpes), HHV-3 (VZV), and Macacine alphaherpesvirus 1 (herpesvirus B or B-virus).
- *Betaherpesvirinae*—HHV-5 (CMV), HHV-6, and HHV-7.
- *Gammaherpesvirinae*—HHV-4 (EBV) and HHV-8 (Kaposi's sarcoma (KS)-associated herpesvirus).

HHV-1 and 2 (herpes simplex)

Virology

The *Alphaherpesviruses* HHV-1 and 2 cause herpes simplex infection, henceforth referred to as HSV-1 and 2. There is considerable overlap in clinical manifestations between the two viruses, but they can be distinguished in the laboratory. Broadly speaking, HSV-1 causes infection in the upper part of the body, with HSV-2 in the lower part. Latency is established in regional nerve ganglions (trigeminal or sacral). While it is generally accepted that infection with one does not confer full immunity to the other, there is debate regarding the susceptibility to infection and severity of the disease course, should dual infection occur. While lifelong IgG is produced following primary infection, the crucial role of cell-mediated immunity necessary to suppress latent virus is amply demonstrated by the susceptibility to invasive disease in populations where it is lacking (e.g. advanced HIV and transplant recipients). Primary infection refers to the first infection (whether symptomatic or not), with subsequent establishment of latency. Reactivation refers to increased viral replication (whether symptomatic or not) of previously acquired (latent) virus. Transmission occurs through breaks in mucosal surfaces via close contact with an individual who is shedding the virus. Asymptomatic shedding is possible.

Epidemiology

- Seroprevalence—90% of people are seropositive to one or both viruses. HSV-1 seroprevalence is around 50–70% by adulthood; HSV-2 around 20%.
- HSV-1 seroprevalence is higher in developing countries and lower socio-economic groups. Primary oral acquisition in childhood is becoming less common.
- HSV-2 seroprevalence is higher in women than in men and correlates with the number of sexual partners. Half of HSV-2 seroconversions are subclinical.

Clinical features

- Wide-ranging and influenced by the site of infection, host age, and immune status. Overlap exists with both viral subtypes, causing manifestations that are not distinguishable on clinical grounds alone. First infections tend to be more severe than reactivation, with more systemic features, longer symptom duration, and a higher rate of complications (particularly with HSV-1).
- Primary infection with either subtype can be asymptomatic (commoner with HSV-2).
- Cutaneous manifestations (➡ see Viral skin infections, pp. 812–14). Painful ulceration with perioral gingivostomatitis with local lymphadenopathy to varying severity is common. PO intake can be limited, warranting hospitalization for IV fluids in severe cases. Genital ulceration involving the penis, labia/vulva, and perineum, and proctitis are possible. Pain and autonomic involvement can cause urinary retention or constipation, which mandate medical intervention. Viral prodromal symptoms are commoner in primary infection and can herald reactivation. Genital reactivation with HSV-2 is more frequent than HSV-1. Other mucocutaneous manifestations of HSV infection are: herpetic whitlow (infection on the fingertips), eczema herpeticum (HSV superinfection on atopic dermatitis or eczema, which can be complicated by bacterial superinfection), and localized dermatomal reactivation that can look similar to VZV/shingles rash.
- Neurological HSV:
  - HSV encephalitis (90% HSV-1) carries a devastating prognosis, with untreated mortality approaching 80% (falls to 19% with treatment) and long-term sequelae common amongst survivors. Bimodal age distribution, with incidence peaks in those aged 5–30 years and those aged over 50 years. These peaks are thought to mirror the concordant route of infection: immediate CNS invasion following primary infection in the young, and viral reactivation in the elderly. The precise pathogenesis is not well understood. Onset is usually acute (may be insidious), with a prodrome of headache, behavioural change, and fever. Other symptoms: focal neurological signs (classically temporal lobe), seizures, and coma. Treatment should be commenced empirically while arranging diagnostics. Demonstration of viral genome by molecular techniques (CSF

PCR 98–99% sensitive) is considered gold standard. False negatives can occur if samples are taken within the first 72h of symptoms (consider repeating). Electroencephalography (EEG) and computed tomography (CT)/MRI may demonstrate characteristic focal features but can be normal early in illness. Brain biopsy for culture and histology is rarely indicated. Paired serum and CSF antibody titres (diagnostic if 4-fold rise) can be performed but are not useful in early disease.
- Meningitis, by contrast, follows a far more benign course. More commonly caused by HSV-2 and can be recurrent (termed Mollaret's meningitis). Cases may complicate genital herpes (women > men), with symptoms following genital lesions by 3–10 days. Diagnosis is clinical and confirmed by molecular analysis of CSF.
- Bell's palsy—HSV is a recognized cause of facial nerve palsy. Empirical steroids are the mainstay, with a possible role for antivirals.
- Ocular HSV—keratitis is a significant cause of blindness globally. Mainly due to reactivation. Presents as pain and visual blurring. Urgent ophthalmological assessment and treatment are paramount.
- Visceral infection—commoner in immunocompromised hosts or at extremes of age. Hepatitis, pneumonitis, and oesophagitis are all described. Mortality is high. Prophylaxis is key in haematology and transplant populations. HSV and other herpesviruses are often detected in respiratory swabs from unwell hospitalized patients (intensive care unit (ICU) settings usually). This is not to say these patients have HSV pneumonitis; it almost always reflects reactivation and may be of no clinical consequence.
- Neonatal HSV can be devastating if not anticipated (unfortunately, the majority of disease cases occur in the absence of maternal history of HSV infection). Most commonly due to HSV-2, but the incidence of HSV-1 is rising. Transmission occurs mainly perinatally (85%) or postnatally (10%), with intrauterine transmission/congenital infection being very rare. The highest risk is primary infection occurring <6 weeks before birth (25–60%). Reactivation or infection in the first half of pregnancy rarely leads to neonatal disease (<2%). These patterns likely reflect the transmission dynamics of protective maternal IgG to the fetus. Congenital infection is devastating and thankfully rare; fetal demise *in utero* can occur, and surviving cases show signs of disseminated HSV disease at birth (microcephaly, hydrocephalus, skin scarring, and eye damage). Peri(post)-natal HSV disease loosely follows three patterns of disease, in order of increasing mortality: cutaneous, CNS only, and disseminated infection. Treatment is syndrome-tailored but centres around prompt diagnosis and antivirals. See HSV guidelines, jointly from British Association for Sexual Health and HIV and Royal College of Obstetricians and Gynaecologists (available at: ℞ https://www.bashhguidelines.org/current-guidelines/genital-ulceration/herpes-in-pregnancy-2014/ and https://www.rcog.org.uk/guidance/browse-all-guidance/other-guidelines-and-reports/management-of-genital-herpes-in-pregnancy/).

Diagnosis
- Herpetic ulcerations can resemble other vesicular rashes. Laboratory diagnosis is important to guide therapy where there is doubt.

- Serology is of little use, given an almost ubiquitous seroprevalence.
- Molecular PCR is the mainstay. It is incredibly sensitive and can differentiate HSV-1 from HSV-2. It can be performed on numerous samples: vesicular fluid, skin swab, blood, CSF, placental biopsies.
- Viral culture is of little use. Occasionally used to detect phenotypic aciclovir resistance, in conjunction with genotypic molecular sequencing.
- Histology may demonstrate giant cells or intranuclear inclusions. Direct fluorescence antibody testing is specific, but almost never done.

Treatment

- (➔ See Antivirals for herpes simplex virus and varicella-zoster virus, pp. 94–5). Almost exclusively revolves around aciclovir or its modified version valaciclovir.
  - PO administration is used to shorten the duration of primary attacks of cutaneous, oral, and genital herpes. It is less effective against recurrent disease but may be given prophylactically where recurrences are frequent and in the immunocompromised.
  - IV administration for encephalitis (see guidelines from British Infection Association, available at: 🕭 https://www.britishinfection.org/guidance/published-guidelines) is for at least 14 days, and patients must be CSF PCR-negative on completion. There s no role for PO antivirals in the treatment of encephalitis. There is no evidence for antiviral therapy in HSV meningitis, although it is frequently given in the acute phase.
  - Neonatal HSV management and treatment should follow local protocols.

HHV-3 (varicella-zoster virus)

Virology

HHV-3 (henceforth referred to as VZV) shows a high degree of genetic similarity to the other alphaherpesviruses. Infection causes two distinct diseases manifestations: primary infection causes varicella (chickenpox), whereas reactivation of latent infection causes zoster (shingles). After attachment and entry, there are two main viraemias. The first is from days 4–6 post-exposure and reflects local site and lymph node replication with disseminated systemic infection. This is followed by a secondary viraemia from day 9 onwards. After primary infection, the virus becomes latent within sensory dorsal root ganglia. Primary reinfection, while common, is mostly subclinical. VZV is spread by aerosolized droplets from mainly symptomatic cases due to the fluid from skin vesicles containing large quantities of virus. Vertical transmission is possible. This one-way chain of transmission can be remembered by the phrase 'you can catch chickenpox from shingles, but not shingles from chickenpox'.

Epidemiology

- In the UK, >90% of people are seropositive by 20 years of age, but in tropical countries, for unknown reasons, the seroprevalence can be as low as 60%. Secondary household attack rates are >90%, with secondary cases showing increasing severity (thought to be due to larger inocula).

- Reactivation, causing shingles, occurs in 20% of the population. Although all ages are affected, the incidence increases with age and in the immunocompromised.
- Mortality is 4–9 per 100 000 (80% will be adults) and is five times more likely to be fatal if it occurs during pregnancy.

Clinical features

Chickenpox

- Largely a benign, self-limiting illness if occurs in early childhood. Disease is more severe and complications commoner if occurs in immunocompromised populations (i.e. pregnancy or neonates).
- Incubation is 10–14 days. Primary infection cases are considered infectious for 48h before rash until all vesicles crust over.
- A 1- to 2-day febrile prodrome (malaise, itch, anorexia) is followed by a vesicular rash. Rash begins as maculopapules (<5mm across), progressing to vesicles that quickly pustulate, forming scabs, which fall off 1–2 weeks later. Lesions appear in successive crops over 2–4 days, starting on the trunk and face and spreading centripetally. May rarely involve the mucosa of the oropharynx and vagina.
- Complications (refer to primary infection only, i.e. not zoster):
  - Pneumonia is the commonest complication in adults and should be actively screened for (will develop in 5–14% of adults). A dry cough and dyspnoea are suspicious. Prompt recognition is crucial; mortality is between 10% and 30% but approaches 50% if mechanical ventilation is required.
  - Secondary bacterial infection of lesions, usually with Gram-positive organisms (*S. aureus* and *Streptococcus pyogenes*).
  - Neurological complications—detection of VZV in CSF during infection is expected and can be asymptomatic. However, encephalitis can occur, of which there are mainly two forms. Acute cerebellar ataxia, which occurs in 1 in 4000 children aged under 15 years, onset 7–21 days after rash and resolves over 2–4 weeks; diffuse encephalitis commoner in adults (0.2% cases), and 5–20% experience progressive neurological deterioration and die.
  - Reye syndrome—a progressive encephalopathy, commonest in children recovering from VZV or another febrile viral illness. Concomitant salicylate administration has been identified as a risk factor.
- Pregnancy poses risks to mother, fetus, and neonate. Timing of infection is critical and reflects the evolving interplay among the risk of *in utero* transmission, maternal antibody transmission, and maturity of the neonatal immune system.
  - Mothers have a higher risk of developing the same complications as non-pregnant adults throughout pregnancy.
  - For the fetus and neonate—*in utero* transmission causing the devastating congenital varicella syndrome (CVS) (30% mortality, cutaneous scarring with neurological, ocular, and limb abnormalities) is rare overall. The risk of developing CVS is greatest between 12 and 20 weeks' gestation (2%). Pre-12 and post-20 weeks' gestation, the risk is much lower. Babies born to mothers who had chickenpox

between 20 and 37 weeks' gestation have a higher incidence of shingles during their first 2 years, reflecting primary infection *in utero*.
- Fetuses exposed to maternal chickenpox 7–20 days before delivery may develop neonatal chickenpox, but it tends to be less severe, reflecting transmission of some maternal antibody to newborn. However, if the mother develops chickenpox in the period of 7 days pre-/post-delivery, then neonatal chickenpox will develop before maternal antibody could be transmitted. This can be devastating. If infection develops past the 10- to 28-day point, outcomes improve again.
- PEP for pregnant women exposed to VZV is recommended (➲ see Chapter 23, VZV, pp. 839–40).

Herpes zoster
- Reflects reactivation of previously acquired latent VZV (shingles). Cases are considered less infectious than in primary infection.
- Typically, unilateral vesicular eruption in a dermatomal distribution (most commonly thoracic and lumbar), often preceded by 2–3 days of pain in the affected area. Maculopapular lesions evolve into vesicles, with new crops forming over 3–5 days. Resolution may take 2–4 weeks.
- Complications:
  - Herpes zoster ophthalmicus is VZV reactivation in the ophthalmic branch of the trigeminal nerve. It is potentially sight-threatening, with lesions on the nose tip (signifying involvement of the nasociliary nerve branch, which also innervates the eye) being a bad prognostic sign. Retinal necrosis is possible. Urgent treatment and ophthalmic assessment are crucial.
  - Ramsay Hunt syndrome refers to reactivation in the geniculate ganglion of the vestibulocochlear nerve. Pain and vesicles in the external auditory meatus, ipsilateral facial palsy, loss of taste to the anterior two-thirds of the tongue.
  - Post-herpetic neuralgia is defined as pain for 90 days post-rash onset; 10–15% overall risk, but age is a significant risk factor, with 50% of cases in those aged over 50 years.
  - Immunocompromised patients—disease is more severe with prolonged lesion formation and recovery with higher risk of cutaneous dissemination and visceral involvement. Rarely fatal.

Diagnosis
- Usually made clinically, but laboratory confirmation useful in atypical rash or in presentations without skin manifestations (e.g. encephalitis, disseminated disease).
- A vesicular scrape involves piercing a vesicle to sample the virus-containing fluid inside, usually on a swab. A dry swab that has not collected fluid is not sufficient.
- Serology—IgG antibodies to VZV indicates prior infection/vaccination and the presence of immunity. IgM is of little use.
- PCR is the mainstay. It is highly sensitive and can be performed on numerous samples: vesicular fluid, skin swab, blood, CSF, placental biopsies.

Treatment

Chickenpox

- General measures—prevent secondary infection of lesions, antihistamines for itch to reduce scratching, paracetamol for fever.
- (Val)aciclovir (➋ see Antivirals for herpes simplex virus and varicella-zoster virus, pp. 94–5)—a 7-day PO course started within 24h of onset reduces the duration and severity of illness. Not recommended for routine use in immunocompetent children aged <12 years, as the clinical impact is modest.
  - Adults—initiate treatment as quickly as possible, particularly if new lesions are still appearing (in previous 24–48h).
  - Children—consider treating those >12 years of age.
  - All immunocompromised patients, pregnant women, and neonatal cases of varicella should be treated.
  - IV aciclovir should be given to treat complications.
  - Use of steroids in VZV pneumonia is unproven and not recommended.

Shingles

- General measures (as discussed under ➋ Chickenpox above), ophthalmic referral if eye involvement.
- PO (val)aciclovir is recommended for those presenting within 72h of symptoms, or longer if lesions are still appearing. Benefits are greatest in those aged >50 years, but treatment can be considered for younger patients. Treatment is for 7 days.
- All immunocompromised patients should be treated without delay, even if after 72h. IV treatment may be necessary.
- There is no evidence supporting the routine use of steroids.
- Post-herpetic neuralgia is unusual beyond 4 weeks, but such cases can be difficult to treat. They usually resolve over 6–24 months. Therapies include tricyclics, counter-irritants, and gabapentin.

Prevention

- VZV vaccines exists for prevention of both primary and recurrent infection.
  - Primary vaccination with a live VZV vaccine against chickenpox is on the routine immunization schedule of some countries (not the UK currently). It is recommended for non-immune HCWs, in addition to household contacts of immunocompromised patients (see *Varicella: the green book*, available at: ⚕ https://www.gov.uk/gov ernment/publications/varicella-the-green-book-chapter-34).
  - Two shingles vaccine are available (a live and a subunit one). The live vaccine is similar to the primary varicella vaccine but contains a far higher quantity of virus. It reduces the incidence of shingles by 51% and reduces post-herpetic neuralgia by 66% in those aged 60–69 years. It is recommended for those aged over 70 years, the age at which its cost-effectiveness is greatest (see *Varicella: the green book*, available at: ⚕ https://www.gov.uk/government/publicati ons/varicella-the-green-book-chapter-34). The subunit vaccine can be used for populations in whom live vaccine use is contraindicated.

- Varicella-zoster immunoglobulin (VZIG) is administered not to prevent infection, but to reduce disease severity. VZIG prophylaxis is offered to seronegative individuals in at-risk groups (immunosuppressed, pregnant women, and neonates) following a significant exposure to VZV. It is ~50% effective at keeping contacts symptom-free, with 15% of cases asymptomatically seroconverting anyway. Most effective if given within 72h, but can be administered up to 10 days post-exposure. It should not be given if a rash is already present (see ⌖ www.gov.uk/government/publications/varicella-the-green-book-chapter-34).
- In some cases (pregnant women at >20 weeks' gestation), prophylaxis with PO aciclovir is an option, which should be given from days 7–14 post-exposure.

HHV-4 (Epstein–Barr virus)

Virology

EBV (like its fellow gammaherpesvirus HHV-8) has oncogenic potential and, like all herpesvirus, is epitomized by establishing latency. It is structurally consistent with other herpesviruses—with an icosahedral nucleocapsid that surrounds a dsDNA linear genome (~172,000bp). This is wrapped in a tegument and encased in an envelope predominantly spiked with a glycoprotein called gp350/220. Molecular sequencing has revealed two viral subtypes termed EBV-1 and EBV-2. The main difference between the types lies in the Epstein–Barr nuclear antigens (EBNAs) (proteins expressed in the nucleus of latently infected cells). While EBV-1 is the most prevalent, there is no firm evidence that the viruses differ in pathogenicity or oncogenic capability. EBV uses the CD21 B-cell receptor, which is the receptor for the C3d component of the complement pathway. Primary infection starts in the oropharynx where squamous epithelial cells are permissive to the full viral replication cycle, with subsequent cell lysis (although, purportedly, EBV binds far less efficiently to them). Latency is achieved through infection of B lymphocytes. It is noteworthy that these B cells become immortalized once infected (multiply indefinitely), which gives EBV its oncogenic potential. Infection is spread by close contact (saliva) with asymptomatic shedding of virus.

Epidemiology

- By adulthood, EBV seroprevalence exceeds 90–95%, although seroconversion is increasingly happening at a later stage in industrialized versus developing countries, reflecting societal behaviours.
- In the UK, 50% seroconvert before the age of 5 years, with a second wave in teenage years, the group in which clinical manifestations are commonest.

Clinical features

- Most primary infection is subclinical, if not asymptomatic.
- Infectious mononucleosis (IM)—usually asymptomatic in young children, although when symptomatic, a wide range of observations; rash, neutropenia, otitis media, or pneumonia are commoner than in adults. In adolescents/adults, 50% of cases are asymptomatic and can

consist of the classic triad of fever, pharyngitis, and lymphadenopathy (symmetrical involvement of cervical, axillary, and sometimes inguinal nodes). A 1- to 2-week prodrome of anorexia and malaise may be present.

- Examination reveals pharyngitis (exudative in 33% of cases, with palatal petechiae in 25–60%), hepatomegaly, splenomegaly (50% of cases—maximal at day 8, resolving over 10 days), periorbital oedema, and lymphadenopathy. Abdominal pain, particularly in the right upper quadrant, may be related to hepatomegaly or splenic enlargement, which may be rapid.
- Complications are rare overall, but airway obstruction/splenic rupture/rash should be borne in mind. Tonsillar enlargement can be so great as to threaten the airway. There is a small risk of splenic rupture with minor trauma or even spontaneously (1–2 cases per 1000). Patients are recommended to avoid contact sports for 3–4 weeks post-symptom onset. Notably, 90–100% of patients with acute EBV infection following inadvertent administration of ampicillin/amoxicillin (but not phenoxymethylpenicillin) will precipitate a florid pruritic maculopapular rash (most commonly administered in an attempt to treat streptococcal pharyngitis). This is not an allergic reaction nor is the patient penicillin-allergic. Numerous rare neurological (GBS, myelitis, ADEM) and haematological manifestations (haemolytic anaemia, haemolytic uraemic syndrome (HUS), thrombotic thrombocytopenic purpura (TTP), DIC) have been described, with acute EBV heralding its disseminated nature. Late-stage complications are exceedingly rare but include chronic active EBV and haemophagocytic lymphohistiocytosis (HLH). If infection occurs in immunocompromised children, complications are encountered more commonly and the risk of fatal disease/malignancy increases.
- Neoplastic disorders:
  - Burkitt's lymphoma—few subtypes, but tissue from >95% of African cases contains the EBV genome. Incompletely understood, but malaria appears to be a key cofactor towards development.
  - Nasopharyngeal carcinoma in southern China is commoner than anticipated, even after accounting for EBV seroprevalence.
  - HIV-associated non-Hodgkin's lymphoma appears to be driven, in part, by EBV.
  - Hodgkin's lymphoma, and both polyclonal B- and T-cell lymphomas appear to be, at least partly, attributable to EBV.
  - Post-transplant lymphoproliferative disorders (PTLDs) are a group of malignancies that occur as a complication of transplant (both solid and haematological) where ~70% of cases are thought to be due to EBV. Iatrogenic immunosuppression is a significant risk factor towards their development. Their prevention and treatment vary by host institution, as well as by subtype, but largely revolve around minimizing duration/intensity of immunosuppression, with surveillance of EBV levels and chemotherapy with rituximab in some cases.
- Congenital/perinatal infection with primary EBV is rare and is not associated with an increased risk of congenital abnormalities.

- Like all herpesviruses, EBV can reactivate in acute/severe illness (e.g. in ICU admission). Detection of viraemia in these cases is almost never clinically relevant.

Diagnosis

- Haematological—during IM, peripheral lymphocytosis is common. Atypical lymphocytes may be seen on a blood film (large, vacuolated, basophilic, eccentric lobulated nucleus), but this is common in acute viral infections and not specific to EBV. Neutropenia (60–70%) and thrombocytopenia (50%) are described.
- Biochemical—LFT abnormalities are common, particularly a hepatitic (aspartate aminotransferase (AST) and alanine aminotransferase (ALT) rise) rather than a cholestatic pattern (90% of cases), mild elevation of bilirubin level (45%), and low-level cryoglobulins (IgG and IgM) in 90% of cases.
- Serology is key to proving IM is due to primary EBV. The heterophile antibody test (where the presence of non-human red blood cell (RBC) agglutination by human antibodies is tested, e.g. Monospot (horse) or Paul–Bunnell (sheep)) is of limited secondary use (particularly unreliable in age <4 years, immunocompromise, autoimmune conditions, and viral co-infections). These tests are replaced by the wider availability of specific EBV serology (see Table 8.1 for interpretation). EBV serology should only be done if primary infection is suspected. It plays no role in assessment of any malignancy/surveillance diagnostics.
- EBV-specific antibodies comprise viral capsid antigen (VCA) IgM/IgG and EBNA. EBV serology is based on the premise that EBNA (IgG) is a marker of latency establishment and appears 5–8 weeks post-onset of symptoms (sometimes sooner) in 95% of people. If EBNA is present, acute EBV is unlikely. Seroconversion of EBNA is the serological gold standard of primary EBV infection. VCA antibodies appear very early in infection, with IgM disappearing after a few months and sometimes IgG persisting. False reactivity with any IgM assay is possible due to concurrent infection/autoimmune illness (like all serological assays).

Table 8.1 Interpretation of EBV serology

VCA (IgM)	VCA (IgG)	EBNA	Interpretation
–	+/–	+	Past infection (not recent)
+	+	–	Likely recent primary EBV infection
+	–	–	Likely primary, but repeat in 4–6 weeks
–	+	–	Unusual, could be distant past (no EBNA) or recent primary, needs repeat
+	+	+	Difficult; primary/false positive/reactivation

EBNA, Epstein–Barr nuclear antigen; EBV, Epstein–Barr virus; IgG, immunoglobulin G; IgM, immunoglobulin M; VCA, viral capsid antigen.

- Molecular—PCR analysis is highly sensitive and can be performed on blood or CSF. It can be both qualitative and quantitative. It plays no role in the diagnosis of acute IM. It is mainly of use in suspected PTLD/surveillance post-transplant/associated malignancies/encephalitis.

Treatment
- Most cases are self-limiting and do not require specific therapy.
- Antiviral drugs—while aciclovir shows activity *in vitro*, it is never used.
- In EBV-driven malignancies, rituximab (monoclonal anti-CD20) is sometimes used to deplete B cells (viral reservoirs).
- Surgical interventions are sometimes necessary for splenic rupture.
- Steroids can be administered for airway compromise in an attempt to avoid a tracheotomy (very rare).
- General malaise can persist for up to 3 months or more. The reasons behind prolonged recovery are not clear. Haematological and hepatic complications settle over 2–3 months.

HHV-5 (cytomegalovirus)

Virology
HHV-5, or CMV, likely represents the largest virus to infect humans (notably excluding case report-level evidence describing large virally infected protozoa). It is a betaherpesvirus (like HHV-6 and 7), with a dsDNA genome (~230 000 bp) encoding around 230 proteins. While numerous strains exist (multiple can be isolated from the same individual), it is generally believed secondary infection (infection in an already seropositive individual) from a different strain is **largely** benign. CMV has a typical herpesvirus structure and expectantly establishes latency. CMV dedicates a significant proportion of its genome towards production of proteins that participate in various immune evasion strategies. The burden and spectrum of disease attributable to CMV are underrecognized and wide. It is the commonest congenitally acquired infection and represents a troubling opportunistic pathogen in immunocompromised cohorts, and yet it is asymptomatic or manifests as a self-limiting mononucleosis illness in immunocompetent hosts. A CMV vaccine has long been a highly desirable and elusive goal. It is spread primarily by close contact, but vertical transmission giving rise to congenital infection is well described, as is iatrogenic transmission through transplants (haematological/organ/blood products).

Epidemiology
- Seroprevalence varies widely (40–100%), with higher rates in developing, rather than developed, countries. However, an individual's age, socio-economic status, ethnicity, and sexuality are all contributory factors.

Clinical features
- A useful distinction is made between 'disease' (i.e. morbidity and the presence of end-organ clinical manifestations) versus 'infection', which is the presence of CMV in the blood (viraemia) which is a(pre-) symptomatic. Disease can be due to primary or secondary infection

(reinfection with different strain) or reactivation of latent virus depending on the seropositivity of the host.

- IM—primary infection in the immunocompetent tends to be asymptomatic or at least subclinical. When symptomatic, it produces an IM phenotype (fever, sore throat, lymphadenopathy). Heterophile tests are usually negative. Differentiating IM due to CMV rather than due to EBV on clinical grounds is difficult. The IM due to CMV disease tends to have more systemic features (typhoidal) and causes less splenomegaly. Lymphadenopathy and sore throat are milder than with EBV. Complications are rare overall and more likely in immunocompromised hosts: GI (colitis, hepatitis), respiratory (pneumonitis), neurological (meningoencephalitis, GBS), haematological (thrombocytopenia, haemolytic anaemia). Myocarditis and rash are described. For reasons that are not completely understood, patients with advanced HIV are at particular risk of CMV retinitis (pizza-pie retinopathy) versus other immunosuppressed populations.
- Transplant cohorts—iatrogenic immunosuppressive regimens render their populations susceptible to CMV disease. The propensity to cause disease is related to the intensity/components of the regimen (use of lymphocyte-depleting agents/antithymocyte globulin are particularly prone) and varies by the organ transplanted: HSCT recipients are worst affected. The result is a delicate balancing act whereby the aim is to administer sufficient immunosuppression to prevent graft rejection, but not so much to facilitate opportunistic infection, in this case CMV disease (due to either primary/secondary infection or reactivation). In all cases of CMV disease, the degree of immunosuppression needs review. In both SOTs and HSCT, the CMV status of both the donor (D+/−) and the recipient (R+/−) is an important consideration. Pre-emptive therapy (routine surveillance with prompt initiation upon detection of viraemia) versus universal antiviral prophylaxis (administration regardless of viraemia or not) are both strategies that are employed to reduce morbidity/mortality. Both have their advantages/disadvantages in terms of drug toxicity/graft survival. Which strategy is employed varies by both transplant type and host institution.
  - Solid organ (liver/lung/kidney)—D+/R− has the highest risk of disease due to direct inoculation of infection. Fever, arthralgia, and cytopenias can precede tissue-invasive/end-organ disease, of which enteritis/colitis, nephritis, pneumonitis, hepatitis, and encephalitis are possible. The presence of CMV disease also increases the chances of graft rejections. Biopsy can be required to differentiate from graft rejection, a complication with the opposite management strategy (intensify immunosuppression). A clear preference between pre-emptive or universal antiviral administration is not clear, except for D+/R− renal transplants where universal prophylaxis is preferred.
  - HSCT—conversely, it is D−/R+ that carries the highest risk of disease due to lack of donor immunity against CMV to protect against host reactivation. Mindful that it is donor cells that post-engraftment form the donor's 'new' immune system and most centres employ a pre-emptive strategy, particularly since the introduction of letermovir.

- Congenital CMV infection—is likely underdiagnosed and is the leading cause of sensorineural hearing loss (SNHL). Numbers regarding transmission/infection/development of sequelae are complex, and cases are managed with local fetal medicine departments. Primary maternal infection is more likely to transmit to the fetus than secondary infection (40% versus 1%), although if transmission occurs, disease outcome will be similar. Chances of fetal transmission is greatest in the third trimester (40% in the first two trimesters versus 60% in the third). Ten per cent of newborns are symptomatic at birth (small for age, thrombocytopenia, jaundice, microcephaly, ventriculomegaly, petechiae), of whom 5% will die. Amongst survivors, 50% will carry no residual defects and the other 50% will display varying rates of motor/SNHL/visual impairments. Of the 90% of newborns who are asymptomatic at birth, 25% will develop sequelae, primarily SNHL, but neurodevelopmental problems are described. Antenatal diagnosis is aided by ultrasound for fetal abnormalities, but these can be non-specific. An interval of 8 weeks between maternal infection and amniocentesis is recommended. Neonatal urine/saliva in first 3 weeks confirms congenital CMV.
- Like all herpesviruses, CMV can reactivate in acute/severe illness (e.g. in ICU admission). Detection of viraemia in these cases is almost never clinically relevant.

Diagnosis

- Serology—IgG seroconversion is diagnostic. The presence of IgM (remains raised for months) or more than 4-fold increase in IgG titre indicates recent infection. IgG avidity (maturation) assays can be useful whereby low IgG avidity suggests infection <3 months ago.
- PCR analysis is highly sensitive and can be performed on blood, amniotic fluid, CSF, urine, or Guthrie cards. It can be both qualitative and quantitative. It plays no role in the diagnosis of acute IM. It is mainly of use in surveillance post-transplant/congenital CMV.
- Biopsy of infected tissue may reveal the distinctive appearance of CMV-infected cells (e.g. inclusion bodies).
- Culture and antigen tests are rarely performed.

Treatment and prevention

- Infection in immunocompetent individuals does not require treatment.
- Ganciclovir, foscarnet, and cidofovir (➔ see Antivirals for cytomegalovirus, pp. 95–8) inhibit CMV DNA polymerase and useful agents. Toxicity limits their use. Letermovir shows promise.
- CMV IgG is rarely used.

HHV-6

Virology

HHV-6 is a betaherpesvirus that is composed of two variants (90% sequence homology): HHV-6A and HHV-6B. They are sufficiently diverse that they could be (but historically are not) classified as separate herpesviruses. While both species infect a variety of host cells, with HHV-6A showing more neurotropism, HHV-6B is the causative agent behind most pathology. Many clinical associations with HHV-6 infection have been asserted (multiple sclerosis, chronic fatigue, myocarditis, neoplasia, synergism with HIV), with little data to support causality, partly due to the ability of HHV-6 to integrate into our genome. The virus has regions very similar to the telomeres of our cells and can insert itself therein. In just under <2% of the population, HHV-6 has integrated into a parental germ line cell, and so every cell in the resultant progeny (individual) will have integrated HHV-6 copies, leading to constitutive expression. This results in consistently high viral loads, which can make the differentiation of pathological reactivation versus inherent integration more challenging.

Epidemiology

- Seroprevalence varies, but most industrialized nations report rates of 75–95%. The period of highest seroconversion is in the first 2 years.

Clinical features

- Incubation is 5–15 days; main transmission through maternal saliva.
- Immunocompetent hosts (majority of cases):
  - infantile fever—in children, a particularly high fever, without rash, which may be associated with seizures (13%);
  - exanthem (sixth disease/roseola—illness in young children; 3–5 days of fever and upper respiratory tract symptoms that cease abruptly, heralding the appearance of a maculopapular rash;
  - mononucleosis syndrome in adults, with rare cases of encephalitis.
- Immunocompromised hosts:
  - Iatrogenic immunosuppression favours reactivation. Encephalitis (most usually), pneumonitis, hepatitis, and marrow suppression have been described. Whether organ or graft rejection can be attributed is still unproven, but delayed haematological engraftment is described. Attributable causation is complicated by reactivation of other herpesviruses (CMV)/pathogens with better established pathological pedigrees.

Diagnosis

- Serology—rarely undertaken due to almost ubiquitous seropositivity.
- PCR—diagnostic, although if detected, comparison with whole blood is usually necessary to differentiate chromosomal integration from reactivation. Consequently, paired CSF/EDTA (ethylenediaminetetraacetic acid) samples are common.

Treatment

- Most cases are self-limiting and need no treatment.
- Precise antiviral therapy is challenging, and evidence is lacking. Similar antiviral sensitivity pattern to CMV. Foscarnet is active against HHV-6A and 6B; ganciclovir is active against HHV-6B (some reports of relative resistance in HHV-6A). As it is a betaherpesvirus, aciclovir is expectantly inactive (➔ see Antivirals for cytomegalovirus, pp. 95–8). There are no controlled trials.

HHV-7

Virology
A betaherpesvirus very similar to HHV-6. First demonstrated in 1990 in an *in vitro* activated CD4+ T cell from a healthy adult. Appears to be shed life-long intermittently from saliva. The extent of its role in human disease is yet to be clearly defined.

Epidemiology
- Seropositivity >95%, although primary infection appears to happen slightly later than HHV-6 at the age of 3.

Clinical features
- Generally asymptomatic. Likely to cause a febrile rash illness in children. Prior to its discovery and availability of molecular diagnostics, many of the clinical manifestations of HHV-6 (particularly in immunocompetent hosts) could be co-attributed.
- Its role in immunosuppressed hosts is not clearly delineated. It may be a cofactor for symptomatic CMV disease in renal transplant recipients.
- Molecular diagnostic tests are not widely available.

Treatment
- Few clinical cases of HHV-7 receive antiviral therapy. It is not a well-researched area. *In vitro* foscarnet, cidofovir, and tenofovir have shown antiviral activity. Notably, it appears to be relatively resistant to ganciclovir.

HHV-8 (Kaposi's sarcoma herpesvirus)

Virology
A gammaherpesvirus with oncogenic potential (like EBV), first identified in Kaposi's Sarcoma (KS); a relatively rare malignancy before the HIV epidemic, where it acts as a cofactor in its development. Like all herpesviruses, latency is established immediately post-primary infection, but it is the environmental cofactors (cellular stress factors, HIV-associated inflammatory cytokines) that induce transition to the lytic phase, with subsequent active viral replication, that are a focus of critical investigation. HHV-8 codes for proteins that control the cell cycle and apoptosis, facilitating its oncogenic potential. Comparisons between the healthy and immunocompromised hosts reveals the importance of cell-mediated immunity (T cells and natural killer cells) in controlling HHV-8. Viral factors will attempt to subvert this (downregulation of MHC and IFN production). Routes of transmission are not well understood and likely vary, depending on the subpopulation in question, but there is ample biological plausibility—mindful of the other herpesviruses—to support sexual, non-sexual (close contact, saliva), and iatrogenic (organ and blood) modes.

Epidemiology
- Reported seroprevalence of HHV-8 show significant variation, based on geography, socio-economic group, and sexuality. Amongst healthy US

adults, ranges from 2% to 30%, and 25–90% in homosexual HIV-positive men without KS. In Africa, seropositivity increases with age, reaching 49% in those aged over 50 years.

Clinical features

- Primary infection—is most likely subclinical but may be associated with a benign febrile rash illness in children. A self-limiting, mononucleosis-like illness, with new-onset lymphadenopathy, has been described in immunocompetent adults, whereas fever, splenomegaly, pancytopenia, and rapid-onset KS have been described in immunocompromised patients.
- KS—four epidemiological types (classic, endemic, HIV-associated, organ transplant-associated). Lesions are vascular, often nodular (0.5–2cm in diameter), and appear on skin, mucous membranes, or viscera (lung and biliary tract in particular). Violaceous or brown/black in pigmented skin. Visceral disease may involve any organ (e.g. GI—can bleed, pulmonary—effusions). Lymphoedema may follow regional lymph node infiltration. Classic KS is a slowly evolving cutaneous proliferative disease seen in elderly Mediterranean and Jewish men, mainly affecting the lower limbs. Endemic KS is more aggressive, with wider dissemination to bone marrow/lymph nodes, and affects immunocompetent children/adults in Africa. HIV-associated KS is the commonest tumour in people with HIV infection. Organ transplant-associated KS is clinically similar to epidemic KS and reflects iatrogenic immunosuppression.
- Primary effusion lymphoma (PEL)—a rare (<5% of lymphoma cases in HIV) aggressive subtype of non-Hodgkin's lymphoma seen in advanced HIV, with a predilection for body cavities. Presents as lymphomatous effusions, arising predominantly in the pleural, pericardial, or peritoneal cavities.
- Castleman's disease—an uncommon lymphoproliferative disorder with fever, spleno(hepato)megaly, and lymphadenopathy. Localized unicentric forms are benign and may be cured by surgical excision. Multicentric Castleman's disease is associated with HHV-8 in 50% of cases, with all HHV-8-associated cases occurring in HIV infection.

Diagnosis

- Serology—rarely undertaken.
- Molecular—PCR is possible, but one must be mindful that HHV-8 viraemia is highly variable (asymptomatic viraemia occurs in 4–20% of cases). Concurrent viraemia certainly supports a diagnosis of KS but is of more diagnostic benefit in PEL/Castleman's disease. Molecular testing of histology samples can be useful for PEL/Castleman's disease.

Treatment

- There is no broadly accepted effective antiviral agent. While numerous agents have demonstrated *in vitro* activity, it is mainly ganciclovir and cidofovir that represent the most used agents *in vivo*.
- Chemotherapy-compatible ART avoiding drug–drug interactions should be commenced if HIV infection is demonstrated.

- Management of KS, PEL, and Castleman's disease require oncology/haematology MDT input.
- KS:
  - limited symptomatic disease—local, rather than systemic, treatment is favoured, comprising intralesional (vinblastine) treatment or radiotherapy. Isolated KS lesions can be observed;
  - extensive cutaneous disease, symptomatic visceral disease, and cutaneous KS that is unresponsive to local therapy warrant systemic chemotherapy (liposomal doxorubicin or daunorubicin). Those who progress on therapy should receive second-line therapy (paclitaxel, pomalidomide). Life-threatening disease may require combination chemotherapy. Experimental therapy includes monoclonal antibodies against vascular endothelial growth factor;
  - forty per cent of transplant-associated KS cases will respond to reduction of immunosuppression alone. This risks graft rejection, and an alternative is to switch immunosuppressive therapy to sirolimus, which has antiangiogenic effects against KS.
- PEL—even with treatment, mean overall survival is 6 months. Where possible, non-HIV-related cases should have any immunosuppressive therapy reduced.
- Castleman's disease—dependent on subtype and disease stage, in addition to co-occurrence of KS. The anti-CD20 agent rituximab and participation in clinical trials are common. Prognosis is variable.

Rotavirus

Virology

Rotavirus in the genus *Rotavirus* is a member of the family *Reoviridae*. It is not enveloped. Unusually, *Reoviridae* have double-stranded, segmented RNA as their genome (most human RNA viruses are single-stranded). Rotavirus has 11 individual segments (~18 000bp in total) that are capable of reassortment (like influenza). This occurs when two rotavirus virions of the same serotype (reassortment cannot occur between serotypes) infect the same cell and segments are exchanged to produce virions different from either 'parent'. There are at least seven serotypes (A–G), based on antibody response to the capsid protein VP6 (viral protein). Sub-serotypes, based on VP7 (G-glycoprotein) and VP4 (P-protease), lend themselves to an influenza-like naming nomenclature (the majority of infections are caused by five genotypes within serotype A; subtype G1P8 is the commonest). The degree and determinants of cross-protective immunity amongst these genotypes are not fully understood, although re-exposure to the same genotype likely manifests in a much-attenuated illness (if not asymptomatic). Pathogenesis of diarrhoea is multifactorial—infection of small intestine luminal enterocytes leads to malabsorption of sugars, which causes an osmotic laxative effect; the non-structural viral protein NSP4 acts as an enterotoxin affecting cellular calcium channels, and rotavirus may directly interfere with the enteric nervous system. On EM, rotavirus has a wheel-like appearance (Latin '*rota*'). Spread is faecal–oral (contaminated food or water, direct contact, or inhalation of aerosol from vomit or faeces).

Rotavirus is very infectious, with a particularly small inoculum needed to establish infection—10–100 virions.

Epidemiology

- Found worldwide, almost universal infection by age 3. Pre-vaccination, it was the commonest cause of severe gastroenteritis in children aged <5 years. Subsequent infection rarely leads to hospitalization.
- Most infection occurs between ages of 6 and 36 months.
- Can show seasonality in temperate climates (UK: January to March), whereas infection occurs year-round in tropical climates. Vaccination, if present, likely modifies this observation.

Clinical features

- Rotavirus is generally accepted as the most dangerous of the viral GI pathogens, with the highest propensity for hospitalization.
- Incubation period of <48h, and virus can be shed for ~10 days, longer in immunocompromised populations. Asymptomatic shedding is possible. Illness overall lasts 3–8 days.
- Infants/young children experience fever, vomiting (duration 2–3 days), and watery (bloodless) diarrhoea (duration 4–5 days).
- Profound dehydration is the most feared complication. This often requires hospital admission for treatment. If this occurs in a healthcare-poor setting, it can easily result in mortality.
- Seizures due to fever/electrolyte disturbance are described.
- Children with immunodeficiency can develop gastroenteritis lasting for many weeks.
- Older children/adults manage GI/fluid loss better due to obvious greater physiological reserve.
- Rotavirus-induced lactase deficiency lasts for up to 2 weeks; beware prompt reintroduction of dairy into the diet.

Diagnosis

- EM is rarely used. Multiple modalities are employed subsequently.
- EIAs are commonly used in faecal samples.
- Molecular techniques—PCR testing of faecal samples is possible, often done as a multiplex with other likely pathogens.

Treatment

- For more information on the management of diarrhoea, ➜ see Infectious diarrhoea, pp. 691–3.
- Fluid replacement is fundamental and the mainstay of care. Should be administered PO in mild and moderate cases. Feeding early in illness (within 24h) promotes enterocyte regeneration and reduces gut permeability. Fruit juices and soft drinks should be avoided. Milk can be given to infants, and lactose-free, carbohydrate-rich foods to older children.
- There is no role for antibiotics nor antimotility drugs, with very limited evidence for the use of (pre-)probiotics.
- Return to most activities once 48h free of symptoms, although should not visit swimming pools for 2 weeks.

Prevention

- Prevention by hygiene alone is difficult. Asymptomatic shedding is common. They are relatively resistant to common handwashing agents and can survive for some time on hard surfaces and in water.
- For management of hospital outbreaks, ➲ see Hospital outbreaks of diarrhoea and vomiting, pp. 194–6.
- There are two live oral vaccines available against rotavirus (see *Rotavirus: the green book*, available at: https://www.gov.uk/government/publications/rotavirus-the-green-book-chapter-27b). Their full efficacy is difficult to measure, but their use has been associated with a 60% fall in death rates due to diarrhoea and a dramatic decrease in hospitalizations. The WHO recommends their addition to immunization schedules in those regions where their efficiency has been demonstrated. They have been in use in the USA since 2006, and were added to the UK schedule in 2013.

Norovirus

Virology

Norovirus is the colloquial name for Norwalk virus (named after the city in Ohio, USA), of which samples from an outbreak in 1968 would show its presence by EM (it is also known as the winter vomiting bug). It is in the genus *Norovirus*, in the family *Caliciviridae*. It is a non-enveloped positive-sense ssRNA virus (linear genome ~8000bp). There is significant genetic diversity, with 10 genogroups and over 50 genotypes; GII.4 is the commonest. Even amongst RNA viruses, there is a very high mutation rate. Immunity post-infection in terms of duration and cross-genotype coverage is poorly understood. It is broadly accepted that it is short-lived and unlikely to be across genogroups. Clinical manifestations are thought secondary to temporary malabsorption of sugar/fat rather than to toxin production per se. Transmission is faecal–oral (contaminated food or water, direct contact, or inhalation of aerosol from vomit or faeces). Like rotavirus, norovirus is very infectious, with a particularly small inoculum needed to establish infection (10–100 virions). It is stable in the environment (as it is non-enveloped), hence its enhanced transmission capabilities.

Epidemiology

- Is the commonest cause of point gastroenteritis globally, especially in countries where rotavirus is on the vaccine schedule. Infection by late childhood is almost universal.
- Leading cause of point foodborne disease outbreaks (e.g. cruise ships, hospitals, prisons, schools, catering).

Clinical features

- Incubation is 24–48h; symptoms last for 2–3 days. Viral shedding lasts for 48h, but longer in immunocompromised.
- Asymptomatic infection is possible/common.
- Vomiting is a dominant feature in most affected people. Very infectious, with high secondary attack rates. Watery diarrhoea follows, with abdominal pain. Sometimes fever is present.
- Some blood groups (O in particular) show increased susceptibility.

Diagnosis/treatment

- Clinically indistinguishable from other acute gastroenteritis, although rapid symptom onset and cluster of cases make norovirus likely.
- Hydration and supportive care are the mainstay.

Prevention

- No antiviral/vaccine exists. Norovirus virions are notoriously resistant to alcohol handwash, low-dose chlorine, and freezing.
- Bleach wash (1000–5000ppm) for surfaces and soap/water for handwashing are recommended.
- Cases should isolate for 48–72h post-symptom resolution.

Sapoviruses

Virology, epidemiology, and clinical features

Sapovirus is a non-enveloped positive-sense ssRNA virus (linear genome of 7500bp) in the family *Caliciviridae* (as is norovirus). It has a 'Star of David'-appearing morphology on EM. It was originally described in samples in the UK, but the prototype strain that has been studied the most comes from samples from an orphanage in Sapporo in Japan in 1982. There are five genogroups, with an increasingly recognized number of genotypes, currently 21. Accurate epidemiology descriptions are lacking, but it is likely underdiagnosed. It causes a similar clinical diarrhoeal phenotype to norovirus (e.g. is capable of individual cases of acute gastroenteritis and carries the potential to cause outbreaks).

Diagnosis and treatment

Diagnosis is normally via molecular testing on a faecal sample. Not all laboratories will have sapovirus on their standard pathogen panel for diarrhoeal illness. Disease is self-limiting, and treatment directed at maintaining hydration.

Astroviruses

Virology, epidemiology, and clinical features

Astrovirus is a non-enveloped positive-sense ssRNA virus (linear genome 8000bp) in the family *Astroviridae*. Currently, there are eight recognized serotypes. The name is derived from its 5- or 6-pointed star appearance when examined by EM. Infection is almost ubiquitous by late childhood, and transmission is faecal–oral. While it is an underrecognized cause of diarrhoeal illness (particularly in children), it is considered to be less pathogenic overall due to asymptomatic infection being well described, in contrast to norovirus. Diarrhoea, malaise and nausea are dominant features, with nausea less common. Incubation is 3–4 days, with symptoms lasting for up to 5 days.

Diagnosis and treatment

Diagnosis is normally via molecular testing or EIA on a faecal sample. Not all laboratories will have astrovirus on their standard pathogen panel for diarrhoeal illness. Disease is self-limited, and treatment directed at maintaining hydration.

Enterovirus and parechovirus

Virology

The word 'enterovirus' (EV) is often used colloquially as a singular term to refer to a number of genera and their many member viruses in the large *Picornaviridae* family. The formal nomenclature in the family has changed (repeatedly), as genetic analysis results prompt more accurate recategorization of its members. Consequently, terms like 'Coxsackie virus' and 'echovirus', while in our daily lexicon, are frequently technically inaccurate (see ℘ https://ictv.global/report/chapter/picornaviridae/picornaviridae/enterovirus). The family *Picornaviridae* is genetically diverse; it contains >60 genera containing almost 150 species (not all are human pathogens). Its members are small, non-enveloped, positive-sense RNA viruses (7000–9000bp). Notable members include polio (⊙ see Poliovirus, p. 460), hepatitis A virus (HAV) (⊙ see Hepatitis A virus, p. 463), and rhinovirus (⊙ see Rhinovirus, p. 415). There are two main genera that are sufficiently clinically similar to discuss here. The genus *Enterovirus* contains all EVs that infect humans and is divided into four species A–D (based on >25% sequence difference in the viral protein (VP1) gene). Members include many of what we used to call 'Coxsackie virus' and 'echovirus'. New additions are named by species and number (e.g. enterovirus D68). The genus *Parechovirus* (PeV) (six species) shares many biological and clinical characteristics with EVs, and the syndromes outlined below can equally be attributed to infections with PeV. Transmission is faecal–oral or respiratory. Vertical transmission is generally accepted to be of little clinical consequence.

Epidemiology

- Infection with EV or PeV is ubiquitous and occurs globally, although the burden of infection occurs in early childhood.
- Found worldwide throughout the year, but in temperate climates, infections peak in summer and autumn months.

Clinical features

- There is a wide spectrum of clinical features, with the majority of infections resulting in either asymptomatic presentation or a self-limiting febrile illness (>90%). Notable clinical entities are discussed individually.
- Neurological syndromes:
  - meningitis—EV is the commonest aetiological agent by a significant margin. Presentation can vary with age, with the very young being more non-specific as meningeal signs are uncommon. Differentiation from bacterial meningitis on clinical grounds can be difficult, even for experienced physicians; hence, CSF analysis is frequently undertaken. In older children/adults, it can manifest as sudden fever (may be biphasic, with a gap as long as 2–10 days), nuchal rigidity, headache,

photophobia, and non-specific features (e.g. vomiting, anorexia, diarrhoea, upper respiratory tract symptoms). In uncomplicated disease, the illness usually lasts for a week. Sequelae are rare in those beyond the neonatal period. Reliable differentiation from other causes of viral meningitis is nigh impossible, except primary VZV where the eponymous rash should be present. As with other viral meningitis, CSF analysis yields a lymphocyte predominance, with a modest increase in protein level and an unchanged glucose level;

- encephalitis—EV is an uncommon cause, relative to herpesviruses (HSV and VZV). Clinical distinction of encephalitis from meningitis is critical, as management differs considerably. Lethargy, drowsiness, seizures, paresis, and coma are commoner in encephalitis. Accurate differentiation between different viral causes of encephalitis is impossible clinically, and CSF analysis is frequently undertaken;
- muscle paralysis (➔ see Poliovirus, p. 460).
- Numerous EV exanthems are recognized:
  - maculopapular eruptions—are very common. Can occur in conjunction with other more predominant symptomatology (e.g. respiratory or neurological disease). Classically non-vesicular in nature (although vesicular manifestations are underrecognized). Resolve spontaneously;
  - herpangina—painful vesicular eruption in the posterior part of the pharynx (soft palate) on the tonsils, causing odynophagia and fever. Commonest in young children. Vesicles are smaller and occur more posteriorly than in classic perioral HSV. Most commonly associated with EV-A species, particularly Coxsackie virus A1–6, 8, 10, and 22;
  - hand, foot, and mouth (HFM)—variably painful vesicular outbreaks on the anterior part of the mouth/buccal mucosa and on the hands and feet. Usually associated with fever. Classically caused by EV-A species, particularly Coxsackie virus A16 and EV-A71.
- Pericarditis—EV can cause (myo)pericarditis that shows considerable variation in both severity and outcome. Again most manifestations are subclinical or resolve without sequelae, but progression to heart failure is described. Numerous other viruses (adenovirus, VZV, HIV), in addition to other infections pathogens, can cause this clinical syndrome. The pathogenesis of viral-induced cardiac injury is poorly understood and heavily debated.
- Respiratory—EV can cause upper respiratory tract symptoms (fever, coryza, cough); these are impossible to differentiate from symptoms caused by the myriad of other respiratory viruses on clinical means alone.
- GI—EV, while capable of causing GI illness (diarrhoea), if detected, may not be the culprit, as incidental detection is common.
- Pregnancy/perinatal—vertical transmission of EV infection is considered rare, although perinatal infection of the mother is linked to an increased incidence of disease in the neonate, which can be severe.

Diagnosis

- As the majority of infections are subclinical and self-resolving, diagnostics are not always undertaken.

- Serology and viral culture are almost never performed outside of a research capacity. Given the ubiquity of infection and the need for paired samples, serology is of particularly little use clinically.
- PCR analysis is the primary method of diagnosing EV infection. It is fast and can be performed on a variety of specimens: blood, CSF, urine, faecal samples, respiratory swabs, and CSF.

Treatment

- As most morbidity is self-limiting, supportive care is the mainstay. Antipyretics and analgesia form the basis of EV meningitis treatment.
- The role of IVIG is debated and likely of little use.
- There are no clinically effective antivirals.

Poliovirus

Virology

PV is a type of enterovirus (EV) (⊙ see enterovirus and parechovirus, pp. 458–60). It is in the family *Picornaviridae*, genus *Enterovirus*, and species C, and has three serotypes (PV1–3). It is a non-enveloped, icosahedral, positive-sense ssRNA virus (7500bp). The majority of cases of paralytic disease is caused by PV-1. Cross-protection between serotypes is incomplete. It is increasingly recognized that other EVs may be capable of causing paralytic disease (e.g. EV-A71, D68, and D70). The virus replicates in the GI tract and adjacent lymphoid tissue. It is highly neurotropic. The CNS is probably infected by retrograde axonal transport from muscle to nerve to cord. The most feared complication is acute flaccid weakness due to anterior horn cell injury. Neurons throughout the grey matter are affected, especially those within the anterior horn of the spinal cord and the motor nuclei of the medulla and pons. Distribution of lesions is similar in all cases—it is their severity that determines clinical disease. Transmission is faecal–oral; hence, PV carries epidemic potential in areas with poor sanitation and suboptimal vaccination rates. Conversely, as humans are the only natural host and there is only a small number of serotypes, improving hygiene standards and an effective vaccination programme make global elimination possible.

Epidemiology

- Polio was largely sporadic in the nineteenth century, affecting mostly children aged <5 years. By 1950, developing world infections were epidemic in nature, with most cases in children aged 5–9 years (one-third in those aged over 15 years). This was attributed to rising standards of hygiene, delaying inapparent infections that previously took place in early childhood, thereby conferring widespread immunity. The resulting pool of older, susceptible individuals facilitated epidemics in a cohort more likely to develop neurological complications.
- Rates fell dramatically after vaccine introduction. Two forms exist: inactivated polio vaccine (IPV) by Salk in 1956 and the attenuated live oral polio vaccine (OPV) by Sabin in 1962. The last naturally occurring UK case was in 1984. In the UK, 40 cases were notified between 1984 and 2002—30 were vaccine-associated, and six had wild-type imported virus, with the source not identified in the remainder.

- The Global Polio Eradication Initiative has seen the number of countries where polio transmission has never been interrupted fall from >125 (1988) to three (Afghanistan, Pakistan, and Nigeria), although many countries remain vulnerable and at risk of outbreaks, especially as economic instability and migration become more prevalent (see GPEI Global Polio Eradication Initiative, available at: ℛ https://polioeradication.org/).

Clinical features

- In addition to being caused by the wild-type virus, disease can be caused by the attenuated virus contained in the live vaccine reverting to a more virulent form. This is termed vaccine-associated paralytic poliomyelitis (VAPP). It was commoner with the PV-2 serotype. Overall, this is an extremely rare occurrence and most likely to occur in immunodeficient individuals (in whom it is contraindicated, like most live vaccines) and in areas of low immunity. There, PV can replicate and transmit, reaching a threshold that gives sufficient opportunity for mutations to occur, reversing its initial attenuation. This is biologically impossible to occur with the inactivated vaccine.
- Infection is largely asymptomatic (>95%); <0.1% develop symptoms of paresis. The ratio of subclinical to paralytic illness can be 1000:1 in children, rising to 75:1 in adults.
- Transmission is primarily faecal–oral, but during epidemics, it can be spread by pharyngeal secretions. Infectious virus can be secreted for many weeks (up to 6) post-illness.
- The incubation period for paralytic illness is 3–21 days (shorter for non-paralytic illness: 3–6 days). An initial prodrome s experienced by 4–8% of patients, which is termed 'minor illness', and correlates with 2–3 days of fever, headache, sore throat, anorexia, vomiting, and abdominal pain. Most will not progress from this. A minority will see relative recovery from the 'minor illness' and progress to CNS involvement with typical meningitis symptomatology, and a minority again will progress to the development of motor weakness.
- Classic paralytic polio is divided into three types, based on the distribution of weakness:
  - spinal polio (80% of cases)—asymmetrical weakness that more commonly affects the legs, rather than the arms, where proximal involvement is more severe than distal. Initial hyperactive reflexes become absent. Bladder paralysis usually accompanies the leg weakness. Sensory loss (consider GBS) or disturbed cognition is unusual;
  - bulbar paralytic polio (1–2% of cases)—paralysis of muscle groups innervated by the lower cranial nerves (IX–X I), resulting in dysphagia and weakness of respiratory, facial, and oropharyngeal muscles. Medullary circulatory and respiratory centres may become involved.;
  - bulbospinal polio (19% of cases)—mixed bulbar and spinal involvement is commoner than isolated bulbar. This represents progression of spinal involvement and shows progression over 2–3 days, halting when the patient becomes afebrile;
  - polioencephalitis—an extremely uncommon form occurring mainly in infants. Presentation is typical for encephalitis.

- Post-poliomyelitis syndrome refers to new or progressive muscle weakness/disability, on average 35 years after the initial infection; 20–30% of patients with existing paralytic polio will experience this syndrome in previously affected muscle groups. This is thought to be due to attrition of motor units in innervated muscle that is already less innervated due to initial disease rather than due to an infectious process. There is no excretion of live virus.
- Prognosis—prior to vaccination, mortality of paralytic disease was 5–10%, rising to 20–60% with bulbar involvement. Mortality increases with age. When paralysis is present, it tends to reach its peak by 72h. The degree of recovery can be assessed at 1 month, at which point most reversible muscle paralysis in spinal disease will have resolved. Any weakness or paralysis present at 12 months is usually permanent and occurs in two-thirds of patients. Complete recovery is rare with severe paralysis, particularly if requiring ventilation. Those surviving bulbar disease show the best recovery, with significant improvement by 10 days and ultimately usually attaining normal function.
- Risk factors for paralysis—prepubertal ♂, pregnancy, B-cell deficiency (increases the risk of OPV-associated disease), strenuous exercise within the first 3 days of major illness, IM injections (paralysis localizes to the limb injected or injured within 2–4 weeks before infection), those who have had a tonsillectomy (eight times the risk of those with tonsils).
- Complications—respiratory compromise requiring ventilatory assistance (involve ICU early), and the eponymous long-term muscle paralysis.

Diagnosis

- Early clinical recognition of infectious flaccid paralysis is key. Notify public health authorities early (see UK polio outbreak guidelines, available at: ℘ https://assets.publishing.service.gov.uk/media/5d888 d10e5274a157558dbdd/National_polio_guidelines_2019.pdf).
- Faeces—molecular detection and sequencing of EV isolated in faecal samples is gold standard. Confirmatory testing and distinction between vaccine-derived or wild-type virus can be performed, and liaison with EV reference laboratory is crucial.
- Serology is of almost no use due to the need for paired sampling and the inability to make a formal diagnosis alone.

Treatment

- No specific antiviral therapy. Management is supportive. No role for IVIG.
- Physiotherapy and MDT planning can start once progression of paralysis has ceased.

Vaccination

- Overall, efficacy rates for the live OPV and inert IPV are comparable. The OPV was widely used historically in mass vaccination campaigns due to ease of use (PO administration) and its ability to induce both humoral and mucosal (GI) immunity (decreases asymptomatic shedding during infection). However, due to the incidence of VAPP (4 out of

1 000 000 vaccinated children, lower since removal of PV-2), its use in developed countries has declined dramatically. It still has a role in endemic countries and during outbreaks. The IPV is the vaccine of choice in most countries, including the UK, but requires trained staff to administer (IM) and does not induce mucosal immunity. It is only available as a combined vaccine (see *Folio: the green book*, available at: 🔊 https://www.gov.uk/government/publications/polio-the-green-book-chapter-26).

Hepatitis viruses

The colloquially named hepatitis viruses (A–E) share only hepatotropism as a characteristic. The individual viral pathogens are a heterogeneous group, each belonging to a completely different virus family. Consequently, fundamental differences emerge: the ability to establish chronic infection (B, C, D, rarely E), differing primary routes of transmission—oral (A, E) versus blood-borne (B, C, D)—and whether they are vaccine-preventable (A, B). Clinically, testing for hepatitis viruses occurs simultaneously (e.g. 'acute viral hepatitis panel') and usually not in isolation unless in chronicity.

Numerous other pathogens can cause liver inflammation: viral (HSV, EBV, CMV, adenovirus, yellow fever (YF), and HIV), bacterial, and protozoal (leptospirosis, syphilis, Q fever, toxoplasmosis, etc.).

Novel hepatitis viruses

Further efforts to identify novel viruses have led to the discovery of other hepatitis viruses, the significance of which are yet to be fully understood.

Hepatitis G

Hepatitis G virus (sometimes called GB virus, the initials of the index patient) is a flavivirus that is best described in blood donor pools. The clinical implications and significance are largely unknown. It appears to be innocuous clinically despite widespread seroprevalence.

Differential diagnosis

Other non-viral infectious diseases may cause acute hepatitis:
- leptospirosis (➋ see *Leptospira* species, pp. 376–8);
- syphilis (➋ see Syphilis, pp. 760–2);
- toxoplasmosis (➋ see *Toxoplasma gondii*, pp. 562–6);
- Q fever (➋ see *Coxiella burnetii*, pp. 332–4).

Hepatitis A virus

Virology

HAV is a non-enveloped* positive-sense ssRNA virus (linear genome 7500bp) in the genus *Hepatovirus*, family *Picornaviridae*. Although there are approximately three genotypes, there is only a single serotype. The

---

* An unusual facet of the HAV replication cycle blurs this orthodox description. In addition to non-enveloped virions excreted in the faeces of infected patients, quasi-enveloped (surrounded by the host membrane) virions are secreted into the bloodstream. Their full role is incompletely understood but likely contributes towards expanding infection within the liver.

liver is the target organ for infection, and although viral replication is non-cytopathic, the induced cytotoxic T-cell response can result in hepatocyte death. The replication cycle is typical of that for a positive-sense RNA virus. Transmission is predominantly faecal–oral; hence, historic descriptions of epidemic jaundice can probably be attributed to HAV. Secondary transmission through close person-to-person transmission (same household), contaminated blood products, or sexual (oral–anal) contact is described.

Epidemiology

HAV is found worldwide, and can be both sporadic and epidemic. It is endemic in countries with poor sanitation where—compounded by overcrowding—it is an illness of childhood. This gives rise to the 'HAV paradox'. Infection in childhood is largely asymptomatic, but improvements in hygiene practices, coupled with incomplete vaccination, lead to infection occurring later in life where HAV-attributable morbidity/mortality are actually higher. In the UK, stringent hygiene practices have seen the incidence fall in children, which, coupled with the HAV vaccine not being in the routine immunization schedule, result in the majority of the adult population being susceptible to infection. Outbreaks have occurred amongst MSM, people who inject drugs (PWID), any communal accommodation areas, and returning travellers from endemic areas.

Clinical features

Incubation is usually 28–30 days but ranges between 15 and 50 days. Cases are infectious throughout the incubation period and for 1 week post-development of jaundice, broadly mirroring viral excretion in the faeces. Disease is usually mild, with fulminant hepatic failure being rare (<1%). Incidence of morbidity/mortality and complications increase with age.
- Subclinical infection—common in children (>90% if aged <5 years).
- Acute hepatitis—symptomatic infection occurs in 70% of adults. An abrupt prodrome of fever, headache, malaise, anorexia, vomiting, and right upper quadrant pain is followed by dark urine, pruritus, and pale faeces. Occasionally diarrhoea, cough, coryzal symptoms, or arthralgia may occur (commoner in children). Physical findings: jaundice, hepatomegaly, splenomegaly (5–15%). LFTs are elevated in a hepatitic fashion (rather than cholestatic), with very high AST and ALT levels (classically >1000IU/L).
- Complications include prolonged cholestasis, relapsing disease, fulminant hepatitis (rare, commoner in older patients), extrahepatic disease, and triggering of autoimmune chronic active hepatitis.

Diagnosis

- Serology—IgM is detectable reliably once symptoms are present and lasts for 3–6 months. IgG becomes positive at 2–3 months and persists for life. It is not possible to differentiate by serology IgG due to natural infection/immunity from IgG due to vaccination.
- PCR—it is possible to test the serum for viraemia, but generally serology and history/clinical features are sufficient.

Treatment

- Acute hepatitis—symptomatic (avoid paracetamol and alcohol); 85% have full clinical/biochemical recovery by 3 months.

- Fulminant hepatitis—cases should be discussed with regional liver transplantation units.
- Acute HAV is a notifiable infection to public health authorities.

Prevention

- Pre-exposure prophylaxis—HAV vaccination. Several inactivated HAV vaccines exist, including co-formulations (HAV with hepatitis B virus (HBV) or typhoid). Administration schedule varies, but they are all highly effective. Indications are numerous but include travellers to endemic areas, patients with chronic liver disease/haemophilia, and regular recipients of blood products (see *Hepatitis A: the green book*, available at: ℘ https://www.gov.uk/government/publications/hepatitis-a-the-green-book-chapter-17).
- PEP—uses a combination of HAV vaccine and human normal immunoglobulin (HNIG). HAV is indicated within 2 weeks of exposure for all contacts of acute HAV. HNIG is occasionally also given to those thought less likely to mount a robust immune response (extremes of age, immunocompromised) or be at high risk of severe disease (chronic liver disease). Full UK guidance on post-exposure hepatitis A is available at: ℘ https://www.gov.uk/government/publications/hepatitis-a-the-green-book-chapter-17

Hepatitis B virus

Virology

HBV is a blood-borne virus—thereby transmitted in three ways: vertically (*in utero*), sexually, and by exposure to infected blood (transfusion or needles). It is not spread by saliva.

HBV is an enveloped, partially double-stranded DNA virus (circular genome 3200bp) in the genus *Orthohepadnavirus* and the archetype member of the *Hepadnaviridae* family. HBV maximizes its coding capacity by using four overlapping reading frames (sections of the genome that are translated). Each corresponds to one of its four genes (surface, core, polymerase, and X) to produce seven proteins (three variants of HBsAg, in addition to HBeAg, HbcAg, HBx, and polymerase). There are approximately eight accepted genotypes (A–H), based on >8% difference in the genome, along with an additional putative two genotypes (I and J), as well as numerous subtypes. There is an association between the genotype and the likelihood of development of hepatocellular carcinoma (HCC) and response to IFN.

The infectious virion (termed a Dane particle) is composed of an outer envelope that contains hepatitis B surface antigen (HBsAg) with a diameter of 42nm. There are three different forms of HBsAg, which differ by size. Beneath the envelope is the nucleocapsid containing hepatitis B core antigen (HBcAg), which surrounds the genome. The precise role of hepatitis B e antigen (HBeAg) is not clear, as it is not necessary for viral replication. It is noteworthy, as it is a component in numerous diagnostic and treatment algorithms because it is crudely attached to disease activity. However, mutations (most commonly G1896A) in the viral promoter (core) driving its transcription can stop its production. This results in 'pre-core mutant' virus whereby patients will appear HBeAg-negative but have high viral loads with high disease activity. The final protein produced is called X (HBx). It is a non-structural protein with numerous purported roles and is incompletely understood. It is essential to viral replication and may play a role in the development of HCC. The loss of HBeAg and the development of hepatitis B e antibody (anti-HBe), known as eAg seroconversion, represent a desirable degree of host immune control response with favourable disease outcomes.

HBV has a unique replication cycle. It replicates exclusively in hepatocytes after gaining entry through a bile salt cell receptor involved in the enterohepatic circulation called NTCP (sodium taurocholate cotransporting polypeptide). Although it is a DNA virus, HBV replicates through an RNA intermediate, mandating the use of RT to turn RNA into DNA. Upon entry into the nucleus, the incomplete double-stranded genome, termed relaxed circular DNA (rcDNA), is repaired by host polymerases to form covalently closed circular DNA (cccDNA). cccDNA exists as an epigenetic minichromosome (separate to host DNA), from which all transcription occurs. Conventional antivirals (➲ see Antivirals for hepatitis B, pp. 101–3) do not have a direct effect on the cccDNA pool, and persistence of cccDNA represents a route by which reactivation of otherwise quiescent disease occurs, in addition to acting as the primary barrier towards achieving a sterilizing cure. The presence of cccDNA has been demonstrated in patients many years after recovery from acute infection. Although some integration into the host genome does occur, this happens infrequently and, unlike HIV, does not represent the transcriptional template for virion production. Integration of HBV DNA may contribute to the oncogenic potential of HBV infection due to interfering with host protein production, depending on the location of insertion into the host genome. During replication, many fold (>1000) smaller, non-infectious particles composed of HBsAg alone are secreted. It is thought these non-infectious particles serve as a decoy to overwhelm the immune system.

The risk of developing chronic infection is inversely related to age. If infected perinatally, the chance of developing chronic infection exceeds 90%; this decreases to between 20% and 60% for those aged between 6 months and 6 years, and declines to under 5% if infection occurs in an adult.

Epidemiology

- HBV infection is a global public health problem, with an estimated 2 billion people having been infected at some point and almost 300 million people showing signs of chronic infection.
  - HBV-attributed liver cirrhosis and HCC cause ~1 million deaths per year.
  - HBV infection carries a 10–25% lifetime risk of HCC and can develop in the absence of cirrhosis (in contrast to HCV infection).
  - Globally, 54% of HCC cases can be attributed to HBV infection.
  - In HBV infection with concomitant cirrhosis, there is a 2% annual risk of developing HCC.
- The global prevalence is ~3.6%, but this burden is shared unequally, ranging from <2% in low-prevalence countries (e.g. the USA, Western Europe) to >8% in parts of China and sub-Saharan Africa. This variation largely reflects differences in age at which infection occurs. Infection in

countries with low prevalence is largely due to migration and contact with contaminated blood, whereas in countries with higher endemicity, infection is due to vertical transmission and early childhood infection.

- HBV is a silent epidemic that is compounded by a lack of disease awareness, with only 10.5% of patients aware of their diagnosis and 16.7% receiving treatment. Even with combined neonatal vaccination and treatment to prevent vertical transmission, it will take centuries to eradicate HBV in the absence of new antivirals.

Clinical features

- HBV is a hepatotropic virus that causes chronic liver disease that can progress to cirrhosis and is a significant risk factor for HCC development. It is often the host inflammatory immune response to the virus that causes repeated flares of hepatitis, during which damage occurs. Extrahepatic manifestations (probably immune complex-mediated) are most commonly in the form of polyarteritis nodosa and glomerular disease.
- Acute hepatitis B (notifiable illness) has an incubation period of 1–4 months; 30–50% of patients are asymptomatic, with 30% developing acute hepatitis. Symptoms include malaise, nausea, abdominal pain, and jaundice. These settle over 1–3 months. Fulminant hepatic failure is rare (0.1–0.5%). Supportive care is the mainstay, with only particularly severe cases considered for antiviral therapy (signs of liver failure, coagulopathy).
- Chronic hepatitis B (presence of HBsAg in blood for >6 months) can be entirely asymptomatic. This poses a major barrier to diagnosis and is often only diagnosed on routine screening (antenatal or new GP registrations). Chronic HBV infection is dynamic, reflecting an interplay between the host immune response and the virus, which is reflected into five disease stages, outlined below (for HBV guidelines from European Association for the Study of the Liver (EASL), see ℬ https://easl.eu/publication/easl-guidelines-management-of-hepatitis-b/). This nomenclature classifies these stages based on the eAg status (present/not present) and infection (minimal liver damage) or hepatitis (liver damage occurring). They serve as a guide to anticipate, and thereby prevent, periods of greatest liver damage, with initiation of suppressive treatment. The disease stages do not always occur in a linear fashion nor will all stages be experienced by every patient:
  - HBeAg-positive infection (immunotolerant phase)—high viral loads (>10⁷IU/mL), with normal ALT levels and minimal liver damage;
  - HBeAg-positive hepatitis (immune reactive)—mainly high viral loads (10⁴–10⁷IU/mL), with raised ALT levels associated with liver damage. These occur as disease flares, with periods of normal ALT levels/low viral loads in between, making differentiation from the previous phase only possible by extended surveillance (>2 years). eAg seroconversion is most likely to occur during this phase;
  - HBeAg-negative infection (inactive carrier)—are usually anti-Hbe positive, with normal ALT levels and low viral loads. Minimal liver damage occurs if the patient remains in this stage;

- HBeAg-negative hepatitis—fluctuating viral loads and ALT levels. Liver damage can occur. These patients may harbour pre-core mutant virus;
- HBsAg negative, also known as occult HBV infection—defined as the presence of replication-competent virus (either as rcDNA in blood or cccDNA in hepatocytes) without HBsAg. Normally represents late-state disease, with very low/undetectable viral loads, with or without anti-HBs.

Diagnosis

Diagnosis is made serologically (see Table 8.2) and confirmed by PCR:

- HBsAg—the first serological marker to appear (1–10 weeks after acute infection). Clearance marks resolution of acute infection. Those who clear infection become negative within 6 months;
- anti-HBs (surface antibody)—the serological marker of immunity. Usually done as a quantitative assay, with >10mIU/mL considered full protection;
- anti-HBc—the antibody to HBcAg. Mainly used in conjunction with anti-HBs to determine if immunity is due to natural infection (present) or vaccination (absent). Specific IgM anti-HBc can be performed if

Table 8.2 Interpretation of HBV serology

A	HBsAg	Negative		No evidence of HBV infection or vaccination, remains susceptible to disease
	Anti-HBc	Negative		
	Anti-HBs	Negative		
B	HBsAg	Negative		Immune due to natural infection
	Anti-HBc		Positive	
	Anti-HBs		Positive	
C	HBsAg	Negative		Immune due to vaccination
	Anti-HBc	Negative		
	Anti-HBs		Positive	
D	HBsAg		Positive	Acute HBV infection
	Anti-HBc (IgM)		Positive	
	Anti-HBc		Positive	
	Anti-HBs	Negative		
E	HBsAg		Positive	Chronic HBV infection
	Anti-HBc (IgM)	Negative		
	Anti-HBc	Negative		
	Anti-HBs	Negative		
F	HBsAg	Negative		Isolated anti-HBc represents an unusual pattern (needs repeat and further discussion)
	Anti-HBc		Positive	
	Anti-HBs	Negative		

acute infection is thought likely. Isolated anti-HBc is unusual and may represent a few scenarios. Possibilities include late-stage disease with burnt-out infection (check e status), weak and non-specific reactivity in the laboratory assay, or resolving acute infection prior to the appearance of anti-HBs;

- HBeAg—a secretory protein that is not required for viral replication. It is used as a crude marker of HBV replication and infectivity. Seroconversion to anti-HBe remains a desirable clinical outcome.

- HBV PCR assays—accurate quantification of HBV DNA in the serum is performed and reported in standarcized IU/mL. Measurement of intrahepatic cccDNA is not undertaken clinically.

Treatment

- General—avoid alcohol; safe sexual practices; hepatitis A vaccination (if non-immune); optimize treatment of comorbidities (treat HIV/HCV co-infection).
- Use of HBV vaccine and immunoglobulin in household, occupational, and sexual contacts, in addition to antenatal care of HBV-exposed babies, in order to prevent infection (for details, see *Hepatitis B: the green book*, available at: ℘ https://www.gov.uk/government/publications/hepatitis-b-the-green-book-chapter-18).
- The decision to commence antiviral therapy is based on the assessment of: serological (e status), virological (serum DNA quantification), biochemical (ALT), and non-invasive estimates of liver damage or inflammation, based on transient elastography (a bedside noninvasive measurement of liver stiffness using ultrasonography). Liver biopsy is rarely performed. See full HBV guidance from National Institute for Health and Care Excellence (NICE) and EASL (available at ℘ https://easl.eu/publication/easl-guidelines-management-of-hepatitis-b/). Summarized treatment indications are:
  - patients with (de)compensated cirrhosis and detectable viral DNA (irrespective of ALT);
  - patients with moderate fibrosis (F2 disease >8kPa on FibroScan) (irrespective of e status), with viral DNA >2000IU/mL and raised ALT levels;
  - patients with viral DNA >20 000IU/mL and raised ALT levels (irrespective of fibrosis score);
  - patients over age 30 with DNA >2000IU/mL and raised ALT levels (irrespective of fibrosis score);
  - patients under age 30 with DNA >2000IU/mL, raised ALT levels, and evidence of fibrosis on biopsy or FibroScan score >6 (irrespective of fibrosis score);
  - patients about to commence immunosuppressive therapy, particularly B-cell-depleting agents.
- Choosing the agent (➔ see Antivirals for hepatitis B, pp. 101–3):
  - IFN is considered first line but is rarely chosen due to its side effect profile and lack of efficacy.
  - Suppressive therapy with a nucleos(t)ide analogue is the mainstay, and treatment should be continued for at least 12 months after HBsAg loss or eAg seroconversion.

- Patients not on therapy still require routine surveillance.
- Screening for HCC with 6-monthly ultrasound scanning is undertaken in select high-risk individuals (family members with HCC, high viral load, age) (see HBV guidelines from NICE and EASL, available at ✆ https://cks.nice.org.uk/topics/hepatitis-b/).

Hepatitis D virus

Virology

Hepatitis delta virus (HDV) is a fascinating entity that is best described as a satellite virus in the genus *Deltavirus*. Although it can replicate (its genome) autonomously, cellular co-infection with HBV is required to assemble and secrete infectious particles. HDV has a small circular negative-sense ssRNA genome (1700bp), which is encased in hepatitis D antigen (HDAg) to form the nucleocapsid. This is surrounded by the envelope, which is made of HBsAg. HDV has a single open reading frame, which produces a single protein (HDAg—although two forms exist) and utilizes host polymerases to replicate. HDV has common modes of transmission with HBV and is acquired either at the same time as (co-infection) or subsequently (superinfection) to HBV. It is currently classified into eight genotypes. HDV superinfection usually results in suppression of HBV replication by poorly described mechanisms.

Epidemiology

HDV is hyperendemic in some geographical areas; ranges of 5–15% amongst HBsAg-positive individuals.

Clinical features

- Co-infection will present identically to mono-infection with acute HBV. Usually HDV will resolve and not become chronic.
- Superinfection can appear as a particularly severe flare of hepatitis in chronic HBV, and progression to chronic HDV infection is expectant. Generally, dual infection accelerates the progression of HBV-associated liver disease.

Diagnosis

- First, diagnose HBV; HDV cannot exist without it. All patients with chronic HBV should be tested for HDV at baseline, with repeat if indicated.
- HDV antibodies—appear late (4 weeks), but >90% of patients will be positive by 2 months.
- Patients with detectable HDV antibody should have a PCR to determine RNA (viral load).

Treatment

- First, diagnose and manage HBV appropriately; HDV cannot exist without it. All patients with chronic HBV should be tested for HDV at baseline, with repeat testing undertaken if indicated.

- While the optimal treatment of HDV is unknown, those with evidence of liver disease due to HDV should be treated with IFNα (➔ see Antivirals for hepatitis B, pp. 101–3), despite low rates of clearance.
- Investigational agents are under review, which include Myrcludex B (an entry inhibitor targeting the NTCP receptor), lonafarnib (prenylation inhibitor, crucial to virion assembly), and REP 2139 (nucleic acid polymer, blocking the release of HBsAg).

Hepatitis C virus

Virology

HCV is an enveloped positive-sense ssRNA virus (linear genome 9600bp) in the genus *Hepacivirus*, family *Flaviviridae*. Two envelope glycoproteins E1/ E2 (important for receptor binding, cell entry, and immune evasion due to a hypervariable region on E2) surround the icosahedral capsid made of core protein, which is wrapped around the genome. Replication takes place in the cytoplasm of hepatocytes (primarily), and the genome is translated from a single open reading frame into a large single polyprotein (3000 amino acids). This is cleaved into three structural proteins (E1, E2, C) and seven non-structural (NS) ones (p7, NS2, NS3 NS4a, NS4b, NS5a, NS5b).

HCV is a highly genetically diverse virus. Globally, there are seven major genotypes (G1–7), the sequence of which can differ by up to 30%, and these may be further grouped into subtypes (e.g. 1a, 1b), of which there are >60. Even within a host, numerous quasispecies will be present, the genetic heterogeneity of which will become increasingly diverse over time. This genetic heterogeneity is, in part, attributable to RNA polymerase lacking a proofreading mechanism. Genotypes show geographical variation and, historically, were important predictors of clinical outcome. G1 and G4 are less responsive to IFN, but this is of less importance since the arrival of directly acting antivirals (DAAs) (➔ see Antivirals for hepatitis C, p. 104). HCV is a blood-borne virus and so can be spread (like HIV/HBV) sexually or by exposure to infected blood (transfusion or needles). In rare circumstances, it can be transmitted vertically (*in utero*) (~5% risk). It is not spread by saliva. There is no vaccine.

Epidemiology

- HCV is found worldwide, with chronic infection occurring in 70 million people and an additional 100 million people showing serological evidence of past exposure. Not all countries bear this burden equally, and rates of endemicity vary from 0.5% to >2% and can be concentrated in certain subpopulations (e.g. PWID). Accurate and contemporary individual country epidemiological data can be lacking. Traditionally, the eastern Mediterranean region, followed by African and European regions, bore the highest prevalence rates, according to WHO figures. Egypt has the highest endemic seroprevalence at almost 15%.
- Chronic HCV is a significant risk factor for the development of chronic liver disease and cirrhosis, in addition to HCC. The precise risk of progression to cirrhosis in patients with chronic HCV infection is difficult to estimate due to a dynamic interplay of numerous host,

environmental, and viral variables (age, gender, ethnicity, co-infection with HBV/HIV, alcohol intake, and diabetes), but ranges from 15% to 30% within 20 years. In contrast to HBV, the majority of HCV-associated HCC cases occur in patients with cirrhosis in whom the risk of developing HCC is estimated at 1–5% per annum.

Clinical features

- Acute HCV—majority (75%) of infection cases are asymptomatic. Clinically symptomatic infection is similar to acute HAV and HBV infections. Jaundice, dark urine, and general systemic symptoms of malaise and nausea. Biochemical tests will reveal LFT dysfunction in a hepatitic pattern (elevated AST/ALT levels). Presents 7–8 weeks (range 2–26 weeks) after exposure. Treatment is supportive. Fulminant hepatic failure is rare and appears to be commoner in HBV co-infection. Of note, there is little to no immunity gained to prevent subsequent reinfection.
- Chronic HCV—~30% (15–45%) will spontaneously clear the virus within 6 months; the rest will develop chronic infection (defined as the presence of HCV RNA in serum >6 months), which is associated with fatigue, malaise, and reduced quality of life indices. Greatly increased risk of developing (de)compensated liver disease, cirrhosis, and HCC. Patients with liver cirrhosis require additional healthcare interventions (regardless of HCV status), including screening for varices and 6-monthly surveillance for HCC. Consultation with a hepatologist is recommended.
- Extrahepatic manifestations are described, with varying incidence—mixed cryoglobulinaemia, membranoproliferative glomerulonephritis, sporadic porphyria cutanea tarda, Mooren's corneal ulcers, Sjögren's syndrome, lichen planus, pulmonary fibrosis, thyroid hormone abnormalities.

Diagnosis

- Serology—detection of anti-HCV antibodies is unable to differentiate between past (cleared) or current (active) infection. Antibody development is slow and averages 60 days, sometimes longer (immunocompromised). Antibodies remain detectable for life; therefore, serology is unable to diagnose reinfection. For occupational exposures, serological follow-up extends to 24 weeks post-incident for this reason. Non-specific reactivity (false positives) can occur, most commonly in pregnancy and in haemodialysis and immunocompromised patients; discussion with local virology laboratories is essential to aid in further diagnostics/interpretation.
- Molecular—HCV RNA is usually detectable 1–3 weeks after infection and almost certainly by the time symptoms develop.
- Genotype testing—usually undertaken before treatment, although several pan-genotypic regimens exist.
- Resistance testing is usually only undertaken when previous treatment (failure) has occurred or if there is clinical suspicion.

Treatment

Treatment for HCV has been transformed by the development of highly effective (>95% cure) DAAs. Most regimens are PO, IFN-free, and well tolerated (➜ see Antivirals for hepatitis C, pp. 104–7).

Hepatitis E virus

Virology

Hepatitis E virus (HEV) is a positive-sense ssRNA virus (linear genome ~7200bp) in the genus *Orthohepevirus* family *Hepeviridae*. The replication cycle is incompletely understood, and t is recognized that some quasi-enveloped virions are secreted into the bloodstream, in addition to non-enveloped virions secreted into the faeces (like HAV). There are approximately four genotypes (G) that show geographical variation—G1–2 only infect humans, but G3–4 can infect animals (pigs, boar, and deer) and humans (i.e. zoonotic potential). While primarly a hepatotropic virus, several extrahepatic manifestations are noted. Reinfection, although possible, likely leads to a greatly attenuated illness due to previous immunity. Transmission is (similar to HAV) predominantly faecal–oral (G1–2) or enteral following ingestion of contaminated food (G3–4). Transmission from blood products is increasingly recognized, which can lead to chronic infection in the immunocompromised. HEV is an infection that is increasingly attracting attention as an underrecognized contributor to global liver morbidity.

Epidemiology

- Overall, the epidemiology is incompletely understood. HEV is endemic in most countries, and infection can be both sporadic and epidemic. Even within countries, infection hotspots can occur.
- Many cases (particularly in resource-rich settings) represent a zoonotic infection (classically, following ingestion of pork produce, in the UK, 85% of pigs show signs of past infection). Although the number of cases reported in the UK is increasing (~1000 annually), it likely represents a significant underestimate as most acute cases will be subclinical.

Clinical features

- Incubation period is 15–60 days. The duration of infectivity is at least 1 week before to 2–5 weeks after symptom onset. Viraemia typically lasts for 3–6 weeks in immunocompetent patients.
- Acute hepatitis/infection—most will have a self-limiting illness that is either entirely asymptomatic or subclinical. Age, comorbidities, and past infection status play a role in determining those that become symptomatic. In symptomatic patients, jaundice occurs in association with fever, nausea, vomiting, and abdominal tenderness. Biochemical tests will show raised LFTs (classically AST/ALT) and raised bilirubin levels. The clinical picture will be indistinguishable from that of other causes of acute viral hepatitis.
- Complications—acute hepatic failure is rare overall (<4%) but is more likely to occur during pregnancy (classically third trimester), in the immunocompromised (organ transplant recipients, HIV), and in

pre-existing chronic liver disease. The rates of developing chronic infection (almost exclusively G3/4) are poorly understood, and chronic HEV infection (defined as RNA in faeces/blood >3 months) should be in the differential of cryptogenic hepatitis in the aforementioned populations. Cholestasis may be prolonged; arthralgia and urticarial rash may occur.

- Extrahepatic neurological manifestations are increasingly recognized, in particular neuralgic amyotrophy, GBS, encephalitis/myelitis, Bell's palsy, peripheral neuropathy, brachial neuritis, and vestibular neuritis.

Diagnosis

- Serology—IgM and IgG responses occur early in infection and are usually detectable by the onset of clinical illness. IgM develops first and is detectable in >90% of cases 1–4 weeks post-infection and wanes within a few weeks. IgG develops 2–4 weeks post-infection. Consequently, samples with IgM alone should be interpreted with caution; repeat serology and molecular analysis should be undertaken. HEV serology is non-specific, and results must be taken in the clinical context. Samples frequently need to be sent to reference laboratories for confirmatory tests. Antigen assays are rarely used.
- Molecular—HEV RNA is detectable in blood (most sensitive) and faeces. PCR is more sensitive that serology. Virus in the serum can be detected 2–6 weeks post-infection, whereas in faeces, it appears 1 week before the onset of illness and persists for 2 weeks. Serial quantitative viral load measurements are possible to assess response to treatments.

Treatment

- Treatment is supportive for acute infection, and most will require no additional therapy.
- In acute infection resulting in fulminant hepatitis, referral to the regional liver transplantation unit is key.
- In SOT recipients who develop chronic infection, the possibility of reducing immunosuppression should be explored initially. Subsequently, ribavirin for 12 weeks is recommended. If RNA is still detectable at this point, the option to extend for a further 12 weeks can be considered. If this fails to clear the infection, there is no clear consensus on what therapy to implement. Pegylated (PEG)-IFN has been used, with some success (for EASL guidance, see ⌖ https://easl.eu/publication/hepati tis-e-virus-infection-guideline/).

Prevention

- Improved sanitation is likely to be important in the control of an infection that is predominantly spread by the faeco–oral route. Travelers to endemic areas should avoid water of unknown purity, uncooked shellfish, etc.
- Pork should be cooked properly to prevent possible zoonotic transmission.
- Patients who develop abnormal LFTs post-transfusion of blood products should be tested for HEV infection.
- Several HEV vaccines are in development, with at least one showing clinical utility (licensed in China).

HIV (virology and diagnosis)

Overview

The topic of HIV traverses the realms of science, geography, medicine, history, and sociology. Virology itself would be unrecognizable without its most prominent retrovirus. It should never be forgotten that although only (relatively) recently described in 1983, a sufficient understanding has been gained. The virology, replication cycle, and diagnosis of HIV will be discussed here. For discussions about HIV epidemiology, ➔ see HIV epidemiology, natural history, and classification; initial evaluation of the HIV patient; skin, oral, cardiovascular, neurological, and pulmonary complications; HIV gastrointestinal, liver, and kidney disease and HIV infection and malignancy, as well as HIV prevention, antiviral treatment, ➔ see Antivirals for HIV, pp. 107–11; and clinical manifestations.

Virology

The family *Retroviridae* contains >60 viral species across 11 genera that can infect numerous host species. The genus *Lentivirus* contains two noteworthy viral species: HIV-1 (henceforth referred to HIV) and HIV-2. HIV is an enveloped icosahedral, positive-sense ssRNA virus (genome ~9800bp). Mature virions are diploid, so they contain two copies of ssRNA. Like all retroviruses, they replicate through a DNA intermediate, requiring the conversion of viral RNA to DNA and back to viral RNA in their viral progeny. This is achieved through a unique polymerase enzyme called reverse transcriptase (RT), which turns RNA into DNA.

HIV-1 is a zoonotic infection that occurred when the simian immunodeficiency virus (SIV) from chimpanzees/gorillas crossed the species barrier to infect humans. This likely occurred at numerous instances in time before establishment of the epidemic human-adapted virus that we recognize today. Retroviruses have an unrivalled predilection for mutation (due to the error-prone nature of RT and lack of a proofreading mechanism) during their replication cycle. Because of this, subsequent phylogenetic analysis has divided the virus into four groups (M, N, O, P), of which M (major) is responsible for 90% of HIV infection. Group M is further subdivided into multiple subtypes, or clades, designated A–K. Clade C is the most prevalent globally, although most infections in Europe and North America are caused by clade B. Clades A, C, and D predominate in Africa. These clades can combine to form recombinant viruses termed circulating recombinant forms (CRFs). More than 100 CRFs are currently described, the nomenclature of which follows a formula—for example, CRF_01AE (a combination of clade A and E viruses). The clinical relevance of these CRFs is debated (differential phenotypical disease characteristics are described), but undoubtedly such genetic heterogeneity places significant barriers to uniform mass effective treatments (e.g. vaccination). Group O ('outlier') strains circulate predominantly in West Africa and account for ~100,000 cases. Group N ('non-M/O') accounts for a few strains (<30 documented cases) in Cameroon. Group P was identified in Cameroon in 2009 and is particularly closely related to SIV.

HIV-2 (1–2 million cases globally) occurs primarily in West Africa (or in countries with historic colonial ties). It is a zoonotic infection that crossed the species barrier to infect human (from the sooty mangabey monkey). It is less readily transmissible than HIV-1, and is associated with lower viral loads, higher CD4 counts, and slower disease progression. Genome sequence homology between both viruses is about 40%. HIV-2 is intrinsically resistant to non-nucleoside reverse transcriptase inhibitors (NNRTIs) and fusion inhibitors, and shows reduced susceptibility to protease inhibitors (PIs). It is likely resistant to CCR5 inhibitors. Thankfully, susceptibility to integrase inhibitors (INIs) remains (➜ see Antivirals for HIV, pp. 107–11). Dual HIV-1/2 infection, while possible, is rare.

Transmission is via the archetypal 'blood-borne' routes—vertical, sexual, or through contact with infected blood (transfusion or needles).

The HIV virion is illustrated in Fig. 8.1. The HIV genome codes for nine genes (three structural (*gag-pol-env*) and six regulatory). These are flanked on either side by long terminal repeat (LTR) regions. These LTRs are responsible for controlling gene expression and are the focus of intense research.

The three structural genes and their products are:

- *Gag* gene products (core and matrix proteins)—p24, p17, p7, p6, p2, p1;
- *Pol* gene products (enzymes)—protease, RT, and integrase;
- *Env* gene products (envelope proteins)—gp120 (surface only) and gp41 (transmembrane).

The virus also encodes six other genes (*vif, vpr, tat, rev, vpu, nef* with *vpu* (HIV-1 only) or *vpx* (HIV-2 only)). These have diverse functions that serve to enhance virulence and bypass/suppress innate host antiviral mechanisms. They broadly act to enhance viral transcription (*tat/rev*), antagonize host innate antiviral defence (*vif* on APOBEC3G), and decrease the expression of MHC-I (*nef*).

HIV replication cycle

- An understanding of the replication cycle allows an understanding of the site of activity of the antiretroviral drugs (➜ see Antivirals for HIV, pp. 107–11).
- Viral entry is preceded by the attachment of the viral surface glycoprotein gp120 to host cells that express a receptor called CD4. CD4 is found on some T cells, macrophages, and dendritic cells (antigen-presenting cells linking innate and adaptive immunity that are mostly present on mucosal surfaces). The binding of gp120 to CD4 results in a confirmational change in gp120 that allows:
  - binding of gp120 to a second cellular receptor, either CCR5 or CXCR4. This is essential to entry and denotes 'tropism' of the virus (R5 versus R4, early infection is primarily R5-tropic). Tropism of a patient's virus can be determined by examination (almost always genotypic) of the V3 loop of gp120;
  - exposure of viral gp41 (somewhat hidden when gp120 is unbound) to the cellular membrane to initiate fusion of viral and cellular membranes, thereby permitting viral entry. This step culminates in the release of the matrix-wrapped nucleocapsid (which is quickly digested) to release viral RNA into the cytoplasm.

- While HIV entry is traditionally an infrequently used ART target, new agents targeting this are emerging. It is noteworthy that ~1% of the population have mutations in their CXCR5 receptor, essentially making them immune to HIV infection. This mutation has been exploited in a few high-profile cases of 'HIV cure' involving stem cell transplantation.
- Reverse transcription is the archetype feature of retroviruses. It involves the conversion of viral RNA to DNA by a virally coded enzyme called reverse transcriptase (RT). RT first converts ssRNA to ssDNA, and then to dsDNA. At least two drug classes target RT: nucleoside reverse transcriptase inhibitors (NRTIs) and NNRTIs. This process takes place in the cytoplasm. This is a notoriously error-prone process (i.e. replication is not 100% faithful and incorrectly matched bases can be incorporated into the growing DNA chains). This is compounded by the fact that RT does not have a proofreading mechanism. Estimates vary considerably (depending on research methodology), but figures of ~1:700 to 1:4000 errors occurring per nucleotide/per replication, which yields 1–2 substitutions per genome replication cycle, are generally accepted. Mindful that up to 10^9 virions can be produced in a person in 1 day—it becomes apparent quickly why the genetic variation in HIV is unrivalled. It is worth remembering that most of these mutations are either disadvantageous or neutral to the virus. However, if replication persists in the presence of a selective pressure (e.g. inadequate drug concentration), the chances of an advantageous mutation occurring increase. This step culminates with the viral dsDNA being taken into the nucleus, led by the viral enzyme integrase.
- Integration of proviral DNA into host DNA is performed by the viral enzyme integrase. This represents a particularly potent site for

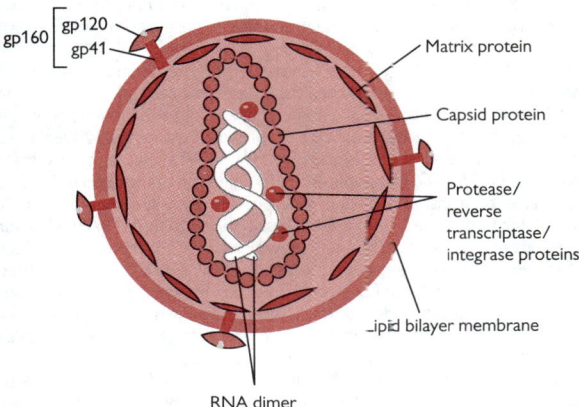

Fig. 8.1 HIV-1 virus structure.

inhibition of HIV replication. Integration of viral DNA into the host DNA genome is what establishes life-long infection and represents the single biggest barrier against a sterilizing cure. This step culminates in the transcription of integrated proviral HIV DNA into mRNA that codes for HIV proteins and pre-genomic RNA (new HIV RNA genome).

- Translation of mRNA in the cytoplasm produces structural and non-structural proteins. What proteins are translated and when are heavily influenced by the virus itself via the activities of many of its non-structural proteins (*tat* and *rev*). This step concludes with the assembly and release of immature non-infectious virions (made of a large polyprotein (*gag*–*pol* components), together with pre-genomic RNA).
- Maturation of these virions is marked by the activity of the viral enzyme protease, which cleaves the gag-pol polyprotein into their functional structural and enzymatic subunits. The resultant infectious virions are now free to infect new cells, and the cycle begins anew.

HIV testing and diagnosis

HIV testing is widespread and streamlined. The barriers to making a diagnosis are bifold. On the healthcare provider's side, there is frequently either a reluctance to perform or an ignorance that a HIV test is warranted. On the patient's side, access to testing has been expanded considerably, whether through postal delivery of dried blood spots, drop-in genitourinary (GU) clinics, or targeted testing at social events. Awareness is the primary stumbling block here, which is often exacerbated by societal perceptions and nescience.

In contrast to untreated (almost uniformly fatal) or delayed treatment of HIV (often associated with significant morbidity), diagnosis and treatment of early infection can result in a normal life expectancy. Additionally, people living with HIV which is well-controlled on treatment cannot transmit the virus (U=U campaign means undetectable = untransmittable). The PARTNER studies showed that across almost 130 000 unprotected sexual occasions between sero-discordant couples (where one member is HIV-positive), no transmission occurred.

As HIV infection is largely asymptomatic until later disease, opportunistic and repeated testing at routine healthcare attendances should be the mainstay. Considerable success has been garnered from the integration of HIV screening into routine antenatal care (all pregnant women at 12 weeks' gestation are offered screening bloods for HIV/HBV/syphilis). It is estimated that in the UK, 5–10% of people with HIV infection do not know they have it (capable of transmission) and 40% present with late-stage illness. For more information, see British HIV Association (BHIVA)/BASHH testing guidelines (available at: ⌖ https://www.bhiva.org/HIV-testing-guidelines).

Oral verbal consent is required to test for HIV. Any HCW who requests laboratory investigations (FBC, renal/liver blood work) can request a HIV test. A lengthy pre-test discussion/written consent is not required. It can usually be incorporated seamlessly into the testing for other infections (HBV, HCV, EBV, CMV, syphilis, specific serologies, or blood cultures).

It can be framed as: '*As part of your medical workup, I would like to exclude some infections that may be causing your symptoms; this will include testing for HIV. This is a routine test for all patients. It is unlikely to come back positive, but if it does—it is an important diagnosis not to miss and it can be managed very effectively. The result will be back in 1–2 days. Is that ok?'*

In patients who lack capacity or are unconscious, clear framework exists for the provision of medical treatment (Mental Capacity Act, 2019). HIV testing can usually be performed. Points to consider are:

- Is capacity present?
- Is it likely to return?
- Is testing in the best interests of the patient?
- Will it optimize current management?
- Will immediate testing prevent harm to the patient?

HIV serology

- The use of fourth-generation assays for HIV diagnosis is now widespread. These assays test for both HIV-1 antigen (p24) as well as antibodies against HIV-1 and 2. These assays differ from their third-generation predecessors by testing for an antigen as well as antibodies. This has reduced the window period (time post-infection where testing is inaccurate) from up to 12 weeks (unlikely in practice) to 4–6 weeks. Most fourth-generation assays can achieve >99% sensitivity and specificity, and most HIV infections will have reactive serology at 4 weeks.
- Clear UK laboratory practice guidelines are in place that guide HIV testing algorithms (for details, see SMI HIV UK, available at: ⌖ https://www.gov.uk/government/publications/smi-v-11-anti-hiv-screening). All initial reactive tests are repeated on a different assay (ideally another fourth-generation), before going onto a tertiary assay to distinguish between HIV-1 and 2. If reactive, a repeat serum blood sample (to repeat the serologies), with an EDTA sample for molecular testing, is requested to confirm the diagnosis of HIV.
- The 12-week window period that is frequently quoted is a remnant of the 'catch-all' window period for pathogens that are frequently tested together. Hepatitis C antibodies, in particular, can be slow to emerge (average 60 days; ➔ see Hepatitis C virus, pp. 471–3).
- Point-of-care assays or analysis of dried blood spots are generally performed on the same assays, with an acknowledgement that sensitivity decreases.
- Like all serological tests, false reactivity is not unusual and is commoner during pregnancy, in the presence of autoimmune conditions, or post-receipt of blood products. A discussion with the local virologist can usually deal with queries rapidly. Usually, the presence of false reactivity can be accurately made based on the lack of antibody evolution on paired samples taken 2 weeks apart.

Viral detection

- Accurate quantitative molecular testing for HIV-1 and 2 RNA by RT-PCR ('viral load') is usually performed on blood but can be performed on CSF where indicated. It is not generally considered of use for initial diagnosis, and its role is almost exclusively in the monitoring of patients with known infection.

- Results are reported as copies/mL or as IU/mL with a local copies/mL conversion. This ensures a standardized, consistent, and accurate quantification of virus in samples.
- The lower limit of detection is ~40 copies/mL.

HIV resistance testing

- HIV resistance testing involves laboratory attempts to determine the presence of virus that would be resistant to components from the major classes of HIV treatment (➔ see Antivirals for HIV, pp. 107–11). This is most commonly undertaken at a genotypic (genetic) level whereby key regions of the HIV genome are sequenced that code for the proteins on which the ART classes act. The RT, protease, and integrase (*pol* gene) regions are looked at most frequently, reflecting likely choices in initial ART regimens ((N)NRTIs, PIs, and INIs). Examination of tropism is possible by looking at the V3 loop of the gp120 region.
- The technology used to determine genetic sequences has changed over the years. There has been a gradual move from Sanger sequencing towards next-generation sequencing (NGS). The primary difference between them is the latter's lower limit of detection. While Sanger sequencing can detect mutations once they make up 20% of a viral population, this figure is closer to 2% for NGS.
- The statistical and bioinformatic analysis required to generate HIV resistance reports is substantial. After the patient's HIV sequence is determined, it is compared with a continually updated and curated database of known HIV mutations and the resultant drug sensitivity is predicted. The Stanford database is the one most commonly used (available at: ✆ http://hivdb.stanford.edu/surveillance/map/).
- HIV infection in an individual does not represent infection with a completely genetically identical virus. A heterogeneous viral population will exist within the host. Combined with the use of NGS to detect mutations at a lower level than ever before, mutations are now being detected that previously would have gone undetected. These are termed minority resistance variants (MRVs), and their clinical significance is hotly debated.
- Overall transmitted drug-resistant HIV is <20% in the UK. Resistance testing is undertaken at baseline and again if viral suppression is not achieved. A serum viral load of 1000 copies/mL is generally needed to achieve a reasonable quality resistance report. Discussion with the laboratory if the viral load is below this is advised, as different techniques can be employed to assist in generating a result.
- Phenotypic assays which involve viral culture in a variable of interest (possible ART drug) are almost never undertaken in a clinical setting.

CD4 T-lymphocyte count

- The CD4 count is used as an indirect measure of immune reconstitution in HIV infection. It is usually determined in the haematology laboratory by flow cytometry on an EDTA sample.
- Normal values are dynamic, and range between 800 and 1500 cells/microlitre.
- Nadir CD4 count is a prognostic sign.

- Prophylactic antibiotics are required at levels of <200 cells/microlitre for *Pneumocystis* pneumonia (PCP) and <50 cells/microlitre for toxoplasmosis.
- Repeated measurement is of extremely limited use and, in the context of a suppressed viral load, should be discouraged.

Human T-cell lymphotropic virus

Virology

The family *Retroviridae* has another genus containing human pathogens *Deltaretrovirus*, which encompasses the viral species called primate T-lymphotropic viruses, to which the human T-cell lymphotropic virus (HTLV) belong. There are currently four HTLV viruses described (notwithstanding that HIV was originally called HTLV-3), but little is known about HTLV-3 and 4. HTLV-1 was the first described retrovirus in 1978, isolated from a patient with leukaemia, and HTLV was described 2 years later. HTLV is an enveloped, linear, diploid (each virion contains two copies) positive-sense ssRNA virus (genome 9000bp). The genome is composed of a typical retrovirus composition and organization: 5'LTR-gag-pro-pol-env-3'LTR. HTLV codes for unique regulatory proteins called Tax, Rex, and HTLV basic zipping factor (HBZ), which all contribute to modifying cell cycle, inhibiting apoptosis, and promoting cellular proliferation, which act cumulatively to promote viral replication. Viral replication itself is consistent with other retroviruses: nuclear in location, genomic RNA being reverse-transcribed to DNA, integration into host DNA (proviral DNA), and transcription into RNA, with subsequent translation of proteins and assembly into infectious virions. In contrast to HIV, cellular infection is not cytopathic and overall viral replication is substantially less. HTLV appears to favour replication of integrated cellular provirus and cell–cell transmission rather than production of new infectious virions; the free virus in plasma is significantly less. Around 0.1–1% of peripheral blood mononuclear cells (PBMCs) carry viral DNA in the host genome in the asymptomatic patient, rising to 30% in disease. Another key difference between HIV and HTLV is the high degree of fidelity with which HTLV replicates; HTLV-1 isolates show 92–97% globally and ~70% sequence homology with HTLV-2. HTLV is a blood-borne virus with the accordant modes of transmission. Breastfeeding appears to be a prominent transmission route.

Epidemiology

- An accurate understanding of the global prevalence is unknown (10–20 million people are infected). Appears endemic in Southern Japan, the Caribbean, Central/West Africa, Melanesia, the Middle East, India, and parts of South America.

Clinical features/treatment

Approximately 5% of HTLV-1 cases will manifest disease. There is an association between HTLV-2 infection and neurological pathology. It is not clear whether it causes other forms of symptomatic disease. The clinical consequences of HTLV infection are hotly debated and represent an under-researched area.

- Adult T-cell leukaemia/lymphoma (ATL)—a clonal proliferative disorder of mature CD4+ T cells. Opportunistic infections are common (PCP and strongyloidiasis). Classified into four types:
  - acute ATL (40–60%)—lymphadenopathy, lymphocytosis, hepatosplenomegaly, skin lesions, pulmonary involvement (potentially opportunistic infections), and hypercalcaemia. Carries the poorest prognosis;
  - lymphomatous ATL (20–30%): lymphadenopathy without lymphocytosis. Prognosis is only slightly better than acute ATL;
  - smouldering ATL (5–10%): notable absence of hypercalcaemia, lymphadenopathy, and hepatosplenomegaly;
  - chronic ATL (5–10%)—raised cell count, with organomegaly and skin or pulmonary involvement, but no effusions, or bone or CNS involvement. Median survival: 24 months;
  - ATL treatment—combination chemotherapy with non-Hodgkin's lymphoma-type regimens. Survival is variable; overall prognosis is poor.
- HTLV-associated myelopathy (HAM)—is the same clinical entity as tropical spastic paraparesis (TSP). An association is increasingly recognized as a complication of HTLV-2. HAM is a chronic, progressive demyelinating disease affecting the spinal cord and white matter of the CNS. It presents insidiously as lower limb weakness (can be either unilateral or bilateral), with features of upper motor neuron disease (spasticity, hyperreflexia, clonus, upgoing plantar reflexes). Back pain, bladder/bowel dysfunction, and variable degrees of sensory loss, with sparing of the upper limbs and cognitive function, are pathognomonic. Radiological findings are variable.
  - HAM treatment—no effective therapy exists, with symptomatic management being the mainstay. Regimens of steroids, IFN, and monoclonals have been attempted, with little definitive success.
- Other disease associations:
  - HTLV-1—arthropathies, uveitis, polymyositis, infectious dermatitis, Sjögren's syndrome, and possibly mycosis fungoides;
  - HTLV-2—unconfirmed associations with rare haematological malignancies and neurodegenerative disorders.

Diagnosis

- Serology is used to screen for HTLV. Molecular testing (PCR) is undertaken to the diagnosis, distinguish subtypes, and measure viraemia/proviral DNA in serum and/or CSF.
- ATL—a combination of clinical features with immunophenotypic analysis of suspected malignant cells (obtained by bone marrow biopsy or from blood).
- HAM—an (often criticized) set of diagnostic criteria exist.

Arboviruses

The term 'arbovirus' refers to any arthropod-borne virus. While this may be of use as a 'catch-all' term clinically (referring to similar epidemiology in their mode of acquisition), it is almost meaningless from a virology perspective as the individual viruses specified are completely distinct. Hantavirus is the most notable exception, as it is transmitted by inhalation of aerosolized particles from rodent faeces (➔ see *Bunyavirales*, pp. 488–90). Symptomatic human arbovirus infections represent a minority of the group, but as climate change progresses and human–vector interactions increase due to overlapping habitats, their incidence will only increase. They have the potential to cause serious disease, with almost no targeted treatment options.

The main human arbovirus infections refer to:
- *Reoviridae* (➔ see *Reoviridae*, p. 483);
- alphaviruses (➔ see Alphaviruses, pp. 483–5);
- flavivirus* (➔ see *Flaviviridae*, pp. 492–4);
- *Bunyavirales** (➔ see *Bunyavirales*, pp. 488–90).

Some arboviruses have viral haemorrhagic fever (√HF) capability (denoted by an asterisk) and will be discussed within that group (➔ see Viral haemorrhagic fevers, pp. 485–7).

Reoviridae

Overview

The non-enveloped, segmented-genome dsRNA family *Reoviridae* contains two genera comprising viral species that cause human disease. *Reoviridae* are a notable exception to the consensus that most human RNA viruses are single-stranded.
- The genus *Coltivirus*:
  - contains the species Colorado tick fever virus, endemic in high-elevation parts of North America. Its vector is the *Dermacentor andersoni* tick and it is linked to causing a febrile illness, which, in most cases, resolve, but meningoencephalitis is described. Diagnosis is by molecular detection in blood of IgM-specific serology, and treatment is supportive.
- The genus *Seadornavirus*:
  - contains the species Banna virus, endemic in South East Asia. It has been isolated from numerous species of mosquito and is linked to febrile meningoencephalitis, but overall it is not well described.

Alphaviruses

Virology

The genus *Alphavirus* in the family *Togaviridae* contains >30 species that infect a range of hosts (birds, reptiles, fish, pigs, and humans) and are predominantly spread by arthropod vectors (predominantly mosquitoes, but also fleas and ticks). They are enveloped positive-sense ssRNA viruses (10 000–12 000bp). As the viral genome is composed of positive-sense RNA, it can act as mRNA and be directly translated from. Expectantly (for an RNA virus), replication takes place in the cytoplasm. Replication is divided into early phases (translation of non-structural proteins) and intermediate-to-late phases (translation of structural proteins).

Epidemiology

- Broadly speaking, human alphavirus species infections are divided
  into two groups: 'New World' (North and South America) which
  predominantly causes encephalitis, and 'Old World' (Europe, Africa,
  and Asia) which predominantly causes fever, rash, and arthropathy (see
  Table 8.3). Their geographical spread is determined by the distribution
  of their vectors, the margins of which are becoming increasingly
  blurred as climate change progresses and the overlap of human–vector
  environments increases.

Table 8.3 Clinical syndromes caused by alphaviruses

Name (vector)	Location	Features
'New World'—encephalitis		
Eastern equine encephalitis (*Culiseta melanura*, but also *Aedes* and others)	Eastern and Gulf Coast (USA), southern Canada, and northern South America	5% of infection cases progress to encephalitis; prognosis is poor, with 30–50% mortality
Western equine encephalitis (*Culex tarsalis*)	North and South America	<1% of infection cases progress to encephalitis, with mortality of 5–10%
Venezuelan equine encephalitis (multiple, including *Culex*; can be spread by aerosols)	South and Central America	<5% of infection cases progress to encephalitis, with mortality rare
'Old World'—fever, rash arthropathy		
Chikungunya (*Aedes aegypti* and *Aedes albopictus*)	Has spread to the Americas	Highly symptomatic polyarthralgia (bilateral, symmetrical) that can cause chronic arthritis. Maculopapular rash is common
O'nyong nyong (*Anopheles*)	Africa	Mortality rare, occurs primarily in sporadic epidemics
Mayaro (*Haemagogus* and others)	South America, the Caribbean	Likely underrecognized as a cause of fever/rash
Sindbis (*Culex*)	Africa, Scandinavia, Asia	Known as Pogosta disease (Finland), Ockelbo disease (Sweden), and Karelian fever (Russia)
Ross River (multiple, including *Aedes*, *Culex*)	Australia, Oceania (up to 50% seroprevalence in Fiji)	Subclinical infection common

Clinical features

- Incubation is 1–12 days following inoculation by an arthropod bite.
- Encephalitis—typical symptoms (fever, confusion, seizures) and CSF findings (lymphocytic picture, with moderately raised protein level).
- Fever, rash, arthritis, and rapid-onset fever (up to 40°C) and chills—may last for several days, remit, then recur (saddleback fever chart). Rash usually appears on day 1 (can be late)—a face and neck pattern evolves to maculopapular lesions on the trunk, limbs, face, and palms/soles, and may be pruritic. Arthralgia is a reliable sign of symptomatic infection. It lasts for a week to a few months, is polyarticular, and affects small joints that may be swollen.

Diagnosis

- Accurate travel history is paramount.
- Molecular testing by PCR can be done on blood/CSF at regional reference laboratories that will perform a multi-species panel based on case epidemiology.

Treatment and prevention

- No specific therapy.
- Prevention depends on vector control and mosquito avoidance.

Viral haemorrhagic fevers

'Viral haemorrhagic fever' (VHF) is a broad clinical term used to refer to a life-threatening syndrome that is caused by a multitude of viral species. VHFs are significant for their high mortality rates and their ability to transmit between humans (causing both nosocomial and community outbreaks). The viral species with sufficient virulence to cause this syndrome share little on a purely virological basis. Notable causative members are listed and cross-references to the other chapters below, but this list is not exhaustive. Haemorrhage is rarely present in early disease.

The diagnosis should be in the differential for a typical 'fever in a returning traveller' presentation (particularly within 21 days of leaving the region). VHF is uncommon, relative to other differential diagnoses, in this presentation (➔ see Imported fever in traveller, pp. 639–40); nevertheless, it must be borne in mind. If the patient is consistently apyrexial and outside the 21-day period, then the risk of VHF is negligible.

Diagnosis and management of suspected viral haemorrhagic fever

Full VHF UK guidance is available and a 1-page algorithm is available at ℘ https://www.gov.uk/government/publications/viral-haemorrhagic-fever-algorithm-and-guidance-on-management-of-patients. Online resources are available, documenting the locations of recent outbreaks, and should be reviewed when risk-assessing. The collaborative workload necessary to efficiently manage these cases is substantial and stretches between front-facing clinical staff (bedside), initial sample processing (bench-side), and transport to tertiary laboratory for diagnostics (roadside).

The algorithm is divided into two risk categories: 'low' and 'high', with corresponding IPC recommendations. Cases are 'high' risk if:
- contact with known cases of VHF/ongoing VHF outbreak;
- returning from a known Lassa/Ebola/Marburg-endemic area;
- returning from known Crimean–Congo haemorrhagic fever (CCHF)-endemic area and the patient had tick exposure.

The overarching aims include:
- early recognition—initial presentation will likely be non-specific and clinically indistinguishable from any other aetiology of fever in a returning traveller;
- appropriate IPC procedures—once symptomatic, patients with VHF are infectious to various extents. All bodily fluids are infectious. Notably, aerosol transmission is not considered significant. Strict IPC aims to prevent secondary infection of other patients, and hospital and laboratory staff. Patients should be in a side room (minimum), ideally negative pressure and en-suite. Limited and pragmatic staff contact is recommended. Recommended PPE requirement is dependent on the estimated risk level—at a minimum ('low' risk): gloves, water-repellent aprons, surgical mask, and eye protection for splash procedures. All waste generated (PPE, sharps) should be considered infectious until VHF result is known;
- prompt diagnosis (or, more likely, exclusion)—rapid malaria diagnosis allows quick stepdown of VHF precautions. Malaria must **never** be missed and is the first diagnosis to be considered. Broad-spectrum antibiotics are often commenced empirically, pending VHF results. Co-infection is unusual, but if pyrexia persists past 72h of appropriate treatment, then the possibility of dual infection should be considered. The balance to be achieved is prevention of VHF transmission while not compromising patient care;
- sample processing—initial blood work should be limited to malaria testing, blood cultures, FBC, LFTs, renal function, clotting, and glucose testing. There is no justification for not processing these samples locally in a timely fashion. Samples from 'low'-risk patients can be performed locally by using containment level 2 laboratory procedures. The laboratory must be informed of all specimens before receipt, so they can be segregated and processed separately with dedicated equipment;
- VHF testing—early liaison with local infection colleagues is paramount, who can then liaise with tertiary testing laboratories if needed. Prompt notification to local IPC and public health teams is integral. After seeking local/regional input, testing of suspected cases (UK) can be arranged with the Imported Fever Service on 0844 778 8990. If VHF testing is positive, patients should be transferred to a high-level isolation unit.

VHF members (ACDP group 4)

Viral species that can cause VHF are broadly derived from four viral families, which are discussed individually. Most are considered group 4 pathogens by the Advisory Committee on Dangerous Pathogens (available at: ⌖ https://www.gov.uk/government/publications/viral-haemorrhagic-fever-algorithm-and-guidance-on-management-of-patients):
- order *Bunyavirales* (➔ see *Bunyavirales*, pp. 488–90):
  - family *Arenaviridae* (➔ see *Arenaviridae*, pp. 487–8): Lassa, Lujo, Sabia, Guanarito, Chapare, Junin, Machupo;

- family *Orthonairoviridae* CCHF;
- family *Filoviridae* (⊘ see *Filoviridae*, pp. 490–2): Ebola and Marburg;
- family *Flaviviridae* (⊘ see Ebola and Marburg are both filoviridae, pp. 490–1): dengue* (⊘ see Dengue and *Flaviviridae*, p. 492), YF* (⊘ see Dengue, pp. 498–9).

Arenaviridae

Virology

The family *Arenaviridae* contains four genera composed of >50 viral species that infect a variety of hosts. The sandy appearance of virions on EM (Latin '*arenus*') gave them their name. Most human arenavirus infections are from the genus *Mammarenavirus*. They are enveloped, segmented (2–3), negative-sense (technically, they are ambisense as they contain a negative-sense majority, with some positive-sense components) ssRNA viruses. Numerous members have the capability to cause VHF (⊘ see Viral haemorrhagic fevers, pp. 485–7) in humans, with more being recognized (particularly New World arenaviruses) in South America.

Arenaviruses with VHF capability are divided into Old and New World, based on traditional geographical distribution:
- Old World (Africa)—Lassa and Lujo (recently described in 2008);
- New World (Americas)—a rapidly emerging group, particularly in South America. Notable members (correspond clinical entity): Junin (Argentinian haemorrhagic fever), Machupo (Bolivian haemorrhagic fever), Chapare, Sabia, and Guanarito (Venezuelan haemorrhagic fever).

All show specific rodent host species reservoirs (chronic asymptomatic infection is described). Transmission is primarily through contact with urine/faeces of the infected host. Person-to-person transmission is recognized, with sporadic reports of sexual transmission.
- Lassa:
  - virology—genome is composed of two segments: large ((L) 7100bp) and small ((S) 3400bp). It is postulated that the presence of an ambisense genome increases the protein-coding ability while exerting greater control of early and late transcription;
  - epidemiology—first recognized following a case in Lassa, Nigeria in 1969. Endemic across West Africa. The host is the multimammate rat. Outbreaks can occur. Seroprevalence rates vary considerably and can be up to 50% in some villages. Sexual transmission from recovered index cases is described infrequently, but it seems prudent that cases should abstain from unprotected intercourse for 3 months post-resolution of symptoms;
  - clinical features—incubation typically 7–12 days, but up to 21. Wide spectrum of clinical manifestations where up to 80% of infection can be mild or subclinical. In hospitalized patients, mortality is between 30% and 50%; it is likely this figure varies considerably, based on the standard of healthcare available and overall health of the patient. Initial symptoms are non-specific, but most notable are fever, chest pain (74%), abdominal pain (50%), cough (50%),

---

* Are classified in the lower group 3 dangerous pathogen category due to availability of treatment or prophylaxis.

vomiting and diarrhoea (25%), pharyngitis (62%), and conjunctivitis. Proteinuria occurs in 43%. When cases progress to life-threatening illness, shock, pulmonary oedema, ascites, and encephalopathy develop, which can be fatal. Zenith viral load appears to correlate with mortality. SNHL is the most commonly reported complication (30%). Haemorrhage occurs in a minority of cases (17%);
- diagnosis and suspect case management——➔ see Viral haemorrhagic fevers (pp. 485–7) for diagnosis/management of suspect cases/testing guidelines;
- treatment—no vaccine is available. Ribavirin does appear to have some benefit in Lassa infection (and, on a smaller scale, in other arenavirus—particularly Junin—infections). It may have a role in PEP, but true efficacy is unknown and is only taken on an individual risk assessment basis.
- Lymphocytic choriomeningitis (LCM) virus:
  - virology—an enveloped, segmented negative-sense ssRNA virus (two segments: L, 7200bp; S, 3400bp) in the genus *Mammarenavirus*, family *Arenaviridae*. Conventional person-to-person transmission (cases acquired by organ transplantation are reported) has not been described. Vertical transmission has been described and is most serious during the first trimester;
  - epidemiology—rodents are the primary host, and LCM zoonotic infection in humans is likely underrecognized. Seroprevalence in both rodents (5%) and humans (2–5%) is a poorly researched area, and estimates vary considerably. It is likely found globally;
  - clinical features—LCM virus infection is primarily a neurological illness, although the overwhelming majority of cases are subclinical. It does not cause VHF. It is a biphasic illness, with an initial non-specific viral prodromal symptoms (fever, malaise, myalgia, nausea, vomiting) occurring 8–13 days after exposure. Following a few days of recovery, neurological manifestations can arise, varying from aseptic meningitis to encephalitis. Clinical course is benign, with <1% of cases fatal;
  - diagnosis and treatment—diagnostic services are extremely limited, particularly in the UK. Serology and molecular testing for PCR is possible in other countries. Treatment is supportive, and as the illness is self-resolving, often diagnostics are not pursued.

Bunyavirales

Overview/virology

A new order containing 12 families and in excess of 400 viral species (still colloquially referred to as bunyaviruses) was created in 2017 by viral taxonomists. They are enveloped negative-sense ssRNA viruses with a segmented genome (2–3 segments, with a total size of 13 000bp; termed large (L), medium (M), and small (S)). The L segment codes for viral polymerase, M segment for the surface glycoprotein, and S segment for the nucleocapsid.

Notable members of the order are listed in Table 8.4, with some members capable of causing VHF (➔ see Viral haemorrhagic fevers, pp. 485–7).

Table 8.4 Notable diseases caused by *Bunyavirales*

Name/genus (vector)	Location	Features
California encephalitis group; main agent is La Crosse virus/*Orthobunyavirus* (Aedes)	Northern America	Meningoencephalitis, symptomatic infection commoner in children; 90% in those aged <15 years. Low mortality
Rift Valley fever/*Phlebovirus* (Aedes). Infected eggs can remain viable for many years	East Africa primarily, but also West Africa. Post-severe rainfall	In addition to vector spread, can be transmitted by aerosols Majority of infection cases result in undifferentiated febrile illness; <1% progress to severe disease, including haemorrhagic jaundice secondary to hepatic failure or encephalitis
Crimean–Congo haemorrhagic fever/*Orthonairovirus* (Hyalomma ticks)	Widespread. Africa, the Middle East, Eastern Europe. Seasonal transmission spikes observed	Vector spread or by contact with infected blood (e.g. crushing ticks). Incubation period is 1–13 days; 90% of cases result in subclinical illness, but progression to a fatal haemorrhagic illness is possible
'Old World': Hantaan, Seoul, Dobrave, Puumala/*Orthohantavirus* (numerous distinct rodent vectors)*	Global, varies with individual species. Transmission is by inhalation of aerosols from faeces/urine	Haemorrhagic fever with renal syndrome (HFRS). Incubation period is 5–40 days. Fever with acute renal failure. Mortality varies; 5% Hantaan and <1% Puumala
'New World': Sin Nombre, New York, Bayou/*Orthohantavirus* (numerous distinct rodent vectors)*	As above	Hantavirus pulmonary syndrome (HPS). Fever and hypoxia due to pulmonary oedema

* The genus *Orthohantavirus* contains >30 species, but human infection follows two main clinical patterns (HFRS or HPS), each caused by different species. These have been referred to as 'Old World' and 'New World' hantaviruses, which is used as the basis for grouping here.

Diagnosis

- Diagnosis can be difficult, and early discussion with local virology and reference laboratories is paramount.
- All healthcare and laboratory staff must be aware that these samples are considered high risk, and appropriate collection and transport arrangements must be made in advance. Some of these organisms are considered group 4 by the ACDP (see ℘ https://www.gov.uk/gov ernment/publications/viral-haemorrhagic-fever-algorithm-and-guida nce-on-management-of-patients).
- Serology for La Crosse and hantavirus infection is diagnostic. Patients are IgM-positive by the time they are symptomatic in primary infection. PCR tests are not widely available, and viral RNA disappears from circulation early on in disease. Viral isolation from CSF in La Crosse infection is rare.
- Molecular tests are being developed and, for CCHF and Rift Valley fever (RVF), represent the diagnostic modality of choice. Antibodies can be detected at 5–14 days, coinciding with clinical improvement.

Treatment and prevention

- There are no vaccines in general use, and prevention is by public health measures to reduce vector numbers and personal avoidance.
- There is no widely accepted antiviral agent recommended.
- Robust evidence that treatment with ribavirin is of benefit in hantavirus-derived infections is lacking. It has been used to slightly more effect in treating hantavirus infection causing haemorrhagic fever with renal syndrome (but not pulmonary syndrome), although studies are conflicting.
- Use of ribavirin in CCHF is not routinely recommended.
- Supportive measures—anticonvulsants, fluids, and circulatory/renal support remain the cornerstone of care.

Filoviridae

Virology

The family *Filoviridae* (named after Latin '*filum*' due to a characteristic filament-like virion morphology) are enveloped, linear negative-sense ssRNA viruses (genome 19 000 bp). The genome codes for seven structural proteins. There are >10 species across six genera. The genus *Ebolavirus* contains the six species *Zaire*, *Sudan*, *Tai Forest*, *Bundibugyo*, *Reston*, and *Bombali*. *Reston* (only documented in animals in the Philippines) and *Bombali* are not yet associated with significant disease in humans.

The genus *Marburgvirus* contains a single species *Marburg marburgvirus*, which is made up of two variants (Lake Victoria and Ravn marburgvirus). There is no serological cross-reactivity between the genera, but cross-reactivity within *Ebolavirus* is recognized. Infection occurs in a variety of cell types, with secondary replication in lymphoid tissue to rapidly produce disseminated infection. A degree of immune paralysis is produced by destruction of dendritic cells, likely due to failure to produce antibodies in a timely manner (attributed to viral proteins (VP)-24, 35, and 40).

Filoviridae transmission is consistent with other VHFs—contact (without PPE) with an infected person's bodily fluid. The risks of transmission are multifactorial (a consequence of the 2014/15 Ebola outbreak was a greater understanding of this). Relative risk of transmission varies with the type of exposure (blood, saliva, aerosol), duration, quantity, stage of illness (asymptomatic, symptomatic late stage, or convalescence), and recipient site (broken versus unbroken skin/mucous membranes). Societal practices of washing cadavers have a devastating potential for transmission. The role of fomites is largely unknown, whereas sexual transmission after the index case has recovered, although described, remains poorly understood (attributed to delayed viral clearance due to immunoprotected sites, e.g. testes). Ebola/Marburg are not spread by arthropod vectors. Infection represents zoonotic spillover. The animal reservoir for Ebola is not conclusively proven but is likely bats. *Rousettus Aegyptiacus*—the Egyptian fruit bat—is the accepted reservoir for Marburg.

Filoviridae are generally considered the most virulent of the zoonotic VHFs in humans (➲ see Viral haemorrhagic fevers, pp. 485–7) and produce similar clinical manifestations, such that they will be discussed collectively. Notably, as with the other VHFs, haemorrhage is not a particularly prominent feature.

Epidemiology

- Marburg virus—identified in 1967 when African green monkeys brought from Uganda to Marburg, Germany and Belgrade developed a haemorrhagic illness subsequently transmitted to humans (seven deaths amongst 31 cases). Most cases due to Lake Victoria variant. Smaller outbreaks have occurred since, the largest in Angola in 2004 (250 cases). Endemic across Central and West Africa.
- Ebola—identified in 1976 following two outbreaks in Zaire and Sudan. Multiple outbreaks in Africa, including the largest one in 2014–16 in West Africa (caused by the *Zaire Ebolavirus* species) where almost 29 000 cases occurred, with >11 000 deaths (see details from WHO and CDC on 2014 Ebola outbreak, available at: ℘ https://www.who.int/emergencies/situations/ebola-outbreak-2014–2016-West-Africa and ℘ https://www.cdc.gov/vhf/ebola/history/2014–2016-outbreak/index.html, respectively). Numerous smaller outbreaks have occurred since.

Clinical features

- Largely consistent between both Ebola and Marburg. Incubation period is 5–10 days (up to 21 days described). Non-specific viral prodrome of fever, myalgia, and headache precedes a maculopapular rash and GI symptoms (diarrhoea commoner than previous y recognized).
- In week 2, patients either become afebrile and improve, or develop shock and multi-organ dysfunction with DIC and renal and liver failure.
- Convalescence is prolonged. The virus is detectable in semen/urine for weeks.
- Mortality rates for both Ebola and Marburg range between 20% and 80%, on average about 50%, but provision of healthcare facilities and background host comorbidities/age are significant variables.

Diagnosis

- For diagnosis/management of suspect cases and testing guidelines, see Viral haemorrhagic fevers, pp. 485–7.

Treatment

- There are no specific treatments; management is supportive, focused on optimal fluid/electrolyte management.
- Monoclonal antibody therapy for *Ebolavirus* infection has proven efficacy (two are available: a three-monoclonal antibody co-formulation called Inmazeb®, and a single-monoclonal antibody formulation called Ebanga®); these target the surface glycoproteins.
- Various other therapies, including convalescent plasma, small interfering RNAs (siRNAs), and numerous antivirals, while under investigation, are of unknown efficacy.
- Two vaccines (a live modified VSV vector and a non-replicating adenoviral base) are available, mainly for use in outbreak settings. Encouraging results have been observed. Others are in development.

Flaviviridae

Virology

The family *Flaviviridae* contains four genera and almost 90 viral species that infect a variety of mammals, including humans (~30 species). They are enveloped, icosahedral, linear positive-sense ssRNA viruses (genome ~12 000bp). The group derives its name from the archetype flavivirus YF virus ('*flavus*' being Latin for 'yellow') (for individual discussion, ➜ Yellow Fever, pp. 496–8). Despite genetic similarities, clinical spectrums can vary (crudely divided into those that show significant neurotropism or not). Replication takes place in the cytoplasm, with translation occurring directly from the genomic RNA as it is positive-sense. Generally, a single polyprotein is produced that is cleaved into three structural proteins (capsid, membrane, and envelope) and seven non-structural proteins.

Many members of the genus *Flavivirus* are arthropod-borne, show significant neurotropism, and are noteworthy causes of encephalitis in humans. Additionally, dengue (➜ see Dengue, pp. 498–9) and YF (➜ see Yellow fever, pp. 496–8) have VHF potential. HCV (➜ see Hepatitis C virus, pp. 471–3) and Zika virus (➜ see Zika, pp. 495–6) are prominent flaviviruses that warrant individual discussions.

Diagnosis/prevention

- An accurate travel history, with compatible timing of exposures and elimination of differentials, is crucial. Testing is often performed on a panel basis (Australasia versus South East Asia) that differ by geographical exposure.
- Molecular testing (PCR)—results must be interpreted with some caution. As humans are accidental hosts in some infections (Japanese encephalitis and West Nile virus), viraemia is minimal and short-lived, which limits the sensitivity of molecular diagnostics of the neurotropic flaviviruses. Successful detection from CSF is possible in early disease, and it may be isolated from tissue samples (brain, spleen, etc.) and from

blood in some cases. Molecular tests for other flavivirus infections (non-neurotropic) remain useful.

- Serology—can be performed on serum and CSF; demonstration of specific IgM (particularly in CSF) or a 4-fold rise in titres is diagnostic. However, caution must be taken with interpretation as cross-reactivity amongst other flavivirus antibodies is possible (previous exposure and vaccination history).
- Close and early liaison with local specialist clinicians is important.
- Many of these illnesses are acquired abroad contemporaneous travel advice is at NaTHNaC (available at: ℘ https://nathnac.net/).

Neurotropic flaviviruses

- Japanese encephalitis:
  - epidemiology—endemic throughout Asia and western Pacific. Transmitted by *Culex* mosquitoes. Incidence can be seasonal in tropical climates or present as outbreaks in temperate climates. Humans are an accidental host, and human-to-human transmission via mosquitoes is not described. Risk to travellers, although low overall, is present; 1 in 150 000 person-months of exposure;
  - clinical features—infection is symptomatic in <1% of cases. Incubation period of 5–15 days. A broad range of clinical neurological manifestations of varying severity is increasingly recognized. A non-specific viral prodrome preceding frank neurological symptoms is possible. The commonest clinical presentation is severe encephalitis (25% fatality, even with intensive care facilities). More unusual presentations, such as flaccid paralysis, psychosis, seizure-predominant or GBS-like illnesses, are described, in addition to milder viral meningitis. Improvement, if it occurs, can be expected within a week of resolution of fever. Mortality rates approach 25%, and long-term neurological sequelae can be expected in a relatively high proportion of symptomatic cases (30%)
  - Treatment—no effective antiviral therapy exists, and treatment is supportive. An inactivated vaccine is available (see *Japanese encephalitis: the green book*, available at: ℘ https://assets.publishing.service.gov.uk/media/5b1aaaed40f0b634abe91283/Greenbook_chapter_20__Japanese_encephalitis_v3.pcf).
- St Louis encephalitis:
  - epidemiology—endemic in North and South America. Transmission by a few species of *Culex* mosquitoes and mirrors that of West Nile virus. Incidence appears to be decreasing, which is attributed to cross-protection and more effective transmission by West Nile virus in birds. Humans are accidental hosts;
  - clinical features—only 0.3% of infections result in manifestations of symptoms. Both the chances of developing symptoms and mortality correlate with age (mortality is >20% in those aged over 60 versus <5% in younger cohorts). The incubation period is 4–21 days. There is a wide range in severity of symptoms from development of the viral prodromal illness to non-specific fever with headache to meningitis to fatal encephalitis;

- treatment and prevention—no effective antiviral therapy exists, and treatment is supportive. No vaccine is available. Environmental sampling of animal vectors is desirable, but underperformed.
- Tick-borne encephalitis (TBE)—the nomenclature surrounding this virus can cause confusion, as it is also the name of a viral species complex, which includes Powossan virus, Omsk haemorrhagic fever, Kyasanur Forest disease, and Louping ill virus.
  - epidemiology—three viral subtypes of TBE are described that correspond to their geographical distribution: European TBE, Siberian TBE, and Far Eastern TBE. Each displays slight variation in neurovirulence. The vector is species of the *Ixodes* tick;
  - clinical features—incubation period of 4–28 days, with up to 75% of people able to remember a tick bite. Symptomatic infection can occur in up to a third of cases. Illness is biphasic and initiated by a prodromal phase (the majority do not progress from this) that improves usually within a week. Those who develop the second neurological phase can present with a range of manifestations that include aseptic meningitis, encephalitis, or acute flaccid paralysis (polio-like illness). Severity correlates with advancing age, and long-term sequelae can be seen in up to 50%;
  - treatment—no effective antiviral therapy exists, and treatment is supportive. An inactivated vaccine is available (see *Tick-borne encephalitis: the green book*, available at: ℘ https://www.gov.uk/gov ernment/publications/tick-borne-encephalitis-the-green-book-chap ter-31).
- West Nile virus:
  - epidemiology—the most widely distributed of the 'arboviruses', with an almost global distribution. Vector is multiple species of *Culex* mosquitoes;
  - clinical features—incubation period of 2–14 days, and about 30% of infections produce symptomatic disease. Produces two main clinical syndromes: West Nile fever (non-specific viral prodromal symptoms, similar clinically to dengue) and West Nile encephalitis (<1% develop neurological disease that ranges from aseptic meningitis to encephalitis to acute flaccid paralysis). Severity correlates with advancing age (mortality of around 10%), and long-term sequelae can be seen in up to 50%;
  - treatment and prevention—no effective antiviral therapy exists, and treatment is supportive. No vaccine is available.
- Murray Valley encephalitis:
  - epidemiology—Australia and New Guinea. Vector is multiple species of *Culex* mosquitoes. Causes sporadic cases and few outbreaks;
  - clinical features—under 0.5% of infections produce symptomatic disease. A viral prodrome precedes the encephalitis that carries a mortality of ~20%;
  - treatment and prevention—no effective antiviral therapy exists, and treatment is supportive. No vaccine is available.

Zika

Virology

Zika virus is a member of the genus *Flavivirus*, family *Flaviridae* (➜ see *Flaviviridae*, pp. 492–4). It is an enveloped, icosahedral, linear ssRNA virus (genome ~10 000bp). It is named after the Zika forest in Uganda where it was first isolated. Transmission is primarily through the bite of an infected mosquito/arthropod (*Aedes*), but it was the feared complications of congenital infection that have gained recent notoriety. Sexual transmission is described.

Epidemiology

- Small outbreaks occurred on Yap Island (2007) and in French Polynesia (2013).
- The 2015/16 outbreak of Zika infection is the largest on record—it primarily took place in Southern and Central America, but imported cases occurred globally. More than 200 000 cases were notified, and sero-surveys show a prevalence of 63% in north-eastern Brazil. The legacy of congenital Zika infection will be long-standing. Our understanding of Zika progressed greatly because of this epidemic.

Clinical features

- Infection results in symptomatic disease in about 20% of cases (the majority of cases are entirely asymptomatic). Incubation period is between 3 and 12 days. Symptoms are usually mild and non-specific, and closely resemble those of dengue infection (➜ see Dengue, pp. 498–9) or chikungunya (➜ see Dengue and chikungunya, p. 484). Fever (65%), rash (>90%), arthralgia (65%), headache (45%), and conjunctivitis (45%) are described. Illness is self-limiting and lasts a week.
- Fetal infection with Zika virus can occur regardless of maternal symptoms. Zika virus shows a clear predilection for neuronal progenitor cells and can cause a range of manifestations, including microcephaly, ocular abnormalities, cranial malformations, and neuromotor disability. Estimates of vertical transmission vary (26–65%) but appear to be greater in the first/second trimesters Estimates of the frequency of fetal disease after transmission are even less reliable (6–40%). Early liaison with fetal medicine is crucial (see UK guidelines, available at: ℛ https://www.gov.uk/government/collections/zika-virus-zikv-clinical-and-travel-guidance).

Diagnosis

- Molecular testing of blood/urine/CSF is sensitive early in disease (<7 days post-symptom onset).
- Detection of viral genome in neonatal CSF/blood/urine within a few days of birth confirms congenital infection. Cranial ultrasound scans can be useful (ventriculomegaly/calcifications/microcephaly).
- Serology is useful in adults.

Treatment/prevention

- No specific antiviral therapy exists. Supportive care is the mainstay. A vaccine is being developed.
- For contemporaneous travel advice, see NaTHNaC (available at: ✍ https://nathnac.net).

Yellow fever

Virology

YF virus is the archetype member of the genus *Flavivirus*, family *Flaviviridae* (➔ see *Flaviviridae*, pp. 492–4). It is an enveloped, icosahedral, linear positive-sense ssRNA virus (genome ~11 000bp). Although there are numerous genotypes, there is a single serotype, which is crucial to vaccine success. Initial local replication occurs in lymphoid tissues before widespread viraemia disseminates infection whereby YF virus shows a predilection for the liver and kidneys. Evolution into VHF is possible (➔ see Viral haemorrhagic fevers, pp. 485–7). Multiple transmission cycles are recognized, which correspond to differing mosquito vectors and locations (➔ see Epidemiology below).

Epidemiology

- Capable of causing both sporadic cases and epidemics. Monkeys are the natural host, with humans as accidental hosts.
- Endemic in Africa and Central/South America. Cross-protective immunity derived from dengue virus infection is postulated as the reason why YF virus is not found in Asia, despite the vector (mosquito) being present.
- Three patterns of transmission are recognized:
  - urban YF (epidemic)—the main viral reservoir is humans, and human–human transmission occurs via *Aedes aegypti* mosquitoes that live in high numbers locally. Occurs in urban areas;
  - an intermediate cycle (savannah)—occurs in urban/forest border areas where initial monkey–human transmission (travels into forest for work) becomes human–human transmission (return to urban home);
  - large outbreaks—potentially epidemics can occur when a savannah-acquired infected human goes to an urban area while viraemic, and gets bitten by a compatible mosquito vector, thereby introducing YF. The result can be explosive if there is a high density of both vector and humans in proximity, which is potentiated by low immunity (poor vaccine coverage);
  - jungle YF (sylvatic)—the reservoir is monkeys with monkey–monkey transmission occurring via *Haemagogus* (South America) and *Aedes* (Africa) mosquitoes.
- YF cases and outbreaks are typically commoner in Africa than in South America due to higher vector burden and less consistent vaccine coverage. This is changing due to better vaccination programmes (Africa) and changing population densities/work practices (South America).

- Person-to-person transmission is theoretically possible in any area where the vector exists, and as climate change worsens, it is a significant cause for concern.
- The estimated risk of death in an unvaccinated traveller to an endemic area is 1 in 5000.

Clinical features

- Incubation period is 3–6 days. Subclinical infection can occur in 5–50% of cases.
- Symptomatic infection is classically divided into three stages:
  - period of infection—non-specific viral prodrome of fever, malaise, etc. Patients are viraemic. Faget's sign (low pulse rate relative to fever) is reported, although it is of likely limited clinical utility;
  - period of remission—occurs with resolution of fever. Most cases resolve at this point;
  - period of intoxication—15% of cases progress to severe disease, which can enter a haemorrhagic phase. Viraemia declines and antibodies appear. LFT derangement follows a slightly unusual pattern (relative to other viral hepatitis) in that AST level is higher than ALT level (due to myocardial/skeletal muscle damage). Fulminant icteric hepatitis (causing multi-site haemorrhage) with renal failure complicates cardiac involvement, before coma and death occurring in 20–50% of cases.

Diagnosis

- Severe YF resembles other VHFs circulating in Africa and South America, so the appropriate patient flow, sample taking, and diagnostic algorithms should be followed (➔ see Viral haemorrhagic fevers, pp. 485–7).
- PCR has a good chance of success due to higher viraemias seen in human hosts, particularly in early disease, and can be performed on numerous samples (blood, CSF, urine, tissue).
- Serology—demonstration of specific IgM or a 4-fold rise in titres in paired samples is diagnostic. However, caution must be taken with interpretation, as cross-reactivity amongst other flaviviral antibodies is possible (previous exposure and vaccination history).

Prevention and treatment

- A live attenuated vaccine exists. For contemporary travel advice, see NaTHNaC (available at: 🔊 https://travelhealthpro.org.uk/factsheet/18/yellow-fever), and for full vaccine specifications, see *Yellow fever: the green book* (available at: 🔊 https://www.gov.uk/government/publications/yellow-fever-the-green-book-chapter-35). A single dose (some immunocompromised cohorts require boosters) confers life-long immunity (efficacy >95%). Travellers to at-risk countries should be vaccinated. A vaccine administration certificate is an entry requirement for some countries. Extreme caution is advised before administration to those aged >60 years or <4 months, or those with a history of thymic disorders who have an increased risk of developing YF vaccine-associated disease (encephalitis or viscerotropic disease). The risk is ~1 per 100,000 doses.

- A specific and effective antiviral therapy against YF does not exist. Research continues, and mindful of the success with HCV, a treatment should be technically within reach.
- Supportive care is the mainstay—fluids, renal and coagulopathy correction, and ICU care. Clearly of limited provision in endemic areas.

Dengue

Virology

Dengue virus is a member of the genus *Flavivirus*, family *Flaviviridae* (➔ see *Flaviviridae*, pp. 492–4). It is an enveloped, icosahedral, linear ssRNA virus (genome ~11 000bp). Four primary serotypes are recognized. Reinfection with a different serotype has the potential to become severe and evolve into VHF—dengue haemorrhagic fever (DHF) (➔ see Viral haemorrhagic fevers, pp. 485–7). This is thought to occur through a phenomenon called antibody-dependent enhancement. The process is not completely understood. Broadly, heterologous antibody to a previously encountered serotype is non-neutralizing (postulated to involve low titres of membrane antibody) and enhances cellular entry of new/current serogroup virions. Thus, past infection with a different serogroup confers not immunity, but instead the potential for worse disease, through an augmented and inappropriate immune response. Primary infection results in lifelong immunity to that serotype, with secondary infections to a different serotype resulting in only partial immunity. More than three or four symptomatic dengue infections in a lifetime is unusual. Transmission is primarily through the bite of an infected mosquito (primarily *Aedes aegypti*, but other species such as *Aedes albopictus* are capable).

Epidemiology

- Once a mosquito is infected, it is capable of transmission for life. *Aedes* are day-biting and easily disturbed, and a single mosquito can infect an entire household. They breed in open water (domestic containers, puddles, etc.)—thus, urban transmission can be very intense.
- Incidence of dengue follows its primary vector (35° North to 35° South). Historically, this was primarily in Asia and the Western Pacific. Sporadic outbreaks are described in Africa and Central/South America, with the southern parts of North America being at risk.
- The potential for widespread distribution is increasing due to climate change, expanding vector habitat, alternate *Aedes* species transmission, and an increase in mosquito–human interactions. Consequently, it is estimated around 3 billion people are at risk of dengue.
- Both endemic (human–human) and sylvatic (monkey–monkey) transmissions are described. It is debated as to whether humans are the main reservoir of infection or not. Endemic transmission occurs in two broad patterns:
  - epidemic—a single viral strain enters a region with sufficient susceptible hosts, causing an epidemic. Attack rates <50%;
  - hyperendemic—multiple serotypes circulate throughout the year, increasing in the rainy season. Incidence varies from year to year, as host immunity changes and new viral strains emerge. Annual attack rates 5–10%. DHF is a risk.

Clinical features

- Differentiation of dengue infection or clinical grounds alone is extremely difficult, nigh impossible conclusively.
- Incubation period is 4–6 days post-bite (up to 14 days), when viraemia begins, which continues until the fever defervesces.
- Most dengue infection cases are subclinical; however, a wide range in severity and the dynamic nature of infection present a challenge to prognosis. This prompted reclassification of symptomatic dengue in 2009 by the WHO into three stages. The goal was to alert the clinician towards early recognition of severe disease, to enable prompt treatment to minimize morbidity and mortality attributed to an increase in vascular permeability:
  - dengue **without** warning signs—fever plus two of nausea/vomiting, rash (maculopapular), headache/eye pain (worse on movement), myalgia/arthralgia, leucopenia/thrombocytopenia, or positive tourniquet test (>10 petechiae per 2.5cm^2 area after inflation of blood pressure (BP) cuff to midpoint between systolic and diastolic BP for 5 minutes);
  - dengue **with** warning signs—as above plus one of abdominal pain, persistent vomiting, bleeding mucosa, plasma leakage, lethargy, clinical fluid accumulation, hepatomegly >2cm, or rising haematocrit;
  - severe dengue—significant plasma leakage (shock, pulmonary oedema, haemorrhage, and organ failure). Most likely to occur in secondary infections >18 months after primary infection.
- Running parallel to these are three disease phases: febrile–critical–recovery. The critical phase is not experienced by all patients.
- Complications—encephalopathy, hepatic failure, renal failure, dual infections (Gram-negative sepsis, parasitic disease).

Diagnosis

- Molecular (PCR)—is the preferred modality due to excellent sensitivity (due to high levels of viraemia, particularly in early symptomatic disease) and specificity (can determine which serotype).
- Serology—demonstration of specific IgM or a 4-fold rise in titres in paired samples is diagnostic. IgG interpretation is difficult and requires paired samples. However, caution must be taken with interpretation, as cross-reactivity amongst other flaviviral antibodies is possible (previous exposure and vaccination history).

Prevention and treatment

- Prevention—bite avoidance and reduction are key (see NaTHNaC, available at: ℘ https://travelhealthpro.org.uk/factsheet/13/dengue). A live vaccine (YF construct with the dengue membrane/envelope proteins) is available (not currently indicated for visiting travellers) that is useful in reinforcing natural immunity. However, its use is limited by unequal efficacy across all four serotypes and an increase in severe dengue in those naïve to primary infection. Further vaccines are in development and are highly desirable.
- Treatment—no specific antiviral therapy exists. Early recognition of severe disease and prompt treatment to maintain fluid status are key (see WHO dengue guidelines, available at: ℘ https://www.who.int/publications/i/item/9789241547871).

Nipah and Hendra

Virology/overview

Within the family *Paramyxoviridae* is the genus *Henipavirus* that contains two particularly notable human zoonotic infections called Nipah and Hendra. These infections differ considerably from the other and somewhat less virulent members of *Paramyxoviridae* (➔ see Measles, pp. 421–3, ➔ Mumps, pp. 423–5, and ➔ see Parainfluenza, p.412), but are noteworthy for their virulence and potential as emerging pathogens. They are enveloped, non-segmented negative-sense ssRNA viruses (genome ~18 000bp).

From a laboratory processing point of view, they are hazard group 4 organisms (see ⌦ https://www.hse.gov.uk/pubns/misc208.pdf).

The reservoir for both infections is the flying fox species of the bat.

- Nipah:
  - epidemiology—first recognized in 1998 in the village of Nipah, Malaysia as a cause of encephalitis in pig farmers. Almost annual outbreaks have occurred in Bangladesh since. Transmission can be person-to-person or by ingestion of contaminated palm sap (bats also feed on it);
  - clinical features—incubation periods of up to 2 months are reported, but in the majority of cases within 14 days. Febrile encephalitis, with a mortality rate of between 30% and 70% (higher rates of mortality noted in Indian outbreaks);
  - diagnosis and treatment—molecular and serology available.
- Hendra:
  - epidemiology—first recognized in 1994 in close contacts of sick horses in the suburb of Hendra, Brisbane, Australia. It is postulated that horses serve as intermediate hosts between bats and humans. Isolated outbreaks have occurred since, and all have had contact with sick horses;
  - clinical features—incubation period is ~21 days. Reported clinical manifestations are limited due to only seven reported cases of human infection (four fatalities). A febrile respiratory illness is reported, but progression to encephalitis is described;
  - diagnosis and treatment—molecular and serology available. A vaccine for use in horses is available.

Rabies

Virology

Rabies virus (Latin 'madness') is one of 17 species (and the archetype member) of the genus *Lyssavirus*, which is in the family *Rhabdoviridae*. The genus is further classified into phylogroups 1–3, based on intragroup cross-neuralization and assumed cross-protective immunity to vaccines/immunoglobulin. In addition to rabies virus, a few other *Lyssavirus* members (European bat lyssavirus 1–2 and Australian bat lyssavirus) are capable of causing a clinically indistinguishable zoonotic disease. Rabies is an enveloped, linear, helical-shaped (bullet) virion containing a negative-sense ssRNA genome (~12 000 bp). *Lyssavirus* genome organization is conserved and codes for five structural proteins; replication takes place in the cytoplasm where large viral inclusion bodies (Negri bodies) are pathognomonic on histology.

Lyssaviruses are neurotropic and travel centripetally towards the CNS following inoculation (hijacking axonal transport systems) and initial local replication in muscle tissue peripherally. Rabies immunoglobulin (RIG) and vaccine can prevent spread at this stage. Once the peripheral nerve is entered, the infection cannot be stopped. The mechanism of CNS damage is unknown, but the viral glycoprotein appears to correlate with virulence. Viral-mediated host immunosuppression occurs, including suppression of IFN responses, and the antibody response develops late in the illness. Transmission is primarily through contact with saliva (typically a bite) from infected animals, although a few reports of organ graft transmission are described—which the reader is highly encouraged to read.

Epidemiology

- Rabies is found worldwide. While an uncommon disease in the developed world, ~59 000 cases occur annually, with up to 29 million people receiving PEP. The developing world shoulders the burden of disease, in particular children.
- Ninety-nine per cent of cases of fatal human rabies infection is acquired from dogs.
- Many terrestrial mammals can carry rabies (cats, skunks, foxes, monkeys) or other *Lyssavirus* species, but as canine vaccination became widespread, bats have become a key vector. A ranking of various animal species susceptibility to rabies virus is provided by the WHO.
- There have been 26 rabies deaths in the UK since 1946; 25 were imported, with a case of endemic European bat lyssavirus 2 in a bat handler in Scotland in 2002. None were known to have had pre- or post-exposure prophylaxis.

Clinical features

- Incubation period is an average of 3 months (75%), although the quoted upper limit of the range extends to years.
- Once symptoms develop, infection is generally accepted to be uniformly fatal. A small body of research regarding cases of recovery/presence of neutralizing antibodies with vaccination exists.
- Risk of rabies transmission correlates with size of the inoculum (multiple bites, skin breach) and site (central carries higher risk than peripheral).
- Initial symptoms—non-specific viral prodrome (4–10 days). Altered sensation at the bite site is suspicious. Percussion myoedema may be observed (fleeting muscle contraction when struck with a tendon hammer).
- Two main clinical presentations:
  - furious (encephalitic) rabies (80%)—hydrophobia (an exaggerated respiratory tract irritant reflex, 50%), aerophobia (similar response to air movement/draft), delirium, agitation (50%), autonomic dysfunction (25%). Autonomic/cardiac abnormalities are described. Patients die of respiratory collapse within 1–2 weeks;

- paralytic (dumb) rabies (20%)—the spinal cord and brainstem are predominantly affected, and patients develop an ascending paralysis that may resemble GBS or a symmetrical quadriparesis. Meningeal signs may develop, then confusion and coma.

Diagnosis

- Accurate history taking focusing on travel/social aspects is vital.
- Early liaison with local/regional reference laboratories is key.
- CSF/radiology are non-specific. Histology is unreliable in real time.
- Immunofluorescence—skin biopsy taken from the nape of the neck (nuchal region), 5–6mm deep containing a minimum of 10 hair follicles.
- Serology—of limited use as antibodies develop late in illness/ administration of immunoglobulin clouds interpretation.
- Molecular testing—three-specimen combination testing of saliva, skin biopsy, and CSF has good sensitivity and specificity (near 100%).

Prevention and treatment

- Prevention—widespread vaccination of animal reservoirs is key.
- PEP—recommended for travellers to endemic areas and those with occupational exposure (vets, bat handlers, and laboratory staff) (see *Rabies: the green book*, available at: ℘ https://travelhealthpro.org.uk/ disease/148/rabies; NaTHNaC, available at: ℘ https://www.gov.uk/ government/publications/rabies-the-green-book-chapter-27).
- Post-exposure treatment (PET)—a commonly encountered clinical query. A risk assessment is performed. Recommendations include no action, vaccination alone, or vaccines and specific RIG administration. RIG is not typically administered if exposure occurred >1 year previously or if a vaccine has been given in the previous 7 days (the magnitude of the quantity of antibody production after vaccination is much greater then that derived from transient RIG). Risk assessment is composed of five main variables:
  - Animal involved—two risk categories exist: terrestrial mammals and bats. Bats are considered high risk globally, except for the UK and Ireland where they are considered low risk;
  - mechanism of injury—physical contact with saliva or not;
  - vaccination history of recipient (full, partial, or none);
  - presence of host immunosuppression, as defined in the green book (available at: ℘ https://www.gov.uk/government/publications/rab ies-the-green-book-chapter-27), can rarely require rabies serology during PET;
  - country of incident—countries are given a risk category;
  - full risk assessment tables and guidance for rabies PET are available at: ℘ https://www.gov.uk/government/publications/rabies-post- exposure-prophylaxis-management-guidelines/rabies-summary-of- risk-assessment-and-treatment
- Treatment—no effective treatment exists. A decision is required about whether to commence palliation or aggressive treatment. There is a lack of robust data on what components should be included in the aggressive treatment protocol because all are experimental. They include IFN, ribavirin, amantadine, intrathecal administration of drugs,

and inducing a coma. Administration of vaccine or RIG is controversial, as the disease process and antigenic stimulation are already under way.
• An experimental protocol called the Milwaukee protocol exists whereby patients are NOT given rabies vaccine nor RIG (➔ see Milwaukee protocol, https://www.ncbi.nlm.nih.gov/pmc/articles/PMC 7670764/, p. 503). It has a success rate of ~4%, but the case numbers are small.

Prion diseases

Overview

Prions are neither viral nor bacterial in origin. They are an independent class of infectious agents. The term 'prion' refers to a small, abnormal particle made of protein that lacks any nucleic acid (major defining feature) which is infectious. The normally occurring cellular prion protein (PrP^C) (which exists predominantly on the cell membrane in an α-helix form) changes its structural confirmation (to a β-sheet-predominant form that now accumulates intracellularly) and becomes resistant to protease degradation. This abnormal prion protein is termed PrP^{Sc} for scrapie (archetype prion disease in sheep). The normal function of PrP^C is not precisely known, but it is highly distributed throughout normal brain tissue. It is normally transcribed from the *PRNP* gene located on chromosome 20, position 13 (20p13). The University of Edinburgh, UK have indispensable resources for Creutzfeldt–Jakob disease (CJD) research/surveillance, with which the reader is encouraged to familiarize themselves with (available at: ✋ https://www.cjd. ed.ac.uk/)

Prion disease manifests itself as a transmissible, rapidly progressive neurodegenerative disease attributed to the accumulation of PrP^{Sc} resulting in cell death. There is no antibody response.

They pose a particular decontamination challenge, as they are resistant to most methods designed to destroy nucleic acid. Prolonged autoclaving is the most readily accessible format.

The nomenclature surrounding prion diseases is confusing, and they are increasingly grouped by aetiology:
• sporadic (90%), three main clinical syndromes—sCJD, sporadic fatal insomnia, and variably protease-sensitive prionopathy;
• genetic (10%), three main clinical syndromes—gCJD, fatal familial insomnia, and Gerstmann–Sträussler–Scheinker syndrome;
• infectious causes (<1%)—variant (v)CJD, atrogenic(i)CJD, and kuru.

Sporadic

• Sporadic Creutzfeldt–Jakob disease (sCJD):
   • epidemiology—90% of prion cases. Early liaison with local neurology/infectious diseases colleagues and the CJD testing laboratory in Edinburgh is highly recommended. Incidence is ~1 case per 1 million people. The origin of the abnormal prion protein PrP^{Sc} is unknown;

- clinical features—average age of onset is 65 years. Patients present with rapidly progressive dementia, psychiatric manifestation, and myoclonus (90%). Cerebellar signs (66%), and extrapyramidal and corticospinal tract signs, such as hyperreflexia and spasticity, are well described. Presentations are broad, and commoner differentials must be excluded. Six clinical phenotypes are recognized, classified by *PRNP* genotyping analysis;
- diagnosis—diagnostic criteria exist and are composed of clinical, radiological, and laboratory criteria;
- radiology—primarily MRI, is of most utility where T1, T2, fluid-attenuated inversion recovery (FLAIR), and DWI protocols and an experienced radiologist are key. Hyperintense signal in the putamen, cerebral cortex, and corpus striatum is commonest, but appearances are variable, even within disease course;
- EEG—between 70% and 95% of patients ultimately develop a typical pattern of slow background waves interrupted by generalized, bilaterally synchronous, biphasic or triphasic periodic sharp wave complexes. They are said to be 91% specific for sCJD and are not seen in variant CJD (vCJD);
- CSF—can be tested for the presence of the 14-3-3 protein (92% sensitive, 80% specific in sCJD, but only 50% and 91%, respectively, in vCJD) and tau protein (best sensitivity and specificity for vCJD). Elevations may be seen in HSV encephalitis, metabolic encephalopathies, and cerebral metastases. A molecular test called real-time quaking-induced conversion (RT-QuIC) looks at real-time induced conformational change of a recombinant PrP which can be accurately measured. This is quickly becoming one of the most useful tools in diagnosis;
- histology—of brain material remains the gold standard: spongiform change, neuronal loss, reactive gliosis, and little inflammatory response. PrP^{sc} can be identified by western blotting of material obtained at autopsy or biopsy;
- treatment—prognosis is poor, as the disease is rapidly progressive and almost uniformly fatal within 12 months (average 4–5 months). Symptom management is crucial, and a few experimental therapies have been investigated, with little overall efficacy, including pentosan polysulfate, flupirtine, and quinacrine.
- Sporadic fatal insomnia—this is where, although sporadic in origin, a disease phenotype almost indistinguishable from genetic fatal familial insomnia manifests (➔ see Genetic below). This has been attributed to an alternate allelic genotype of a valine substitution at codon 129, in conjunction with the expected D178N mutation.
- Variably protease-sensitive prionopathy—a clinically milder form of illness resembling frontotemporal dementia that is attributed to a more protease degradation-sensitive form of PrP^{sc}.

Genetic

- Genetic Creutzfeldt–Jakob disease (gCJD):
  - epidemiology—numerous mutations (>30 currently recognized, although almost certainly more exist) in the *PRNP* gene corresponding to a clinical phenotype that overall closely resembles

sCJD. Despite being inherited in an autosomal dominant fashion, a family history is not always present (50%). Our understanding of factors affecting penetrance is incomplete and will likely depend on the precise mutations present. The most commonly described mutation is a missense substitution of lysine for glutamine at codon 200;
* clinical features/diagnosis/treatment—as for sCJD, although it is likely that individual mutation patterns will have somewhat unique clinical courses that are as yet not fully described.
* Fatal familial insomnia:
  * epidemiology—first described in Italian families and displays autosomal dominant inheritance. Is due to the D178 missense mutation (aspartic acid for asparagine) occurring in conjunction with a methionine substitution at codon 129. Sporadic cases involving a different allelic substitution are described;
  * clinical features—patients typically present earlier than in CJD (age 56 on average). Sleep disturbance is a prominent feature, along with autonomic pathology (hypertension, abnormal sweating, and disorganized thermoregulation). Motor symptoms develop later. Spongiform change is rare. PrP^{Sc} concentrations are significantly lower than in CJD;
  * diagnosis—radiology and CSF analysis can be unhelpful. Even 14-3-3 and RT-QuIC molecular testing is not reliable. Genetic testing is central;
  * treatment—average disease duration is 13 months.
* Gerstmann–Sträussler–Scheinker syndrome—an extremely rare prion disease (<10 cases/100 million people per year), predominantly familial in nature. A multitude of concordant genetic mutations are described in the *PRNP* gene, most commonly P102L and a repeat insertion. The key feature is spinocerebellar degeneration (parkinsonism-like), with dementia developing at a mean age of around 43–48 years. Diagnosis centres around genetic testing.

Infectious

* Variant Creutzfeldt–Jakob disease (vCJD):
  * epidemiology—vCJD is attributed to consumption of cattle infected with bovine spongiform encephalopathy (BSE) (archetype prion disease in cattle). A large outbreak of BSE in the UK in the 1980s/ 90s was attributed to cattle being fed feed composed of scrapie-infected sheep carcasses. This continued until the introduction of a ban on ruminant feed in 1988. Five million animals were slaughtered in an effort to halt the epidemic. By November 2019, 178 human cases of definite or probable vCJD had been reported in the UK. vCJD appears to show a particular predilection for lymphoid tissue, which makes transmission via blood products possible (four known cases). Numerous bans on people with epidemiological links to blood products in the UK in the 1980/90s exist. The true impact of vCJD and potential cases yet to appear remains a worrying unknown entity, but thankfully cases continue to decrease. *PRNP* mutations are not present in vCJD;

- clinical features—typically affecting much younger patients (mean age 29 years), with a longer illness (14 months). Psychiatric and sensory symptomatology is prominent and tends to herald the onset of expectant neurological manifestations (cerebellar signs progressing to cognitive impairment);
- diagnosis—EEG and CSF analysis are broadly unhelpful, except for ruling out differential diagnosis; MRI shows pulvinar sign (symmetrical hyperintensity of the posterior thalamus) with numerous plaques. CSF RT-QuIC is not usually positive. The PrP^{sc} protein in vCJD appears remarkably conserved, and so tonsillar biopsy for western blot analysis is the test of choice. A multitude of diagnosis criteria exist;
- treatment—slightly longer prognosis of 14 months, but still no effective treatment exists.
- Iatrogenic CJD (iCJD)—refers to transmission of CJD secondary to medical intervention, and cases have been reported secondary to dural grafts/corneal transplants/transfusion-related/contaminated surgical instruments. The reader is referred to UKHSA guidelines for minimizing transmission of CJD in healthcare settings (available at: ✎ https:// www.gov.uk/government/publications/guidance-from-the-acdp-tse- risk-management-subgroup-formerly-tse-working-group).
- Kuru—originally endemic within a specific tribal group of Papua New Guinea; epidemiological studies suggested it was transmitted through ritual cannibalism, and there have been no further cases since the practice was abandoned. No mutations in the *PRNP* gene have been identified. Kuru appears to occur in a somewhat ordered clinical course. A prodromal phase of headache and arthralgia is followed by progressive neurological decline (ataxia, tremor, choreoathetosis, myoclonus) and dementia. Cranial nerve abnormalities, weakness, and sensory loss occur late in the disease, if at all. Laboratory tests are unhelpful, and EEG does not share the characteristic features of those seen in some cases of CJD. The pathologically distinct feature of kuru is the presence of PrP^{sc} plaques, predominantly in the cerebellum (similar, but not identical, to those seen in vCJD).

Fungi

Overview of fungi

Fungi are aerobic eukaryotes with limited anaerobic capabilities. They have chitinous cell walls and ergosterol-containing plasma membranes (human cell walls contain cholesterol). They may grow as yeasts (single-celled, reproduce by budding), moulds (form multicellular hyphae, which grow by branching and extension), or both—dimorphic, growing as yeasts *in vivo* and at 37°C *in vitro*, but as moulds at 25°C; 'mould in the cold and yeast in the beast'.

Reproduction

Fungal reproduction may be sexual or asexual. Virtually all fungi can produce asexual spores by mitosis. Sexual spores are formed by the fusion of two haploid nuclei, followed by meiotic division of the diploid nucleus. Certain fungi can only sexually reproduce with other colonies of a different compatible mating type (e.g. *Histoplasma* spp.).

Pathogenesis

Fungal infections may be cutaneous (e.g. dermatophyte infection), subcutaneous (e.g. following traumatic inoculation—sporotrichosis), or systemic (see Table 9.1). Systemic mycoses usually follow inhalation-acquired primary lung infection but may be caused by normal flora in an immunocompromised host (e.g. *Candida albicans*). Disease may be a consequence of toxin production (e.g. aflatoxin) or the host immune response to an infecting agent. Organism characteristics facilitating infection include: good growth at 37°C, production of substances such as keratinases by dermatophytes (digest keratin in skin, hair, and nails), the ability to change form (exist in nature as moulds, but take on yeast forms in a host, allowing them to spread and become pathogenic), the ability to adhere to surfaces (e.g. *C. albicans*, *Candidozyma auris*), antiphagocytic capsules (*Cryptococcus neoformans*), or persisting following phagocytosis, allowing dissemination via macrophages. Generally, hosts have a high level of innate immunity to fungi—most infections are mild and self-limiting. This resistance derives from the fatty acid content and pH of the skin, mucosal surfaces, and body fluids, epithelial turnover, competition

Table 9.1 Overview of common fungi causing human disease

Phylum	Organism	Syndrome				Comment
		D	O	SC	SU	
Basidiomycota	**Yeasts**					
	Cryptococcus neoformans	✓	✓			Mild lung granuloma in healthy
	Trichosporon beigelii		✓		✓	May disseminate
	Rhodotorula spp.		✓			
	Malassezia furfur		✓		✓	Pityriasis versicolor

Table 9.1 (Contd.)

Phylum	Organism	Syndrome				Comment
		D	O	SC	SU	
Ascomycota	Candida spp.		✓		✓	
	Pneumocystis jirovecii (previously carinii)		✓			
	Dimorphic fungi					
	Histoplasma capsulatum	✓				Histoplasmosis
	Blastomyces dermatitidis	✓				Blastomycosis
	Sporothrix schenkii	✓	✓	✓		Acquired by local trauma. Rare dissemination
	Coccidioides immitis, Paracoccidioides brasiliensis	✓				In the Americas
	Taloromyces marneffii		✓			Disseminate in immunosuppressed
	Moulds					
	Aspergillus spp.	✓	✓		✓	Allergic, localized and invasive disease
	Epidermophyton spp., Trichophyton spp., Microsporum spp.				✓	Dermatophytes—infect skin, hair, and nails
	Fusarium spp.		✓		✓	Disseminate in immunosuppressed
	Scedosporium boydii		✓	✓		Mycetoma. May also infect any organ or disseminate
	Madurella spp., Acremonium spp., Exophiala spp., etc.			✓		Mycetoma
Zygomycota	Mucor spp., Rhizopus spp.	✓	✓			Rare invasion (e.g. mucormycosis)

D, disseminated infection; O, opportunistic infection; SC, subcutaneous infection; SU, superficial infection.

with the normal bacterial flora, transferrin, and cilia of the respiratory tract. Cell-mediated immunity (CMI) is important in controlling fungal infection. Humoral responses play a part, but patients with defects in CMI experience more severe fungal infections than those with humoral defects.

Epidemiology

- Host factors—immunocompromise leads to a general increase in opportunistic fungal infections.

Certain conditions predispose to specific organisms:
- diabetic ketoacidosis and rhinocerebral mucormycosis;
- uncontrolled HIV and histoplasmosis;
- antibiotics, and candidal vaginitis.
- Environment—affects the pattern of fungal disease. Some are worldwide, but seen mostly in individuals whose lifestyles place them at risk of exposure (e.g. a gardener experiencing s/c inoculation of *Sporothrix schenckii* through minor trauma). Others are more likely to be seen in people living in, or visiting, specific regions (e.g. *Coccidioides immitis* in the desert of south-western USA).

Candida species

Mycology and epidemiology

- Small ovoid cells that reproduce by budding. Both sexual and asexual forms exist. Of the over 150 *Candida* spp., only 10 are frequent human pathogens—*Candida glabrata* (now called *Nakaseomyces glabrata*) and *C. albicans* account for 70–80% of cases of invasive candidiasis. The others are: *Candida guilliermondii* (now called *Meyerozyma guilliermondii*), *Candida krusei* (now called *Pichia kudriavzevii*), *Candida parapsilosis*, *Candida tropicalis*, *Candida pseudotropicalis*, *Candida lusitaniae* (now called *Clavispora lusitaniae*), *Candida dubliniensis*, and *C. auris*.
- *C. albicans* is ubiquitous and may be found in soil, food, and hospital environments. They are normal commensals of humans (skin, sputum, GI tract, ♀ genital tract, etc.). The vast majority of human infections are of endogenous origin.
- *C. krusei* (now called *Pichia kudriavzevii*) is found in many environmental sites. It is fluconazole-resistant and often found colonizing patients receiving fluconazole prophylaxis.
- *C. parapsilosis* (adheres well to synthetic materials) and *C. tropicalis* are now commoner causes of intravascular catheter (IVC) infections and endocarditis than *C. albicans*.
- *C. glabrata* (now called *Nakaseomyces glabrata*) infections of intensive care unit (ICU) patients are associated with a low survival rate.
- *C. auris* is an emerging pathogen isolated globally and frequently associated with infections in ICU patients. Delayed identification by using conventional diagnostics and variable antifungal resistance profiles have led to widespread outbreaks.[2]
- Many species have been renamed recently (Table 9.2).

Pathogenesis

The rise in *Candida* spp. infection relates to the increase in medical interventions: use of antibiotics (suppressing normal bacterial flora and permitting

Table 9.2 New names of fungi, following widespread application of molecular technologies in taxonomy, which allowed correction of past classification errors

Previous name	New name
Candida krusei	Pichia kudriavzevii
Candida glabrata	Nakaseomyces glabrata
Candida guilliermondii	Meyerozyma guilliermondii
Candida lusitaniae	Clavispora lusitaniae
Candida rugosa	Diutina rugosa

the proliferation of *Candida* organisms), IVCs (providing a route of entry) or prosthetic implants, and GI tract surgery. Immune suppression mediated by disease (e.g. HIV) or therapies, such as steroids, are also associated with increased rates of infection. The immune response to *Candida* infection is mediated by humoral and cellular mechanisms (cf. patients with uncontrolled HIV who demonstrate high susceptibility to cutaneous infection). *Candida* spp. virulence factors include surface molecules that permit organism adherence to other structures (human cells, extracellular matrix, prosthetic devices), acid proteases, and the ability to convert to a hyphal form.

General points on diagnosis and management

- Many patients will require early treatment in the absence of a conclusive microbiological diagnosis. Those at risk (e.g. the neutropenic) who remain febrile, despite broad-spectrum antibiotic therapy, should be suspected of having systemic candidiasis. Therapy should be started early and empirically in such patients.[1] Always consider positive culture results from sterile sites to be significant. *Candida* may contaminate blood cultures (BCs), but treatment is usually indicated, as distinguishing contamination from infection is very difficult. BCs are positive in 50–60% of cases of disseminated disease. Serology is rarely useful.
- **Culture**—strict aerobes that grow well when present in biopsy specimens. Unfortunately, BCs in proven candidaemia are positive in only around 60% of cases (usually within 48–96h). Yeast forms (Gram-positive) and hyphae may be found or microscopy of clinical specimens (facilitated by 10% potassium hydroxide (KOH)). Appear as smooth, white colonies on agar. Presumptive identification of *C. albicans* is possible by inoculating organisms from a colony into a small tube of serum—germ tubes should form within 90min, which tend not to be seen with the other species (relatively high rates of false positives and false negatives). Germ tubes may also appear as 'whiskers' forming a star-shaped colony. Accurate speciation relies on physiological characteristics (e.g. fermentation, nitrate utilization) and can be demonstrated on commercial indicator agar preparations (ChromAgar™) and with multiparameter kits and matrix-assisted laser desorption/ionization time-of-flight mass spectroscopy (MALDI-TOF).

- *Candida* spp. are uncommon laboratory contaminants.
- **Fungal antigen detection assays**—are useful adjuncts in the diagnosis and monitoring of invasive fungal infection:
  - 1-3 beta-*D*-glucan—a cell wall component in a wide variety of fungi, except *Cryptococcus* and the mucoromycota. It is a broad-spectrum assay that detects *Aspergillus*, *Candida*, *Fusarium*, *Acremonium*, *Pneumocystis*, and *Saccharomyces* spp. Its negative predictive value is useful, but its positive predictive value is limited by the ubiquitous nature of glucan. Specificity of the assay is improved by two consecutive positive results. *Candida* mannan assay—sensitivity ranges from 31% to 90% (less for non-*albicans* spp.).
- **Sensitivity testing**—*in vitro* susceptibility testing can help guide treatment of candidiasis to a greater extent than of the other fungi. Knowledge of the infecting species is highly predictive of likely susceptibility and can be used to guide therapy. Susceptibility testing is important in managing deep infections of non-*albicans* spp., particularly if the patient has been previously treated with an azole. *C. albicans* is rarely resistant to azoles, whereas certain non-*albicans* spp. may show intrinsic resistance to these and certain other antifungal agents (see Table 9.3).
- **Treatment** duration will depend on the source, presence of indwelling prosthetic material, and host immune status. In the case of invasive infection, removal of prosthetic material (e.g. IV lines) is recommended and all patients should have fundoscopy and transthoracic echocardiography (TTE) to exclude seeding of infection.
- **Infection control** precautions in *Candidozyma auris* infections. Patients known to be infected or colonized with *C. auris* should be isolated in a single room with en suite facilities and should undergo regular longitudinal screening while in hospital and on readmission.[2]

Superficial Candida infections

For details of the cutaneous manifestations of candidal infection, see Fungal skin infections, *Candida*, p. 810.

Mucous membrane infection

Thrush

A form of oral candidiasis characterized by white, creamy patches on the tongue and oral mucosa. Scraping removes the lesions, leaving a sore bleeding surface. Diagnosis can be confirmed by using a KOH smear or Gram staining to demonstrate hyphae and yeast forms. Other manifestations include acute atrophic candidiasis (affecting the tongue), chronic atrophic candidiasis (associated with denture use), angular cheilitis (not caused solely by *Candida*), and *Candida* leukoplakia (white plaques affecting the cheek, lips, and tongue; may be pre-cancerous). Oral thrush is associated with the use of inhaled steroids (often resolves spontaneously, even without reduction in steroid use, or with TOP therapy), malignancy, and uncontrolled HIV. Treatment is usually TOP (systemic where this fails).

Table 9.3 Treatment of *Candida* infections

Presentation	First-line treatment	Duration	Comment
Candidaemia in non-neutropenic adults	Echino or flucon (alternatives: liposomal amphotericin or voricon)	14 days after first negative BC and resolution of symptoms	Echino if moderate/severe or recent azole exposure
Candidaemia in neutropenic adults	Echino or LFAmB (alternatives: flucon or voricon)	Duration uncertain, but at least 14–21 days after first negative BC, resolution of symptoms, and resolved neutropenia	Voricon if mould coverage desirable. Flucon can be used once sensitivities confirmed
Suspected candidaemia in neutropenia	LFAmB, caspo, or voricon (alternative: flucon if no prior exposure)	Uncertain	Consider antifungals in neutropenia after 4 days of fever unresponsive to antibiotics
Chronic disseminated candidiasis	Flucon if stable, LFAmB if unwell (alternative: echino)	Until resolution or calcification of radiological lesions (usually months)	Flucon may be given after 1–2 weeks of AmB therapy if stable or improved
Candidal cystitis	Flucon (alternatives: AmB-d or 5-FC). Modify once culture results available	2 weeks	Remove/replace stents/catheters. High-risk patients should be treated as disseminated, even if asymptomatic
Pyelonephritis	Flucon (alternative: AmB-d with/without 5-FC)	2 weeks	If suspected dissemination, treat as such
Endocarditis	LFAmB with/without 5-FC (alternative: echino). Flucon step-down if sensitive	Variable, depending on surgical outcome	Valve replacement is nearly always necessary. Long-term suppression with flucon if this is not possible
Meningitis	LFAmB with/without 5-FC	Several weeks	Flucon follow-on therapy

(Continued)

Table 9.3 (Contd.)

Presentation	First-line treatment	Duration	Comment
Endophthalmitis	AmB-d with 5-FC (alternative: flucon or LFAmB)	At least 6 weeks, as determined by repeated eye exam	Vitrectomy is usually necessary if vitritis present
Oropharyngeal candidiasis	Clo or nystatin or flucon PO (alternative itracon, voricon, or AmB PO suspension)	7–14 days after	Topical for mild, flucon for moderate/ severe
Oesophageal candidiasis	Flucon PO (alternatives: echino, AmB-d, itracon, voricon)	14–21 days	IV therapy may be required in severe cases

AmB-d, amphotericin B deoxycholate; caspo, caspofungin; clo, clotrimazole; echino, an echinocandin; 5-FC, 5- flucytosine; flucon, fluconazole; itracon, itraconazole; LFAmB, liposomal amphotericin B; voricon, voriconazole.

Prophylaxis with fluconazole has been effective in the prevention of oral *Candida* infections in patients with cancer or uncontrolled HIV, but remains controversial.

Candida oesophagitis

The majority of cases are associated with immunosuppressed patients. May occur in the absence of oral disease. Symptoms include dysphagia, retrosternal chest pain, nausea, and vomiting. Symptoms may be mild, even in extensive disease. Diagnosis is made by endoscopy and biopsy. In practice, diagnosis is often made presumptively in those with uncontrolled HIV or malignancy, on the basis of oral thrush and symptoms of oesophagitis. Extensive disease may result in intraluminal protrusions and partial obstruction. Perforation is rare. Severely immunocompromised patients may be co-infected with cytomegalovirus (CMV) or herpes simplex virus (HSV). Fluconazole has been demonstrated to have greater efficacy than ketoconazole in patients with uncontrolled HIV with *Candida* oesophagitis.

Gastrointestinal candidiasis

Usually associated with malignant disease, the commonest manifestation being focal invasion of benign stomach ulcers. Diffuse gastric mucosal involvement is rare. Small and large bowel infection also occurs, with white plaques, erosions, pseudomembrane, and ulceration visible on endoscopy.

Vulvovaginitis

Candida is the commonest cause of vaginitis, and 75% of women have at least one episode in their lives. Predisposing factors include diabetes, antibiotic therapy, and pregnancy. Oedema and vulval pruritus may be accompanied by discharge that may be scanty or thick. Secondary infection of perineal skin and the urethra can occur.

Invasive Candida

Candidaemia/candidiasis

Patients at risk of dissemination include those with malignancy (particularly acute leukaemia), burns patients, and those with complicated post-operative courses (e.g. organ transplants, GI tract surgery). Multiple organs tend to be affected. The pathological features are small abscesses with diffuse microabscesses with a granulomatous reaction. While it **may** represent colonization of a venous catheter, *Candida* in a BC should be treated with antifungals, and the patient examined carefully for manifestations of disseminated disease. Presentation varies from mild fever to severe sepsis, and it can spread haematogenously to multiple organs. Always check for endocarditis and eye involvement (chorioretinitis or vitritis in ~25%), and consider: skin (pustules/nodules), renal/muscle abscess, prosthetic vascular devices, and CNS infection. Disease may be more extensive than symptoms suggest. Management always involves removal of lines or prosthetic material. BCs are positive in <60% of those with proven candidaemia, and diagnosis is often very late or at post-mortem. Tests for *Candida* antigen have a high rate of false-negative results—diagnosis is largely clinical. Cultures should be repeated several times, and catheters removed or replaced. Speciation and isolate sensitivity should be confirmed. Therapy should be continued for at least 2 weeks after the first negative BC/line removal.

CNS candidiasis

May infect both brain substance and meninges Around 50% of *Candida* meningitis cases occur in the context of disseminated disease. Meningitis may present non-specifically or with features typical of meningism. Parenchymal infection takes the form of scattered multiple microabscesses and can have extremely variable clinical presentations. Infection may follow trauma, neurosurgery, or colonization of a ventricular shunt. The CSF may show lymphocytosis, with low glucose levels, but these findings are not consistent. Organisms are visible on Gram staining in 40% of cases. The mortality rate is very high without therapy. Complications include hydrocephalus.

Candida endocarditis and other cardiac involvement

Candida endocarditis usually affects the aortic and mitral valves. Associations include valve disease, chemotherapy, implantation of prosthetic heart valves, prolonged use of IVCs, heroin addiction (*C. parapsilosis* is the commonest cause), and pre-existing bacterial endocarditis. Around 50% of cases follow cardiac surgery (associated with the length of the post-operative course, reflecting the use of IV lines and antibiotics). Most cases present within the first 2 months post-operatively; <40% of cases are caused by non-*albicans* spp.; >70% of patients have positive BCs. Prior to antifungal therapy, mortality was 90%. Combined prolonged (6–10 weeks) medical and early surgical treatment has brought this to around 45%. There is a high risk of relapse. Patients should be followed up for at least 2 years post-operatively. It may be appropriate to use long-term suppressive therapy (e.g. fluconazole). Other cardiac manifestations include myocardial microabscesses and pericarditis.

Urinary tract infection

Either follows extension of vaginitis in women or is sexually acquired by a man from a woman with thrush. Recent antibiotic use is common. *Candida* cystitis is associated with prolonged catheterization, and bladder perforation may occur in severe cases. Renal infection may occur haematogenously or, less commonly, by retrograde spread (particularly in association with renal tract obstruction or diabetes), causing papillary necrosis, fungal balls, and perinephric abscesses. Surgery may be required to remove fungal balls. Renal tract imaging is advised and prosthetic material within the tract should be removed.

Candiduria per se (particularly in those with urinary catheters) may represent colonization. Asymptomatic candiduria should be treated in certain patient groups (e.g. renal transplant patients, neutropenic patients, low-birthweight infants, those undergoing urinary tract interventions such as nephrostomy).

Bone and joint infection

Candida osteomyelitis may affect the vertebrae and discs, wrist, femur, scapula, humerus, and costochondral junctions. BCs are usually negative. Diagnosis is by aspiration of the affected area. Most cases follow haematogenous spread but may occur secondary to spread from the skin. Surgery may be required. Septic arthritis due to *Candida* occurs in the context of disseminated *Candida*, trauma, surgery, and intra-articular injection of steroids. It may be a complication of uncontrolled HIV and rheumatoid arthritis. *C. albicans* is the commonest cause in the context of disseminated infection. Non-*albicans* spp. are commoner when infection is local.

Intra-abdominal infection

Candidal peritonitis may complicate peritoneal dialysis (PD), GI perforation, and surgery. Infection tends to remain localized—dissemination is rare in cases associated with PD, and in around 25% of cases secondary to GI perforation. Other GI organs that can be affected include the gall bladder, spleen, liver, and pancreas. Hepatosplenic infection occurs in the severely immunocompromised. *Candida* PD peritonitis can be treated by local instillation of amphotericin B (can be painful) or fluconazole. Catheter removal may be indicated. *Candida* from long-standing post-operative drains may represent colonization—its presence does not equate with infection, and treatment is not always required. Isolation from radiologically guided biopsy or ascites suggests infection that must be treated. The failure rate for treatment of liver and spleen infection is high.

Candidiasis of the biliary tract may require drainage.

Other

- Respiratory tract candidiasis—may cause a diffuse infiltrate, following haematogenous spread (resembling heart failure or *Pneumocystis* pneumonia (PCP) in early stages), or bronchopneumonia due to

local inoculation from the bronchial tree. While *Candida* is frequently recovered from bronchoalveolar lavage (BAL) in ICU patients, it is an extremely rare cause of pneumonia in those with an otherwise normal immune system. Definitive diagnosis depends on biopsy.
- Ocular infection—➔ see Uveitis, pp. 796–8.

Treatment of Candida

Key points
- Source control: remove infected IV lines, and replace infected valves, if possible.[1]
- Non-*albicans* spp. are often fluconazole-resistant, while remaining sensitive to newer azoles and echinocandins (see Table 9.4). Thus, knowledge of the infecting species is predictive of likely susceptibility. Susceptibility testing is recommended for all invasive isolates.
  - *C. albicans* is generally sensitive to fluconazole. Resistance may occur in immunosuppressed patients with prolonged fluconazole exposure.
  - *C. glabrata* (now called *Nakaseomyces glabrata*) is less susceptible to azoles (increased drug efflux) and amphotericin (use higher doses). Cross-resistance amongst all azoles is common. Echinocandins generally remain effective.
  - *C. krusei* (now called *Pichia kudriavzevii*) is intrinsically resistant to fluconazole (due to altered P450 isoenzyme) and less susceptible to voriconazole and amphotericin (use higher doses). It is sensitive to echinocandins.
  - *C. lusitaniae* (now called *Clavispora lusitaniae*) is susceptible to azoles, but uniquely amongst *Candida* spp., frequently resistant to amphotericin.
  - *C. parapsilosis* remains susceptible to most antifungals, but the minimum inhibitory concentration (MICs) with echinocandins are higher than for other species.
  - *C. auris* has variable resistance profiles. Empirical treatment is with an echinocandin; however, these drugs have limited CNS/urinary infection penetration and combination therapy may be needed. Discussion with a national reference laboratory is recommended.
- Echinocandin or amphotericin is first line in most disseminated and deep organ infection—**especially** if there is a risk of fluconazole resistance. Most strains are sensitive, and lipid formulations are less nephrotoxic. Used in combination with flucytosine for invasive disease (e.g. meningitis).
- Susceptibility testing is important in managing deep infections of non-*albicans* spp., particularly with previous azole exposure.
- Azoles are a useful continuation therapy for *C. albicans* infections initially controlled with other agents.

References
1 Pappas PG, Kauffman CA, Andes D, *et al.*; Infectious Diseases Society of America. Clinical practice guidelines for the management of candidiasis: 2009 update by the Infectious Diseases Society of America. *Clin Infect Dis.* 2016;**62**:e1–50.
2 UKHSA *C. auris* guidance (2017). https://www.gov.uk/government/collections/candida-auris

Table 9.4 Candida sensitivity to different antifungal agents

	Candida albicans	Candida glabrata (now called Nakaseomyces glabrata)	Candida krusei (now called Pichia kudriavzevii)	Candida lusitaniae (now called Clavispora lusitaniae)	Aspergillus	Aspergillus terreus	Mucor
Fluconazole	✓	*	✗	✓	✗	✗	✗
Voriconazole/itraconazole	✓	✓	✓	✓	✓	✓	✗
Posaconazole/isavuconazole	✓	✓	✓	✓	✓	✓	✓
Micafungin/anidulafungin/caspofungin	✓	✓	✓	✓	✓	✓	✗
Amphotericin	✓	✓	✓	✗	✓	✗	✓

✓ Has activity against the species.

✗ Does not have activity against the species.

* C. glabrata (now called Nakaseomyces glabrata) has less susceptibility to fluconazole.

Malassezia

These are lipophilic yeasts (e.g. they grow in the presence of certain fatty acids). They are oval or round in shape. They first colonize the skin in late childhood and are seen as normal commensals. They can cause skin or line infections (e.g. newborns receiving lipid infusions).

Pityriasis versicolor

Superficial skin infection characterized by hypopigmented lesions usually confined to the trunk and proximal limbs. Usually caused by *Malassezia globosa* or *Malassezia furfur*.

- **Pathogenesis**—clinical infection is usually associated with yeasts transforming to hyphal forms from their round/oval appearance. Although seen at greater frequency in those with Cushing's syndrome, there is no clear association with T-cell suppression. Commoner in the tropics and may be precipitated by sun exposure. A carboxylic acid produced by the yeast may lead to depigmentation.
- **Clinical features**—non-itchy macules develop on the trunk and proximal limbs, and may be hypo- or hyperpigmented. They can coalesce, forming scaly plaques.
- **Diagnosis**—direct microscopy of the lesions will reveal yeasts and hyphae. They may fluoresce under ultraviolet (UV) light. Organisms are best seen in skin scrapings after ink and KOH staining.
- **Treatment**—some lesions resolve spontaneously. Otherwise, TOP treatment for 2 weeks with an azole, terbinafine cream, selenium lotion, or 20% sodium thiosulfate is usually effective. Severe cases may require a course of an oral azole.

Malassezia folliculitis

TOP therapy may be effective. Systemic treatment is often necessary. Three clinical presentations:
- itchy papules/pustules on the back and upper chest, sometimes appearing after sun exposure;
- multiple small papules across the back and chest in patients with seborrhoeic dermatitis. Lesions may display erythema and scaling;
- multiple pustules across the trunk and face in patients with HIV.

Seborrhoeic dermatitis

The cause is not known, but *Malassezia* has been implicated in its pathogenesis. There is no evidence that direct invasion precipitates the appearance of seborrhoeic dermatitis, but most cases resolve with a course of azole.

Line sepsis

Infections are treated with line removal, and with either amphotericin or an azole (if found to be sensitive). There have been reports of successful treatment with line removal alone, as well as with antifungal treatment alone.

Other yeasts

Trichosporon **species**

Trichosporon beigelii can be part of the commensal flora of humans. It can cause invasive infections in the immunocompromised and has also been identified in prosthetic valve infections. Trichosporonosis is an acute, febrile infection, with dissemination to multiple organs. The means of acquisition is not clear. Diagnosis is by biopsy and culture. BCs tend to be positive late in the course of illness. Amphotericin has been used in treatment.

Rhodotorula **species**

Three species are recognized rare human pathogens: *Rhodotorula mucilaginosa* (accounting for 74–75% of cases), *Rhodotorula glutinis*, and *Rhodotorula minuta*. Infection is commonest in immunocompromised patients, including those with uncontrolled HIV, burns patients, peritoneal dialysis patients, IV drug users, and haematological malignancy patients. The yeast has a predilection for adhering to plastic surfaces and is often seen with central venous catheter (CVC) use.

Cryptococcus

An encapsulated yeast-like organism that reproduces by budding.[2] The cell is round or ovoid (4–6 micrometres in diameter), and surrounded by a capsule of variable size. There are four capsular serotypes (A to D). Genotypic differences have led to reclassification: *C. neoformans* belong to A and D (var. *grubii* and var. *neoformans*, respectively) and cause infections in immunodeficient patients. Serotypes B and C are now considered as a separate species (*Cryptococcus gattii*) and are more likely to cause infections in the immunocompetent.

Epidemiology

C. neoformans is a ubiquitous environmental saprophyte found worldwide. It has been isolated from pigeon droppings and from contaminated soil and fruit. Infections caused by *C. gattii* are largely restricted to tropical and subtropical areas, and has been cultured from eucalyptus trees. Infection occurs by inhalation of aerosolized organisms, but there is no evidence of person-to-person transmission or laboratory-acquired infection. Rare routes of transmission include organ transplantation from infected donors or cutaneous inoculation. There is no evidence of zoonotic transmission. Cryptococcosis occurs more commonly in patients with defects in T-cell-mediated immunity: uncontrolled HIV (80–90% of cryptococcal infections, CD4 <100 cells/mm³), prolonged glucocorticoid treatment, post-transplantation (peak period 4–6 weeks), malignancy, and sarcoidosis.

Pathogenesis

A number of potential virulence factors have been identified: capsular polysaccharide, melanin/mannitol production, and a lack of soluble anticryptococcal factors in the CSF. The inflammatory response to infection is variable. The characteristic lesion consists of cystic clusters of fungi spread throughout the brain, with no inflammatory response. Less commonly, focal inflammatory lesions (cryptococcomas) are found. In severe infections, the leptomeninges are thickened, with distension of the subarachnoid by a white gelatinous material (capsular polysaccharide).

Clinical features

- Cryptococcal meningitis—acute or chronic, and symptoms may be mild and non-specific. Fever and neck stiffness may be minimal or absent. Papilloedema (30%), cranial nerve palsies (20%), blindness. Seizures occur late. Differential diagnosis: other mycoses, TB meningitis, viral meningoencephalitides, meningeal metastases.
- Pulmonary cryptococcosis—asymptomatic or dyspnoea, cough, chest pain. Physical signs are unusual. May be rapidly progressive in uncontrolled HIV. Differential: tumour, PCP, pulmonary TB, histoplasmosis.
- Other sites—skin lesions, bone lesions, oral lesions, vulvar lesions, post-transplant pyelonephritis, prostatic cryptococcosis.

Laboratory diagnosis

- **CSF**—elevated opening pressure (>50cmCSF), low glucose level, high protein level, high WCC (>20/mm³, lymphocyte predominance). CSF abnormalities may be minimal in uncontrolled HIV. Check cryptococcal antigen.
- **India ink smear**—India ink or nigrosin staining of the CSF deposit shows a capsule, a double cell wall, and refractile inclusions in the cytoplasm in 20–50% of HIV-negative cases and in around 75% of patients with uncontrolled HIV.
- **Fungal culture**—samples include CSF, sputum, and urine. Grows on Sabouraud agar within 3–7 days. Smooth, convex, yellow/tan colonies on solid media, or brown on birdseed agar (melanin production). Unlike other yeasts, it does not produce pseudomycelia on cornmeal or Tween agar. Confirmation is by MALDI.
- **Cryptococcal antigen test**—latex agglutination tests have sensitivities of ≥90% and can be performed on CSF or serum. False-positive tests occur, but titres are usually ≤1:8 (may result from infection with *T. beigelii* and *Capnocytophaga*).
- **Histopathology**—methenamine silver or periodic acid–Schiff (PAS) staining shows a yeast-like organism with narrow-based buds. Mayer's mucicarmine stain stains the capsule rose red.
- **MALDI-TOF**—can be used to discriminate between *C. neoformans* and *C. gattii* complexes.

Treatment

- **Meningitis**—antifungal therapy, combined with aggressive management of raised intracranial pressure (ICP), is associated with better outcomes. Those with raised ICP at diagnosis, or developing symptoms suggestive of it, should have daily lumbar punctures (LPs) to reduce the pressure to <20cmCSF or to 50% of the opening pressure. Those requiring LPs after 4 weeks probably need a shunt.
    - **Induction**: amphotericin and flucytosine. Rapidly fungicidal. Continue for 2 weeks (4–6 weeks if using amphotericin alone, in non-HIV/non-transplant hosts or if cryptococcomas). Some authorities recommend repeat LP after induction, to ensure sterilization of CSF.

- **Consolidation**: high-dose fluconazole (400mg daily) for 8–10 weeks.
- **Maintenance therapy**: fluconazole (200mg daily) for at least a year in patients with ongoing risk (e.g. low CD4). Consider monitoring cryptococcal antigen until CD4 >200 cells/mm³.
- Selected patients with uncontrolled HIV who have mild, asymptomatic CNS cryptococcosis have been treated successfully with a long course of high-dose PO fluconazole (<1g/day) and flucytosine—however, many have significant problems with drug side effects (GI and bone marrow toxicity).
- **Pulmonary disease**—mild to moderate infections in the immunocompetent can be treated with PO fluconazole alone. Those with severe disease or multi-organ involvement should be treated as for meningitis. Surgical excision may be curative.

Prognosis

Prognosis depends on severity of the illness at presentation and the nature of any underlying disease. Relapse is rare in those HIV patients who respond to treatment, continue suppressive therapy, and experience improved immune function on antiretroviral therapy (ART). Note that immune reconstitution inflammatory syndrome (IRIS) may occur in the early weeks of ART. Steroids may be indicated in severe cases.

Pneumocystis jirovecii

For many years, *Pneumocystis carinii* was thought to be a protozoan, but ribosomal RNA (rRNA) analysis suggests that it is more closely related to fungi. The human-derived organism was renamed *Pneumocystis jirovecii*, whereas the rat-derived organism remains named as *Pneumocystis carinii*. The first cases of pneumonitis in humans were recognized in malnourished European children during the Second World War.

Microbiology

P. jirovecii is an unusual fungus, lacking ergosterol in its cell wall, and therefore not susceptible to certain antifungals. It is extremely difficult to culture *in vitro*, so biochemical and metabolic studies of the organism have been limited. Three developmental stages exist: the trophic form, the sporocyte, and the spores.

Epidemiology

P. jirovecii is ubiquitous in the environment and has a worldwide distribution. Acquisition is via the airborne route. It was originally believed that primary infection occurred in childhood, with the organism persisting in a latent state. It is now thought that frequent clearance and reinfection are more likely. Cluster outbreaks have occurred in hospitals, suggesting person-to-person transmission is commoner than previously thought. Risk factors for disease include:
- debilitated infants and those with severe protein malnutrition;
- primary/acquired immunodeficiency (e.g. HIV with CD4 count <200 cell/mm³);
- immunosuppressive drugs (e.g. glucocorticoids)—especially in organ transplantation or malignancy.

Pathogenesis

Once inhaled, the trophic form attaches to the alveolar type I cell and undergoes proliferation. Impaired humoral and T-cell-mediated immunity contributes to its uncontrolled proliferation. The host immune response results in the production of inflammatory cytokines (e.g. tumour necrosis factor (TNF)-α and interleukin (IL)-1), which contribute to lung damage. The main histological finding is a foamy eosinophilic alveolar exudate. There may be hyaline membrane formation, interstitial fibrosis, and oedema.

Clinical features

- **Pneumonia**—HIV patients tend to experience an insidious onset of fever, dyspnoea, non-productive cough, and reduced exercise tolerance over days/weeks. There may be sputum production, haemoptysis, or chest pain. Non-HIV cases are more likely to present with fulminant respiratory failure that may occur following a **decrease** in immunosuppression. Examination reveals tachypnoea, tachycardia, exercise-induced hypoxia, and crackles (in <30% of adults). Infants may be cyanosed, with respiratory distress. CXR may show diffuse bilateral interstitial ground-glass infiltrates, but lobar or nodular changes can occur.
- **Extrapulmonary disease**—this occurs mainly in the context of advanced HIV infection and is rare. The most commonly affected sites are the lymph nodes, spleen, liver, bone marrow, GI tract, eyes, thyroid, adrenal glands, and kidneys. Clinical findings may vary from incidental findings at autopsy to severe progressive disease.

Laboratory diagnosis

- Microscopy—*P. jirovecii* is rarely found in expectorated sputum; induced sputum is much more sensitive (50–90%). BAL increases the diagnostic rate to >90% in HIV cases, especially if multiple lobes are sampled or the procedure is directed to the sites of radiographic involvement. Yield is lower in non-HIV cases and in those receiving aerosolized pentamidine (decreased organism burden) Transbronchial biopsy may provide further information but is associated with complications. Open lung biopsy may be helpful. A variety of stains have been used to identify *P. jirovecii* (e.g. methenamine silver, Wright Giemsa). Commercial immunofluorescence tests and immunohistochemistry are more sensitive, but expensive.
- Molecular diagnostics—PCR amplification and detection of *P. jirovecii* DNA have proved highly sensitive and reasonably specific. It is of particular use in non-HIV infected cases. However, detection of a PCR product in a clinical specimen may represent subclinical infection.
- Antigen detection—beta-D-glucan is present in all fungal cell walls so, while not specific for PCP, may have a role in diagnostic evaluation.

Treatment

The treatment of choice is high-dose co-trimoxazole (120mg/kg/day in four divided doses) for 14–21 days. Side effects: skin rash, fever, cytopenias, vomiting, hepatitis, pancreatitis, nephritis, hyperkalaemia, acidosis, CNS symptoms. Alternatives: atovaquone (mild/moderate disease), clindamycin with primaquine (test for glucose-6-phosphate dehydrogenase (G6PD) deficiency), IV pentamidine. Adjunctive corticosteroids are recommended for HIV-positive patients with pO_2 <70mmHg, and should be considered in hypoxic non-HIV patients (less data on their efficacy). Start ART within 2 weeks if HIV-positive.

Prognosis

Untreated PCP in immunocompromised patients is fatal. Poor prognostic factors include hypoxia (PaO_2 <7kPa), high alveolar–arterial oxygen gradient (>45mmHg), and extensive pulmonary infiltrates. Short-term mortality (1–3 months) in HIV-infected patients has fallen to 10–20%, whereas mortality in HIV-negative patients remains 30–50%. Patients who recover are at risk of developing recurrent episodes or pneumothoraces.

Prevention

- **HIV-infected patients**—primary prophylaxis with co-trimoxazole is recommended in HIV-infected patients with a CD4 count <200 cells/mm³. Secondary prophylaxis is recommended for life but may be discontinued in patients with CD4 counts consistently >200 cells/mm³. Alternative regimens: dapsone ± pyrimethamine + folinic acid or IV pentamidine isethionate.
- **HIV-negative patients**—chemoprophylaxis should be considered in all patients with predisposing conditions (⊕ see Epidemiology above):
- Risk factors for disease include:
  - debilitated infants and those with severe protein malnutrition;
  - primary/acquired immunodeficiency (e.g. HIV with CD4 count <200 cell/mm3);
- immunosuppressive drugs (e.g. glucocorticoids)—especially in organ transplantation or malignancy.
- Co-trimoxazole is the agent of choice, as there is limited clinical experience in HIV-negative individuals with other regimens.
- There has been a suggestion that PCP may be acquired through hospital admission events, with outbreak management focused on transmission-based precautions. These include isolation of all patients with PCP in a single en-suite room until resolution of symptom/discharge from hospital. During an outbreak, all immunocompromised patients should wear single-use, fluid-resistant masks during transport to clinical wards to reduce cross-transmission. Healthcare staff do not need to wear respiratory protection, as there is no evidence of acquisition from patients.

Aspergillus

A mould capable of causing a wide range of disease in both healthy and immunocompromised individuals.

Mycology

- Many species cause invasive disease in humans. The most frequently identified are *Aspergillus fumigatus* (around 90%), *Aspergillus flavus*, and *Aspergillus niger*.

- Pathogenic species grow better on routine mycological media at 37°C than non-pathogenic species, most of which cannot grow at this temperature. Colonies become apparent at 36–90h. Sporulation (required for speciation) occurs up to 2 days later, longer with less common species.
- Identification of common species is by microscopic and colonial appearance. Detailed identification requires more specialized methods.
- Microscopy of pathological specimens may reveal hyphae (best seen on silver stains), but sporulation is not often seen (except in specimens taken from air-containing areas such as the lung); thus, the organism cannot be distinguished from other pathogenic moulds by this means.

Epidemiology

Found worldwide, favouring decomposing vegetable material (e.g. potted plants, spices, farms). Molecular techniques have demonstrated that colonized individuals and those with aspergilloma tend to pick up several different genotypes over time. Most invasive infections are caused by a single genotype.

Pathogenesis

- Disease spectrum is wide. Time from exposure to disease in invasive aspergillosis ranges from 36h to months. Disease may follow infection by organisms that have already colonized an individual (e.g. in neutropenia).
- Many factors influence disease form and severity—organism growth rate (*A. fumigatus* being the fastest), spore size (*A. fumigatus*' small spores allow them to pass deep into the lung) the hydrophobic coat of conidia (protection from host defence), the ability to adhere to epithelial surfaces (achieved by *A. fumigatus* much more effectively than other species), enzyme/toxin production (e.g aflatoxin produced by *A. flavus*).
- Host defences include lung macrophages (capable of ingesting and killing conidia), T lymphocytes (appear to be important in chronic and allergic disease), complement proteins, and neutrophils (damage hyphae). Corticosteroids impair macrophage and neutrophil killing.

Clinical features

Non-invasive disease

- Superficial—cutaneous infections are rare (usually in neutropenic patients or burns). Commoner is otomycosis—growth of *A. niger* in those with chronic otitis externa, which may cause itch and discomfort. Cleaning and TOP therapy with 3% amphotericin or clotrimazole are curative.
- Allergic bronchopulmonary aspergillosis (ABFA) occurs in those with asthma or cystic fibrosis (CF) and hypersensitivity to airway colonization by *Aspergillus*. Presents with worsening asthma or lung function. Patients may have eosinophilic pneumonia or airway sputum impaction. Blood tests may reveal eosinophilia early in disease. Oral corticosteroids can help exacerbations, and inhaled steroids may prevent episodes from occurring. PO itraconazole may help those requiring long-term steroids.

Aspergillus may also cause allergic sinusitis, best managed by aeration of the affected sinus.

- Aspergilloma—pulmonary aspergilloma follows *Aspergillus* colonization of pre-existing cavities or cysts left from TB, sarcoidosis, or PCP. TB cavities measuring 2cm or larger have a 15–25% risk of developing an aspergilloma. Some patients are asymptomatic; most have productive cough, haemoptysis, weight loss, wheeze, and clubbing. Culture of sputum may reveal the organism, and immunoglobulin G (IgG) precipitins may be detected in the serum. Radiological imaging demonstrates the hyphal mass as a cavity surrounded by a rim of air. Complications: massive haemoptysis (may be fatal—consider embolization or surgery), spread of infection to pleurae or vertebrae, dissemination. Aspergilloma must be distinguished from chronic invasive disease requiring systemic therapy. Treatment: 10% of cases resolve spontaneously; surgical resection has a role in the treatment of isolated lesions in those with good lung function; amphotericin has been injected into cavities, with some effect; PO itraconazole provides symptomatic relief. Sinus aspergilloma may develop in the ethmoid or maxillary cavities. Surgical drainage is usually sufficient in those with no evidence of mucosal involvement. Medical therapy should be used in combination with surgery in those with invasive disease or involvement of the frontal or sphenoid sinus.
- *Aspergillus* keratitis (less commonly endophthalmitis) may occur following ocular trauma or haematogenously (e.g. people who inject drugs (PWID), endocarditis). Early recognition and treatment are essential for a good outcome. Corneal smears may reveal hyphae, and cultures are usually positive. Keratitis may be treated with TOP amphotericin (27% response when given hourly). Superficial infections may be treated with TOP clotrimazole. PO itraconazole is effective in up to 75% of cases. Surgery is required where medical therapy fails or where there is a threat of ocular perforation or formation of a descemetocele (herniation of the posterior limiting layer of the cornea). Vitrectomy may be required to establish the diagnosis, and intraoperative examination of the specimen for hyphae allows immediate administration of intravitreal amphotericin. Systemic therapy is also recommended.

Invasive disease

Uncommon, occurring most frequently in the setting of iatrogenic immuno-suppression (haematological malignancy, transplantation).

- Invasive pulmonary disease—over 80% of patients with invasive disease have pulmonary infection. The immunocompromised tend to experience few symptoms but progress rapidly, whereas the less immune-impaired have more symptoms with a slowly progressive, chronic course.
  - Acute invasive pulmonary aspergillosis—early stages: dry cough and mild fever (25% have no symptoms); later stages: pleuritic chest pain, haemoptysis, breathlessness in those with bilateral disease who can become hypoxic. May resemble pulmonary embolism (PE) or mucormycosis. CXR changes can be non-specific (consolidation, cavities, wedge-shaped lesions, lower lobe shadowing) or

absent (10% of cases). High-resolution CT images aid in prompt diagnosis: early disease—nodules with the 'halo' sign (a zone of ground-glass attenuation surrounding a nodule or mass); in later disease, with neutrophil recovery, these may cavitate, producing the 'air-crescent' sign (crescenteric and radio ucency around nodules). Focal or nodular disease has a better prognosis than diffuse or bilateral infection. In focal disease, the danger is that of massive haemoptysis that may occur with no warning.

- Chronic invasive pulmonary aspergillosis—less frequent than acute. Predisposing conditions: uncontrolled HIV, alcoholism, diabetes mellitus, chronic granulomatous diseases, corticosteroid therapy for chronic pulmonary diseases. Some patients have no identifiable predisposing factors. Presentation: weeks of chronic productive cough. Other symptoms: haemoptysis, fever, weight loss. Infection may extend to the chest wall, spine, or brachial plexus. CXR shows cavitation and consolidation. May resemble aspergilloma (previous images demonstrating the presence of a pre-existing cavity may help distinguish between the two). Definitive diagnosis is by positive culture of a biopsy specimen. Patients usually have strongly positive serum *Aspergillus* antibodies (with the possible exception of uncontrolled HIV patients).

- Airways—commoner in lung transplant and patients with uncontrolled HIV. *Aspergillus* tracheobronchitis varies from mild inflammation to severe ulcerative disease; 80% experience symptoms (cough, fever, breathlessness, pain, haemoptysis), which become more severe with progression. Complications: stridor, tracheal perforation, dissemination, airway occlusion, death. Diagnosis by bronchoscopy. CXR usually normal in early disease.

- Sinus—invasive *Aspergillus* sinusitis can be acute or chronic:
  - acute—fever, cough, nosebleeding, headaches, discharge, sinus discomfort. Decreased blood flow to the affected nasal areas results in loss of sensation, and ultimately ulceration. Infection may extend to the palate, orbit, and brain. CT or MRI identifies the extent of disease. Culture or hyphal identification within tissues confirms the diagnosis;
  - chronic—early symptoms: nasal congestion, discharge, loss of smell, headache. Clinically indistinguishable from other causes of sinusitis. As disease extends, proptosis, loss of vision, ocular pain, and features of stroke may develop. Radiological features are similar to those of acute disease. Obtaining a positive culture may require multiple samples.

- Brain—10–20% of cases of disseminated disease develop cerebral aspergillosis. It is rare in the immunocompetent when it is usually secondary to neurosurgery. Severely immunocompromised individuals have a non-specific presentation with confusion and seizures, and death following a few days later. Less severely immune-impaired patients tend to have headache and focal neurological features. Fever may occur. Meningitis is rare. Contrast CT appearances are of infarction or of a ring-enhancing abscess with oedema. Lesions may be deep and surgically inaccessible. Diagnosis rests on culture and microscopy of a biopsy or an aspiration sample. This may not be possible, and diagnosis can be made presumptively in those with invasive disease elsewhere and typical radiological appearances.

- Other—endocarditis (BCs usually negative, and valve replacement is necessary to achieve cure), pericardial, intestinal, oesophageal, renal, vascular graft, bone.

Diagnosis in invasive disease

- A diagnostic approach for all invasive fungal disease (IFD) (see Box 9.1)—includes appropriate imaging and non-invasive tests (sputum, galactomannan testing). If positive in the correct clinical context, this may be sufficient to guide therapy. Otherwise, BAL (with sample tested for galactomannan) or lung biopsy, if safe and technically feasible, may be needed. Culture from a sterile sample or from histology demonstrating invasion provides a definitive diagnosis. However, culture is insensitive. Treatment should not be withheld from those at risk with suggestive features.

Invasive *Aspergillus* disease

- Radiology—perform CT assessment of the lungs and sinuses or MRI of the brain within 24h if clinical suspicion of invasive aspergillosis.
- Airway disease—bronchoscopic biopsy is rarely positive in focal lung disease. A needle biopsy or surgical resection (superior to open biopsy) is appropriate for peripheral pulmonary lesions. Focal lesions near the great vessels should prompt urgent resection (risk of massive haemoptysis). Positive BAL cultures support the diagnosis in the context of at-risk patients with suggestive radiological features. Antigen tests can be performed on BAL fluid.
- Histology—organisms may be observed, but several filamentous fungi have similar appearances, and culture is important for confirmation.
- Antibody testing—*Aspergillus* precipitin antibodies, while useful in diagnosing ABPA and aspergilloma, have no role in invasive disease.

Box 9.1 Possible, probable, and proven definitions for invasive fungal disease

- **Proven invasive fungal disease (IFD)** requires detection of the fungus in a tissue sample or culture of a specimen obtained from a normally sterile site.
- In the case of cryptococcosis, detection of cryptococcal antigen in blood or the CSF is also sufficient to prove diagnosis. For pneumocytosis, its detection in BAL fluid or expectorated sputum by using conventional or immunofluorescence staining is considered to prove a diagnosis of *Pneumocystis* pneumonia.
- **Probable IFD** requires the presence of at least one host factor, one clinical feature, and one mycological criterion.
- **Possible IFD** requires the presence of a host factor and a clinical feature, but this should not be applied to endemic mycosis because host factors and clinical signs and symptoms are not sufficiently specific.

- Serum antigen tests—galactomannan is a fungal exoantigen released by all pathogenic *Aspergillus* spp. during growth. The assay has moderate accuracy for diagnosis of invasive aspergillosis in immunocompromised patients. Useful in the setting of suspected disease (in which the higher prevalence leads to a better positive predictive value). Sensitivity/ specificity for proven invasive disease in those with haematological malignancy or haematopoietic cell transplantation is 71–89%. Less useful in solid organ transplant recipients and paediatric patients with primary immunodeficiencies. May become positive a week before clinical disease manifests. NB Sensitivity is reduced if the patient is receiving mould-active antifungals; false positives may follow absorption of galactomannan from the gut (e.g. mucositis) or use of the antibiotic piperacillin–tazobactam; other fungi also produce galactomannan (*Fusarium*, *Histoplasma* spp.). The 1-3 beta-*D*-glucan test has a high negative predictive value that may help exclude invasive disease in adults (⮕ see *Candida* species, pp. 510–12).

Treatment

(See The Fungal Infection Trust.)[3]

- Primary prophylaxis (e.g. with voriconazole) is effective in at-risk groups.
- Invasive aspergillosis is fatal if untreated in virtually all cases. Good outcomes require aggressive diagnosis in at-risk groups, early presumptive treatment, early changes in treatment if response is poor, and early surgical resection of lung lesions located near the hilum/ great vessels. Evaluating the response takes longer in those with less immunocompromise.
- Invasive aspergillosis—voriconazole is the treatment of choice. Alternative: liposomal amphotericin or ech nocandin. If invasive mould infection is suspected, but the organism is not confirmed, empirical treatment with amphotericin is preferred, as it is also active against mucormycosis (intrinsically resistant to voriconazole). Consider measuring voriconazole levels; standard dosing results in low levels in some patients. Duration: generally continued until all symptoms and signs have resolved; longer (many months) in those with persistent immune deficits. Consider secondary prophylaxis in those at risk of relapse (e.g. those continuing to receive chemotherapy). An echinocandin may be used in combination therapy if there is no response to first-line treatment. Be aware of interactions between azole drugs and chemotherapeutic agents. *Aspergillus terreus* is less susceptible to amphotericin. Some *A. fumigatus* isolates have increased MICs for azoles.
- Acute invasive sinusitis—first-line treatment is amphotericin. Itraconazole is not as effective for this form of disease.
- Chronic invasive sinusitis—surgical debridement and prolonged medical therapy. Relapse is common.
- Cerebral disease—surgery is useful only for diagnosis, unless the lesion is superficial and isolated. Otherwise, antifungal therapy is key.

- Surgery—indicated for focal invasive pulmonary disease, persisting lung shadows prior to bone marrow transplant (BMT) or aggressive chemotherapy, significant haemoptysis, or lesions near great vessels and airways.
- See European Organization for Research and Treatment of Cancer (EORTC) guidelines for full treatment guidance.[4]

References

3 The Fungal Infection Trust. *Aspergillus and aspergillosis*. Available at: ℅ https://www.aspergillus.org.uk

4 Donnelly JP, Chen SC, Kaufflan CA, *et al*. Revision and update of the consensus definitions of invasive fungal disease from the European Organization for Research and Treatment of Cancer and the Mycoses Study Group Education and Research Consortium. *Clin Infect Dis*. 2020;**71**:1367–76.

Mucormycosis

Mucormycosis is a clinical syndrome caused by a number of fungal species belonging to the order *Mucorales* (class *Zygomycetes*).

Mycology

Spores form and grow rapidly in the mould form in both tissues and the environment. Common species causing mucormycosis include *Rhizopus*, *Rhizomucor*, and *Mucor*. Microscopy allows a degree of speciation, and the hyphae of *Mucorales* are sufficiently different (broad, aseptate, and irregularly branched, usually at right angles) to allow them to be distinguished from *Aspergillus* (narrow, septate, and regularly branched, at more acute angles).

Epidemiology

All members of the order are widespread in decaying matter. As testament to their ubiquitous nature, they have been isolated from wooden tongue depressors, and infection has resulted from their use as splints in neonates. Clinical disease is limited largely to the immunocompromised, transplant patients, those with diabetes mellitus, and trauma patients. Infection may be rhinocerebral, respiratory, cutaneous, disseminated, or localized to specific organs.

Pathogenesis

Infection is acquired via the respiratory tract or in primary cutaneous infection via the inoculation of spores into skin abrasions. Spore germination follows in hosts whose immune response is deficient. Macrophages and neutrophils are important in preventing growth, and normal human serum is fungistatic. Invasive disease is favoured by hyperglycaemia and acidosis, and in patients receiving desferrioxamine (an agent which enhances fungal growth experimentally). Cases are not as significantly raised in those with uncontrolled HIV as it might otherwise be expected. Hyphae invade tissues, penetrate blood vessel walls, and may grow along the vessel, contributing to thrombosis and necrosis.

Clinical features

- Rhinocerebral disease—a disease of the immunosuppressed, seen in diabetic patients (particularly if acidotic) and neutropenic leukaemia patients on antibiotics. Almost invariably fatal, causing septic necrosis and infarction of the tissues of the nasopharynx and orbit. Patients develop facial pain or headache with fever, and may have orbital cellulitis, with proptosis and conjunctival swelling, evolving cranial nerve defects, and black, crusty material apparent in the nasopharynx. Fungal invasion of vessels may lead to retina artery thrombosis and visual impairment. Other complications: ptosis/pupil dilatation (secondary to cranial nerve lesions), cerebral abscess, cavernous sinus/internal carotid artery thrombosis. X-ray of the sinuses may show mucosal thickening, and fluid and bone destruction may be apparent on CT. Endoscopic evaluation of the sinuses should be performed to assess the appearance and obtain tissue. Features may recur after apparently successful therapy—patients should be monitored.

- Pulmonary disease—usually secondary to neutropenia and seen in BMT or leukaemia patients receiving chemotherapy. Symptoms are initially mild: fever, mild shortness of breath, and cough. With progression, haemoptysis may develop and erosion of a blood vessel can cause severe pulmonary haemorrhage. CXR may show infiltration, consolidation, and cavities. Infection may start in one lung segment but often disseminates in late stages (e.g. multiple lung areas, spleen, kidney). Diabetics may develop a milder chronic form of pulmonary infection.
- Cutaneous disease—outbreaks have been associated with colonized bandages. The appearance is that of cellulitis, but, if unrecognized, the organism penetrates deeper into the skin and necrosis may follow vascular invasion. Dissemination may follow. May take the appearance of a chronic ulcer. Cases have occurred with minor trauma (e.g. in gardeners), major trauma, burns, insect bites, and dissemination from a distant site.
- GI disease—seen in those suffering from malnutrition, although cases have occurred in renal transplant recipients. Any part of the tract may be infected, and it is rapidly fatal. Symptoms include abdominal pain, fever, nausea, and vomiting.
- CNS disease—rare and usually due to direct invasion from infected sinuses. Cases have occurred in leukaemia patients with no obvious route of acquisition and as a result of open head trauma. Presentation is with decreasing levels of consciousness and multiple focal neurological deficits.
- Other—endocarditis, osteomyelitis, renal infection, allergic sinusitis.

Diagnosis

- Clinical suspicion should be raised by the presence of vascular invasion and tissue necrosis that may manifest as black eschars and discharge. These are markers of advanced disease, and the earlier the diagnosis, the better the outcome. Lesions may be apparent only on the nasal mucosa and palate.
- Diagnosis rests on identifying the organism in tissue biopsy. Swabs are insufficient. There is usually an associated neutrophilic infiltrate, and tissue necrosis may follow blood vessel invasion with inflammatory vasculitis. Organisms rarely appear in BCs. The differential includes *Aspergillus* infection, rapidly progressive orbital tumour, cavernous sinus thrombosis, PE, and acute leukaemia.

Treatment
- Good outcomes rest on early diagnosis and correction of any predisposing factors (e.g. acidosis, hyperglycaemia, immunosuppression). Overall mortality is around 50%.
- Invasive disease—high-dose amphotericin B, in combination with aggressive surgical debridement of necrotic tissue. Reconstructive surgery may be necessary once recovered. Duration: until clinical resolution (usually several weeks/months). Posaconazole has been used in salvage or for PO step-down therapy. The other azoles and echinocandins are ineffective (reference RAG table).
- Primary cutaneous disease—local debridement and TOP amphotericin. Treatment duration should be guided by response.

Eumycetoma

Mycetoma is a chronic, slow-growing, destructive infection, usually involving the hands or feet and characterized by spread of the infecting organism from its subcutaneous site of implantation to adjacent structures. Serous discharges contain small grains of organism colonies.
- Actinomycetoma—caused by filamentous branching bacteria.
- Eumycetoma—caused by fungi.

Epidemiology
Found in tropical regions—most commonly in India, Mexico, parts of sub-Saharan Africa, and Yemen, amongst others. Rare in temperate areas but may be seen in south-western USA. Causative organism varies with geography—*Madurella mycetomatis* accounts for most cases worldwide; *Madurella grisea* is a common cause in South America; *Scedosporium boydii* is common in the USA; *Leptosphaeria senegalensis* and *Leptosphaeria tompkinsii* are common causes in West Africa. Geographical distribution of the causative agents is related to local climate (e.g. rainfall).

Pathogenesis
Soil fungi enter tissues of the foot or hand after local trauma. Infection spreads along tissue planes, destroying connective tissue and bone. Multiple sinuses and tracts form between the surface, each other, and deep abscesses. Inflammation and scarring lead to enlargement and disfigurement of the infected area. Histologically, the appearance is that of a suppurative granuloma, with grains embedded in abscesses. Grain appearance is often characteristic of the specific organism.

Clinical features
Seen most frequently in men aged 20–40 years, often farmers and rural labourers. The foot is the most commonly affected area; other regions include the hand, leg, arm, head, thigh, and even the back (carrying contaminated sacks). Early manifestation is a small, painless nodule. This quickly increases in size (faster in actinomycetoma) and ruptures, forming a sinus. Additional nodules appear in adjacent areas, as some areas heal. The cycle of swelling, discharge, and scarring leads to a swollen mass of deformed tissue with multiple discharging fistulae. Lymphatic spread to regional nodes

may occur. The cortex of bone may be invaded. Osteolytic lesions can be seen on X-ray. Pathological fractures are less common than would be expected. Constitutional symptoms are rare. Fever implies secondary bacterial infection.

Diagnosis

The appearance is fairly typical: indurated swelling, deformity, with multiple sinus tracts draining grainy pus. Grains may be black, white, yellow, red, or pink, depending on the causative organism (e.g. white to yellow grains with *Acremonium* spp., *Aspergillus nidurans*, *A. flavus*, *Cylindrocarpon cyanescens*, *S. boydii*, and *Fusarium* spp.; black grains with *Corynespora cassiicola*, *Curvularia* spp., and *M. mycetamatis*) They can be difficult to spot in tissue sections. Tissue Gram staining can detect fine-branching hyphae of actinomycetoma, but other stains are better for detection of eumycetoma grains (e.g. PAS stain). A good idea of the causative organism can be drawn from grain characteristics. They can be cultured for a more exact diagnosis—biopsy specimens are best, to avoid contamination. Serological diagnosis is possible in some centres.

Treatment

Mycetoma at all stages is usually amenable to medical therapy. Surgery usually leads to recurrence or mutilation that is more severe than that pre-existing. Treatment success depends on identification of the causative organism. All cases of actinomycetoma are treated with a combination of streptomycin sulfate and a second agent determined by the causal species (e.g. dapsone for *Actinomadura madurae*). Eumycetoma caused by fungi is treated with azoles, usually itraconazole, ketoconazole, or voriconazole (preferred for *S. boydii*). Fluconazole cannot be used due to intrinsic resistance. Treatment continues in all cases for at least 12 months, longer with extensive bone involvement. There is a role for surgery in combination with effective medical treatment (e.g. for bulk reduction).

Dermatophytes

A group of fungi capable of invading the dead keratin of skin, hair, and nails, causing dermatophytosis (tinea). Also known as 'ringworm', several species infect humans and belong to the genera *Epidermophyton*, *Microsporum*, and *Trichophyton*. Clinical classification is by the body area involved: tinea capitis (scalp hair and the commonest in children), corporis (trunk and limbs), manuum and pedis (palms and soles, and the commonest overall worldwide), cruris (groin), barbae (beard area and neck), faciale (face), and unguium (nail—also known as onychomycosis and affecting 2.7–4.7% of adults in the UK).

Mycology

- May be anthropophilic, zoophilic (causing incidental human infection), or geophilic (found primarily in soil and infrequent causes of human infection outside certain specific tropical regions). All favour humid or moist skin. Cases occur worldwide, but the incidence is highest in hot, humid regions.

- The commonest anthropophilic species is *Trichophyton rubrum*, a common cause of tinea pedis or tinea cruris in temperate regions, and tinea corporis in the tropics. Spread is through contact with infected desquamated skin scales (e.g. through sharing common washing facilities).
- *Epidermophyton floccosum* may cause tinea cruris and foot infections, either sporadically or in outbreaks in institutions.
- *Trichophyton concentricum* is a cause of tinea corporis in remote parts of the humid tropics, often affecting infants shortly after birth.
- Some species have specific geographical distributions: *Trichophyton tonsurans* is the main cause of tinea capitis in the UK and USA, and *Trichophyton violaceum* in India.

Pathogenesis

Infection is transmitted by hardy arthrospores formed by dermatophyte hyphae. Direct contact between individual people is not necessary. Fungal cells adhere to keratinocytes where they germinate and invade. Host susceptibility to infection appears to be influenced by genetic factors, local moisture, and CMI. Risk factors: moist conditions, communal baths, athletic activities leading to abrasions (wrestling, judo, etc.), atopy, genetic predisposition, impaired CMI (e.g. Cushing's disease, uncontrolled HIV—may lead to severe infection, e.g. extensive disease, abscess, dissemination).

Clinical features

The key feature is an annular scaling patch, with a raised margin showing a degree of inflammation and the centre usually less inflamed than the edge. The precise appearance varies with the affected site, the fungal species involved, and the host immune response. Inappropriate application of topical steroids may lead to an infection showing none of the classical signs. Differential diagnosis: seborrhoeic dermatitis, psoriasis, eczema, erysipelas, impetigo.

- Tinea capitis—a disease of childhood (medium chain-length fatty acids in sebum inhibit growth in post-pubertal adults). Found worldwide. Endemic infections affecting a large number of children tend to be caused by anthropophilic organisms, and sporadic cases by zoophilic fungi. Those infections in which the arthrospores are found on the hair surface are termed ectothrix infections, and those in which the spores develop within the hair are called endothrix infections. Clinical findings: scalp scaling and hair loss; may resemble dandruff. In ectothrix infections, the hair tends to break a few millimetres above the skin, in contrast to endothrix infections where the hair breaks at the skin surface. Inflammation is variable and may be severe with pustules and an exudative crust. Untreated, it usually remits spontaneously after puberty.
- Tinea corporis ('ringworm')—several causes. Anthropophilic species produce only mild inflammation and consequently a less well-defined skin lesion (e.g. *T. rubrum*), whereas zoophilic species produce more inflamed lesions that may contain pustules (e.g. *Microsporum canis*). Tinea barbae affects only the beard area with scaly plaques, pustules, and vesicles. Tinea imbricata is a variant caused by *T. concentricum*, characterized by a rash composed of concentric rings of scales. It is

endemic in parts of South East Asia, the South Pacific, Central America, and South America.

- Tinea pedis—seen in children and young adults, and usually due to infection with *T. rubrum* or *Trichophyton mentagrophytes*. Toe-web fissures, maceration, scaling of the soles, erythema, vesicles/pustules, bullae. 'Athlete's foot' is typical, but infection with other organisms may produce a similar appearance.
- Tinea cruris—*T. rubrum* or *E. floccosum*. Erythematous lesions with central clearing and raised borders in the groin and, less commonly, the scrotum. Usually seen in young men.
- Tinea unguium (onychomycosis)—often associated with infection of adjacent skin. Nail usually invaded from the distal and lateral aspects with onycholysis (separation of the nail from the nail bed), thick, discoloured (white, yellow, brown, black), dystrophic nails. Commoner with increasing age. Causes: *Scopulariopsis brevicaulis*, *Acremonium* spp., *Fusarium* spp.

Diagnosis

Skin scrapings, nail specimens, or plucked hairs are treated with KOH and examined by direct microscopy. Samples should be taken from the edge of the lesion. Look for hyphae and arthrospores around the hair shaft. Fungal cultures may be performed (culture on Sabouraud agar containing antibiotics and antifungal agents to selectively suppress the growth of environmental fungi—growth may take at least 2 weeks). Examination of the lesions under UV light may help in the diagnosis of tinea capitis—hairs infected with *Microsporum audouinii* and *M. canis* fluoresce yellow-green, and those infected with *Trichophyton schoenleinii* dull green. It is important to identify the organism causing scalp infection—the presence of an anthropophilic species should prompt screening of classmates and the family of affected children. Zoophilic infections rarely spread from child to child.

Treatment

- Tinea capitis—TOP therapy ineffective. PO treatment with griseofulvin, terbinafine, or itraconazole.
- Tinea pedis, corporis, and cruris—TOP ketoconazole 2%, miconazole 2%, or clotrimazole 1%, rubbed into the affected area daily for 2–6 weeks. Extensive or unresponsive disease may need systemic therapy.
- Infections confined to the palms/soles may respond to keratolytic agents such as Whitfield's ointment (compound benzoic acid ointment BP).
- Nail infections—topicals rarely work. Terbinafine PO is first line (70–80% cure for fingernails after 6 weeks' treatment, and for toenails after 12 weeks). Well tolerated, but there is a low risk of hepatic injury (1 in 70 000). Check baseline LFTs. Itraconazole is an alternative.[5]

References

5 National Institute for Health and Care Excellence (2013). *Fungal skin infection: body and groin*. Available at: ℛ https://cks.nice.org.uk/topics/fungal-skin-infection-body-groin/

Other moulds

Scedosporium

The genus *Scedosporium* consists of two medically important species: *Scedosporium apiospermum* (and its sexual state *Pseudallescheria boydii*) and *Scedosporium prolificans*. *S. apiospermum*/*P. boydii* and *S. prolificans* are present in soil, sewage, and polluted waters.

S. apiospermum/Pseudallescheria boydii

It causes two distinct diseases: mycetoma (⊃ see Eumycetoma, pp. 532–3) and pseudallescheriasis (all other infections). Pseudallescheriasis may affect the lung, bone, joints, CNS, skin, and soft tissue. Infection may be acquired by inhalation or through skin trauma. Weeks or months may pass between a local fungal inoculation and the development of symptoms.

- Immunocompetent—subacute/chronic infection (e.g. osteoarticular). Cerebral abscesses have occurred as a result of near drowning in pond water (probably due to spread from infected paranasal sinuses).
- Immunocompromised—acute and severe, including invasive pulmonary disease reminiscent of pulmonary aspergillosis. Commonly isolated from patients with CF, bronchiectasis, or old TB. Cerebral abscesses may develop in association with lung infection.
- There have been cases of indolent meningitis.
- Isolation of the organism from sterile sites is diagnostic. It is rarely cultured from blood. Effective antifungal therapy has not been established. Resistance to amphotericin B and voriconazole has been reported. Successful treatment regimens have utilized surgical debridement.

Scedosporium prolificans

An uncommon cause of human infection, with several dozen cases reported worldwide. Immunocompetent patients experience focal disease, usually osteoarticular. Immunocompromised patients may develop disseminated infection. Fungaemia, skin lesions, myalgia, pulmonary infiltrates, and cerebral lesions have all been reported. Diagnosis is made by culture. The organism is intrinsically resistant to most antifungals. Most therapy successes have involved debridement. Disseminated disease carries high mortality.

Fusarium species

Found in soil and, in the healthy, causes disease only rarely, usually through traumatic inoculation. *Fusarium* spp. may cause endophthalmitis, skin infection, musculoskeletal infections, and mycetoma. May disseminate in the immunocompromised. Systemic fusariosis occurs most commonly in patients with acute leukaemia and prolonged neutropenia, and those undergoing BMT. Presentation is with fever and myalgia unresponsive to antibiotics. Skin lesions are seen in up to 80% of cases, often starting as macules and progressing to necrotic papules. Infection may progress rapidly to death in the severely neutropenic. Once neutrophils recover, infection is more subacute and progresses slowly, or is controlled and cured. Diagnosis is by culture. Unlike aspergillosis, BCs are often positive (50% cases). High-dose amphotericin is the drug of choice. Overall mortality ranges from

50% to 80%, and survival is nearly always associated with recovery from neutropenia.

Dark-walled fungi

Phaeohyphomycosis is a loose term designating infection with moulds with dark walls in culture, but not always in tissue. These organisms are a cause of brain abscess (e.g. *Cladophialophora bantiana*), allergic fungal sinusitis (e.g. *Bipolaris*, *Exserohilum*), and cutaneous disease.

Sporothrix schenckii

A dimorphic fungus and the cause of sporotrichosis. May take the form of cutaneous infection, granulomatous pneumonitis, or disseminated disease.

Mycology

- Dimorphic. Demonstrating the temperature-dependent conversion is a useful means of identification. Hyphal colonies are initially white and later turn brown/black, as they produce pigment.

Epidemiology

- Found across the world—most human infections occur in tropical and subtropical parts of the Americas.
- Animal-to-human transmission has been described. Human-to-human transmission is rare.
- Identified in soil, plants, straw, and wood, and outbreaks have occurred in association with exposure to mine timbers, hay, thorned plants, etc.

Clinical features

- Cutaneous sporotrichosis—fungus is inoculated into the skin at sites of minor trauma, with disease usually arising in cooler body areas such as distal extremities. There are no systemic symptoms. Lesions may take the form of either a fixed plaque, which does not spread and may spontaneously resolve, or painless, smooth or verrucous, erythematous papulonodular lesions (0.5–4cm in diameter) which often ulcerate and can be followed by secondary lesions along the line of proximal lymphatics.
- Extracutaneous sporotrichosis—**osteoarticular** is commonest, involving the extremities (e.g. elbow, knee, hand, foot). Most present with primary involvement of a single joint (swollen, painful, with an effusion and possibly a sinus tract). Other joints may become involved without therapy. There are few systemic features. Repeated joint aspiration and culture or synovial biopsy may be necessary to make a diagnosis. **Pulmonary sporotrichosis**—one-third of patients are alcoholic, one-third have a pre-existing illness (e.g. diabetes, sarcoidosis), and one-third are healthy. They may be asymptomatic, but productive cough, fever, and weight loss are common, as are raised inflammatory markers. CXR reveals cavitation with or without hilar lymphadenopathy and effusions. Sputum Gram staining and culture are usually diagnostic, but long-term follow-up with repeated cultures may be necessary for diagnosis. Untreated disease leads to progressive

respiratory decline. **Other**—meningitis (CSF: high lymphocytes, high protein, low glucose), endophthalmitis, sinuses, kidney, testes.
- Multifocal extracutaneous sporotrichosis—in healthy people, lesions tend to be single-site. Multifocal disease with systemic features is usually seen in those with immunosuppression. Untreated infection is fatal.
- Patients with HIV—those with low CD4 counts are at greater risk of widespread ulcerative skin lesions and systemic dissemination. Presentation may be with arthritis and resemble seronegative arthropathies such as reactive arthritis (previously known as Reiter's syndrome). Visceral involvement occurs: meningitis, lung abscess, liver and spleen, endophthalmitis, bone marrow, sinus invasion, etc.

Diagnosis
- Culture—success may require multiple samples taken from affected sites at different times. A positive BC indicates multifocal disease. Although culture of skin lesion fluid may be positive, biopsy is best.
- Histology—a pyogranulomatous response is usually apparent and, in the presence of yeast forms, can be diagnostic. Again, multiple samples may be necessary. Yeast may be cigar or oval in shape.

Differential diagnosis
- Cutaneous disease—fixed lesions: bacterial pyoderma, foreign body granuloma, dermatophyte infections, cutaneous TB, and other granulomatous conditions; lymphocutaneous lesions: nocardiosis, leishmaniasis, mycobacterial infections (e.g. *Mycobacterium chelonae*, *Mycobacterium marinum*).
- Osteoarticular disease—TB, gout, rheumatoid arthritis.
- Pulmonary disease—TB and other mycobacteria, histoplasmosis, coccidioidomycosis.

Treatment
- Cutaneous disease—itraconazole or saturated potassium iodide (5–10 drops PO tds, increased slowly to 40 drops per dose; side effects include anorexia, diarrhoea, and parotid gland enlargement). Treatment course is usually 6–12 weeks. Prognosis is good. There have been cases described in which simply warming the lesion has been curative, reflecting the organism's temperature sensitivity.
- Osteoarticular disease—itraconazole is used as initial therapy. Amphotericin is curative in two-thirds of cases. Duration is at least 12 months. Relapse is common, and functional outcomes often poor.
- Pulmonary disease—prior to cavitation, amphotericin may be effective. Advanced disease requires surgical resection of cavities and a course of lipid-formulation amphotericin. PO itraconazole can be used as step-down therapy. Total duration is at least 12 months.
- Meningitis—varying response to amphotericin, and some advocate combination therapy with 5- flucytosine. Step down to itraconazole, once initial therapy is complete. At least 12 months' treatment required.
- Immunocompromised patients may require lifelong itraconazole therapy for multifocal extracutaneous disease.

Further reading

Kauffman CA, Bustamante B, Chapman SW, Pappas PG; Infectious Diseases Society of America. Clinical practice guidelines for the management of sporotrichosis: 2007 update by the Infectious Diseases Society of America. *Clin Infect Dis.* 2007;**45**:1255–65.

Chromomycosis

A localized chronic fungal infection of cutaneous and subcutaneous tissue, caused by several species and producing verrucous lesions.

Mycology

- Several different species cause chromomycosis—all take the appearance of dark brown cells, occurring singly or in small clusters. Culture colonies are dark, with a grey/green or brown/black surface.
- Agents grow slowly, and culture may take 6 weeks.
- Organisms include *Fonsecaea pedrosoi* (the most commonly isolated agent), *Fonsecaea compacta*, *Phialophora verrucosa*, *Cladosporium carrionii* (common in Australia, South Africa, and Venezuela).

Epidemiology

- Occurs worldwide, but commonest in tropical/subtropical areas amongst barefoot workers.
- Found in soil, decaying vegetation, etc., and inoculated into the skin by minor trauma; thus, feet and legs are the most commonly affected areas.

Clinical features

- Lesions can appear a long time after inoculation.
- Primary lesion usually a small pink papule that may itch and is followed (possibly many months later) by crops of either warty, violaceous nodules or firm tumours. These tend to enlarge and form groups with ulceration and dark haemopurulent material on the surface. Satellite lesions may occur.
- Some people develop annular, papular lesions, with active edges and healing in the centre, which can become scarred or form keloid. Fibrosis and oedema of the affected limb may occur in severe cases.
- Complications: secondary infection, lymphoedema (elephantiasis), fistula formation, haematogenous spread (rare), squamous carcinoma in long-standing lesions, late recurrence (years later sometimes).
- Differential diagnosis—blastomycosis, yaws, tertiary syphilis, leishmaniasis, mycetoma, sporotrichosis, *M. marinum* infection, leprosy.

Diagnosis

- All forms of disease produce characteristic sclerotic bodies, which may be identified on biopsy, along with pyogranulomata and microabscesses. Microscopy of exudates may reveal hyphal strands.
- Culture is necessary to confirm identity and may take 6 weeks.

Treatment
- Early small lesions—surgical excision or cryotherapy is effective.
- Late disease—most cases present late with large lesions. Local heat and several antifungals have been reported as effective (e.g. itraconazole). Treatment duration may last well over a year. It has been used in combination with flucytosine in cases of relapse.

Histoplasma capsulatum

A dimorphic fungus and an emerging infection in parts of the Americas.

The organism
- A member of the class *Ascomycetes*. Recognized as a fungus in the 1930s, leading to the re-evaluation of many TB cases in the USA, the diagnosis of which had been made on CXR alone.
- *H. capsulatum* contains between four and seven chromosomes. Restriction fragment length polymorphism (RFLP) of certain genes permits strains to be placed in one of six groups that correlate with virulence and geographical location.
- Mating types exist: (+) and (−). These are found in equal ratio in soil, but the (−) type predominates in clinical isolates.
- It is dimorphic—the mycelial phase grows at ambient temperatures, and the yeast phase at 37°C. The mycelial phase exists in two forms: macroconidia (<15 micrometres) and microconidia (<5 micrometres; the infective form being small enough to reach terminal bronchioles).

Epidemiology
- Found throughout the world, but commonest in warm, humid environments (e.g. southern USA; estimated 500 000 cases a year). It is associated with the presence of bat and bird guano. Birds do not carry the organism—bats can and shed it in their droppings.
- Infection tends to occur when soil disruption (e.g. excavation) releases fungal elements that are then inhaled.
- Disease develops in men more often than in women (4:1), which may reflect the association of chronic pulmonary disease with smoking (previously commoner in men).

Pathogenesis
- Microconidia settle in terminal airways, are phagocytosed by neutrophils and macrophages, and then switch to the yeast phase over hours/days. They migrate to the local lymph nodes and beyond. The resulting inflammatory response produces caseating or non-caseating granulomas, consisting of fungal elements, mononuclear cells, T cells, and calcium deposits. Excessive granuloma formation may be followed by fibrosis.
- Macrophages are the key mediator of resistance to *H. capsulatum*. T cells (CD4+ in particular) are important in acquired immune defence—B cells and antibodies have little role in resistance. CD4+ cells seem to be vital for the activation of mononuclear phagocytes through cytokine release. CMI limits, but does not eliminate, infection—infected people

contain dormant organisms for years. These pose a risk only if the individual subsequently becomes immunosuppressed.

Clinical features

Pulmonary histoplasmosis

- Acute primary infection—incubation is 1 week to a few months. Most patients are asymptomatic. Around 10% become very unwell. Severity affected by inoculum size, age (the young and the elderly), underlying disease, and presence of immunodeficiency. Symptoms: high fever, headache, dry cough, substernal chest pain, malaise, weakness, arthralgias, erythema nodosum, and erythema multiforme. Examination: added respiratory sounds, hepatosplenomegaly (rare). CXR: hilar lymphadenopathy and patchy pneumonitis, which may calcify with time (differential includes sarcoidosis, haematological malignancy, and TB). Most symptoms settle by day 10 but may persist in those with a large initial inoculum. Laboratory tests are non-specific. Diagnosis is by antibody/antigen testing and/or BAL (diagnostic in 40%).
- Cavitary (chronic) pulmonary histoplasmosis—seen in men aged over 50 years with existing lung disease (e.g. chronic obstructive lung disease). Symptoms: low-grade fever, cough, weight loss, night sweats, and chest pain. Any existing pulmonary impairment may be exacerbated. CXR: cavitating lesions, mostly in the upper lobes (90%) near a bulla. Resolves spontaneously in up to 60%. Diagnosis by serology and sputum/BAL culture. Avoid biopsy due to the potential for complications in this patient group. Healing leads to fibrosis, with consequent respiratory impairment. Recurs in 20%. Death is rare.
- Complications—histoplasmoma: a mass lesion resembling a fibroma and a rare complication of primary infection. Usually located in the lung. Enlarges slowly over years, forming a calcified mass. Mediastinal granuloma: granulomatous inflammation in response to infection leading to massive enlargement of the mediastinal lymph nodes (up to 10cm) that may cause airway impingement. Fibrotic tissue formed during healing can distort airways (leading to pneumonia and bronchiectasis), the oesophagus, or the superior vena cava. Large nodes may penetrate the airways, creating sinuses or fistulae to the pericardium or oesophagus. Rarely, mediastinal fibrosis can develop, affecting all structures within the mediastinum. Diagnosis is by histology and antibody testing, as there are rarely any viable organisms. Pericarditis: seen in 5–10% of patients and probably an immune response to adjacent infected lymph nodes. Ocular histoplasmosis (uveitis or panophthalmitis) occurs rarely.

Progressive disseminated histoplasmosis

Occurs in 1 in 2000 acute infections. Risk factors: age, immunosuppression (uncontrolled HIV, primary immunodeficiency, steroids, TNF-α inhibitors, etc.). Most cases probably represent reactivation of quiescent fungi, although progressive disseminated histoplasmosis (PDH) may result from primary infection or reinfection with a large inoculum. Diagnosis is made through a combination of antigen tests (urine, serum, CSF, BAL), histology, antibody tests, and culture. Urinary antigen is positive in 95% of immunocompromised patients. Serum antibody tests are positive in 90% of immunocompetent patients.

- Acute PDH—associated with a fulminant course and seen in children and the immunosuppressed (HIV and haematological malignancies). Symptoms: abrupt onset of fever, cough, weight loss, and diarrhoea. Children: chest features predominate; also hepatosplenomegaly, cervical lymphadenopathy, mouth ulcers, jaundice, anaemia (90%), and low platelet count and WCC. CXR may show enlarged hilar lymph nodes and patchy pneumonitis. Untreated, mortality is 100%, and, prior to antifungal therapy, children died around 6 weeks after symptom onset as a result of disseminated intravascular coagulopathy (DIC), haemorrhage, or secondary infections. Adults with HIV: before antiretrovirals, up to 25% of patients with uncontrolled HIV in an endemic area could develop infection. Findings: hepatosplenomegaly, lymphadenopathy, cutaneous signs (rash, bruising, petechiae), anaemia, low platelet counts. Rarer manifestations: colonic masses, perianal ulcers, meningitis, encephalitis. Untreated, fatality is 100%; with therapy, 80% survive. Reactive haemophagocytic syndrome, a rare severe form, is often fatal despite therapy.
- Subacute PDH—symptoms are prolonged. Hepatosplenomegaly is common, but fever, weight loss, and laboratory abnormalities are less pronounced. Infective lesions may occur in the GI tract (ulceration), CNS (chronic meningitis, cerebritis, and mass lesions), adrenal glands (affected in 80%, but overt Addison's seen in only 10%), and vascular structures (endocarditis and infection of aortic aneurysms). CSF in chronic meningitis shows lymphocytosis, elevated protein level, and low glucose level. Basilar meninges are badly affected, and hydrocephalus may develop.
- Chronic PDH—seen exclusively in adults. It is distinguished from subacute disease by the mild chronic nature of the symptoms. Malaise and lethargy are the key complaints. Fever is less common. The commonest physical finding is painless mouth ulceration (may appear malignant). Yeasts and macrophages can be identified on biopsy from the centre of the lesion.

African histoplasmosis

H. capsulatum var. *duboisii* is found in Africa, along with var. *capsulatum*. Infection has a distinct clinical presentation, with the skin and bone being the most frequently affected organs (perhaps reflecting cutaneous inoculation). Patients develop ulcers, nodules, and rashes that may resemble psoriasis. Osteolytic lesions develop in the skull, ribs, and vertebrae. Infection can become disseminated and affect multiple organs, resembling infection with *C. immitis* (perhaps due to the larger size of the var. *duboisii* yeast form, compared to var. *capsulatum*).

Diagnosis

- This is a Category 3 organism
- Culture—isolation of *H. capsulatum* is the only sure way to confirm a diagnosis of histoplasmosis. Sensitivity varies: 10–15% for sputum from patients with acute pulmonary histoplasmosis, 60–90% from patients with cavitatory disease, and 65% from CSF with meningitis. Rates higher

with repeated sampling. Specimens are cultured for 6 weeks at 30°C in brain–heart infusion agar with blood, antibiotics, and cycloheximide; 90% of positives grow fungus by day 7. In endocarditis, BCs are often negative; heart valves are frequently positive. The organism is rarely found in pleural or pericardial fluid—best grown from the pleura or pericardium.

- Antigen detection—galactomannan assays performed on urine or serum are positive in 90% of patients with progressive disseminated disease, and in 20% of those with acute pulmonary histoplasmosis. May also be performed on BAL samples. Useful for detecting relapses in those with PDH and more sensitive than serology. It is sensitive and fairly specific in the diagnosis of meningitis from CSF samples. Cross-reactivity with *Blastomyces* and *Coccidioides* spp. causes false-positive results.
- Serology—use only in those with a compatible clinical presentation. False negatives in 50% of immunosuppressed patients. Complement fixation tests (CFTs) are more sensitive, but less specific, than immunodiffusion. One to 5% of healthy people living in endemic areas have positive serology.
  - Complement fixation—a 4-fold rise or a titre of 1:32 suggests active infection (75% of patients 6 weeks after inoculation). Rising titres in the previously treated imply relapse. Less than 15% false-positive rate due to other fungi (coccidioidomycosis, blastomycosis), TB, and sarcoidosis.
  - Immunodiffusion test detects antibodies to the H and M fungal glycoproteins in patient sera. Anti-M antigen is detected in 80% of cases but does not distinguish active disease from previous infection. The presence of anti-H antigen suggests active infection but is not sensitive.
- Histology—rapid identification of fungus from tissues and body fluids. It may be positive in up to 40% of blood smears from patients with acute PDH.
- PCR—assays are rapid and specific, but sensitivity is currently poor.

Treatment

- Acute pulmonary histoplasmosis—most cases do not require treatment. Moderate illness and those with symptoms after 4 weeks can be treated with itraconazole (6–12 weeks). Give liposomal amphotericin for the first 2 weeks of therapy in severe disease, and consider steroids.
- Mediastinal granuloma—if symptoms, treat as above. Amphotericin may be preferable if rapid resolution of symptoms is required.
- Mediastinal fibrosis—antifungal therapy is not recommended. Surgery is often difficult, and fibrosis may recur. Obstructed vessels can be stented.
- Histoplasmoma—surgical excision if enlarging; 2–3 months' therapy with an azole may be beneficial afterwards.
- Cavitary pulmonary histoplasmosis—treatment should be given to those with progressive infiltrates, thick-walled cavities, or persistent cavities impairing respiratory function. Itraconazole 400mg daily for

6 months leads to improvement in up to 85% of patients. Amphotericin should be used in the immunosuppressed or if disease progresses on therapy. Relapse is seen in up to 20%, and surgical resection may be necessary.

- Acute PDH—life-threatening PDH should be treated with early liposomal amphotericin. Most patients show significant improvement in the first week. Mild disease can be treated with a 12-month course of itraconazole. Patients with uncontrolled HIV and those on long-term immunosuppressive therapy should receive lifelong itraconazole.
- Subacute and chronic PDH—itraconazole 400mg daily gives a 90% success rate. Alternative: amphotericin.
- Meningitis—treatment is with liposomal amphotericin for 4–6 weeks, followed by 12 months of itraconazole (poor CNS penetration). Assess with weekly LPs. Relapses are common. Around 50% are cured (higher rates in the immunocompetent, lower rates in the immunocompromised).
- Endocarditis—amphotericin and surgical removal of the infected valve.
- Pericarditis—may be seen after acute PDH. The pericardium is rarely infected. Bed rest, NSAIDs, and possibly steroids (beware of exacerbating active histoplasmosis lesions) usually suffice. Cardiac tamponade is uncommon.
- See Infectious Diseases Society of America (IDSA) guidelines for further details on treatment of histoplasmosis.[6]

Prevention

There is no vaccine available at present. Prevention relies on educating those who work in areas where there is a risk of acquiring infection (e.g. workers in buildings and other environments that have served as bat habitation). In HIV-infected patients who have had histoplasmosis, secondary prophylaxis is given until the CD4 count is consistently above 200 cells/mm^3.

References

6 Wheat LJ, Freifeld AG, Kleiman MB, *et al.*; Infectious Diseases Society of America. Clinical practice guidelines for the management of patients with histoplasmosis: 2007 update by the Infectious Diseases Society of America. *Clin Infect Dis.* 2007;**45**:807–25.

Blastomyces dermatitidis

A dimorphic fungus and the cause of systemic pyogranulomatous disease.

Mycology

Grows in the mycelial form at room temperature and as a yeast at 37°C. The mycelial form grows on plates by 3 weeks and produces the infectious conidia (2–10 micrometres in diameter). Yeast cells are multinucleate with thick cell walls and have a similar appearance *in vitro* as in clinical specimens. *B. dermatitidis* is the asexual stage of *Ajellomyces dermatitidis*, the sexual form which requires opposite mating types for reproduction.

Epidemiology

Limited information, as there is no sensitive skin test. Endemic areas: south-eastern USA, parts of South America, the Middle East, and India. African strains are serologically distinct from American strains. Favours decaying wood material in moist areas. Symptomatic disease occurs in <50% of infections.

Pathogenesis

Infection is acquired via the lungs. Conidia are inhaled and convert to the yeast phase. A non-caseating granulomatous response usually follows, although respiratory disease may not be apparent. The organism may disseminate to other sites. The histology of cutaneous disease is distinct, producing pseudoepitheliomatous hyperplasia with microabscesses. In appearance, it may resemble other skin lesions (e.g. squamous cell carcinoma). Mucosal involvement of the mouth and larynx may take a similar appearance. Protection from infection is mediated primarily by natural resistance (e.g. alveolar macrophages—rates are not greatly increased in those with immunocompromise) and cellular immunity (antibodies confer no protection).

Clinical features

Almost any organ can become infected. Some patients present with an acute pneumonia, but most experience a more chronic course.

- Acute infection—following exposure, there is an incubation period of 4–6 weeks before the development of non-specific flu-like symptoms: fever, arthralgia, and cough (initially non-productive but may later produce purulent sputum). CXR may demonstrate an area of consolidation. There have been reports of spontaneous resolution of such acute pneumonias.
- Chronic pulmonary infection—chronic pneumonia with productive cough, pleuritic chest pain, haemoptysis, weight loss, and low-grade fever. CXR may show infiltrates, mass lesions (which may resemble malignancy), and cavities, but effusions are rare. Miliary disease or diffuse pneumonitis is unusual—both have high mortality.
- Skin—commonest extrapulmonary manifestation, seen in up to 80% of cases. May occur in the absence of respiratory features. Lesions may be verrucous or ulcerative—both may occur in the same patient. Verrucous lesions resemble squamous cell carcinoma. Where there is discharge, microscopy may reveal yeast forms. Subcutaneous nodules represent cold abscesses and are usually seen in acutely ill patients with severe pulmonary or extrapulmonary disease at another site.
- Bone and joint—long bones, vertebrae, and ribs. Extension may lead to arthritis. Organisms are seen in synovial aspirates.
- Genitourinary (GU) tract—around 25% of men have GU involvement, usually of the prostate.
- CNS—uncommon in the normal host. More likely (e.g. as abscess or meningitis) in patients with uncontrolled HIV who develop blastomycosis.

- The immunocompromised—an unusual opportunistic pathogen in HIV patients. Disease is more severe and more likely to be fatal in those with late-stage uncontrolled HIV. CNS infection is seen in 40% of cases. Similar severity is seen in patients with immunocompromise due to steroid therapy and chemotherapy. Up to 40% of cases are fatal. Treat suspected cases early—most deaths occur within a few weeks. Relapse is common if immunodeficiency remains, and long-term suppression should be considered.

Diagnosis

- This is a Category 3 organism.
- Microscopy of secretions—the characteristic yeast cell may be seen in a wet preparation of sputum or pus. Body fluids, such as urine or pleural fluid, should be centrifuged, and the sediment examined. BAL may be useful in patients who are not producing sputum. When organisms are sparse, they may be more easily identified on Papanicolaou preparations.
- Histology—visualized by Gomori's methenamine silver and PAS stains.
- Culture—material should be inoculated on Sabouraud or more enriched agar and incubated at 30°C. The mycelial form is not diagnostic, and ideally conversion to yeast at 37°C should be demonstrated. This is not always possible, and nucleic acid probes can confirm identification.
- Serology—complement fixation, immunodiffusion, and enzyme-linked immunoassay (EIA)-based tests are available, but sensitivity and specificity vary widely. A negative test does not rule out disease, and a positive does not, on its own, warrant therapy (cross-reactivity with endemic mycoses)—rather it should fuel the hunt for the organism.
- Antigen detection—a commercial assay is available, but its modest specificity (79%) limits its utility.

Treatment

All patients should receive therapy. A small number of cases do resolve spontaneously, but these cannot be predicted at presentation. Surgery has a role in drainage of large abscesses and resection of necrotic bone tissue, in combination with medical therapy.

- Mild to moderate pulmonary/disseminated disease—itraconazole for 6 months (12 months in osteoarticular). Relapses do occur, and patients should be followed up for 2 years.
- Severe pulmonary/disseminated and the immunosuppressed—liposomal amphotericin 1–2 weeks, then itraconazole ~12 months. Relapse is commoner in those with immunocompromise.
- CNS disease—liposomal amphotericin for 4–6 weeks, then PO azole for 1 year. Voriconazole may be best (good activity and CNS penetration), but limited data.
- Echinocandins have intermediate to poor *in vitro* activity and should not be used to treat blastomycosis.
- See IDSA guidelines for full details on management of blastomycosis.[7]

Emmonsia

New species of Emmonsia-like dimorphic fungi, with phylogenetic and clinical similarities to Blastomyces and Histoplasma, have emerged as causes of systemic human mycoses worldwide. They cause disseminated infections, predominantly in immunocompromised patients. Case-fatality rates are high.

References

7 Chapman SW, Dismukes WE, Proia LA, *et al.*; nfectious Diseases Society of America. Clinical practice guidelines for the management of blastomycosis: 2008 update by the Infectious Diseases Society of America. *Clin Infect Dis*. 2008;**46**:1801–12.

Coccidioides immitis

A dimorphic fungus found in certain regions of the Western hemisphere and a cause of respiratory illness.

Mycology

May exist as a mycelium or a spherule (a structure unique to this organism). The mycelial form is seen on routine laboratory agar and in soil. Mature cells can develop a hydrophobic outer layer that renders them capable of prolonged survival (arthroconidia). Once airborne these may be inhaled and deposited in the lungs where they begin to multiply. The resultant spherule consists of a thin wall containing many endospores. This wall eventually ruptures, allowing the spread of endospores.

Epidemiology

Endemic to certain regions of the Western hemisphere with an arid climate, hot summers, and alkaline soil (e.g. regions of southern USA, Mexico, Central America, parts of South America). Arthroconidia transport (e.g. in dust storms) has resulted in infections in non-endemic areas. Infections tend to occur when the soil is dry towards the end of summer. The organism is most easily isolated after the winter rains. The number of new infections varies greatly from year to year; 30% of people living in endemic regions of the USA show evidence of prior exposure.

Pathogenesis

Most infections follow inhalation of arthroconidia. There are rare cases of cutaneous infection (which tend to resolve without treatment). Inflammation follows its conversion to a spherule. The resulting pulmonary lesion consists of neutrophils and eosinophils and, if infection becomes chronic, granulomas with lymphocytes and multinucleated giant cells. Both acute and chronic lesions may be found at different sites in the same individual. Control of infection relies on the T-cell response, and those with deficient T-cell immunity are at risk of severe disease. The innate immune response appears to be important against arthroconidia and endospores.

Clinical features

Up to two-thirds of infections produce only mild or subclinical disease, and of those producing respiratory symptoms, most follow a self-limiting course. Complications may occur up to 2 years later and do not correlate with the severity of the original infection.

- Early respiratory infection—symptoms develop 1–3 weeks after exposure: cough, pleuritic chest pain, breathlessness, and fever. Onset is usually slow but can be abrupt. Inhalation of a large number of arthroconidia may result in early symptoms. Weight loss and migratory arthritis can occur, and some develop skin rashes, ranging from a fine papular rash early in illness to erythema multiforme and nodosum (particularly in women). Laboratory tests may reveal peripheral blood eosinophilia and raised inflammatory markers. Around 50% of patients have CXR changes: effusions, infiltrates, hilar lymphadenopathy, and cavities. Most infections resolve without complications over several weeks. There are rare cases of severe diffuse coccidioidal pneumonia (due to either massive exposure or haematogenous seeding), leading to respiratory failure and septic shock, with high mortality. One-third of coccidioidal infections in HIV-positive patients (typically those with CD4 counts <100 cells/mm^3) present in this manner.
- Pulmonary nodules and cavities—4% of lung infections result in a nodule that may reach up to 5cm in diameter. Although usually asymptomatic, a biopsy may be necessary to distinguish it from a neoplastic lesion. Nodules may liquefy and drain via a bronchus to form a cavity. Cavities are usually peripheral, and although half close within 2 years, some may cause pain, cough, and haemoptysis, as well as provide a focus for the development of mycetoma. Peripheral cavities can rupture, causing a pyopneumothorax.
- Chronic fibrocavity pneumonia—associated with diabetes or pre-existing lung fibrosis; some people develop chronic fibrotic pneumonia with widespread pulmonary infiltrates and cavities involving >1 lobe. Patients may experience night sweats and weight loss.
- Dissemination—rare (0.5% of cases overall). Those with immunodeficiency (solid organ transplants, late-stage HIV infection, high-dose steroids, Hodgkin's disease) are at greater risk. Many with disseminated disease do not develop respiratory features and have normal CXRs. Sites of dissemination: skin (causing maculopapular lesions, verrucous ulcers, and abscesses, with a predilection for the nasolabial fold), joints (knee, hand, wrist, feet), bone (particularly the vertebrae—which may progress to develop a paraspinous abscess), and meningitis—the most serious manifestation. Meningitis develops a few weeks to a few months after initial infection and is usually fatal within 2 years of diagnosis. CSF findings: elevated pressure, raised protein level, low glucose level, raised eosinophil count. The basilar meninges are usually involved, and hydrocephalus is a common complication in children.

Diagnosis

- This is a Category 3 organism.
- Clinical features of coccidioidal infection are not specific, and laboratory tests are required to establish the diagnosis. Travel history is vital—exposure can be subtle (e.g. changing planes within an endemic area). Complications are usually apparent within 2 years of exposure, but infection may have occurred many years previously in the

immunodeficient. Most diagnoses are made serologically, with culture in severe cases.

- Isolation of the organism—definitive diagnosis is by culture of, or identifying fungal elements within, clinical specimens (e.g. biopsy, sputum). *Coccidioides* spp. are never normal flora. Stains, such as silver, PAS, and haematoxylin and eosin (H&E), will reveal spherules. *C. immitis* grows on standard microbiological media in aerobic conditions and typically takes the form of a white mould at around 1 week. At this point, it is highly infectious. Unlike the spherule, the mycelial form is not unique, and reference laboratories make identification either antigenically or by the detection of specific rRNA.
- Serology—most patients are not very symptomatic, and diagnosis is by serology. Serology is important in the diagnosis of coccidioidal meningitis, as the CSF is usually culture-negative. Tests are highly specific, and even borderline positive results should be treated seriously. Antibodies may only become detectable weeks/months after illness onset, and negative tests do not exclude infection. The tube precipitin (TP) antibody (IgM) test detects a fungal cell wall polysaccharide and is positive in 90% of patients by the third week of illness; complement fixing antibodies (predominantly IgG) are detected later and for longer than TP antibodies, and their presence in the CSF is important in the diagnosis of coccidioidal meningitis; EIA tests for IgG and IgM are highly sensitive and specific or both the CSF and serum; immunodiffusion tests are the most specific assays. Some laboratories screen with EIA and confirm with immunodiffusion. Immunodiffusion tests can be reported qualitatively, allowing assessment of treatment response.
- Antigen detection—a urinary antigen test is available. Sensitivity is 71%, thus best used as part of a wider diagnostic strategy.
- Skin testing—for delayed-type hypersensitivity to coccidioidal antigens, is useful epidemiologically, but limited as a diagnostic tool.

Treatment

- Uncomplicated primary disease—newly diagnosed patients should be assessed for the extent of disease and factors that increase the risk of dissemination or future complications. If otherwise well, those with mild disease do not need therapy but should be followed up for a year.
- Consider treatment with an azole antifungal for 3–6 months in those with:
  - moderate/severe pulmonary infection—weight loss of over 10%, night sweats for 3 or more weeks, infiltrates that are either bilateral or involve more than half of a lung, persistent hilar lymphadenopathy, symptoms persisting for over 2 months;
  - risk of dissemination—the immunosuppressed, pregnant women;
  - severe pulmonary disease (e.g. pre-existing lung fibrosis);
  - amphotericin is the preferred agent in cases of severe pulmonary disease or those who are deteriorating. Surgery may be required in some patients (e.g. cavities that do not resolve). Debridement and drainage of infected sites are essential in extensive bone infection, and in cases of vertebral infection, stabilization may be required.

- Persistent fibrocavitary pneumonia—treatment is usually started with PO azoles. Up to 60% respond, with improved symptoms and CXR. Those who do not may respond to amphotericin.
- Meningitis—treat initially with fluconazole (response rate of 70%). Voriconazole may be an alternative. Consider intrathecal amphotericin if no response or in the first trimester of pregnancy. Hydrocephalus may require shunting. Cerebral abscesses may need draining.
- Other forms of dissemination can usually be treated with PO azoles, except in those who are showing rapid deterioration or have infection in critical places when amphotericin is preferred. Treatment is continued for at least a year, and for 6 months beyond the end of recovery. Relapses occur in one-third of cases. Lifelong suppressive therapy may be required.
- See IDSA guidelines for further details on the management of coccidioidomycosis.[8]

References

8 Galgiani JN, Ampel NM, Blair JE, et al.; Infectious Diseases Society of America. Coccidioidomycosis. *Clin Infect Dis*. 2005;**41**:1217–23.

Paracoccidioides brasiliensis

A cause of chronic progressive systemic mycosis in South America.

Mycology

P. brasiliensis is a dimorphic fungus (at 37°C a yeast, below 28°C a mycelium). At 37°C, colonies take around 10 days to appear and have a creamy, soft appearance. Mould-form colonies take up to a month to develop.

Epidemiology

Limited to South America, from Argentina to Mexico, causing infections in forest regions with high year-round humidity and mild temperatures. Brazil has the highest number of reported cases. It has been isolated from soil. Human infection is probably acquired by inhalation. Most cases occur in men over 30 years of age. Agricultural workers, smokers, and alcoholics are at greater risk.

Clinical features

Most primary cases are subclinical. The organism can remain dormant for prolonged periods, with disease becoming apparent only in states of debilitation or immunosuppression. Causes subacute severe disease in the young and chronic disease in adults, in whom it has a better prognosis with therapy.

- Lung—breathlessness, and CXR may reveal nodular infiltrates which are often bilateral. Lesions concentrated in the mid and lower zones; apices are usually clear. Cavities, fibrosis, emphysema, and right ventricular hypertrophy become more likely, as disease becomes chronic.
- Mouth and upper respiratory mucosa—ulcerated lesions of the mouth, lip, gums, tongue, and palate. Other features: tooth loss, dysphonia, nasal lesions.

- Cutaneous lesions—warty, ulcerated lesions over legs and orifices.
- Other—lymphadenopathy (sometimes with fistulae), diminished adrenal function, spleen, liver, gut, vascular system, bone, CNS.

Diagnosis

- This is a Category 3 organism
- Microscopy with KOH—reveals the organism (identified by its distinctive multiple budding) in >90% of cases where sputum or exudates are available.
- Biopsy—often diagnostic. Histology shows granuloma with multinucleated giant cells that may contain fungi. Ulcerated lesions may show a pyogenic reaction, and skin lesions may have intraepithelial microabscesses.
- Culture—on Sabouraud–dextrose agar (keep for 6 weeks).
- Serology—immunodiffusion is most reliable. Remains positive after successful treatment. CFTs cross-react with *H. capsulatum*.

Treatment

- Mild/moderate—PO itraconazole for 6–12 months.
- Severe—amphotericin or co-trimoxazole IV. Voriconazole may be an alternative. Switch to a PO agent once improved (20–40 days). Duration may need to be >2 years if co-trimoxazole is used or CNS involvement.
- Relapse may occur in <5% of those with chronic disease treated with itraconazole, and in <25% of those treated with co-trimoxazole. Immunocompromised patients are at particular risk. Serological testing and radiological follow-up may guide decisions on duration.

Talaromyces (Penicillium) marneffei

Previously known as *Penicillium marneffei*, this is a thermally dimorphic fungus that may cause severe disseminated infection.

Epidemiology

Limited to South East Asia and southern China. Humans and bamboo rats are the only known hosts. The exact route of transmission is unknown but is thought to be inhalation or, rarely, inoculation. Infection is commonly seen in young adults with HIV (fourth commonest opportunistic infection in Thai patients). Cases are seen in immunocompetent children and adults. Occupational exposure to soil is a risk factor.

Clinical features

Occurs in uncontrolled HIV infection (CD4 count <100 cells/mm³). Systemic infection is known as talaromycosis. Patients present with around 1 month of fever, weight loss, and skin lesions (pustules, papules, ulcers, or abscesses on the face, upper trunk, or extremities). Pharyngeal and palatal lesions are common in those with HIV. Most have anaemia and weight loss, with around half presenting with fungaemia or lymphadenopathy. Hepatomegaly, splenomegaly, haemoptysis (secondary to cavitating lung lesions), joint infections, and pericarditis may occur. The diagnosis should be considered in those with immunocompromise and a history of travel to an affected area. Disease may present many years after travel.

Diagnosis

- This is a Category 3 organism
- Histology—a presumptive diagnosis may be made on smear (skin lesion, sputum) or biopsy (lymph node, bone marrow) in the appropriate setting. Microscopic examination may reveal yeast forms extracellularly and within phagocytes. Histology may demonstrate either a granulomatous (in the immunocompetent), suppurative, or necrotizing (in the immunocompromised) response.
- Culture—treatment may need to be initiated, while culture is ongoing. Typically takes 4–7 days, but occasionally weeks. At 25°C, grows as a mould with sporulating structures. May convert to yeast form at 37°C.
- Serological assays are not widely used due to limited data on their accuracy.

Treatment

May need to be initiated prior to culture completion. Beware of interactions between azoles and antiretrovirals. Consider therapeutic drug level monitoring.[9]

- Severe or CNS involvement—2 weeks IV amphotericin, followed by 10 weeks PO itraconazole. Voriconazole may also be effective.
- Mild—PO itraconazole for 8 weeks.
- HIV-infected patients—should be started on ART within 2–4 weeks of commencing antifungal treatment. Secondary prophylaxis with PO itraconazole should continue until CD4 counts >100 cells/mm³ for at least 6 months.

References

9 Panel on Opportunistic Infections in HIV-Infected Adults and Adolescents. *Guidelines for the prevention and treatment of opportunistic infections in HIV-infected adults and adolescents: recommendations from the Centers for Disease Control and Prevention, the National Institutes of Health, and the HIV Medicine Association of the Infectious Diseases Society of America.* Available at: ℘ https://pubmed.ncbi.nlm.nih.gov/19357635/ https://aidsinfo.nih.gov

Microsporidia

Microsporidia are a diverse group of obligate intracellular, spore-forming parasites that belong to the phylum *Microspora*, order *Microsporida*. Comparative molecular phylogenetic studies have identified microsporidia as fungi, having previously been identified as protozoa. Over 1400 species exist, and 15 species have been implicated in human disease, with *Enterocytozoon bieneusi* and *Encephalitozoon* spp. being the commonest pathogens.

Epidemiology

Human infection has been reported worldwide (except in Antarctica). Most severe infections are associated with immunocompromise (e.g. HIV infection, organ transplantation, corticosteroid therapy). However, infections are becoming increasingly recognized in immunocompetent patients (e.g.

residents of, or travellers from, tropical countries). Routes of transmission include food-borne, waterborne, person-to person spread, inhalation/aerosol, or zoonotic spread.

Pathology

Microsporidia can infect many different organs:
* eye—punctate epithelial keratopathy;
* respiratory tract—rhinitis, sinusitis, nasal polyposis, tracheitis, bronchitis, bronchiolitis ± pneumonia;
* GU tract—chronic and granulomatous interstitial nephritis, acute tubular necrosis, microabscesses, granulomas, necrotizing ureteritis and cystitis, prostatic abscess;
* GI and hepatobiliary tract—enteritis, ulceration, mucosal invasion, granulomatous hepatitis, and cholecystitis;
* CNS—ring-enhancing lesion with central areas of necrosis filled with spores/macrophages, surrounded by microsporidia-filled astrocytes;
* musculoskeletal system—myositis, muscle fibrosis.

Clinical features

The clinical manifestations of microsporidiosis can be divided into two groups, according to the host's immune status.

Immunocompetent patients
* Intestinal infections caused by *E. bieneusi* or *Encephalitozoon intestinalis* are commonest. Present with watery diarrhoea, nausea, abdominal pain, and fever, and is usually self-limiting.
* Ocular infections are rare and may present with corneal stromal infection or keratoconjunctivitis.
* Cerebral infections, endocarditis, and myositis have also been reported.

HIV-infected patients
* *E. bieneusi* typically causes intestinal infections with chronic diarrhoea, anorexia, weight loss, and malabsorption. CD4 counts are typically <100 cells/mm³. Patients may also develop cholecystitis or cholangitis, with fever, nausea, vomiting, and abdominal pain.
* *E. intestinalis* causes intestinal and systemic infections that appear similar to those caused by *E. bieneusi*. Disseminated disease, particularly to the kidneys, may occur.
* *Encephalitozoon hellem* and *Encephalitozoon cuniculi* can both cause keratoconjunctivitis sicca. Patients often have laboratory evidence of disseminated infection and may present with bronchiolitis, sinusitis, nephritis, cystitis, urethritis, prostatitis, hepatitis, peritonitis, cerebral infection, or nodular skin infections.
* Myositis may be caused by various microsporidial species (e.g. *Pleistophora* spp., *Trachipleistophora hominis*, *Brachiola vesicularum*).

Diagnosis

* Faeces microscopy requires special stains to detect microsporidia (e.g. modified trichrome stain, calcofluor white stain, indirect immunofluorescence stains).

- Cytology is used for diagnosis of microsporidiosis in other organs. Various stains may be used (e.g. Weber, Gram, Giemsa, Steiner silver, trichrome blue, chemifluorescence stains).
- Histology remains important in the diagnosis of microsporidiosis. Various stains may be used (e.g. modified Gram, Giemsa, PAS, Steiner silver stains).
- Electron microscopy can be used to identify microsporidia to genus or species level.
- Nucleic acid amplification assays—several PCR-based assays have been developed for species-specific diagnosis and are becoming increasing widespread in clinical practice.
- Immunofluorescent detection methods using polyclonal antisera can detect microsporidia (except *E. bieneusi*) in most clinical specimens. Sensitivity is poor in faeces specimens.
- Serology is unhelpful in the diagnosis of microsporidiosis.
- Tissue culture is only available in a few specialist laboratories.

Treatment

- GI infection—albendazole is effective against most microsporidia species, particularly *Encephalitozoon* infections, but has minimal activity against *E. bieneusi*. Fumagillin is used for *E. bieneusi* infection (side effects: nausea, vomiting, bone marrow toxicity). Nitazoxanide may also be effective for *E. bieneusi* infections in HIV-infected patients.
- Ocular infections—TOP fumagillin is used, and concomitant albendazole is warranted, particularly if there is evidence of systemic infection. TOP voriconazole has been used in keratitis.

Prevention

Meticulous handwashing and adherence to existing guidelines for the general prevention of opportunistic infections in HIV-infected patients are pertinent. As yet, there are no clinical trial data to support antimicrobial prophylaxis. ART may be important in preventing microsporidiosis.

Protozoa

Protozoa

Protozoa is an informal term for single-celled protists, which are defined as eukaryotic organisms that are not an animal, fungus, or plant that feed by heterotrophy (i.e. they cannot produce their own food). The taxonomy is complex, but in general, protozoa are motile and may be free-living or parasitic. They live in a variety of environments and may reproduce sexually or asexually.

Parasitic protozoa can cause a wide spectrum of disease in humans. In general, they are either vector-borne (such as *Plasmodium* and *Babesia* spp.) or ingested from the environment (such as *Cryptosporidium* and *Giardia* spp.).

Plasmodium species (malaria)

Malaria, an infection caused by *Plasmodium* spp., has affected mankind for millennia. The word malaria is derived from 'bad air' in Italian and refers to the association between the illness and the 'bad air of the marshes'. It was not until the late 1890s when the British Army surgeon Sir Ronald Ross proved the *Anopheles* mosquitoes, which breed in the wet ground, are the vector. Malaria remains a major global health problem in tropical countries where it causes an estimated 228 million cases and 405 000 deaths per year. Imported infections occur sporadically in the UK, with between 1300 and 1800 cases per year.

Plasmodium species

Five *Plasmodium* spp. cause human infection:
- *Plasmodium falciparum* can invade red blood cells (RBCs) of all ages, may be drug-resistant, and is responsible for most severe, life-threatening infections. It does not produce dormant liver stages (hypnozoites) or cause relapse.
- *Plasmodium vivax* and *Plasmodium ovale* cause clinically similar, milder infections. They produce hypnozoites and may cause relapse months after the initial infection.
- *Plasmodium malariae* rarely causes acute illness in normal hosts and does not produce hypnozoites, but may persist in the bloodstream for years.
- *Plasmodium knowlesi* causes malaria in macaques and has recently been recognized as a cause of human malaria in South East Asia. Microscopically, it resembles *P. malariae* but can cause fatal disease (like *P. falciparum*).

Mixed infections may occur in 5–7% of patients.

Life cycle

Humans acquire malaria from sporozoites transmitted by the bite of the female *Anopheles* mosquito. Sporozoites travel through the bloodstream and enter hepatocytes. Here they mature into tissue schizonts, which rupture and release merozoites into the bloodstream. These invade RBCs and mature into ring forms, then trophozoites, and finally schizonts, before rupturing to release merozoites. Alternatively, some erythrocytic parasites develop into gametocytes (sexual forms), which are ingested by the mosquito and complete the sexual life cycle. In *P. vivax* and *P. ovale* infections,

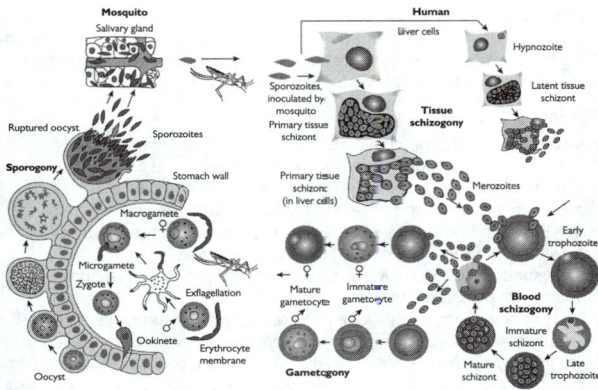

Fig. 10.1 Life cycle of malaria parasite.

Reproduced from Morrow, R.H., Moss, W.J., Malaria, in Detels *et al.* (eds.), *Oxford Textbook of Public Health*, Fifth Edition, Oxford University Press, Oxford, UK, Copyright © 2009, by permission of Oxford University Press.

some parasites remain dormant in the liver as hypnozoites for months, before they mature into tissue schizonts. (See Fig 10.1.)

Epidemiology

The epidemiology of malaria varies and depends on a number of factors: climate, *Plasmodium* spp. and life cycle, efficiency of transmission by vectors, and drug resistance. Thus, in sub-Saharan Africa, *P. falciparum* can survive as a result of the year-round presence and efficient transmission by its mosquito vectors (*Anopheles gambiae* and *Anopheles funestus*). In contrast, *P. vivax*, which is found in more temperate zones, requires hypnozoites to sustain its transmission.

Pathogenesis

The following mechanisms contribute to the pathogenesis of severe falciparum malaria:

- **cytoadherence**—adherence of parasitized RBCs to the vascular endothelium is mediated by *P. falciparum*-infected erythrocyte membrane protein 1 (PfEMP1), which binds to specific endothelial receptors (e.g. thrombospondin, CD36, ICAM-1 (intercellular adhesion molecule 1), VCAM-1 (vascular cell adhesion molecule 1), and ELAM-1 (endothelial leucocyte adhesion molecule 1)). This results in peripheral sequestration of parasites, which protects them from removal from the circulation via the spleen. It also causes microthrombi, which can lead to end-organ dysfunction such as in cerebral malaria;
- **rosetting**—PfEMP1 also binds to complement receptor 1, resulting in clustering of unparasitized red cells around parasitized red cells;

- **hyperparasitaemia** (>5%)—is associated with a greater risk of death, particularly in non-immune patients. *P. falciparum* is able to reach higher parasite counts than the other species, which leads to significant metabolic effects such as hypoglycaemia and lactic acidosis.

Clinical features

- Incubation period for all malaria species is at least 6 days.
- Fevers (cyclical or continuous with intermittent spikes).
- Malarial paroxysm—chills, high fever, sweats. Patterns of malaria paroxysms give rise to the terms 'tertian malaria' (fever every third day or 48h) seen in *P. falciparum*, *P. vivax*, and *P. ovale*, and quartan malaria (fever every fourth day or 72h) seen in *P. malariae*.
- Non-specific features, such as nausea, vomiting, headaches, and abdominal pain, are common.
- Signs of severe malaria include impaired consciousness or seizures, renal impairment, acidosis, hypoglycaemia, pulmonary oedema/acute respiratory distress syndrome (ARDS), anaemia, spontaneous bleeding/ disseminated intravascular coagulopathy (DIC), shock, haemoglobinuria, and parasitaemia of >10%.

Laboratory diagnosis

- Thick (for increased sensitivity of parasite detection) and thin (for improved species identification) blood smears are stained with Field's stain or Giemsa stain, and examined under light microscopy. Giemsa stain is better for species identification, whereas Field's stain is felt to have increased sensitivity for detection of parasites.
- Malaria rapid diagnostic tests (RDTs) can be used as a rapid bedside diagnostic test. The majority detect plasmodial lactate dehydrogenase (pLDH), and some tests enable distinction of species via detection of specific antigens—histidine-rich protein II (HRP II) in the case of *P. falciparum*.
- Molecular methods, such loop-mediated isothermal amplification (LAMP), are increasingly used in hospital settings and have been shown to have comparable sensitivity and specificity to a thick film with an experienced microscopist. PCR remains the gold standard test but is only performed in a limited number of centres in the UK.
- Laboratory findings—haemolytic anaemia, thrombocytopenia (common), uraemia, hyperbilirubinaemia, abnormal LFTs, and coagulopathy may be present. (See Box 10.1.)

Treatment

- **Antimalarials** (⊕ see Antimalarials, pp. 120–1)—remain the mainstay of therapy, but successful treatment is threatened by increasing drug resistance. The main classes of drugs are:
  - quinoline derivatives (chloroquine, quinine, mefloquine, halofantrine);
  - antifolates (pyrimethamine, sulfonamides);
  - ribosomal inhibitors (tetracycline, doxycycline, clindamycin);
  - artemisinin derivates (artemisinin, artemether, artemotil, artesunate); they are the treatment of choice and show rapid parasite clearance and have low toxicity and limited resistance (in South East Asia). Despite superior efficacy to quinine, IV artesunate is not licensed in

the UK but is recommended for use on a 'named patient' basis for all patients with severe or complicated falciparum malaria.

- **Supportive therapy**—good supportive therapy, with careful management of seizures, pulmonary oedema, acute renal failure, and lactic acidosis, is essential in severe malaria. Exchange transfusion may be helpful in hyperparasitaemia.
- **Adjunctive therapies**—adjunctive therapies for severe malaria have proved disappointing. Monoclonal antibodies directed against tumour necrosis factor alpha (TNF-α) reduced fever but showed no effect on mortality and may have increased morbidity. Dexamethasone has been shown to increase the duration of coma and was associated with poorer outcome in cerebral malaria. (See Box 10.1.)

Box 10.1 Malaria treatment and prevention guidelines

Treatment
- UK guidelines:
  - Lalloo D, Shingadia D, Pasvol G, *et al*. UK malaria treatment guidelines. *J Infect*. 2016;**72**:635–64
  - Public Health England (2019). *Guideline for malaria prevention in travellers from the UK*. Available at: ✍ https://www.britishinfection.org/guidance/published-guidelines and UKHSA guidance: https://www.gov.uk/government/collections/malaria-guidance-data-and-analysis
  - See also *British National Formulary*. *Malaria prophylaxis*. Available at: ✍ https://bnf.nice.org.uk/treatment-summary/malaria-prophylaxis.html
- US guidelines:
  - Centers for Disease Control and Prevention (2020). *Treatment of malaria: guidelines for clinicians*. Available at: ✍ https://www.cdc.gov/malaria/diagnosis_treatment/clinicians1.html
  - Centers for Disease Control and Prevention (2024). *CDC Yellow Book 2024*. Chapter 4: Travel-related infectious diseases. Available at: ✍ https://wwwnc.cdc.gov/travel/page/yellowbook-home
- World Health Organization:
  - World Health Organization (2023). *WHO guidelines for malaria*. Available at: ✍ https://www.who.int/teams/global-malaria-programme/guidelines-for-malaria

---

Prevention

- **Insecticide-treated bed nets**—have been shown to reduce intradomiciliary vector populations and protect against infection.
- **Insect repellents** such as diethyltoluamide (DEET)—reduce the risk of transmission in areas where mosquitoes are active before bedtime.
- **Chemoprophylaxis**—taken rigorously, is efficacious in reducing the incidence of malaria in travellers.

- **Vaccines**—a number of candidate vaccines using various antigens have been developed. Two are approved by WHO for use in children living in areas of moderate to high transmission: RTS,S/AS01 and R21/Matrix-M.

Babesia

Babesiosis is a zoonotic infection caused by *Babesia* spp., a malaria-like parasite that parasitizes erythrocytes of animals and causes fever, haemolysis, and haemoglobinuria. It typically causes mild illness in humans, but fulminant disease may occur in asplenic or immunosuppressed patients.

The parasite

There are >70 *Babesia* spp. worldwide that infect a wide range of mammals and birds. *Babesia* spp. have traditionally been classified into four clades:
- clade 1—contains *Babesia microti* spp. that cause disease in the USA and Japan;
- clade 2—contains *Babesia duncani* and *B. duncani*-like organisms that cause disease in western USA;
- clade 3—contains *Babesia divergens* that causes disease in cattle in Europe, *B. divergens*-like organisms that cause disease in humans in Europe and the USA, and *Babesia venatorum* that causes human disease in Europe;
- clade 4—contains *Babesia bovis* and *Babesia bigemina* that rarely cause disease in humans.

Babesia spp. vary in length from 1 to 5 micrometres, and are pear-shaped, oval, or round; their ring conformation and peripheral location in erythrocytes may lead to their misidentification as *P. falciparum*. *Babesia* spp. are transmitted from their animal reservoir to humans via a tick vector—*Ixodes scapularis* (USA) or *Ixodes ricinus* (Europe). The tick has three developmental stages (larva, nymph, and adult) and requires a blood meal, often from different mammalian species (e.g. deer, rodent) to mature to the next stage.

Epidemiology

The first fatal human case of babesiosis was reported in 1996. Since then, >2700 cases have been reported worldwide, most from the north-eastern coastal regions of the USA and sporadically in mainland Europe. The first UK acquired case was identified in 1979 in Scotland, and a further case was identified in 2020 in Devon, England. Based on seroprevalence data, most infections appear to be subclinical. Rarely, transfusion, transplacental, and perinatal transmission has been known to occur.

The clinical features of babesiosis vary markedly across regions. Virtually all of the European cases have been caused by *B. bovis* or *B. divergens*, have occurred in splenectomized patients, and have had a fulminant and usually fatal course. In contrast, epidemiological data from the USA suggest that most infections are caused by *B. microti* and are mild or subclinical; clinical infections are more likely in asplenic and immunosuppressed patients, the elderly, and patients with concomitant Lyme disease. Risk factors for severe disease include age >50 years, splenectomy, poorly controlled HIV, immunosuppression, and therapy with anti-TNF agents (infliximab, etanercept) or anti-CD20 antibody (rituximab).

Clinical features

- Clinical features are relatively non-specific and include fever, chills, malaise, fatigue, anorexia, headache, myalgia, arthralgia, nausea, vomiting, abdominal pain, dark urine, depression, and emotional lability. Photophobia, conjunctival injection, retinal infarcts, sore throat, and cough have also been described.
- Clinical features of severe disease include ARDS, congestive cardiac failure (CCF), acute kidney injury, liver failure, and DIC.
- Laboratory abnormalities include haemolytic anaemia, reticulocytosis, normal or low WCC, thrombocytopenia, raised ESR, positive direct Coombs' test, abnormal LFTs, renal impairment, and reduced serum haptoglobin levels.
- Urinalysis reveals haemoglobinuria and proteinuria.

Laboratory diagnosis

- Microscopy—examination of thick and thin blood smears stained with Giemsa or Wright stain show parasitized erythrocytes, sometimes with diagnostic tetrads ('Maltese cross') of merozoites. *Babesia* spp. can be distinguished from *P. falciparum* by its lack of haemozoin and the absence of schizonts and gametocytes.
- Serology—indirect immunofluorescent antibody titre for *B. microti* is available from CDC Atlanta. A titre of ≥1:256 is considered diagnostic for acute *B. microti* infection.
- Molecular methods—a PCR-based assay may be used for the detection of low levels of parasitaemia.

Treatment

- Atovaquone plus azithromycin for 7–10 days is the preferred regimen as it is generally well tolerated.
- Quinine plus clindamycin given for 7–10 days is the alternative.
- Longer durations of therapy may be required for severe disease—up to 6 weeks in immunosuppressed patients.
- Exchange transfusion can be considered in critically ill patients with high-grade parasitaemia (≥10%).
- Repeat blood films are recommended in immunocompetent patients while they are symptomatic, to ensure falling parasitaemia. In immunocompromised patients, blood films should be repeated until parasitaemia is undetectable, even in the absence of symptoms.
- A return of non-specific symptoms post-treatment should be investigated for babesiosis, as recurrence is relatively common.

Prevention

- Avoid exposure to ticks in endemic areas between May and September.
- Wear light-coloured, long-sleeved clothing, and tuck trousers into socks or boots.
- Use insect repellent (e.g. DEET) on skin and clothes.
- Carefully remove any ticks.

- Discourage blood donations from donors in endemic areas between May and September, donors with fevers 2 months prior to donation, and donors with a history of tick bite.

Further reading

Centers for Disease Control and Prevention (2023). *Parasites: babesiosis*. Available at: ℘ https:// www.cdc.gov/parasites/babesiosis/index.html

Toxoplasma gondii

Toxoplasmosis is a zoonotic infection caused by *Toxoplasma gondii*, a coccidian parasite of cats that affects humans and other mammals as intermediate hosts. Although infection with *T. gondii* is common, it rarely causes disease, apart from in congenitally acquired infection and in patients with cell-mediated immunodeficiency, especially poorly controlled HIV.

Classification

T. gondii belongs to subphylum *Apicomplexa*, class *Sporozoa* and exists in three forms: the oocyst (which releases sporozoites), the tissue cyst (which contains bradyzoites), and the tachyzoite.

Life cycle

Oocysts are produced in the cat's intestine and shed in its faeces. Once outside the cat, the oocysts sporulate and develop sporozoites. Oocysts are ingested by other animals and release sporozoites, which develop into tachyzoites. These infect a wide variety of cells, multiply rapidly to form rosettes, lyse the cells, and spread to other cells or parts of the body. In the tissues, formation of tissue cysts may occur, with slowly replicating bradyzoites inside them. Cats become infected by ingesting tissue cysts from the intermediate host, completing the life cycle (see Fig. 10.2).

Epidemiology

Toxoplasmosis is a worldwide zoonosis infecting a wide variety of mammals. Human infection occurs through ingestion of:

- tissue cysts in raw or undercooked meat;
- food or water contaminated with oocysts;
- transplacental transmission from mother to fetus;
- rarely, organ transplantation from a seropositive donor, contaminated blood transfusion, or needlestick injury.

In HIV-infected patients, cerebral toxoplasmosis is usually due to reactivation of latent infection due to advanced immunosuppression (CD4 count <100 cells/mm^3). The incidence of toxoplasmosis amongst HIV-infected individuals is directly related to the seroprevalence of *T. gondii* antibodies in the general population. Thus, rates are higher in Western Europe and Africa than in the USA. However, the introduction of antiretroviral therapy (ART) and use of co-trimoxazole prophylaxis for *Pneumocystis* pneumonia (PCP) have resulted in a dramatic fall in the incidence of toxoplasmosis in the developed world.

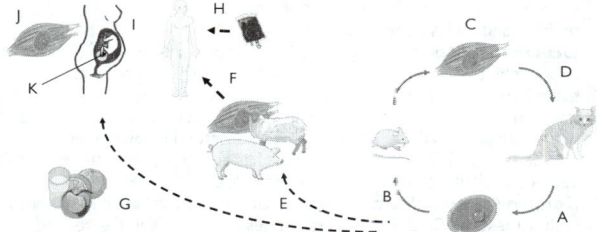

Fig. 10.2 Life cycle of *Toxoplasma gondii*. Unsporulated oocysts are shed in cat faeces, become infective after 1–5 days in the environment, and are ingested by intermediate hosts such as birds and rodents. Oocysts transform into tachyzoites, localize in neural and muscle tissue, and develop into tissue cyst bradyzoites. Cats become infected after consuming intermediate hosts with tissue cysts present. Animals bred for human consumption may also become infected by environmental sporulated oocysts. Humans may become infected by eating infected animal meat or consuming food or water infected with oocysts. Blood transfusion or organ transplantation can also be a route of transmission to humans. Infection can happen transplacentally from mother to fetus. Diagnosis is normally via serology, but tissue cysts may be observed in biopsy specimens. Diagnosis of congenital infections can be done via detecting *T. gondii* DNA in amniotic fluid via PCR.

Pathogenesis

T. gondii penetrates intestinal epithelial cells and multiplies intracellularly. Organisms spread to the regional lymph nodes before being carried to distant organs in the lymphatics and blood. Infection with *T. gondii* induces both humoral and cellular immune responses, which are important for early clearance of organisms from the blood and limit the parasite burden in other organs. Cyst formation is responsible for persistent or latent infection; the main sites are the brain, skeletal and cardiac muscle, and the eye. In immunocompetent individuals, initial infection is often asymptomatic; chronic/latent infection is not clinically significant, and immunity is lifelong. In immunosuppressed patients, toxoplasmosis may be caused by primary infection but is usually due to reactivation of latent infection.

Clinical features

- **Immunocompetent patients**—10–20% of infections are symptomatic. Clinical features include lymphadenopathy and/or an infectious mononucleosis-like syndrome. Rarely, severe disseminated disease (myocarditis, pericarditis, pneumonitis, ARDS, polymyositis, hepatitis, encephalitis) may occur.
- **Immunodeficient patients**—toxoplasmosis in HIV-negative patients is associated with organ transplants and lymphoma, and presents with CNS, myocardial, or pulmonary involvement. In patients with uncontrolled HIV, cerebral toxoplasmosis is the commonest diagnosis and presents subacutely with focal neurological symptoms. It commonly presents as multiple brain abscesses (but may be single) and can be complicated by hydrocephalus. Other manifestations include spinal

cord involvement, pneumonitis, chorioretinitis, pituitary abnormalities, orchitis, and GI involvement.

- **Ocular toxoplasmosis**—*T. gondii* is an important cause of chorioretinitis. Congenitally acquired infection usually presents in the second or third decade of life, with bilateral disease, macular involvement, and old retinal scars. Postnatal infection usually presents in the fourth to sixth decade of life, with unilateral involvement and macular sparing. Ocular toxoplasmosis has also been reported in HIV-infected patients, especially those from Brazil.

- **Congenital toxoplasmosis**—the incidence of fetal infection varies with trimester: 10–25% in the first trimester, 30–54% in the second trimester, 60–65% in the third trimester. The risk of severe congenital infection is highest in the first and second trimesters (weeks 10–24). Clinical features include: chorioretinitis, strabismus, blindness, seizures, microcephaly, intracranial calcification, hydrocephalus, anaemia, jaundice, rash, encephalitis, pneumonitis, diarrhoea, and hypothermia. In contrast, infants who acquire infection in the third trimester may be born with subclinical infection but, if untreated, may go on to develop disease (e.g. chorioretinitis, developmental delay).

Laboratory diagnosis

- Serology—this remains the mainstay of diagnosis. The main issue is that a high proportion of patients have had previous exposure to toxoplasmosis and therefore will be seropositive, and this may persist for years. There is no single test that can be used to differentiate acute from chronic infection. A combination of tests is often used and discussion with a reference laboratory is advisable:
  - IgM antibodies appear within a week of acute infection but may persist for months to years, limiting their use as the sole marker of acute infection;
  - IgG antibodies usually appear within 1–2 weeks, peak at around 8 weeks, and persist for life;
  - IgA assays are used predominantly as a marker of acute toxoplasmosis infection in pregnancy;
  - IgG avidity testing can be helpful to distinguish between acute and chronic infection;
  - the most widely used methods are: enzyme-linked immunoassays (EIAs), immunosorbent agglutination assay (ISAGA), and the Sabin–Feldman dye test.

- PCR—the detection of *T. gondii* DNA in body fluids and tissues has been used to diagnose all forms of *Toxoplasma* infection, but is primarily used in samples from immunocompromised patients. Sensitivity is 15–85% in blood, and 11–77% in CSF, although specificity is >95%.

- Isolation—direct culture of *T. gondii* is possible from clinical specimens but is rarely performed.

- Histology—demonstration of tachyzoites in tissues or body fluids is diagnostic of acute infection. Direct visualization of tachyzoites can be achieved via use of Giemsa or Wright stain. Various immunostaining methods may also be used on histological specimens.

Radiological features

Radiological imaging is helpful in patients with CNS disease. In neonates with congenital toxoplasmosis, ultrasound scanning (USS) or CT may demonstrate intracranial calcification and ventricular dilatation. In immunodeficient adults with cerebral toxoplasmosis, MRI appears to be more sensitive than CT and is the imaging modality of choice. Imaging typically shows multiple ring-enhancing lesions, often associated with oedema. However, scans may be normal or show solitary lesions or cortical atrophy. The main differential is CNS lymphoma, and nuclear imaging techniques, such as single-photon emission computed tomography (SPECT), can be helpful in distinguishing lesions radiologically.

Treatment

Currently recommended drugs act primarily against the tachyzoite form and do not eradicate the encysted form. Pyrimethamine is the most effective agent and should be given with folinic acid to prevent bone marrow suppression. A second drug, sulfadiazine or clindamycin, is also given. Alternative agents include co-trimoxazole or pyrimethamine plus one of azithromycin, clarithromycin, atovaquone, or dapsone. (See Nelson *et al.*, 2011.)[1,2]

- **Immunocompetent adults**—do not usually require treatment, unless symptoms are severe and persistent, visceral disease is overt, or infection is parenterally acquired.
- **Immunodeficient patients**—acute/primary therapy with pyrimethamine and sulfadiazine is recommended for 3–6 weeks, followed by maintenance therapy (at lower doses) until the CD4 count is >200 for 6 months. Patients with cerebral toxoplasmosis usually respond clinically within 2 weeks; those who do not should be investigated for other alternative diagnoses (e.g. CNS lymphoma).
- **Ocular toxoplasmosis**—treatment may not be required for small peripheral retinal lesions in immunocompetent adults but is generally indicated for lesions that threaten or cause visual loss.
- **Toxoplasmosis in pregnancy**[2]—patients with suspected acute toxoplasmosis in pregnancy should be referred to a specialist unit for further investigation and management. Treatment with spiramycin reduces the risk of transmission to the fetus. As spiramycin does not cross the placenta, if fetal infection occurs, treatment should be changed to pyrimethamine (not in the first trimester) and sulfadiazine.
- **Congenital toxoplasmosis**—infants with congenital toxoplasmosis should be referred to a specialist unit. Treatment is with pyrimethamine and sulfadiazine for up to 12 months.

Prevention

- Prevention of primary infection in susceptible individuals (e.g. pregnant women, immunosuppressed patients) is by education:
  - avoid contact with cat faeces in gardens and cat litters;
  - avoid ingestion of undercooked meat.
- For HIV-infected patients with CD4 count <200 cells/mm^3, primary prophylaxis with co-trimoxazole has been shown to reduce the

incidence of cerebral toxoplasmosis. Prophylaxis may be discontinued when CD4 count remains >200 cells/mm³ for 3 months.
- Some countries (e.g. France, Austria) advocate monthly screening of seronegative pregnant women during pregnancy.

References

1 Nelson M, Dockrell DH, Edwards S; BHIVA Guidelines Subcommittee (2011). *BHIVA and BIA guidelines for the treatment of opportunistic infection in HIV-seropositive individuals 2011*. Available at: ℘ https://www.gov.uk/guidance/infectious-diseases-during-pregnancy-screening-vaccination-and-treatment

Cryptosporidium

Cryptosporidium is an intracellular protozoan, first described in 1907 in mice and thought to be rare and clinically insignificant for 50 years. It has since been recognized as a common enteric pathogen and is associated with waterborne outbreaks and diarrhoea in children and adults. It infects and replicates in epithelial cells of the digestive and respiratory tracts of most vertebrates. Twenty species are recognized; *Cryptosporidium parvum* is the primary infecting species in humans, and *Cryptosporidium hominis* also causes disease.

Life cycle

Ingestion of oocysts is followed by encystation, usually following exposure to digestive enzymes or bile acids, then by release of four sporozoites, which attach to the epithelial cell wall. Sporozoites mature asexually into meronts and release merozoites intraluminally. Some of these reinvade the host cells (autoinfection), whereas others mature sexually into oocysts which are excreted in the faeces.

Epidemiology

Cryptosporidium is a ubiquitous enteric pathogen of all age groups. Transmission occurs by person-to-person, animal-to-person, waterborne, or, less commonly, food-borne spread. The prevalence of faecal oocyst excretion varies from 1–3% in industrialized countries to 5–10% in Asia and Africa. Seroprevalence data indicate that cryptosporidiosis is commoner than what surveys of faecal oocyst excretion demonstrate (e.g. 25–35% seroprevalence in Europe and North America). Alongside sporadic outbreaks in immunocompetent individuals, it is also a major cause of diarrhoea and malnutrition in the developing world. It is also an important cause of diarrhoea in patients with HIV/uncontrolled HIV. Risk factors for severe disease include: immunoglobulin deficiencies, haematological malignancies, diabetes mellitus, and secondary to immunosuppressive agents taken after organ transplantation.

Clinical features

- Symptoms usually develop 7–10 days after ingestion of oocysts:
  - GI symptoms—diarrhoea (may be copious), cramping abdominal pains, anorexia, nausea, vomiting, toxic megacolon (rare);
  - other symptoms—low-grade fever, weakness, malaise, fatigue, cholecystitis (especially HIV patients), hepatitis, pancreatitis, reactive

arthritis, respiratory symptoms, disseminated disease. Recovery depends on the immune status of the patient—immunocompetent patients tend to have self-limiting disease.

Diagnosis

- Faeces microscopy—examination of three faecal samples from separate days may be required due to intermittent shedding, to ensure the diagnosis is not missed. Most laboratories use a faecal concentration method, followed by microscopy by using a modified acid-fast stain—oocysts stain red/pink (carbol fuchsin) against a blue (methylene blue) or green (malachite green) counterstain. Other stains include safranin–methylene blue, methenamine silver–nigrosin acridine orange, auramine–rhodamine, and auramine–carbol fuchsin.
- Antigen detection—direct immunofluorescence assays (DFAs) and EIA tests are commonly used for *Cryptosporidium* diagnosis. Many kits have superior sensitivity relative to microscopy and circumvent the need for multiple faecal samples.
- Faecal multiplex PCR assays now commonly contain *Cryptosporidium* primers and are highly sensitive and specific.
- Serology is rarely used outside epidemiological studies.
- Histology has low sensitivity and is now rarely used.

Treatment

- Disease is usually self-limiting in immunocompetent patients, and supportive therapy (hydration, parenteral nutrition) is key.
- When specific treatment is required in immunocompetent patients, nitazoxanide is the preferred agent.
- In HIV-infected patients, ART is the key intervention. For patients with severe symptoms, antidiarrhoeal agents and enteral/parenteral nutrition may be considered. The benefit of nitazoxanide or paromomycin in HIV-infected patients has not been established.

Prevention

- Prevention of exposure in 'at-risk' individuals (e.g. water filters, avoiding exposure to human and animal faeces, boiling water during outbreaks).
- Prophylaxis against *Cryptosporidium* in HIV-infected patients is not recommended; one report suggested that clarithromycin or rifabutin given as *Mycobacterium avium* complex (MAC) prophylaxis may be beneficial.

Cystoisospora

Cystoisospora belli (formerly known as *Isospora belli*) is a coccidian GI parasite, first described in 1915.

Epidemiology

C. belli is found worldwide but predominantly causes infections in tropical and subtropical climates. Infection may occur in immunosuppressed (HIV infection, human T-cell lymphotropic virus 1 (HTLV-1) infection, lymphoblastic lymphoma, T-cell leukaemia, non-Hodgkin's lymphoma) and immunocompetent patients. Transmission is by the faeco-oral route with ingestion of sporulated oocysts in contaminated food and water.

Clinical features

It causes a self-limiting diarrhoeal illness in immunocompetent patients but may cause chronic or severe diarrhoea in immunocompromised individuals, especially HIV-infected patients. Rare presentations include disseminated disease, cholecystitis, and reactive arthritis.

Laboratory diagnosis

In cases of heavy infection, oocysts may be seen in a wet mount of the faecal sample. However, shedding may be intermittent, requiring examination of several faecal samples and use of acid-fast stains or immunofluorescence techniques. Real-time PCR assays have been developed but are not widely available.

Treatment

- Supportive therapy with fluid resuscitation and nutritional support may be required for patients with severe diarrhoea.
- Treatment is with co-trimoxazole for 7–10 days for immunocompetent patients.
- For immunosuppressed patients, treatment with co-trimoxazole for 10 days, followed by a dose three times a week, has been shown to be beneficial. Alternative agents include ciprofloxacin (inferior efficacy), pyrimethamine, and nitazoxanide.

Cyclospora

Epidemiology

Cyclospora cayetanensis was first described in humans in Papua New Guinea in 1977. Since then, it has emerged as a worldwide cause of diarrhoea in travellers, children, and HIV-infected patients. Transmission is by contaminated food and water. Most of the early cases were described in Nepal, Peru, and Haiti. More recently, outbreaks have been associated with the importation of fruits and vegetables from endemic areas.

Clinical features

The clinical features of the disease vary significantly. In endemic areas, infection may be asymptomatic or mild and self-limiting. In non-endemic areas, clinical features include anorexia, fatigue, nausea, abdominal pain, diarrhoea, fever, and weight loss. Symptoms may last 10–12 weeks, and relapse is common. In immunocompromised/HIV-infected patients, symptoms may be severe and persist longer.

Laboratory diagnosis

Diagnosis is by microscopic detection of oocysts in faeces (after concentration techniques), by using modified acid-fast or safranin stain. The parasite is shed intermittently, so three faecal specimens from different days need to be examined before infection can be excluded. Commercial PCR platforms are available for *Cyclospora* and are highly sensitive and specific.

Treatment

Treatment is with co-trimoxazole for 7 days for immunocompetent patients. For patients with HIV or other immunosuppression, the initial treatment course is longer, followed by lifelong suppressive therapy (until the CD4 count is consistently >200 cells/mm^3).

Trypanosoma

The genus *Trypanosoma* consists of 720 species of protozoa. They are common animal pathogens that cause severe disease in domestic animals. Three species infect humans:

- *Trypanosoma cruzi*, which causes Chagas' disease;
- *Trypanosoma brucei gambiense*, which causes West African sleeping sickness;
- *Trypanosoma brucei rhodesiense*, which causes East African sleeping sickness.

Trypanosoma cruzi

Chagas' disease is a zoonosis caused by the protozoan parasite *T. cruzi*. The disease is endemic in wild and domestic animals in Central and South America, and is estimated to infect 8–10 million people. It is transmitted by triatome or 'kissing' bugs. Humans are considered accidental hosts. Transmission of *T. cruzi* may also occur through vertical transmission, blood transfusion, organ transplantation, oral transmission (contaminated food), and laboratory exposure.

Life cycle

The parasites multiply in the midgut of the insects as promastigotes (see Fig. 10.3). In the hindgut, they transform into trypomastigotes, which pass out in the faeces during blood meals. Transmission to a second mammalian host occurs when breaks in the skin, mucous membranes, or conjunctivae are contaminated with bug faeces. The parasites enter host cells, transform into amastigotes, and multiply and differentiate into trypomastigotes. The cell ruptures, releasing the parasites which invade local tissue and spread haematogenously. The triatome bug then ingests trypomastigotes during a blood meal to complete the life cycle.

Pathogenesis

In acute Chagas' disease, the inflammatory lesion that develops at the site of entry is called the chagoma. Trypomastigotes released by cell rupture may be detected by microscopic examination of the blood. Muscles are the most heavily parasitized tissues, resulting in chronic complications (e.g. cardiac and GI disease).

Clinical features

There are five main clinical presentations:

- **acute Chagas' disease**—is usually an illness of children. An inflammatory lesion, called a chagoma, develops at the site of entry in around 25% of patients. The Romaña's sign (painless periorbital oedema) may be seen if the site of entry is the conjunctivae.

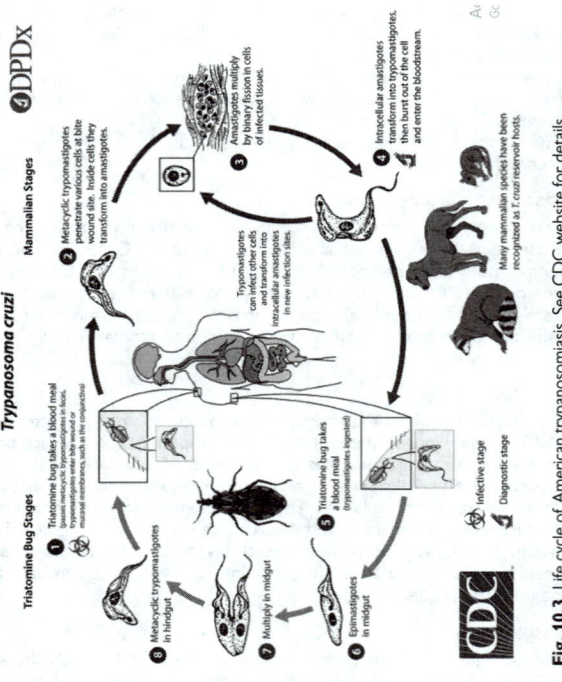

Fig. 10.3 Life cycle of American trypanosomiasis. See CDC website for details.
🔗 https://www.cdc.gov/dpdx/trypanosomiasisamerican/index.html

Localized signs may be followed by fever, malaise, anorexia, oedema, lymphadenopathy, and hepatosplenomegaly. CNS involvement is rare but carries a poor prognosis. Severe myocarditis with CCF may also occur. Acute illness usually resolves over 4–8 weeks, and the patient enters the asymptomatic phase;

- **indeterminate form (latent disease)**—is characterized by the absence of symptoms and signs of infection, a normal ECG, and normal radiological investigations (e.g. CXR, barium studies), with serological/parasitological evidence of chronic *T. cruzi* infection. No formal guidelines exist for monitoring patients with asymptomatic infection; 30–40% progress to chronic disease after 10–30 years;
- **chronic cardiac cardiomyopathy**—the heart is the commonest site for chronic disease, with cardiac failure and conduction abnormalities being the primary manifestations. Clinical features include dizziness, syncope, chest pain, pulmonary and systemic emboli, and stroke. Cardiac examination may reveal apical heave, prominent mitral or tricuspid regurgitation, and splitting of the second heart sound. The CXR shows cardiomegaly, and the ECG typically shows right bundle branch block. Death occurs within months of developing cardiac failure;
- **GI disease**—this usually affects 10–15% of patients with chronic Chagas' disease and presents between the ages of 20 and 40 years. Patients present with symptoms of achalasia and megaoesophagus (e.g. dysphagia, odynophagia, cough, chest pain, regurgitation). Aspiration pneumonitis is common and may be fatal. An increased incidence of oesophageal cancer has been reported. Patients with megacolon present with constipation, abdominal pain, intestinal obstruction, or bowel perforation;
- **disease in immunosuppressed patients**—reactivation of *T. cruzi* may occur in immunosuppressed patients (e.g. solid organ transplantation, advanced HIV infection). Clinical presentation is similar to acute Chagas' disease but may be more severe with CNS involvement.

Diagnosis

Diagnosis of Chagas' disease is based on:

- history of exposure to *T. cruzi* (e.g. residence or travel to an endemic area, blood transfusion in an endemic area);
- acute Chagas' disease—wet prep or Giemsa smear for detection of circulating trypomastigotes. In immunocompromised patients, other specimens may need to be examined (e.g. lymph node, bone marrow aspirates, pericardial fluid, CSF). If the smear is negative, culture of blood or specimens in liquid media or xenodiagnosis may be attempted, but both methods are slow and have low sensitivity;
- chronic Chagas' disease—is diagnosed by detection of IgG antibodies to the parasite, with a suggestive history. The presence of amastigotes on tissue histology (such as bowel or cardiac) is also diagnostic;
- PCR assays have been developed over the past 20 years. Sensitivity is usually >90% (range 47–100%).

Treatment

Current treatment of Chagas' disease is far from ideal.

- Indications for treatment—acute infection, early congenital infection, children with chronic *T. cruzi* infection, reactivated infection in immunosuppressed patients.
- Benznidazole, a nitroimidazole derivative, is the preferred agent, as it is better tolerated than nifurtimox. Side effects include rash, peripheral neuropathy, insomnia, and bone marrow suppression. Concurrent alcohol use can result in disulfiram effects and should be avoided. Suggested duration is 90 days.
- Nifurtimox, a nitrofuran derivative, is an alternative agent and is better tolerated in children. Side effects include nausea, vomiting, abdominal pain, weight loss, and neurological symptoms. Suggested duration is 60 days.
- Both agents are contraindicated in pregnancy, as well as in patients with severe renal and hepatic dysfunction.
- Chronic infection—treatment is supportive. Pacemakers are helpful in patients with bradyarrhythmias. Cardiac transplantation is considered in those with significant cardiac failure, but immunosuppression can promote reactivation, and periodic PCR is often used to monitor for this. Megaoesophagus may be treated with balloon dilatation/ myomectomy of the lower oesophageal sphincter. Megacolon is managed with high-fibre diet and laxatives/enemas. Surgery may be required for complications.

Trypanosoma brucei complex

Human African trypanosomiasis (HAT), or sleeping sickness, is caused by protozoan parasites that belong to the *T. brucei* complex:

- *T. brucei rhodesiense* that causes East African trypanosomiasis;
- *T. brucei gambiense* that causes West African trypanosomiasis.

They are morphologically indistinguishable and transmitted by tsetse flies (*Glossina* spp.), but the clinical features of infection differ in presentation and prognosis. A third species *Trypanosoma brucei brucei* is an animal pathogen.

Life cycle

Tsetse flies ingest trypomastigotes during a blood meal from an infected mammalian host (see Fig. 10.4). Once in the midgut, the short, stumpy trypomastigotes transform into long, slender, procyclic trypomastigotes. After several cycles of replication, they migrate to the salivary glands where they differentiate into epimastigotes and continue to multiply. The epimastigotes transform into infective trypomastigotes, which are ingested by tsetse flies at their next blood meal. African trypanosomes differ from *T. cruzi* in that they exhibit antigenic variation and are thus able to evade the host immune response.

Pathogenesis

The pathogenesis of African sleeping sickness is complex and incompletely understood. An acute inflammatory lesion (trypanosomal chancre)

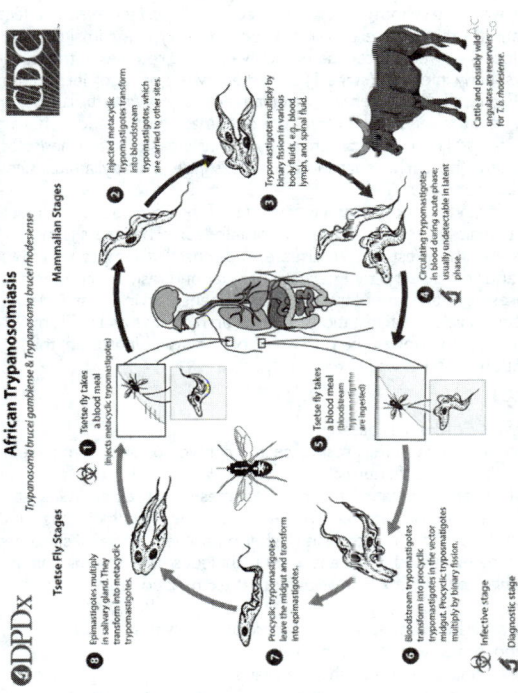

Fig. 10.4 Life cycle of African trypanosomiasis. See CDC website for details.
https://www.cdc.gov/dpdx/trypanosomiasisafrican/index.html

develops at the site of the tsetse fly bite. Multiplication of the parasite occurs in this lesion, resulting in inflammation, oedema, and local tissue destruction. The parasites spread to the local lymph nodes and then disseminate in the bloodstream. In stage 1 disease (haemolymphatic), there is widespread lymphadenopathy and histiocytic infiltration, followed by fibrosis. The heart may be involved. Stage 2 disease (meningoencephalitic) is characterized by CNS invasion.

Clinical features

- West African trypanosomiasis is caused by *T. brucei gambiense*. Infected humans are the main reservoir of infection. A trypanosomal chancre develops 1–2 weeks after the tsetse fly bite and resolves within several weeks. Early infection (stage 1) is marked by the onset of intermittent high fevers, posterior cervical lymphadenopathy (Winterbottom's sign), hepatosplenomegaly, transient oedema, pruritus, and rash. Late infection (stage 2) is characterized by the insidious onset of neurological symptoms (headache, somnolence, listless gaze, extrapyramidal signs) and CSF abnormalities.
- East African trypanosomiasis is caused by *T. brucei rhodesiense*. Infected wild animals are the main reservoir of infection. The illness is more acute than the West African disease, with onset of symptoms a few days after the insect bite. Intermittent fever and rash are common features—lymphadenopathy is less prominent than in West African disease. Cardiac manifestations, such as arrhythmias and CCF, may result in death prior to the onset of CNS disease. Untreated, this condition is fatal in weeks to months.

Diagnosis

The diagnosis of HAT is based on:
- history of exposure (e.g. residence in, or travel to, an endemic area);
- compatible clinical features;
- blood smear examination for trypanosomes (wet prep and Giemsa stain)—is more likely to be positive in the haemolymphatic stage and in East African trypanosomiasis (higher parasitaemia). Serial specimens should be examined. Concentration techniques such as a mini-anion exchange column (MAEC) or buffy coat examination may increase sensitivity;
- tissue aspirate examination of chancre fluid or lymph nodes for trypanosomes (wet prep and Giemsa stain);
- CSF examination—which shows increased WCC, raised pressure, elevated protein levels, and elevated IgM levels. A patient with any CSF abnormalities should be regarded as having CNS disease;
- bone marrow aspiration—may be helpful in patients whose other tests are negative;
- serology—antibody tests for *T. brucei gambiense* are available but have variable sensitivity and specificity. The test that is most frequently used in the field is the card agglutination tests for *T. gambiense* trypanosomes (CATT). Antigen detection EIAs have been developed but are not commercially available;
- molecular tests—have been used for subspeciation in research settings.

Treatment

A number of drugs are available to treat African trypanosomiasis (see Table 10.1):

- melarsoprol (see Antiprotozoal drugs, p. 130);
- pentamidine (see Antiprotozoal drugs, p. 132);
- suramin (see Antiprotozoal drugs, p. 132);
- eflornithine (see Antiprotozoal drugs, p. 125);
- fexinidazole (see Antiprotozoal drugs, p. 129).

Treatment of African trypanosomiasis depends on the infecting species, drug resistance patterns, and stage of disease. Seek expert advice.

Table 10.1 Treatment of African trypanosomiasis

	Stage 1 disease	Stage 2 disease
Trypanosoma brucei gambiense	Fexinidazole OR pentamidine	Nifurtimox–eflornithine combination therapy OR pentamidine
Trypanosoma brucei rhodesiense	Suramin	Melarsoprol

Prevention

Prevention of HAT relies on two strategies—vector control (aerial insecticide spraying, tsetse fly traps, reduction of wild animal populations) and surveillance (with early treatment of identified cases). Travellers to endemic areas are advised to avoid areas where tsetse flies are endemic, wear protective clothing, and use insect repellents. There is no vaccine.

Leishmania

Leishmaniasis is caused by various *Leishmania* spp. that vary in their geographical distribution and clinical features. There are three clinical syndromes, each of which may be caused by several species:

- visceral leishmaniasis (kala-azar);
- cutaneous leishmaniasis;
- mucosal leishmaniasis (espundia).

The parasite

Leishmania spp. are transmitted by female phlebotomine sandflies (see Fig. 10.5). In the New World (South and Central America), *Leishmania* spp. are transmitted by *Lutzomyia* genus and in the Old World (Europe, Africa, and Asia) by the *Phlebotomus* genus. The sandfly becomes infected by ingesting amastigotes of infected mammalian hosts. Amastigotes develop into flagellated promastigotes in the gut and migrate to the proboscis of the sandfly, where they are injected into the host on feeding. Promastigotes are ingested by macrophages where they develop into amastigotes. The amastigotes are then spread via the reticuloendothelial system where they continue to multiply or are ingested by a sandfly bite, completing the life cycle. Transmission has also likely occurred via needle sharing amongst

Life Cycle

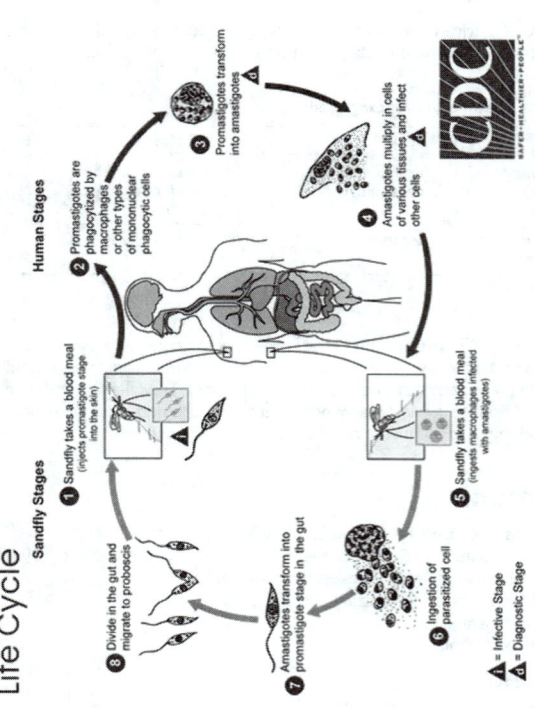

Fig. 10.5 Life cycle of leishmaniasis. See CDC website for details.

https://www.cdc.gov/dpdx/leishmaniasis/index.html

people who inject drugs and through organ transplantation. *Leishmania* spp. cannot be differentiated on the basis of morphology. Speciation was initially based on epidemiological and clinical features; several molecular assays are now used.

Epidemiology

- Visceral leishmaniasis has a wide geographical distribution and is caused by the three species from the *Leishmania donovani* complex. It is caused by *Leishmania donovani* spp. (India, Pakistan, Nepal, East Africa, Eastern China), *Leishmania infantum* spp. (Middle East, Mediterranean, Balkans, Central and South West Asia, North and West China, North and sub-Saharan Africa), and *Leishmania chagasi* spp. (Latin America). Rarely, *Leishmania amazonensis* or *Leishmania tropica* may cause visceral leishmaniasis.
- Cutaneous leishmaniasis is also widely distributed. Old World cutaneous leishmaniasis is found in the Middle East, the Mediterranean, Africa, India, and Asia. It is usually caused by *Leishmania major*, *L. tropica*, *Leishmania aethiopica*, and occasionally *L. donovani* and *L. infantum*. New World cutaneous leishmaniasis is endemic in Latin America. It is caused by *Leishmania braziliensis*, *Leishmania mexicana*, *Leishmania panamensis*, and occasionally *L. chagasi*.
- Mucosal leishmaniasis (espundia) mainly occurs in Latin America and is usually caused by *L. braziliensis*.

Clinical features

- **Visceral leishmaniasis**—the incubation period is usually 3–8 months but has been noted 10 years after exposure. Many infections are subclinical. Onset is usually insidious but may occasionally be acute. Symptoms include abdominal enlargement, fever, weakness, anorexia, and weight loss. Examination may reveal pallor, hepatosplenomegaly ± lymphadenopathy. The skin may become dry, thin, scaly, and discoloured (kala-azar = black fever). Haemorrhage may occur at various sites. Secondary infections are common in advanced disease and may lead to death. Laboratory findings include renal impairment, anaemia, leucopenia, and hypergammaglobulinaemia. Uncontrolled HIV is a strong risk factor for active visceral leishmaniasis (>100 times risk relative to HIV-negative individuals). It may present atypically and represent reactivation of latent infection.
- **Cutaneous leishmaniasis**—the incubation period varies between 2 weeks to several months. A wide variety of skin lesions may occur, from small, dry, crusted lesions (usually *L. tropica*) to large, deep ulcers with a granulating base and an overlying exudate (usually *L. braziliensis*). Lesions may be single or multiple, and tend to occur on exposed areas. Secondary bacterial infections and lymphadenopathy may occur.
- **Mucosal leishmaniasis**—a small proportion of patients with cutaneous leishmaniasis develop mucous membrane involvement of the nose, oral cavity, pharynx, and larynx months to years after their skin lesions have healed. Symptoms include nasal stuffiness, discharge, or epistaxis. The nasal septum may be destroyed, resulting in nasal collapse. Perforation may occur through the nose or soft palate.

Occasionally, patients may be unable to eat or may develop aspiration pneumonia.

- **Post-kala-azar dermal leishmaniasis (PKDL)**—is a complication of visceral leishmaniasis and is characterized by the development of rash following seemingly effective treatment. The rash classically starts around the mouth, may be macular or papular, and progressively spreads over the face, trunk, and limbs. The rash may become nodular or hypopigmented as time progresses. The lesions may contain amastigotes on biopsy. It is seen most commonly following visceral leishmaniasis in Sudan (50% cases) and India (10% cases). Though PKDL may resolve without specific treatment, treatment is usually advised with miltefosine, pentavalent antimonial compounds, or liposomal amphotericin B.

Diagnosis

- **Visceral leishmaniasis**—tissue biopsy of the spleen (highest sensitivity), bone marrow, lymph node, or liver may confirm the diagnosis. Amastigotes may be seen in Wright- or Giemsa-stained smears. Specimens should be inoculated into special media (e.g. Novy, McNeal and Nicoll medium, Schneider insect medium) and cultured at 22–26°C. Motile promastigotes develop after days to weeks. Anti-leishmanial antibodies (e.g. EIA, immunofluorescence antibody test (IFAT)) have high specificity and sensitivity in immunocompetent patients but may be falsely negative in HIV-infected patients. False-positive reactions may occur with leprosy, Chagas' disease, malaria, schistosomiasis, toxoplasmosis, and cutaneous leishmaniasis. The direct agglutination test (DAT) on serum is >95% sensitive and specific, but may be falsely positive in an endemic population and remains positive post-successful therapy. Urinary antigen tests against polypeptide fraction K39 of the *Leishmania* antigen is >95% sensitive and specific in visceral leishmaniasis, and does not remain positive post-treatment, which may be helpful in monitoring treatment efficacy.
- **Cutaneous leishmaniasis**—skin biopsies taken from the edge of a lesion may show amastigotes on Wright or Giemsa staining. Lesions may also be injected and aspirated with saline and examined for amastigotes. Samples may be cultured by using special media (see bullet point above). Anti-leishmanial antibodies may be present in some patients. The leishmanin (Montenegro) skin test becomes positive during the course of the disease but is no longer used clinically. PCR-based assays are highly sensitive for the diagnosis of cutaneous leishmaniasis.
- **Mucosal leishmaniasis**—a definitive diagnosis is made by tissue biopsy, either via identification or culture of amastigotes or via PCR. However, the diagnosis is often presumptive and based on the presence of characteristic clinical findings.

Treatment

- **Visceral leishmaniasis**—liposomal amphotericin B has the highest therapeutic efficacy and the lowest toxicity profile. Conventional amphotericin B is used but carries a risk of renal toxicity. Pentavalent antimonial compounds (e.g. sodium stibogluconate and meglumine antimoniate) have been used for decades. Side effects include cardiotoxicity, pancreatitis, myalgia and arthralgia, nausea, vomiting, abdominal pain, headache, fatigue, rash, elevated LFTs, anaemia, leucopenia, and thrombocytopenia Alternative agents include PO miltefosine or IV or IM paromomycin. Observational studies and small trials suggest that combination therapy is the way forward, but published data are sparse.

- **Cutaneous leishmaniasis**—many lesions will resolve without treatment. Uncomplicated disease is treated with local therapy (e.g. cryotherapy, thermotherapy, intralesional pentavalent antimony compounds, topical paromomycin, photodynamic therapy). Complicated disease is treated with systemic therapy (e.g. PO fluconazole, ketoconazole, or miltefosine). Parenteral systemic therapy is sometimes indicated—options include pentavalent antimony compounds, amphotericin, and pentamidine.

Prevention

Prevention strategies include:

- control of sandfly vectors (insecticides, bed nets);
- control of animal reservoirs (difficult);
- treatment of infected humans.

Although there is no effective form of immunoprophylaxis, there are on-going efforts to produce a vaccine.

Giardia lamblia

Giardia lamblia, a flagellated intestinal protozoan, is a common cause of diarrhoea throughout the world, particularly in areas of poor sanitation.

The pathogen

The differentiation of *Giardia* spp. has traditionally relied on the morphological features and identity of the host. However, they may now be classified on the basis of antigen, isoenzyme, and genetic analysis. *G. lamblia* is the only species that infects humans. The life cycle consists of two stages: trophozoite and cyst.

Epidemiology

G. lamblia has a worldwide distribution and is the most commonly identified intestinal parasite. It is usually acquired by ingestion of contaminated water or food but may also be spread from person to person (children in day-care centres, institutionalized people, sexual transmission). Natural or experimental infections with *Giardia* spp. have been documented for many mammalian species; whether these act as reservoirs for transmission to humans is less clear.

Pathogenesis

Infection occurs after ingestion of as few as 10–25 cysts. After encystation, trophozoites colonize and multiply in the small bowel. The production of GI secretory immunoglobulin A (IgA) antibodies appears to be key in preventing and clearing infection. The cellular immune response is also important in clearing infection, by coordinating IgA secretion and cellular cytotoxicity. Susceptibility to giardiasis has been seen in patients with common variable immunodeficiency, X-linked agammaglobulinaemia, previous gastric surgery, and reduced gastric acidity.

Clinical features

- Incubation period—symptoms develop 1–2 weeks after ingestion of cysts; detection of cysts in the faeces may take longer.
- Clinical features include asymptomatic cyst passers (5–15%), diarrhoeal syndrome (25–50%), and subclinical infection (35–70%).
- Symptomatic giardiasis is characterized by diarrhoea, abdominal cramps, bloating, flatulence, malaise, nausea, anorexia, and weight loss. Initially, faeces may be profuse and watery, but later may become greasy and foul-smelling and may float (steatorrhoea). Vomiting, fever, and tenesmus are less common.
- Unusual features include urticaria, reactive arthritis, biliary disease, and gastric infection (achlorhydria a key risk factor).
- Severe volume depletion may occur in young children and pregnant women, necessitating hospital admission.

Diagnosis

The diagnosis should be considered in all patients with chronic diarrhoea, particularly if associated with malabsorption or weight loss.

- Faeces examination—a wet mount of fresh liquid faeces may show motile trophozoites; iodine staining may reveal cysts. Formol-ether concentration techniques may increase the yield. Due to intermittent excretion, three faecal samples on separate days should be taken to exclude infection.
- A variety of antigen detection assays can detect *G. lamblia* by direct fluorescence or EIA. They are increasingly used as the first-line diagnostic technique due to high sensitivity relative to microscopy and circumvent the issue of intermittent excretion of the parasite.
- The duodenal string test (Entero-Test) may be helpful in difficult cases.
- Duodenal aspirate and biopsy are more invasive but may help to exclude other diagnoses.
- Antibody tests are not widely available but are useful in distinguishing acute from past infection, and in epidemiological surveys.
- *In vitro* culture and molecular assays are available in research settings.

Treatment

- Treatment is recommended for symptomatic individuals. Acquired lactose intolerance occurs in 20–40% of cases, so patients should be advised to avoid lactose-containing foods for a month after treatment.
- Metronidazole antibiotic is the drug of choice and has an efficacy of 75–100%. Drug resistance can be induced *in vitro* and may occur *in vivo*. Side effects—metallic taste, nausea, dizziness, headache, disulfiram reaction (with alcohol), neutropenia (rare). Concerns about teratogenicity mean that it is contraindicated in pregnancy (first trimester) and is not recommended in children.
- Tinidazole (➔ see Antiprotozoal drugs, pp. 128–33), another nitroimidazole, can be given as a single dose and has fewer side effects and an efficacy of >90%.

- Nitazoxanide antibiotic has been found to be at least as effective as metronidazole, with an efficacy of 81–85%.
- Albendazole and mebendazole (➔ see Anthelmintic drugs, pp. 133–4) have been shown to have similar efficacy to metronidazole, and fewer side effects than metronidazole and tinidazole.
- Paromomycin antibiotic has been shown to have an efficacy of 55–90%. It has poor intestinal absorption and is used for patients in whom other agents are contraindicated (including pregnancy). Side effects—nausea, diarrhoea, and abdominal pain.
- Furazolidone (➔ see Nitrofurans, pp. 70–1) a nitrofuran, has a lower efficacy rate (80%) but is available as a liquid suspension. Side effects— GI symptoms, brown discoloration of urine, mild haemolysis (in glucose-6-phosphate dehydrogenase (G6PD) deficiency).
- Quinacrine antibiotic is an alternative and has an efficacy of 90%. Side effects—nausea, vomiting, abdominal cramps, yellow discoloration of skin, urine, and sclerae (rare), exfoliative dermatitis (rare).

Prevention

- Good sanitation, with proper treatment of public water supplies.
- Boiling or purification of water with chlorine- or iodine-based preparations in endemic areas.
- Prevention of person-to-person spread by good personal hygiene/ handwashing/avoidance of orogenital or orc-aral sex.
- Breastfeeding reduces the risk of *Giardia* infection in infants in developing countries.

Trichomonas vaginalis

Trichomonas vaginalis, a flagellated protozoan, is the commonest non-viral sexually transmitted infection (STI).

The pathogen

On microscopic examination of genital specimens, *T. vaginalis* is a pear-shaped organism (10×7 micrometres) with twitching motility. There are four anterior flagellae that arise from a single stalk and a fifth flagellum which is embedded in the undulating membrane.

Epidemiology

The incidence appears to be declining in Western Europe and the USA. Trichomoniasis is usually sexually transmitted, and its incidence is highest in women with multiple partners, in patients with other STIs, and in HIV-infected patients. Trichomoniasis is occasionally acquired non-venereally (e.g. in institutionalized patients) or by vertical transmission during delivery.

Pathogenesis

All areas of the cell surface are capable of phagocytosis and can ingest bacteria, leucocytes, erythrocytes, and epithelial cells. Trichomonads appear to damage the genital epithelium by direct contact, which is mediated by surface proteins, and cause micro-ulceration. Specific virulence factors have not been defined, and the immune response is incompletely understood.

T. vaginalis activates the alternative complement pathway and attracts neutrophils which may kill the protozoan.

Clinical features

- The incubation period is 5–28 days.
- Symptoms often begin or worsen during periods and include vaginal discharge (may be smelly or itchy), dyspareunia, dysuria, and lower abdominal discomfort.
- Signs include vulvar erythema, yellow/green or frothy vaginal discharge, vaginal inflammation, and punctate haemorrhages on the cervix ('strawberry cervix').
- Most infected men are asymptomatic, but those who are symptomatic may have urethritis that is clinically indistinguishable from other causes of non-gonococcal urethritis.
- Complications of vaginal trichomoniasis include vaginitis emphysematosa (gas-filled blebs in the vaginal wall), vaginal cuff cellulitis after hysterectomy, premature labour, and low-birthweight infants.
- *Trichomonas* may cause inflammation of the vaginal epithelium, which increases the risk of transmission of HIV.

Diagnosis

- Diagnosis relies on identification of the organism in genital specimens.
- The wet mount will identify organisms in 48–80% of infected women and in 50–90% of infected men.
- Various staining methods (e.g. Gram, Giemsa, Pappenheim, acridine orange) are less sensitive than the wet mount.
- Other methods (e.g. direct fluorescent antibody staining, latex agglutination, EIA, DNA probe, PCR-based assays) are more sensitive than wet prep, but less sensitive than culture.
- Culture remains the most sensitive technique, and trichomonads can be cultured on a variety of media; modified Diamond's media is the best.
- Serological diagnosis is hampered by low sensitivity and poor specificity, particularly in high-risk populations.

Treatment

- Metronidazole (➔ Nitroimidazoles, pp. 69–70) is the treatment of choice and can be given as a single 2g dose or in divided doses for 7 days. The main disadvantage of a single dose is the risk of reinfection if the partner is not treated simultaneously.
- Alternative drugs include tinidazole (single dose).
- Patients should be advised to avoid alcohol because of the risk of a disulfiram reaction with metronidazole and tinidazole.

Prevention

- General advice about prevention of STIs.
- Use of barrier contraceptive methods (e.g. condoms, spermicides).

Entamoeba histolytica

Entamoeba histolytica is a common cause of diarrhoea worldwide, particularly in the tropics. It can also cause extraintestinal disease (e.g. abscesses in the liver, lung, heart, brain).

The parasite

E. histolytica, *Entamoeba dispar*, and *Entamoeba moshkovskii* are known to reside in the large intestine of the human host. They are morphologically identical, but only *E. histolytica* causes disease in humans, whereas the other two species are regarded as non-pathogenic. *E. histolytica* exists in two forms: the trophozoite (10–60 micrometres with a single nucleus ± ingested erythrocytes) and the cyst (5–20 micrometres with four nuclei). Ingestion of the cyst results in excystation in the small bowel and trophozoite infection of the colon, causing symptoms. When conditions are no longer favourable, the trophozoite encysts and is passed out in the faeces. Cysts remain viable for weeks or months in moist environments.

Epidemiology

Ten per cent of the world's population is estimated to be infected with *E. histolytica*. Over 80% are asymptomatic but may asymptomatically shed the organism, perpetuating infection. There is a wide geographical variation in prevalence, ranging from ≤5% in developed countries to 20–30% in the tropics. Risk factors for amoebiasis in endemic areas include low socio-economic status, poor sanitation, and overcrowding. In low-prevalence countries, certain groups are at higher risk: immigrants or travellers from endemic regions, institutionalized individuals, and within the men who have sex with men (MSM) communities. Factors associated with severe disease include neonates, pregnancy, corticosteroid therapy, and malnutrition.

Clinical features

The clinical features of amoebiasis can be divided into intestinal and extraintestinal syndromes.

- Intestinal manifestations include asymptomatic infection, symptomatic non-invasive infection, amoebic dysentery (gradual onset, abdominal pain/tenderness, bloody diarrhoea), fulminant colitis (rare but carries high mortality), toxic megacolon and chronic colitis, amoeboma (annular lesion of the colon), and perianal ulceration.
- Amoebic liver abscess—this is the commonest extraintestinal manifestation and typically presents 8–20 weeks after return from an endemic area. Clinical features include fever, right upper quadrant pain, anorexia, malaise, weight loss, cough, and hiccough. Rupture of the abscess can cause pleural infection or peritonitis.
- Pleuro-pulmonary infection—risk factors include malnutrition, alcoholism, and atrial septal defect. Clinical features include serous pleural effusion, amoebic empyema, consolidation, lung abscess, and hepato-bronchial fistula.
- Cardiac infection—this is very rare and occurs after rupture of a liver abscess into the pericardium. It presents with chest pain, cardiac failure, and pericardial tamponade.
- Brain abscess—results from haematogenous spread.

Diagnosis

- Faeces microscopy remains the cornerstone of diagnosis, but sensitivity is poor and multiple specimens (at least three) should be examined. Fresh liquid faeces (within 15 minutes) should be examined by wet mount for motile trophozoites. A formol-ether concentrate with examination of iodine-stained deposit increases the likelihood of seeing cysts. The presence of cysts alone cannot distinguish between *E. histolytica* and the non-pathogenic *E. dispar*. Trophozoites of *E. histolytica* may be diagnostic if they contain ingested erythrocytes. Trophozoites may be seen within aspirates from amoebic liver abscesses.

- Colonoscopy and biopsy may be helpful in confirming the diagnosis in patients with colitis. Endoscopic features include punctate haemorrhages and ulcers, but may appear normal in early disease.
- Antigen testing—faeces and serum antigen tests are rapid, sensitive, and specific, and can distinguish between *E. histolytica* and other species.
- Serological tests, such as EIAs, are helpful in both the diagnosis of invasive intestinal amoebiasis (70% sensitive) and extraintestinal amoebiasis (95% sensitive). However, titres may be negative in early disease and remain high for years, which needs to be taken into account when interpreting the result.
- Molecular methods, such as real-time and multiplex PCR, can detect *E. histolytica* with high specificity and sensitivity.
- Imaging studies (e.g. USS, CT, MRI) are useful in assessing patients with suspected amoebic liver abscess (➲ Chapter 16, Liver abscess, pp. 714–16), though often they cannot distinguish definitively from a pyogenic abscess. Aspiration of the abscess yields a brown, odourless sterile liquid, which is said to resemble anchovy sauce, though it is not usually performed due to the risk of peritoneal spillage/peritonitis.

Treatment

Treatment of amoebiasis is complicated by a number of factors, including a variety of clinical syndromes, varying sites of action of different drugs, and availability of different drugs in different countries.

- Intraluminal carriage (e.g. asymptomatic cyst passers) should be treated because of the risk of invasive disease. Possible regimens include: paromomycin, diloxanide furoate, or iodoquinol.
- Invasive intestinal disease (e.g. dysentery, colitis) should be treated with metronidazole or tinidazole, followed by a luminal agent (see bullet point above). Surgery may be required for colonic perforation, abdominal abscess, or toxic megacolon.
- Extraintestinal amoebiasis (e.g. liver abscess) should be treated by metronidazole, followed by an intraluminal agent (see above). Indications for aspiration include diagnostic uncertainty, failure to respond to medical therapy, and suggestion of an impending rupture on imaging. Surgical attempts to correct amoebic bowel perforation or peritonitis should be avoided.
- Nitazoxanide has been shown to be an effective luminal and extraintestinal amoebicide and is generally well tolerated.

Prevention

- Avoid ingestion of contaminated water and food.
- In endemic areas, vegetables should be treated with a detergent and soaked in acetic acid or vinegar. Water should be boiled, as purification with chlorine or iodine may not be sufficient to kill cysts.
- Avoid sexual practices that involve faeco-oral contact.
- Development of oral and parenteral vaccines is in progress.

Free-living amoebae

Human infection with free-living amoebae is infrequent but may be severe and life-threatening. Three clinical syndromes occur:

- primary amoebic meningoencephalitis, caused by *Naegleria fowleri*;
- granulomatous amoebic encephalitis (GAM), caused by *Acanthamoeba* spp. and *Balamuthia mandrillaris*;
- amoebic keratitis, caused by *Acanthamoeba* spp.

Naegleria fowleri

- **Epidemiology**—*N. fowleri* is a free-living thermophilic flagellate amoeba found throughout the world in soil and particularly in warm freshwater such as rivers and lakes. Very rarely, *N. fowleri* causes primary amoebic encephalitis in children and young adults who have usually had recent freshwater exposure.
- **Pathogenesis**—amoebae penetrate the olfactory mucosa and enter the CNS through the cribriform plate, resulting in diffuse meningoencephalitis, purulent leptomeningitis, and cortical haemorrhages.
- **Clinical features**—symptoms occur 1–7 days after exposure. Patients may initially report changes in smell or taste, followed by an abrupt onset of fever, anorexia, nausea, vomiting, headache, meningism, and altered mental status. Patients rapidly progress to coma and death within a week.
- **Diagnosis**—is based on clinical suspicion and confirmed by demonstration of trophozoites in the CSF. A variety of molecular assays have been developed. Serological tests are not helpful, as the majority of adults tested in endemic areas (e.g. Florida) have antibodies.
- **Treatment**—the optimal treatment is unknown, with a case fatality rate of around 95%. Amphotericin is known to be active against the protozoa and is often used in treatment. Other agents that may be active are fluconazole, azithromycin, rifampicin, and miltefosine.

Acanthamoeba species

- **Epidemiology**—*Acanthamoeba* spp. are ubiquitous amoeba which have been isolated from soil, water, and air. Serological surveys indicate that exposure is common, and the organism may be isolated in pharyngeal swabs from healthy people. Encephalitis tends to occur in debilitated or immunosuppressed patients (e.g. HIV infection, liver disease, diabetes mellitus, chronic renal failure, systemic lupus erythematosus, malignancy, chemotherapy, organ transplantation, corticosteroid therapy). In contrast, keratitis occurs in healthy patients.
- **GAM**—has an insidious onset and presents with focal neurological deficits. Clinical features include altered mental status, seizures, fever, headache, hemiparesis, meningism, visual disturbance, and ataxia. The duration of CNS illness until death is 7–120 days. Other clinical syndromes include skin lesions, pneumonitis, adrenalitis, leucocytoclastic vasculitis, and osteomyelitis.
- **Amoebic keratitis**—is strongly associated with contact lenses and occasionally ocular trauma. Clinical features include foreign body sensation, followed by severe pain, photophobia, tearing,

blepharospasm, conjunctivitis, and blurred vision. The diagnosis is often delayed because of initial misdiagnosis or periods of temporary remission. A classic white 'ring infiltrate' is often seen on examination.

- **Diagnosis**—GAM is usually diagnosed post-mortem but may be diagnosed ante-mortem by brain biopsy. CT head has shown multiple lucent, non-enhancing lesions. Lumbar puncture is often contraindicated because of the risk of herniation. When performed, CSF examination has been non-diagnostic, with elevated WCC and protein levels and decreased glucose levels. The diagnosis of amoebic keratitis depends on the demonstration of *Acanthamoeba* in corneal scrapings, contact lenses, or contact lens fluid by histology or culture. Corneal scrapings may be examined by wet mount for motile trophozoites, or fixed and stained using a variety of stains, including Giemsa. PCR on corneal material is often used to confirm diagnosis.

- **Treatment**—the optimal treatment for GAM is unknown. Drugs that are active *in vitro* include propamidine, pentamidine, ketoconazole, miconazole, paromomycin, neomycin, 5- flucytosine, and, to a lesser extent, amphotericin. Combination therapy with miltefosine, fluconazole, and pentamidine isetionate has been recommended. Co-trimoxazole, metronidazole, and a macrolide may be added. The first-line treatment of amoebic keratitis is often polyhexamethylene biguanide (PHMB) and chlorhexidine eye drops. Surgical debridement may be required in severe disease. Corneal transplant may be required if secondary corneal perforation or scarring occurs.

Balamuthia mandrillaris

- **Epidemiology**—*B. mandrillaris* is a soil inhabitant which contaminates fresh water. It causes GAM in both immunocompetent and immunocompromised hosts.

- **Clinical features**—some patients present with a skin lesion (non-ulcerated plaque), followed by neurological symptoms, whereas others present with meningoencephalitis. Clinical features include fever, malaise, headache, nausea, vomiting, seizures, and focal neurological signs. Death occurs 1 week to several months after onset of symptoms.

- **Diagnosis**—CT head may show multiple hypodense lesions with mass effect. CSF abnormalities include mononuclear pleocytosis (10– 500 cells), raised protein levels, and low glucose levels. Brain biopsy specimens may demonstrate the cyst and trophozoite. Previously, *B. mandrillaris* was difficult to distinguish from *Acanthamoeba* spp., but an immunofluorescence assay and a cell-free growth medium have been developed.

- **Treatment**—the optimal treatment is unknown. Survivors have been treated with a combination of pentamidine, 5- flucytosine, fluconazole, and a macrolide.

Microsporidia

➔ See Chapter 9, *Microsporidias*, pp. 552–4, as these have now been classified as a fungi.

Helminths

Helminths: overview

Overview

Helminth is a term derived from the Greek word for worm, which describes a broad group of multicellular organisms which are parasitic to humans. The vast majority of adult stages of helminths are visible to the naked eye and produce eggs during reproduction. Transmission can occur via contaminated food, water, or soil or may be vector-borne such as via arthropods. The life cycles of helminths are varied and can involve direct inoculation via the faecal–oral route (such as soil-transmitted helminths) or involve intermediate hosts (such as *Schistosoma* spp.). All helminths have an outer coat known as a cuticle (or tegument). The majority of parasitic helminths are divided into two distinct phyla: nematodes (roundworms) and platyhelminths (flatworms).

Nematodes

Nematodes are elongated, cylindrical, non-segmented organisms, with a smooth cuticle and a body cavity containing a digestive tract and reproductive organs.

Platyhelminths

Platyhelminths are symmetrical, non-segmented, flat organisms. They possess no circulatory or respiratory organs, and therefore, their flat shape aids diffusion, on which they rely for respiration. Platyhelminths can be further subdivided into cestodes (tapeworms) and trematodes (flukes).

Neglected tropical diseases

Soil-transmitted helminths (i.e. *Ascaris lumbricoides*—often known just as *Ascaris*, whipworm (*Trichuris trichiura*), and hookworm (*Ancylostoma duodenale* and *Necator americanus*)) are examples of neglected tropical diseases (NTDs). They are found mainly in areas of poor sanitation and hygiene, and infection occurs in warm and moist climates, including in temperate zones during warmer months. They can theoretically be controlled or eliminated, but still result in huge disability and suffering. Other NTDs include dengue, rabies, and trachoma. See ℘ https://www.who.int/health-topics/neglected-tropical-diseases for a full list.

> For clear life cycle images, please search the Centers for Disease Control and Prevention website for the names of parasites and parasite biology (e.g. ℘ https://www.cdc.gov/dpdx/ascariasis/index.html).

Nematodes

Nematodes (or roundworms) are elongated, cylindrical organisms of varying length. There are >60 species of nematodes or roundworms that infect humans, some of which are shown in Table 11.1. They are the commonest human parasites and are a major public health burden, particularly geohelminths (or soil-transmitted helminths) in the developing world.

Table 11.1 Medically important nematodes

Type	Disease	Species
Intestinal	Ascariasis	*Ascaris lumbricoides*
	Trichuriasis	*Trichuris trichiura*
	Hookworm	*Ancylostoma duodenale*
		Necator americanus
	Strongyloidiasis	*Strongyloides stercoralis*
	Pinworm	*Enterobius vermicularis*
Tissue	Trichinosis	*Trichinella spiralis*
	Dracunculiasis	*Dracunculus medinensis*
	Filariasis	*Wuchereria bancrofti*
		Brugia malayi
		Brugia timori
	Onchocerciasis	*Onchocerca volvulus*

Intestinal nematodes

Intestinal nematodes are the largest group of human helminths. The commonest intestinal nematodes (A. lumbricoides, A. duodenale, N. americanus, and T. trichiura) cannot reproduce in humans and are referred to as geohelminths, as their eggs have to develop in the soil. The exceptions are *Strongyloides stercoralis* and *Enterobius vermicularis*, which can be transmitted from person to person.

Tissue nematodes

Tissue-dwelling roundworms are also a major public health problem, particularly in the tropics. Some affect humans only, whereas others have an animal reservoir. All of the parasites have a complex life cycle involving intermediate hosts, except *Trichinella* spp. Adult worms do not multiply in humans, so the worm load and severity of disease depend on intensity of exposure.

Ascaris lumbricoides

Ascariasis is the commonest helminthic infection in humans, with an estimated prevalence of around 800 million. It is caused by A. lumbricoides (roundworm) and is found worldwide, most commonly in the tropics.

The parasite

The adult worms (usually white, 15–30cm in length, 3–6mm in diameter) live in the small intestine and have a lifespan of 10–24 months. Each ♀ produces up to 200 000 ova/day, which pass out in the faeces. When ingested, the eggs hatch in the small intestine, penetrate the intestinal wall, migrate through the venous system to the lungs where they break into the alveoli and migrate up the bronchial tree, before they are swallowed and develop into mature worms in the intestine (see Fig. 11.1).

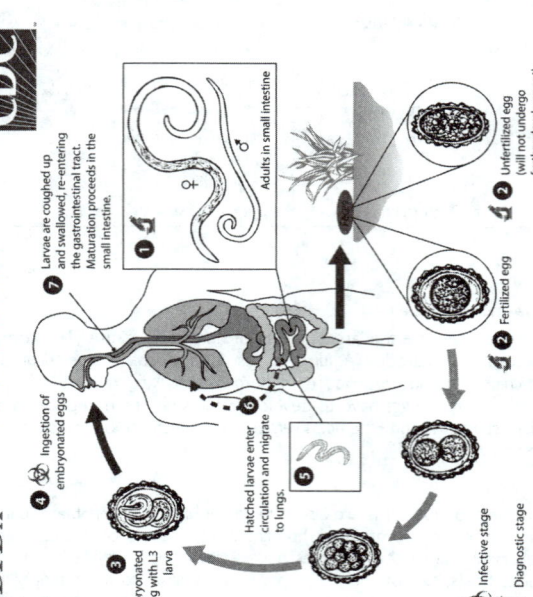

Fig. 11.1 Life cycle of ascariasis. See CDC website for details.
https://www.cdc.gov/dpdx/ascariasis/index.html.

Epidemiology

Ascaris infection is commonest in young children but can occur at any age. Transmission is by the faeco–oral route and is enhanced by the high output of ova and their ability to survive unfavourable environmental conditions. In endemic areas, most people have light to moderate worm burdens.

Clinical features

Most infected patients are asymptomatic. Clinical features depend on the site and intensity of infection:

* **pulmonary manifestations**—occur during larval migration through the lungs. Patients may present with Löeffler's syndrome (respiratory symptoms, pulmonary infiltration, peripheral eosinophilia) (see Box 11.1);

Box 11.1 Common causes of Löeffler's syndrome (respiratory syndromes and eosinophilia due to migration through the lungs)

* Ascariasis
* Hookworm (*Ancylostoma duodenale* and *Necator americanus*)
* Strongyloidiasis

---

* **GI manifestations**—include malnutrition, malabsorption, steatorrhoea, and intestinal obstruction (particularly in children);
* **biliary obstruction**—may cause abdominal pain, cholangitis, pancreatitis, and obstructive jaundice;
* **ectopic infections**—occur rarely (e.g. umbilical or hernial fistulae, fallopian tubes, bladder, lungs, heart).

Diagnosis

* Faecal sample microscopy—may be negative until 40 days after infection.
* The eggs are brown and oval-shaped, with a thick, mamillated shell, and measure 45–70 micrometres (length) by 35–50 micrometres (breadth) (see Fig. 11.1). Sometimes an adult worm is passed.
* Eosinophilia—may be seen in early infection when the larvae migrate through the lungs. Serum IgE and IgG levels may also be raised.
* Serology is rarely useful outside of epidemiological studies.

Treatment

* Albendazole (400mg stat) or mebendazole (500mg stat) is the treatment of choice.
* Alternative agents include nitazoxanide and levamisole.
* Endoscopic or surgical intervention may be required for biliary/intestinal obstruction.

Trichuris trichiura (whipworm)

Trichuriasis is one of the most prevalent helminthic infections—it is estimated that 500 million people carry the parasite. Infection is mainly asymptomatic, but heavy infection may cause anaemia, bloody diarrhoea, growth retardation, or rectal prolapse.

The parasite

T. trichiura principally infects humans, residing in the caecum and ascending colon. The mean lifespan of adult worms is 1 year, and each ♀ worm produces 2000–20 000 eggs per day. After excretion, embryonic development occurs over 2–4 weeks. The embryonated egg is ingested, and the larva escapes its shell, penetrating the small intestinal mucosa, before migrating down into the caecum or colon. The anterior whip-like portion remains embedded in the mucosa, whereas the shorter posterior end is free in the lumen (see Fig. 11.2).

Epidemiology

T. trichiura has a worldwide distribution but is commoner in most tropical environments. Infection results from ingestion of embryonated eggs by

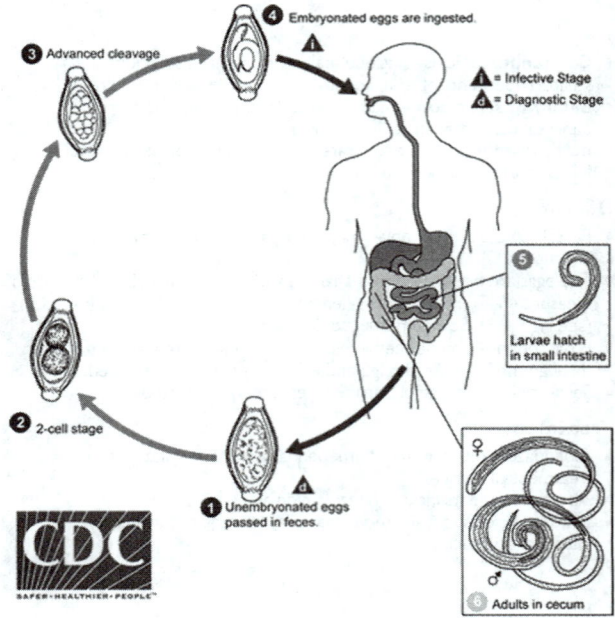

Fig. 11.2 Life cycle of *Trichuris*. See CDC website for details.
🔗 https://www.cdc.gov/dpdx/trichuriasis/index.html

direct contamination of hands, food, or drink, or indirectly through flies or other insects. The intensity of infection is usually light; heavy infection is commoner in children.

Clinical features

Infection is asymptomatic in most patients, but heavy infection may present with a variety of symptoms:

- **iron deficiency anaemia**;
- **acute GI symptoms**—diarrhoea (often containing mucus and/or blood) and nocturnal soiling;
- **chronic colitis with growth retardation**;
- ***Trichuris* dysentery syndrome**—which is associated with rectal prolapse, and also associated with heavy worm burden.

Diagnosis

- Faecal sample microscopy reveals characteristic lemon-shaped ova (50–55 × 20–25 micrometres) (see Fig. 11.1). They are thick-shelled and exhibit characteristic polar plugs. The Kato–Katz technique can be used to quantify egg numbers, which tend to correlate with worm burden.
- Eosinophilia is uncommon.
- Proctoscopy or colonoscopy may demonstrate adult worms protruding from the bowel mucosa.

Treatment

- Mebendazole 500mg stat is the treatment of choice. Albendazole 400mg stat or nitazoxanide is an alternative.

Ancylostoma duodenale and *Necator americanus* (hookworm)

Human hookworm infection is estimated to affect over 700 million people worldwide. It is caused by two species *A. duodenale* and *N. americanus*.

The parasite

Adult hookworms are small, cylindrical (1cm long), and greyish-white in colour. They live in the upper small intestine, attached to the mucosa. Adult worms produce about 7000 eggs per day. They pass out in the faeces and hatch into larvae. Skin penetration requires contact with contaminated soil. The larvae are carried in the venous circulation to the lungs where they migrate up the respiratory tree to be swallowed and carried to the small intestine (see Fig. 11.3).

Epidemiology

The prevalence of hookworm infection is highest in sub-Saharan Africa, Asia, Latin America, and the Caribbean. Transmission requires human faecal contamination of the soil, favourable conditions for larvae (warmth, moisture, and shade), and contact of human skin with

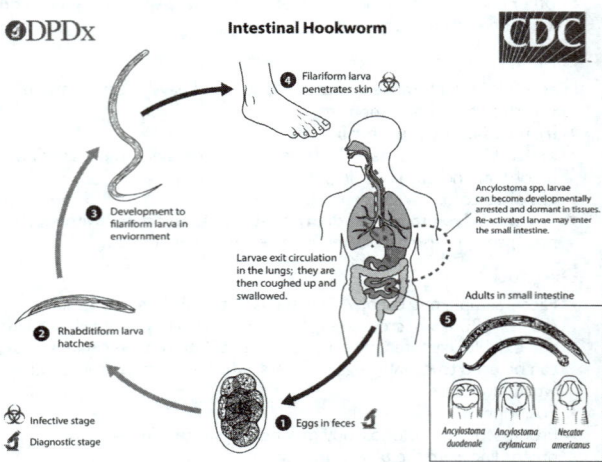

Fig. 11.3 Life cycle of hookworm. See CDC website for details.
℗ https://www.cdc.gov/dpdx/hookworm/index.html.

contaminated soil. Transmission may also occur from mother to child, either transplacentally or during breastfeeding.

Clinical features

- **Skin rash**—patients may present early in the disease with 'ground itch', intense pruritus, erythema, and a papular/vesicular rash at the site of larval penetration.
- **Pulmonary manifestations**—Löeffler's syndrome (respiratory symptoms, pulmonary infiltration, and eosinophilia; see Box 11.1) is caused by migration of larvae through the lungs.
- **Acute GI symptoms**—include nausea, vomiting, diarrhoea, and epigastric pain.
- **Chronic iron deficiency anaemia**—is the commonest manifestation due to attachment of the hookworm to the intestinal mucosa. The average daily blood loss is 0.15mL/day/worm and tends to present in conjunction with a lack of dietary iron or heavy menstrual bleeding.

Diagnosis

- Faecal sample microscopy for ova is diagnostic, but not very sensitive, so serial tests may be required. The ova are ovoid and thin-shelled, and measure 58×36 micrometres. The eggs of the two species are indistinguishable microscopically (see Fig. 11.1).
- Eosinophilia is usually mild and varies during the course of the disease.

Treatment

- Albendazole (400mg stat) or mebendazole (500mg stat) is the treatment of choice. Levamisole is an alternative.
- Iron replacement therapy for iron deficiency anaemia.
- Association with poverty, inadequate hygiene, and sanitation. Co-infection with other geohelminths is common.
- Hygiene measures, including safe drinking water properly cleaning and cooking food, handwashing, and wearing shoes.
- Regular anthelminthic therapy for at-risk populations (e.g. children, pregnant women, women of childbearing age in endemic countries). World Health Organization (WHO)—annual treatment where the prevalence is between 20% and 50%, and biannual treatment where the prevalence is over 50%.
- For mass community therapy in developing countries, a combination of ivermectin plus albendazole or mebendazole is used.
- Development of a human vaccine is under way.

Strongyloides stercoralis

Strongyloidiasis, caused by the helminth *S. stercoralis*, is estimated to infect between 30 and 100 million people worldwide. It can cause a spectrum of infection, from asymptomatic eosinophilia to life-threatening disease. It is also unusual in that it can cause autoinfection, resulting in chronic infections which can persist long after the initial exposure.

The parasite

S. stercoralis worms can survive as parasitic forms in humans or free-living forms in the soil. Adult worms inhabit the small intestine where the ♀ deposit ova. Eggs hatch in the mucosa, releasing larvae, and enter the intestinal lumen where they pass out in the faeces. The usual route of infection is through skin contact with contaminated soil. Humans can also be infected via the faeco-oral route. The larvae migrate through the bloodstream to the lungs where they migrate up the respiratory tree to be swallowed to the small intestine. Autoinfection may occur where larvae may penetrate the large intestinal mucosa and migrate to other organs, perpetuating the life cycle (see Fig. 11.4).

Epidemiology

S. stercoralis infection is found worldwide, though it is endemic in tropical and subtropical regions and occurs only sporadically in temperate climates, often in immigrants, travellers, military personnel, and institutions.

Clinical features

- Asymptomatic infection occurs in around 50% of patients.
- **Skin rash**—patients may present with a pruritic papulo-vesicular rash at the site of larval penetration (ground itch), usually on the patient's feet, but may occur anywhere in contact with soil, including the buttocks, thighs, or abdomen.
- **Larva currens**—is a pathognomonic manifestation of intradermal migration during autoinfection with strongyloidiasis. It is characterized

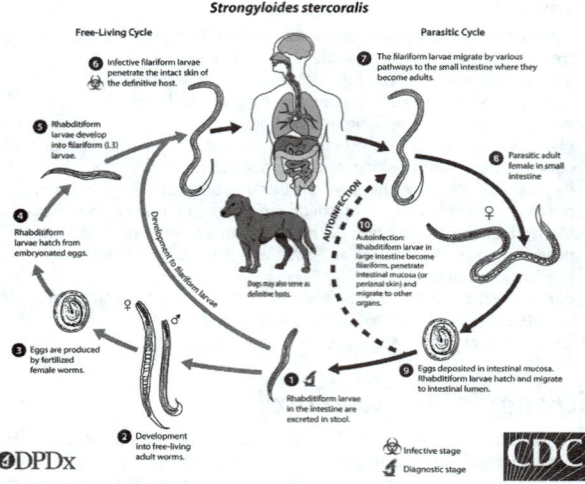

Fig. 11.4 Life cycle of *Strongyloides*. See CDC website for details.
🔗 https://www.cdc.gov/dpdx/strongyloidiasis/index.html.

by a serpiginous rash with associated urticaria which is intensely itchy and tends to occur on the trunk or buttocks or perianally. It can be differentiated from cutaneous larva migrans by its rapid migration (inches/hour), distribution (cutaneous larva migrans affects the site of inoculation such as the feet), and wider band of urticaria.

- **Pulmonary manifestations**—patients may present with Löeffler's syndrome (respiratory symptoms, pulmonary infiltration, and eosinophilia; see Box 11.1) caused by migration of larvae through the lungs.
- **Abdominal symptoms**—are common and include colicky abdominal pain, diarrhoea, passage of mucus, nausea, vomiting, weight loss, malabsorption, and protein-losing enteropathy.
- **Hyperinfection syndrome**—massive larval invasion may occur with autoinfection, particularly in immunocompromised hosts (e.g. patients with leukaemia, lymphoma, or lepromatous leprosy, those receiving corticosteroids or with HIV or human T-cell lymphotropic virus 1 (HTLV-1) infection). Other associations include malnutrition, cytotoxic therapy, poorly controlled diabetes, and anti-tumour necrosis factor (TNF) receptor therapy.
- Clinical features include shock, fever, severe abdominal pain, and vomiting and diarrhoea, with pulmonary infiltrates and haemoptysis. Widespread petechial purpuric eruptions can be seen. Complications can include meningitis (particularly with Gram-negative organisms such as *Escherichia coli*) or secondary septicaemia. Mortality is high.

Diagnosis

- **Faecal sample microscopy**—this is notoriously insensitive (<50%) for detection of rhabditiform larvae which are excreted intermittently. Please note that eggs are not seen in faecal samples.
- **FBC**—commonly demonstrates eosinophilia in acute infection but can be intermittent or absent in chronic disease.
- **Duodenal aspirates**, or the string test (Entero-Test)—sometimes used in patients with negative faecal samples
- **Molecular tests**—PCR tests to detect *Strongyloides* in faecal samples are not widely available.
- **Serology**—EIA tests are useful for diagnosing strongyloidiasis in immunocompetent individuals but may be negative in immunocompromised patients.
- **Endoscopy**—this is rarely required to diagnose strongyloidiasis but may be performed in the investigation of patients with GI symptoms. Larvae may be seen on mucosal biopsies.

Treatment

- Ivermectin is the treatment of choice for uncomplicated infections. It is usually administered as two single 200 micrograms/kg doses, either on three consecutive days or 1 week apart. Immigrants from areas of Africa that are endemic for loiasis should be screened for this prior to treatment, as ivermectin may precipitate encephalopathy in patients with high levels of microfilaraemia.
- Albendazole (400mg twice daily (bd) for 3 days, repeated 2 weeks later) is also effective against strongyloidiasis.
- Disseminated disease/hyperinfection syndrome—the optimal treatment is uncertain. Treatment is with ivermectin, alone or in combination with albendazole, until symptoms resolve and faecal sample tests have been negative for 2 weeks. For patients who cannot tolerate PO therapy, alternative (unlicensed) regimens include s/c vermectin or a parenteral veterinary formulation. In immunocompromised patients, reduction of immunosuppressive therapy is an important adjunct to anthelminthic therapy.

Prognosis

The prognosis of strongyloidiasis is good apart from in patients with disseminated infection/hyperinfection syndrome, which has a high case fatality rate.

Prevention

Prevention of disease is by wearing shoes and avoiding contact with infected soil in endemic areas.

Enterobius vermicularis (threadworm)

Infection with *E. vermicularis* (also known as threadworm or pinworm) is highly prevalent in both temperate and tropical climates. Pinworm infection is commonest in children and institutionalized populations.

The parasite

E. vermicularis is a small, white, thread-like worm, around 1cm long, which inhabits the caecum and ascending colon in humans; ♀ worms contain about 11 000 ova and live for 11–35 days. The gravid ♀ migrate at night to the perianal region where they deposit their eggs. The eggs embryonate within hours and are transferred from the perianal region to clothing, bedding, dust, and air. The commonest route of transmission, however, is via the patient's hands.

Epidemiology

The prevalence of pinworm is highest in children aged 5–10 years. Pinworm is primarily a family or institutional infection, with no particular socioeconomic associations. As the lifespan of the worm is relatively brief, and eggs can only survive out of the body for 20 days, long-standing infections must be due to continuous reinfection.

Clinical features

- Most infected patients are asymptomatic.
- Perianal/perineal pruritus (frequently intense and worse at night) and disturbed sleep are the commonest symptoms.
- Occasionally, migration of the worms may cause ectopic disease (e.g. appendicitis, salpingitis, oophoritis, vulvovaginitis, ulcerative bowel lesions, peritoneal inflammation).

Diagnosis

- A 'sellotape slide' is used to collect worms from the perianal region. Sellotape should be applied to the anus first thing in the morning.
- The ova are oval-shaped, but flattened on one side, and measure 56 × 27 micrometres (see Fig. 11.5).
- The number of examinations is correlated with the rate of detection. Perianal swabs are also used for this purpose. (e.g. 50% for a single examination, 90% for three examinations).
- All family members of an affected individual should be screened for infection.

Treatment

- Mebendazole (100mg stat, repeated at 2 weeks) is the treatment of choice. Albendazole and pyrantel pamoate are alternatives. All medications are given 2 weeks apart to prevent reinfection from adults born from eggs subsequent to the initial therapy.

Prevention

- Recurrence is common and highly likely due to reinfection rather than drug resistance, which is very uncommon. Strict hand hygiene measures

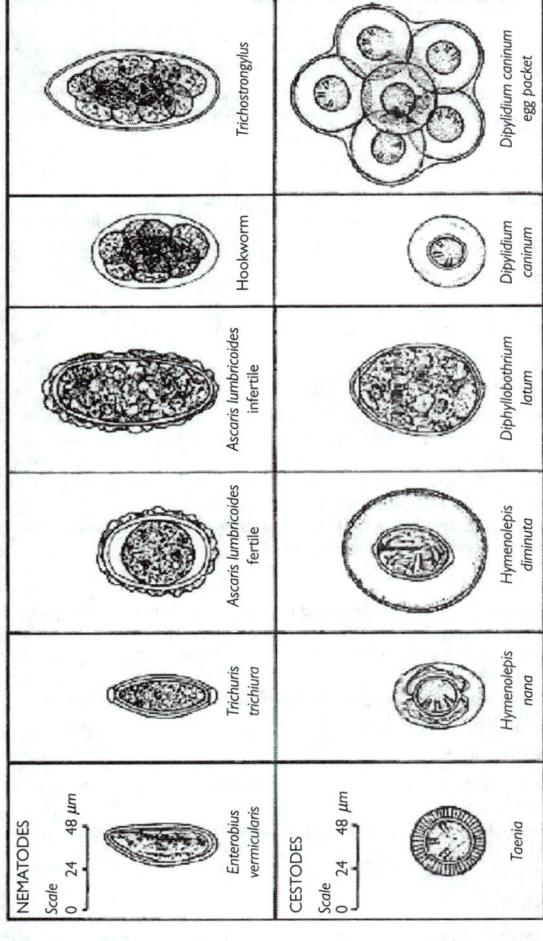

Fig. 11.5 Identification of helminth ova (nematodes and cestodes).
Reproduced from CDC. Image is in the Public Domain.

should be advised, and treatment of household contacts should be considered. Exclusion from schools is not necessary.

Cutaneous larva migrans

Cutaneous larva migrans (creeping eruption) is characterized by an erythematous, pruritic, serpiginous skin lesion. It is usually caused by the cat or dog hookworm *Ancylostoma braziliense* or *Ancylostoma caninum,* for which humans are an accidental host. Other worms that can cause similar findings include *Unicinaria stenocephala*, *Bunostomum phlebotomum*, and *Gnathostoma spinigerum*.

The parasite

The larvae infect dogs or cats by burrowing through the skin. The adults live in the host's intestine and shed eggs in the faeces, which develop into larvae in the sandy soil.

Epidemiology

Infections are commonest in warmer climates, especially in holidaymakers who visit tropical sandy beaches. Infection is commoner in children than in adults.

Clinical features

- Cutaneous disease—the larvae penetrate the skin of humans, usually via the feet, but occasionally via the abdomen, back, or thighs, causing tingling, itching, and vesicle formation. They then migrate through the skin, causing a characteristic raised, erythematous, pruritic, serpiginous track. In severe infections, many tracks may be seen.
- Pulmonary disease—haematogenous dissemination to the lungs is rare and may present with chronic cough.

Diagnosis

- The diagnosis is usually made based on the clinical history (walking or lying on sand) and characteristic serpiginous rash. The main differential diagnosis is larva currens (strongyloidiasis) (➔ see *Strongyloides stercoralis*, pp. 595–7).
- Skin biopsy may show an eosinophilic inflammatory infiltrate, but the migrating parasite is rarely found.

Treatment

- Cutaneous larva migrans is self-limiting, and the migrating larvae usually die within 6 weeks.
- Ivermectin 200 micrograms/kg stat or albendazole 400mg od stat is the treatment of choice.
- Antihistamines may be helpful for pruritus.

Prevention

- Travellers should be encouraged to wear footwear on the beach. Dogs have been excluded from the beach in some countries, such as Australia, but this is difficult to enforce.

Toxocariasis

Toxocariasis is caused by the dog roundworm *Toxocara canis* or, less commonly, the cat roundworm *Toxocara cati.*. Clinical presentations include visceral larva migrans (VLM) and ocular toxocariasis, or ocular larva migrans (OLM).

The parasite

The life cycle of *T. canis* and *T. cati* occurs in dogs and cats, respectively. Eggs are shed in the faeces of the definitive host, and humans become an accidental host by ingestion of eggs in faecally contaminated soil or encysted larvae in the tissues of infected hosts. Following ingestion, the eggs hatch and larvae penetrate the intestinal wall before migrating to other tissues (e.g. liver, heart, lungs, brain, eyes, and muscles].

Epidemiology

Toxocariasis has a worldwide distribution and is commonest in tropical rural populations. The prevalence of infection is unknown, but epidemiological surveys show seroprevalence rates of up to 80% in children in poorer communities in tropical regions. Most seropositive people are asymptomatic. VLM is commoner in children, whereas OLM may occur in children or adults.

Clinical features

- Most infections are asymptomatic, particularly in adults.
- VLM—presents with hepatitis and pneumonitis, as the larvae migrate through the organs. May also result in fever, anorexia, malaise, irritability, and pruritic urticarial rash. CNS manifestations are rare but include eosinophilic meningoencephalitis, space-occupying lesion, myelitis, and cerebral vasculitis.
- OLM—may present with uniocular visual impairment, with possible associated leukocoria, ocular pain, and strabismus, though symptoms range from asymptomatic routine finding on eye examination to monocular blindness. As larvae migrate through the eye, a granuloma is formed and can cause endophthalmitis, uveitis, or chorioretinitis, depending on its location.

Diagnosis

- The diagnosis is usually made clinically in a child with typical clinical features and a history of exposure to dogs (typically puppies).
- A definitive diagnosis is made by finding larvae in the tissues on histological examination.
- Laboratory abnormalities include eosinophilia, leucocytosis, and hypergammaglobulinaemia.
- Serological tests (e.g. EIA) may help to confirm the diagnosis (but may also be positive in asymptomatic patients). Serology may be falsely negative in OLM. PCR assays are not routinely available.
- Eosinophils may be detected in bronchoalveolar lavage (BAL) fluid and the CSF in patients with pulmonary and CNS involvement, respectively.
- Imaging studies—hepatic, pulmonary, and cerebral lesions may be detected by USS (liver lesions), CT, and MRI.

Treatment

- The optimal treatment is unknown, and patients with mild symptoms may recover without anthelminthic therapy.
- VLM—for patients with moderate/severe symptoms, treatment with albendazole (400mg bd for 5 days) may be warranted. In cases with pulmonary, cardiac, or CNS involvement, concomitant corticosteroids should be given.
- OLM—corticosteroids (topical or systemic) are the mainstay of management. Use of concurrent anthelminthic therapy is controversial.

Prevention

Prevention measures include good hygiene practices, routine deworming of pets, timely disposal of pet faeces, and handwashing after contact with pets.

Trichinella species

Trichinellosis (trichinosis) is a parasitic infection caused by nematodes of the genus *Trichinella*. Most infections are asymptomatic, but heavy exposure may cause fever, diarrhoea, periorbital oedema, and myositis.

The parasite

The genus *Trichinella* comprises eight species, seven of which cause human disease: *Trichinella spiralis* (commonest), *Trichinella nativa*, *Trichinella nelsoni*, *Trichinella britovi*, *Trichinella pseudospiralis*, *Trichinella murrelli*, and *Trichinella papuae*. The cysts are ingested in undercooked meat, and the larvae liberated by acid–pepsin digestion of the cysts in the stomach. The larvae invade the small bowel mucosa where they develop into adult worms. The ♀ adult worms may then release larvae, which disseminate in the bloodstream and seed skeletal muscles where they encyst.

Epidemiology

Trichinella spp. have a worldwide distribution and infect a wide range of animals (e.g. pigs, rats, horses, bears, foxes, wild boar, big cats). The prevalence of human infection is highest in China, Thailand, Argentina, Bolivia, Mexico, the former USSR, and Romania.

Clinical features

- The severity of infection correlates with the number of ingested larvae—the incubation period is 7–30 days.
- Mild infections may be subclinical.
- In heavy infections, two clinical stages occur. The intestinal stage occurs 1–7 days after ingestion and may be asymptomatic or present with abdominal pain, nausea, vomiting, and diarrhoea. This is followed by the muscle stage 2 weeks later when larvae disseminate and become encysted in the host muscle. This is associated with myositis, fever, weakness, and classically periorbital oedema. Respiratory involvement with a dry cough and secondary bacterial pneumonia has been described.

- Complications are uncommon but include cardiac (myocarditis and arrhythmias) and neurological (meningitis and encephalitis) manifestations.
- Renal involvement is very rare and only occurs in severe disease.

Diagnosis

- The diagnosis should be suspected in any patient who presents with fever, periorbital oedema, and myositis, particularly if there is a history of ingestion of undercooked meat.
- Routine laboratory tests may show eosinophilia raised ESR, elevated creatine kinase (CK), and lactate dehydrogenase (LDH) levels.
- Serology—antibodies are detectable 3 weeks after infection. Various assays may be used (e.g. EIA, immunofluorescence, indirect haemagglutination, precipitin, bentonite flocculation assays).
- Molecular tests—multiplex PCR assays have been developed for a number of *Trichinella* spp. but are not widely available.
- Muscle biopsy—is diagnostic but is not usually required, unless there is diagnostic uncertainty.

Treatment

- Most *Trichinella* infections are mild and self-limiting within 8 weeks and therefore do not require anthelminthic treatment. Most patients are treated symptomatically with bed rest and analgesics.
- Management of severe disease (CNS, cardiac, or pulmonary involvement) consists of anthelminthic therapy and corticosteroids. Albendazole (400mg bd for 8–14 days) or mebendazole (200–400mg three times daily (tds) for 3 days, then 400–500mg tds for 10 days) is the treatment of choice. Prednisolone should be administered concomitantly (30–60mg/day for 10–15 days).

Prevention

The most effective way to prevent trichinosis is to cook meat properly. Freezing at –15°C for 3 weeks or irradiation of packed meat will also kill larvae.

Dracunculus medinensis

Dracunculiasis (guinea worm infection) occurs after drinking water containing copepods infected with the larvae of *Dracunculus medinensis*.

The parasite

The life cycle begins with ingestion of the copepods (small crustaceans), which act as the intermediate host, from a contaminated water source. The larvae are released in the stomach, pass into the small intestine, penetrate the mucosa, and reach the retroperitoneum where they mature and mate. About a year later, the ♀ worm migrates to the subcutaneous tissues of the legs. The overlying skin ulcerates, and a portion of the worm protrudes. On contact with water, large numbers of larvae are released where they are ingested by copepods, completing the life cycle.

Epidemiology

D. medinensis is found in sub-Saharan Africa where water supplies are used for both drinking and bathing. Due to a successful WHO-led eradication programme, only 53 cases were reported worldwide in 2019. Seven nations have yet to be certified as dracunculiasis-free—Angola, Chad, Democratic Republic of Congo (DRC), Ethiopia, Mali, South Sudan, and Sudan.

Clinical features

- No symptoms are apparent until the worm reaches the skin surface.
- Initially a stinging papule develops on the lower leg.
- Some patients may develop generalized symptoms such as urticaria, nausea, vomiting, diarrhoea, and dyspnoea.
- Over the next few days, the lesion vesiculates and ruptures, and forms a painful ulcer. If the area is rinsed with water, a milky fluid containing larvae wells up.
- Discharge continues intermittently over weeks, and the worm is slowly absorbed or extruded, after which the ulcer heals.
- Multiple ulcers may occur, and secondary infection is common.

Diagnosis

The diagnosis is mainly clinical, but larvae may be seen on microscopic examination of the discharge fluid.

Treatment

- Treatment consists of removal of the worm by gradually rolling it around a small stick. Unerupted worms may be removed by minor surgery under local anaesthesia.
- Secondary bacterial infections should be treated with antibiotics.

Prevention

Boiling, chlorinating, or sieving drinking water, alongside educational programmes, have dramatically reduced the number of dracunculiasis cases.

Filariasis

Filariasis (also known as lymphatic filariasis to distinguish from subcutaneous filariasis caused by *Loa loa* and *Onchocerca volvulus*) is caused by three species of nematodes (roundworms) that primarily inhabit the lymphatic system: *Wuchereria bancrofti*, *Brugia malayi*, and *Brugia timori*.

The parasite

After the bite of an infected mosquito, larvae enter the lymphatics and lymph nodes where they mature into white, thread-like adult worms and can live for 5 years. The adults mate, and ♀ discharge microfilariae into the bloodstream. Microfilariae circulating in the blood show periodicity, with peak microfilaraemia classically at around midnight. In the South Pacific, the peak is less pronounced and may occur during the day.

Epidemiology

It is estimated that 120 million people are infected with these parasites.
- *W. bancrofti* occurs throughout the tropics and subtropics, and is responsible for at least 90% of infections worldwide.
- *B. malayi* occurs mainly in South East Asia.
- *B. timori* is restricted to Timor in Indonesia.

Humans are the only host for *W. bancrofti*, but *B. malayi* has been found in felines and primates. Only a small proportion of people who are bitten by infected mosquitoes develop clinical disease.

Clinical features

- Most patients are asymptomatic, despite microfilaraemia.
- Acute infection may present with acute adenolymphangitis (ADL), an inflamed lymph node with surrounding lymphangitis, or acute dermatolymphangioadenitis (DLA) which can resemble cellulitis and can be associated with lymphangitis and oedema. Isolated filarial fever and tropical eosinophilia can also be presenting features.
- Chronic manifestations include lymphoedema (which may progress to elephantiasis) and hydrocele (which may be unilateral or bilateral).
- Renal involvement with discharge of lymph into the renal pelvis causes chyluria, which can result in anaemia and hypoproteinaemia.

Diagnosis

- Blood smear—a blood sample should be taken between 10 p.m. and 2 a.m. (apart from if the patient is from the South Pacific when they may be taken in the daytime), and stained with Giemsa or Wright's stain. Microfilariae are occasionally seen in hydrocele fluid, chylous urine, or lymph node aspirates.
- Circulating filarial antigen (CFA) assays are available for *W. bancrofti* infections and can be performed at any time of the day. These tests have high sensitivity and specificity, and can be performed as a point-of-care test.
- Serological tests may be positive but do not distinguish current from past infection. A *Brugia malayi*-specific IgG4 has been developed.
- Molecular tests—species-specific PCR tests are only available in the research setting.
- Ultrasonography of lymphatic vessels in the spermatic cord may show motile adult worms.
- Evaluation for co-infection with onchocerciasis and loiasis should occur prior to treatment in areas where these diseases are endemic. Severe inflammatory reactions may occur with diethylcarbamazine (DEC) use and co-infection with onchocerciasis in particular

Treatment

- DEC (❷ see Diethylcarbamazine, p.134) (6mg/kg/day for 12 days) is the treatment of choice for lymphatic filariasis. Side effects: fever, headache, nausea, arthralgia.
- Doxycycline (200mg/day for 4–6 weeks) has macrofilaricidal activity and reduces pathology in mild to moderate disease.

- Patients with concomitant infection with onchocerciasis (➔ see *Onchocerca volvulus*, pp. 607–9) should be treated with ivermectin (150 micrograms/kg stat), followed by standard treatment for filariasis.
- Patients with concomitant loiasis should be managed according to the circulating concentration of *L. loa* microfilariae (➔ see *Loa loa*, pp. 606–7).
- Mass drug treatment of populations in endemic areas use yearly single doses of ivermectin (200 micrograms/kg) in conjunction with DEC (6mg/kg), and albendazole (400mg) in countries without endemic onchocerciasis. In areas with endemic onchocerciasis, single doses of albendazole (400mg) and ivermectin (200 micrograms/kg) are used.

Prevention

Mass drug administration to reduce the reservoir of microfilariae has been the cornerstone of prevention. Vector control using insecticide-treated bed nets has been useful in areas where anopheline mosquitoes transmit *W. bancrofti*. Travellers to endemic areas should be advised to avoid mosquito bites (protective clothing, insect repellent).

Loa loa

Loiasis is caused by *L. loa* and characterized by transient subcutaneous swellings (Calabar swellings). Occasionally, worms can migrate through the subconjunctivae, causing conjunctivitis.

The parasite

The white, thread-like worms measure 30–70 × 0.3mm and migrate through connective tissues. The microfilariae measure 300 × 8 micrometres and appear in the blood during the day.

Epidemiology

L. loa is endemic in West and Central Africa. It is transmitted to humans by the bite of the *Chrysops* fly (tabanid fly, horse or deer fly) that inhabits tropical forests in the region.

Clinical features

- Many patients are asymptomatic but often have eosinophilia.
- The characteristic feature is transient, oedematous swellings (Calabar swellings), which are caused by worms migrating through the subcutaneous tissues. They are usually preceded by localized pain and itching, are solitary and commonly found around joints, and may last for days to weeks.
- Occasionally, a worm may migrate across the subconjunctivae, causing conjunctivitis.
- Other complications may include proteinuria and haematuria, cardiomyopathy, retinopathy, encephalopathy, peripheral neuropathy, arthritis, lymphadenitis, and pleural effusions.

Diagnosis

- The diagnosis is often clinical, based on finding typical clinical features in a patient from West or Central Africa.

- Detection of organisms—the diagnosis is confirmed by demonstrating characteristically sheathed microfilariae in subcutaneous tissues, the eyes, or a peripheral blood smear taken between 10 a.m. and 2 p.m. Quantification in microfilariae per millilitre (Mf/mL) is then required to direct treatment (see below).
- Serology—may be helpful in travellers and expatriates, but not in residents of endemic areas.
- Other tests—a quantitative real-time PCR-based assay has been developed but is not widely available. Tests that detect circulating *L. loa* antigens are under development.

Treatment

- DEC is the treatment of choice but is contraindicated in those with high microfilaraemia loads (risk of encephalopathy) and those with O. *volvulus* co-infection (risk of severe eye lesions thus must be treated first). Seek expert advice. See Anthelmintic drugs, pp. 133–6.
- Those with levels <2000mf/ml can be treated with DEC. Those with higher levels can be pre-treated with albendazole to reduce acute symptoms and microfilaraemia prior to definitive treatment with DEC.
- Steroids and antihistamines can be used around the initiation of therapy to reduce the possibility of a transient increase in symptoms.
- Albendazole has macrofilaricidal activity, causing sterilization or death of adult worms; it has no significant effect on microfilariae.
- Ivermectin is no longer a preferred treatment. It has rapid microfilaricidal activity and can precipitate encephalitis and/or shock, particularly in patients with high levels of microfilaraemia.

Prevention

- Avoid insect bites (protective clothing, insect repellent) in endemic areas.
- Mass treatment with DEC or ivermectin interrupts transmission in endemic areas.
- Temporary visitors to endemic areas may take prophylactic DEC (300mg weekly).

Further reading

Centers for Disease Control and Prevention (2020). *Loiasis*. Available at: ⅋ https://www.cdc.gov/parasites/loiasis/health_professionals/index.html#tx

Onchocerca volvulus

Onchocerciasis (river blindness) is caused by the nematode *O. volvulus* and characterized by blindness and skin disease.

The parasite

O. volvulus is transmitted to humans by the *Simulium* blackfly, which lives in tropical forested regions. After a bite, the larvae penetrate the skin and migrate into connective tissues where they develop into filiform adults. The worms are often found tangled in nodules of subcutaneous tissue. Each ♀ can live for around 12 years and produce large numbers of microfilariae that migrate through the skin and connective tissues *Simulium* flies then take up microfilariae during blood meals, completing the life cycle.

Epidemiology

Onchocerciasis is the second leading infectious cause of blindness world-wide. It is estimated that 20.9 million people are infected, with 1.15 million with associated visual loss. It occurs in West, Central, and East Africa, with scattered foci in Central and South America.

Clinical features

- Subcutaneous nodules—adult worms form fibrous nodules (onchocercomata), classically over bony prominences, from where they produce microfilariae which cause the other manifestations.
- Onchocercal skin disease—generalized itching is often the first symptom, which may be associated with a maculopapular rash. This may progress to pruritic inflammatory papules, nodules, and plaques. The skin may become hyperpigmented and, over time, may become lichenified, atrophied, and depigmented. Lymphadenopathy may develop, particularly in the inguinal region. Fibrosis of lymph nodes may result in lymphatic obstruction and elephantiasis.
- Ocular onchocerciasis—this may initially present with conjunctivitis, lacrimation, and itching. Prolonged infection can cause significant pathology to various tissues, including punctate keratitis, sclerosing keratitis, uveitis, chorioretinitis, and optic atrophy. All these features can cause eventual blindness as early as the age of 20 years.

Diagnosis

- Bloodless skin snips—detection of microfilariae is diagnostic, but skin snips may be negative in early disease. A minimum of two, and ideally six, snips should be taken and incubated in saline for 24h prior to examination, especially if microfilariae are not seen initially.
- Slit-lamp examination—this may demonstrate microfilariae in the anterior chamber of the eye.
- Antigen tests—a luciferase immunoprecipation system (LIPS) assay, which detects four onchocerca antigens, has shown high sensitivity and could potentially be used as a point-of-care diagnostic method.
- Serology—serological tests have been developed to antigen OV16, though they are not commercially available.
- Molecular tests—highly sensitive PCR assays have been developed but are not routinely available.
- Imaging—USS may identify adult worms within subcutaneous nodules.
- Mazotti test—this consists of a 50mg PO dose of DEC (➔ see Anthelmintic drugs, pp. 133–6), which results in microfilarial death and exacerbation of symptoms. It is now rarely used, given the alternative diagnostic methods. It is contraindicated in heavily infected individuals because of the risk of severe reactions.
- Patch test—a topical preparation of DEC can be administered to the skin to assess for a local skin reaction. It is a useful alternative to skin snips in low-prevalence areas, as it is cheap, non-invasive, and more sensitive than skin snips.

Treatment

- Ivermectin (➔ see Anthelmintic drugs, pp. 133–6) is the treatment of choice—it kills microfilariae and has some effect on adult worms (macrofilariae). Side effects include fever, pruritus, headache, and arthralgia. A single dose of ivermectin annually has been shown to be effective for population-based treatment. It should be used with caution where *L. loa* is endemic, as it can cause serious systemic side effects in patients with co-infection.

- Doxycycline (⮕ see Tetracyclines, pp. 61–3) is active against *Wolbachia*, the endosymbiotic bacteria within *O. volvulus*, and thus is macrofilaricidal. Doxycycline (100mg/day for 6 weeks), followed by a single dose of ivermectin (150 micrograms/kg stat), has been shown to be effective. Rifampicin and azithromycin also have activity against *Wolbachia*.
- Other agents—moxidectin is a veterinary deworming agent, which was approved for human use by the Food and Drug Administration (FDA) in 2018. It has been shown to give a more sustained reduction in microfilarial load, compared to ivermectin.

Prevention

- The Expanded Special Project for Elimination of Neglected Tropical Diseases (ESPEN) includes onchocerciasis elimination. This has significantly reduced onchocerca transmission worldwide and predominantly relies on regular ivermectin administration and post-treatment surveillance.
- Vector control has now become secondary to population treatment.

Angiostrongyliasis

The nematode parasite *Angiostrongylus* have two species that can rarely affect humans: *Angiostrongylus costaricensis* which causes abdominal angiostrongyliasis, and *Angiostrongylus cantonensis* which causes neural angiostrongyliasis, a cause of eosinophilic meningitis (⮕ see Chronic meningitis, pp. 770–2). The definitive host is the rat where the parasite lives in the intestine (*A. costaricensis*) or lungs (*A. cantonensis*). Eggs are excreted in the faeces, before being ingested by a slug intermediate where a similar cycle occurs. Humans may be infected by accidental ingestion of foods contaminated by larvae or slugs.

Abdominal angiostrongyliasis

Epidemiology
A. cantonensis infection usually affects children in Central and South America, and rarely Africa.

Clinical features
Patients usually complain of abdominal pain, fever, and vomiting. Physical findings include fever, abdominal tenderness, and a right lower quadrant mass (50%).

Diagnosis
The syndrome resembles appendicitis, apart from the presence of eosinophilia. Radiological features are non-specific. Serology and PCR techniques are not routinely available.

Treatment

Most patients undergo laparotomy and removal of infected tissue. Use of anthelminthic therapy is relatively controversial, though PO mebendazole and albendazole have been used successfully.

Anisakiasis

Anisakid nematodes are parasites of marine mammals (e.g. dolphins, seals, whales). *Anisakis simplex* (herring worm) is the most commonly implicated organism, which occurs in ocean fish. The eggs are excreted in the faeces and hatch as free-swimming larvae that are ingested by crustaceans and then by fish and squid. Humans are accidental hosts following ingestion of raw or poorly cooked seafood.

Epidemiology

Infection occurs most frequently in countries where raw fish is consumed (e.g. Japan, the Netherlands), though cases have been seen worldwide.

Clinical features

Symptoms usually occur a few hours after ingestion and are caused by worms attempting to burrow through the GI mucosa. The anisakids die in the lumen, causing a local inflammatory reaction. Extraintestinal manifestations are possible, but rare. Gastric anisakiasis is characterized by abdominal pain, nausea, and vomiting. Small intestinal involvement is characterized by lower abdominal pain and signs of obstruction. Symptoms may become chronic, with the development of abdominal masses. Acute allergic symptoms (e.g. urticaria, anaphylaxis) may also occur with anisakiasis, with or without abdominal symptoms.

Diagnosis

The diagnosis should be suspected in any patient with a history of ingestion of raw fish and abdominal symptoms. Leucocytosis or eosinophilia may be seen. Gastric anisakiasis is confirmed by upper GI endoscopy and histological examination of biopsy specimens. Intestinal anisakiasis is confirmed by radiological features of obstruction and detection of eosinophils in aspirated ascites, with a compatible history. Serological tests are not routinely available.

Treatment

Symptoms usually improve without specific therapy but may resolve more quickly if gastric worms are removed by endoscopy. Occasionally, removal of an intestinal mass may be required.

Prevention

Anisakiasis may be prevented by cooking or freezing fish for 24h prior to ingestion.

Capillariasis

Capillaria philippinensis larvae are found in freshwater fish and are known to be infectious to humans and birds. After ingestion of raw fish, the larvae invade the jejunum and ileum, and adult ♀ worms produce both eggs and larvae. Eggs may hatch within the intestine, leading to a hyperinfection syndrome.

Epidemiology

Infections are rare and usually occur in the context of raw fish consumption in South East Asia such as the Philippines and Thailand.

Clinical features

These are consistent with malabsorption and protein-losing enteropathy, and include abdominal pain, vomiting, diarrhoea, abdominal distension, borborygmi, malaise, weight loss, and peripheral oedema.

Diagnosis

This is confirmed by detecting ova or larvae in the faecal sample or via biopsy of the small intestine. There are no serological tests.

Treatment

Treatment is with mebendazole or albendazole. Mortality rates of up to 30% have been reported in untreated patients.

Cestodes

Human cestode (tapeworm) infections occur in one of two forms: mature tapeworms residing in the gut, or larval cysts in tissues. The form that the infection takes depends on the species. Medically important cestodes are summarized in Table 11.2.

Parasite structure

Parasitic cestodes are flatworms (platyhelminths). The worms consist of several parts: a head (scolex, which has suckers and sometimes hooks), a short neck, and a strobila (a segmented tail made of proglottids). The proglottid has both ♂ and ♀ sexual organs, and is responsible for egg production. They become gravid and eventually break free of the tapeworm, releasing eggs in the faeces or outside the body.

Parasite life cycle

Cestodes divide their life cycle between two animal hosts: the definitive carnivorous host and the intermediate herbivorous/omnivorous host. Mature tapeworms reside in the intestinal tract of the definitive host and shed eggs into the faeces. The eggs may be embryonated (can immediately infect the intermediate host) or non-embryonated (require development outside the body). The intermediate host is infected by ingestion of eggs that hatch in the intestine, releasing an oncosphere. This penetrates the gut mucosa and spreads through the circulation to the tissues where it forms a larval cyst. The life cycle is completed when the carnivorous host ingests the cyst-infected tissues of the intermediate host.

Table 11.2 Medically important cestodes

Type of cestode	Disease	Species
Intestinal	Tapeworm	*Taenia saginata*
		Taenia solium
		Diphyllobothrium spp. (*Diphyllobothrium latum, Diphyllobothrium nihonkaiense, Diphyllobothrium dendriticum, Diphyllobothrium stemmacephalum, Diphyllobothrium balaenopterae*)
		Hymenolepis nana
Invasive	Cysticercosis, echinococcosis	*Taenia solium*
		Echinococcus spp. (*Echinococcus granulosus, Echinococcus multilocularis, Echinococcus vogeli, Echinococcus oligarthrus*)

Taenia saginata (beef tapeworm)

- The parasite—adult worms are long (up to 10m in length) and contain >1000 proglottids, each capable of producing thousands of eggs.
- Epidemiology—transmitted to humans (who are the definitive host) by ingestion of larval cysts in rare or undercooked meat from infected cattle (who are the intermediate host).
- Common in cattle-breeding areas of the world, such as Central and Eastern Asia and Central and Eastern Africa, where cattle-rearing areas may be contaminated with human faeces and the prevalence of infection may be >10%. Areas of lower prevalence (<1%) include Europe, South East Asia, and Central America.
- Clinical features—patients are usually asymptomatic, but a minority complain of nausea, anorexia, and abdominal pain. The proglottids are motile and may be seen on the perineum or clothing.
- Diagnosis is confirmed by examination of proglottids (with 15–20 lateral uterine branches). The eggs are morphologically indistinguishable from those of *Taenia solium* (see Fig. 11.1).
- Treatment is with praziquantel (5–10mg/kg) or niclosamide (2g) PO stat. Faecal samples should be re-examined at 1 and 3 months to ensure clearance.

Taenia solium (pork tapeworm)

- The parasite—*T. solium* tapeworms may live for 10–20 years and grow up to 8m in length.
- Epidemiology—humans can be definitive or intermediate hosts for *T. solium*. Individuals who ingest larval cysts in raw or undercooked pork acquire pork tapeworm as the definitive host in a similar way to *Taenia saginata*. However, when humans ingest proglottids, onchospheres hatch in the stomach and then disseminate via the bloodstream and encyst in various organs (➔ Cysticercosis, pp. 613–14).
- *T. solium* infection is endemic in sub-Saharan Africa, Central and South America, and South East Asia, including the Philippines.
- Clinical features—most patients are asymptomatic, unless autoinfection with parasite eggs occurs.
- Diagnosis—infection is readily diagnosed by detection of eggs in the faeces (morphologically indistinguishable from those of *T. saginata*). Definitive diagnosis is by examination of the proglottids—with 7–13 lateral uterine branches) (see Fig. 11.6).
- Treatment—praziquantel (5–10mg/kg) or niclosamide (2g) PO stat. Faeces should be re-examined at 1 and 3 months to ensure clearance.

Cysticercosis

- The parasite—cysticercosis is an infection with proglottids or eggs of the cestode *T. solium* (➔ see *Taenia solium* (pork tapeworm), p. 613). Ingested eggs develop into oncospheres in the stomach, which

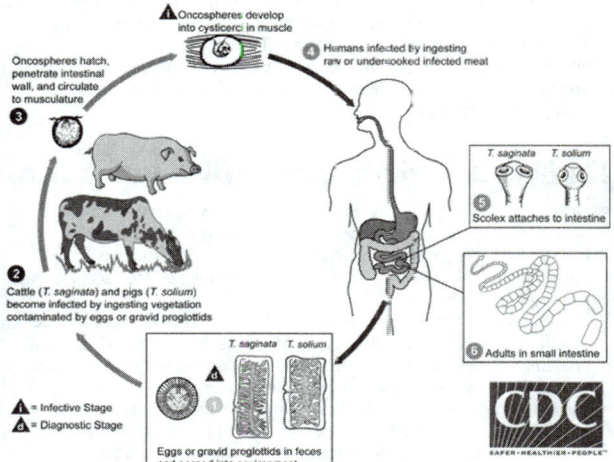

Fig. 11.6 Life cycle of *Taenia* spp. See CDC website for details. ➔ https://www.cdc.gov/dpdx/taeniasis/index.html

disseminate via the circulation to various sites—classically striated muscle, the CNS, the heart, and eye tissue.

- Epidemiology—infection is acquired by consumption of *T. solium* eggs and occurs wherever *T. solium* infection is prevalent (➔ see *Taenia solium* (pork tapeworm), p. 613). The cumulative risk of infection increases with age, the frequency of pork consumption, and poor household hygiene.
- Clinical features—infected individuals may harbour multiple cysts throughout the body but are often asymptomatic. Occasionally, patients may develop painless subcutaneous nodules. Symptoms may develop because of local inflammation at the site of infection, usually as cysts degenerate. Serious disease is rare but occurs with cardiac or CNS involvement (neurocysticercosis; ➔ see Neurocysticercosis, pp. 776–7). The latter may present with focal symptoms, seizures, chronic meningitis, or spinal cord compression. Neurocysticercosis is the commonest cause of seizures in Central America. Racemose cysticercosis is an aggressive form of basilar neurocysticercosis, resulting in coma and death.
- Diagnosis—asymptomatic patients may be diagnosed incidentally by detection of calcified cysts on plain radiographs. Extraneural and extraocular cysticercosis very rarely requires specific therapy, and cysts usually regress over time. The conduction system of the heart is an exception, where treatment may be considered.
- Neurocysticercosis may be diagnosed by CT or MRI scan, which show multiple enhancing and non-enhancing unilocular cysts. Diagnosis may be supported by a positive EIA, indicating prior exposure to *T. solium* antigens, but patients infected with other helminths may have cross-reactive antibodies. Immunoblotting techniques using purified glycoprotein from cyst fluid may be more sensitive/specific.
- Treatment may involve a combination of antiparasitics (usually albendazole or praziquantel), corticosteroids, anti-epileptic medication, and neurosurgical intervention. This is often discussed at a national multidisciplinary team meeting.

Diphyllobothrium species (fish tapeworm)

- *Diphyllobothrium* spp. are a family of cestodes which have marine life cycles, and transmission occurs by ingestion of undercooked freshwater fish containing cysts. *Diphyllobothrium latum* is the commonest pathogen, but increasingly other species are recognized as causing human infection.
- Epidemiology—areas of endemic infection (>2% prevalence) include Siberia, Scandinavia and other Baltic countries, North America, Japan, and Chile where there is stable zoonotic transmission through other animal hosts (e.g. seals, cats, bears, foxes, wolves).
- Clinical features—infection is usually asymptomatic, but patients may report weakness, dizziness, salt cravings, diarrhoea, or intermittent abdominal discomfort. Prolonged/heavy infection may lead to megaloblastic anaemia caused by vitamin B_{12} deficiency ± folate deficiency.

- Diagnosis—faecal sample examination shows operculated eggs (45–65 micrometres). Recovery of proglottids (with a characteristic central uterus) also confirms the diagnosis.
- Treatment—is with praziquantel (5–10mg/kg) or niclosamide (2g) PO stat. Mild vitamin B_{12} deficiency resolves with eradication of the tapeworm; severe deficiency requires parenteral treatment.

Hymenolepis nana (dwarf tapeworm)

- The parasite—*Hymenolepis nana* is the only tapeworm that can be transmitted directly from human to human, as the egg is immediately infectious after excretion, without an intermediate host. Adult tapeworms measure 15–50mm. Some estimate it to be the commonest cestode infection worldwide.
- Epidemiology—areas of endemic infection (up to 26%) include Asia, southern and eastern Europe, Central and South America, and Africa. Infection is commoner in children and institutionalized patients.
- Clinical features—heavy infection may be associated with abdominal cramps, nausea, diarrhoea, and dizziness.
- Diagnosis—is made by identification of eggs (30–47 micrometres, with a characteristic double membrane) in the faecal sample (see Fig. 11.5.
- Treatment—is with praziquantel (25mg/kg PO stat) or niclosamide (2g PO daily for 1 week).

Echinococcosis (hydatid disease)

- The parasite—the tapeworms *Echinococcus* spp. inadvertently infect humans, causing visceral cysts. *Echinococcus granulosus* causes cystic echinococcosis, and *Echinococcus multilocularis* causes alveolar echinococcosis. Two other species *Echinococcus vogeli* and *Echinococcus oligarthrus* rarely cause polycystic echinococcosis. The definitive host for *E. granulosus* are dogs and other canids such as wolves, whereas *E. multilocularis* has a number of potential definitive hosts, including foxes, dogs, and cats.
- Life cycle—adult echinococcosis species live in the gut of the definitive carnivorous host. Gravid proglottids are released and excreted in the faeces where they are ingested by the intermediate host (sheep, cattle, pigs, and other herbivores in the case of *E. granulosus*, and small rodents in the case of *E. multilocularis*). After ingestion, embryonated eggs hatch and release oncospheres that penetrate the intestinal wall and migrate to various organs where they form a thick-walled hydatid cyst. The definitive host ingests the cysts containing protoscoleces, which eventually develop into adult stages in the gut, completing the life cycle. Humans are accidental hosts but may become infected after ingestion of proglottids and eventual hydatid cyst formation in a similar way to intermediate hosts.
- Epidemiology—*E. granulosus* is prevalent in South America, some sub-Saharan African countries, China, the former Soviet Union, the Middle East, and Southern and Eastern Europe (with cases also reported in northern Wales). *E. multilocularis* is found in Central Europe, much of

Russia, the Central Asian republics, north-eastern, north-western, and western China, the north-western portion of Canada, and Western Alaska.

- Risk factors—aside from geographical risk factors, livestock ownership (particularly sheep in the case of *E. granulosus*), agricultural work, and poor hygienic living conditions are associated with echinococcosis.
- Clinical features—the hydatid cysts of *E. granulosus* usually affect the liver (50–70%) or lungs (20–30%), but may affect any organ of the body (e.g. heart, kidneys, bones, CNS, eyes). They are often asymptomatic and found incidentally on radiological imaging. Symptoms may occur as a result of expansion or rupture into adjacent organs. Cyst rupture may cause a severe allergic reaction or seeding to distant organs. Alveolar cyst disease caused by *E. multilocularis* may be asymptomatic or present with malaise, weight loss, and right upper quadrant pain. Complications include biliary disease, portal hypertension, and Budd–Chiari syndrome. Extrahepatic disease is rare.
- Diagnosis—infection is detected by radiological imaging (USS, CT, or MRI); may be confirmed serologically by EIA or western blot assay. This confirms exposure to the parasite and is more sensitive for *E. multilocularis* than for *E. granulosus* infections. Biopsy is usually only considered in diagnostic uncertainty, due to concern of seeding along the biopsy tract.
- Treatment—asymptomatic cysts may be monitored, whereas symptomatic cysts should be treated. The optimal treatment should be discussed by an experienced multidisciplinary team. Options include surgical resection of the whole cyst 30 minutes after instillation of a cysticidal agent (e.g. 30% saline, iodophor, or 95% ethanol). Perioperative anthelminthic agents (e.g. albendazole 400mg bd or mebendazole 40–50mg/kg/day in three divided doses) may be given, and care must be taken to prevent cyst rupture or spillage during surgery. The PAIR procedure (puncture, aspiration, injection, and re-aspiration) is increasingly used as an alternative to surgery. For inoperable cysts, medical therapy improves symptoms (55–79%), although cure rates are low (29%). In patients treated surgically, an antiparasitic agent, preferably albendazole, is continued for at least 2 years. In inoperable patients, treatment is considered for years, and possibly lifelong.

Trematodes (flukes)

Flukes are parasitic worms of the class *Trematoda*. They are usually oval-shaped and vary in length (from 1mm to several centimetres). Structurally, they have an oral sucker, a ventral sucker (usually), a blind bifurcate intestinal tract, and prominent reproductive organs. The human flukes belong to the digenetic group, in which sexual reproduction is followed by asexual multiplication. Most human parasites are hermaphrodites, except *Schistosoma* spp. Medically important trematodes are summarized in Table 11.3. Morphology of the ova directs identification (Fig. 11.7).

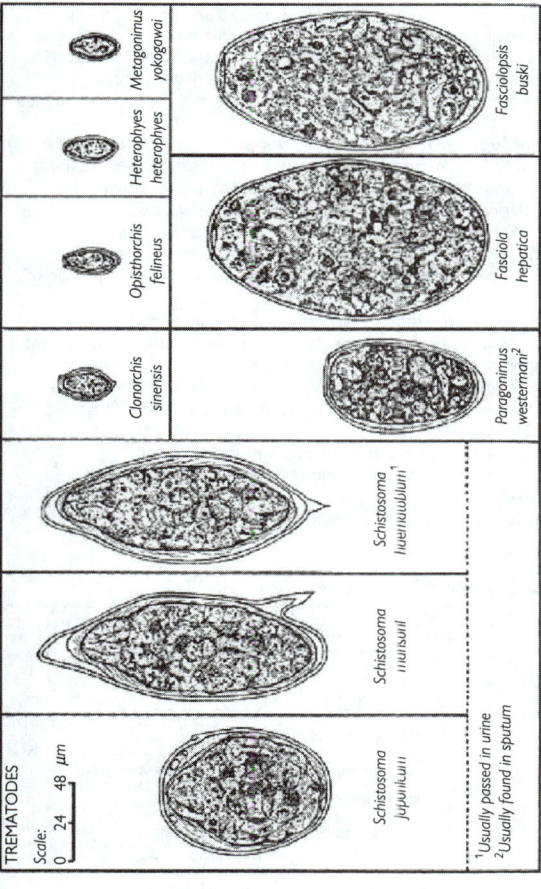

Fig. 11.7 Identification of trematode eggs.
Reproduced from CDC/ Dr. Mae Melvin. Public Health Image Library (adapted from Melvin, Brook, and Sadun, 1959). Image is in the Public Domain.

Schistosoma species

- Humans are the principal host of the five *Schistosoma* spp. (see Table 11.3). Adult worms live in the venous plexus of the urinary bladder (*Schistosoma haematobium*) or the portal venous system (*Schistosoma mansoni*, *Schistosoma japonicum*) where they mate and shed their eggs. Eggs are passed out in the urine or faeces and hatch in fresh water, releasing miracidia that enter the snail (intermediate host). The miracidia multiply asexually in the snail and eventually release cercariae. These infective forms penetrate human skin and migrate through the lungs and the liver, before passing to their preferred venous system (see Fig. 11.8).
- **Epidemiology**—240 million people worldwide are estimated to be infected with *Schistosoma* spp. Each species has a specific geographical location: *S. haematobium* (Africa, the Middle East), *S. mansoni* (Arabia, Africa, South America, the Caribbean), *S. japonicum* (the Far East), *Schistosoma mekongi* (South East Asia), and *Schistosoma intercalatum* (West and Central Africa). Two factors are responsible for endemicity—the presence of the snail vector and contamination of fresh water by human waste.
- **Pathogenesis**—the disease syndromes that characterize schistosomiasis coincide with the three stages of parasite development:
  - cercariae penetrate the skin to cause a rash;
  - weeks following primary infection, the mature worms deposit their eggs; this may be accompanied by acute schistosomiasis (Katayama fever);
  - production of large numbers of eggs results in chronic granulomatous inflammation and fibrosis of the urinary tract or portal venous system.
- **Clinical features** of schistosomiasis include:

Table 11.3 Medically important trematodes

Type of fluke	Disease	Species
Blood	Schistosomiasis	*Schistosoma haematobium*
		Schistosoma japonicum
		Schistosoma mansoni
		Schistosoma mekongi
		Schistosoma intercalatum
Liver	Clonorchiasis	*Clonorchis sinensis*
	Opisthorchiasis	*Opisthorcis felineus*
		Opisthorcis viverrini
	Fascioliasis	*Fasciola hepatica*
Intestine	Fasciolopsiasis	*Fasciolopsis buski*
	Heterophyiasis	*Heterophyes heterophyes*
Lung	Paragonimiasis	*Paragonimus westermani*

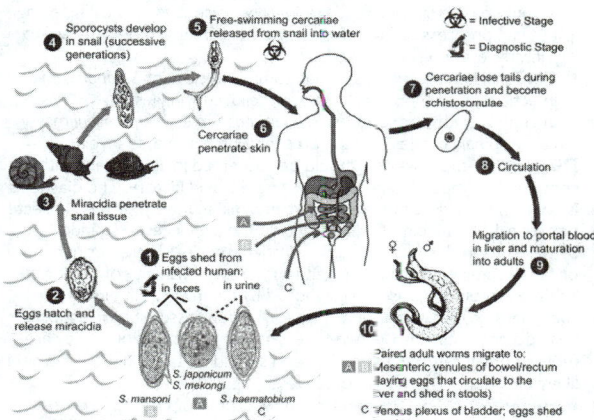

Fig. 11.8 The life cycle of flatworms of the genus *Schistosoma*, the causal agents of the parasitic disease schistosomiasis.

Reproduced from CDC/ Alexander J. da Silva, PhD; Melanie Moser. Public Health Image Library. Image is in the Public Domain.

- swimmer's itch—a papular, pruritic dermatitis that occasionally occurs 24h after penetration of the skin by cercariae. It appears to be a sensitization phenomenon, as it rarely occurs on primary exposure;
- acute schistosomiasis or Katayama fever—occurs 4–8 weeks after infection and is characterized by fever, chills, sweating, headache, cough, hepatosplenomegaly, and lymphadenopathy. Peripheral eosinophilia is common. Symptoms usually resolve within a few weeks, but rarely death may occur;
- chronic schistosomiasis—generally occurs in patients with heavy infestation;
- intestinal schistosomiasis, caused by *S. mansoni*, *S. japonicum*, *S. intercalatum*, or *S. mekongi*, may present with fatigue, colicky abdominal pain, diarrhoea, dysentery, chronic granulomatous bowel lesions, mucosal ulceration, or anaemia;
- hepatic schistosomiasis—also caused by *S. mansoni*, *S. japonicum*, *S. intercalatum*, or *S. mekongi*; may present with hepatomegaly, portal hypertension, splenomegaly, oesophageal varices, or decompensated liver disease;
- urinary schistosomiasis—caused by *S. haematobium*, causes granulomatous inflammation in the bladder and ureters. Patients may complain of dysuria and terminal haematuria. Haematospermia is common. Progression of disease may cause urinary obstruction with hydronephrosis and hydroureter;

- female genital schistosomiasis (FGS) is increasingly recognized as a manifestation of *S. haematobium* infiltration and subsequent granuloma formation. Tends to initially present as cervical bleeding but can progress to infertility and pelvic pain. It can be resistant to therapy, especially if delayed.
- CNS schistosomiasis—rare, but complicates 3% of *S. japonicum* infections. It may present with a space-occupying lesion, encephalopathy, or seizures. *S. haematobium* and *S. mansoni* may cause spinal cord lesions and present with transverse myelitis.
- **Diagnosis**—the diagnosis should be suspected in any patient with compatible symptoms and an appropriate travel history. The diagnosis is confirmed by detection of eggs in a terminal urine specimen collected between 12 and 2 p.m. (*S. haematobium*), or in faeces examined by the Kato thick smear procedure (other species). Three urinary or faecal samples should be taken to improve sensitivity of testing. Schistosomiasis may also be diagnosed by finding eggs in biopsy specimens of rectal, intestinal, liver, or bladder tissue. Serodiagnostic tests do not distinguish between recent and past infection—they are most useful in returning travellers and should be taken 6–8 weeks after likely exposure (➔ see Imported fever, pp. 639–40).
- **Management**—praziquantel is the treatment of choice. The dose is 20mg/kg, followed by a further dose 6h later for *S. haematobium* and *S. mansoni* or three doses 20mg/kg over 1 day for *S. japonicum*. Side effects are mild—abdominal discomfort, fever, and headache. Drug resistance may become a problem in endemic areas with mass treatment. Adjunctive treatment with corticosteroids is given in Katayama fever and CNS disease.

Clonorchiasis

- *Clonorchis sinensis* (Chinese or oriental liver fluke) is a parasite of fish-eating mammals in Eastern Asia. The adult flukes are flat, elongated worms (15 × 3mm) that inhabit the distal biliary capillaries where they deposit small, yellow, operculated eggs (30 × 14 micrometres). The eggs pass out in the faeces and are ingested by snails, inside which they hatch into miracidia. Miracidia multiply into cercariae that pass into water and penetrate the flesh of freshwater fish where they encyst as metacercariae. Humans are infected by ingestion of raw or undercooked fish. Once ingested, the metacercariae excyst in the duodenum and migrate to the bile ducts where they mature.
- **Epidemiology**—millions of humans are estimated to be infected, mainly in China, Hong Kong, Korea, and Vietnam.
- **Clinical features**—most infected people are asymptomatic. Heavy infection may result in cholangitis and cholangiohepatitis. Infection has been associated with an increased risk of cholangiocarcinoma.
- **Diagnosis**—infection is confirmed by demonstration of characteristic operculated, embryonated eggs in the faeces (see Fig. 11.7).
- **Management**—praziquantel or albendazole is the drug of choice for treatment. Surgery is needed rarely to relieve biliary obstruction.

Opisthorciasis

- *Opisthorcis felineus* and *Opisthorcis viverrini* are common liver flukes of cats and dogs that are occasionally transmitted to humans. The life cycle is similar to that of *C. sinensis*.
- **Epidemiology**—*O. felineus* is endemic in Russia and Eastern Europe, whereas *O. viverrini* is found in Thailand.
- **Clinical features**—mild or moderate infection is usually asymptomatic. Biliary tract symptoms and ultrasonographic signs are commoner in patients aged 20–40 years with heavy infection. There is a strong association between *O. viverrini* infection and cholangiocarcinoma.
- **Diagnosis**—this is confirmed by detection of eggs in the faeces (see Fig. 11.7).
- **Management**—praziquantel is the drug of choice.

Fascioliasis

- *Fasciola hepatica* is a liver fluke of sheep and cattle that can infect humans. The adult worms are large, flat, brown, and leaf-shaped, (2.5 × 1cm), and live in the biliary tract of their mammalian host. The large, oval, yellow-brown, operculated eggs (140 × 75 micrometres) pass out in the faeces and complete their development in water. The miracidia hatch and enter the snail intermediate host where they multiply into unforked-tail cercariae. These emerge and undergo encystment into metacercariae on aquatic plants, grasses, and sometimes soil. After ingestion, the metacercariae excyst, releasing larvae that penetrate the intestinal wall, peritoneum, and liver capsule to migrate to the biliary tract.
- **Epidemiology**—infection is commoner in sheep- and cattle-rearing areas (e.g. South America, Europe, Africa, China, Australia).
- **Clinical features**—*F. hepatica* infection has two distinct clinical phases:
  - acute hepatic migratory phase over 3–5 months, characterized by fever, right upper quadrant pain, hepatomegaly, and peripheral eosinophilia. Nodules or linear tracks may be seen on USS, CT, or MRI;
  - chronic biliary phase, which may be asymptomatic or present with biliary obstruction or cirrhosis several years after exposure.
- **Diagnosis**—this is confirmed by detection of characteristic ova in the faecal sample or bile (see Fig. 11.7). Serological testing is available and may be helpful, particularly in early infection, as it may take 3–4 months before eggs are produced.
- **Management**—triclabendazole 10mg/kg PO one dose is the treatment of choice. Alternatives: nitazoxanide (500mg bd for 7 days).

Fasciolopsiasis

- *Fasciolopsis buski* is a large intestinal fluke (2–7.5cm in length), which is endemic in South East Asia and the Far East. It inhabits the duodenum and jejunum, producing large, operculated eggs (135 × 80 micrometres), which are excreted and hatch into miracidia in fresh water. These enter the snail intermediate host where they multiply and develop into cercariae, which encyst into metacercariae on aquatic plants. Humans are infected by ingestion of contaminated plants. The metacercariae excyst in the intestine and develop into adult worms.
- **Clinical features**—fasciolopsiasis is usually asymptomatic, but heavy infection may present with diarrhoea, abdominal pain, or malabsorption.
- **Diagnosis**—this is confirmed by detection of eggs in the faeces (see Fig. 11.7).
- **Management**—praziquantel 25mg/kg tds for 1 day.

Heterophyiasis

- *Heterophyes heterophyes* is a tiny intestinal fluke (<2mm in length), which is endemic in the Nile Delta, South East Asia, and the Far East. The life cycle is similar to that of *F. buski* (➔ see Fasciolopsiasis, p. 622), except that the metacercariae encyst in fish. Humans are infected by consumption of undercooked fish.
- **Clinical features**—infection may present with abdominal pain and diarrhoea. Rarely, eggs can enter the vascular system and cause infections at ectopic sites, including cardiac muscle, valvular tissue, and the CNS.
- **Diagnosis**—adult worms produce small, operculated eggs (30 × 15 micrometres), which may be detected in the faeces (see Fig. 11.7).
- **Management**—praziquantel 25mg/kg tds for 2 days.

Paragonimiasis

- *Paragonimus westermani* is a lung fluke that is widely distributed (West Africa, the Indian subcontinent, the Far East, Central and South America). An estimated 20 million people are infected, with around 5 million felt to be symptomatic.
- **Life cycle**—adult worms inhabit the lungs and produce golden brown, operculated eggs that pass into the bronchioles and are coughed up or swallowed and pass out into the faeces. In fresh water, the eggs mature and release miracidia that infect the snail intermediate host. After 3–5 months, cerceriae are released and infect freshwater crustaceans (crayfish and crabs) where they encyst in muscles. Humans are infected by ingestion of raw or pickled crustaceans. The metacercariae excyst in the intestine, penetrate the intestinal wall, enter the peritoneal cavity, and migrate through the diaphragm and pleural cavities to the lungs. Worms may also lodge in the peritoneal cavity or the brain.
- **Clinical features**—infection may be asymptomatic or present with cough, brown sputum, intermittent haemoptysis, pleuritic chest

pain, and peripheral eosinophilia. Complications include lung abscess and pleural effusion. Ectopic infection is rare and may present with abdominal masses, epilepsy, or focal neurological signs.
- **Diagnosis**—this is confirmed by detection of characteristic eggs in the sputum or faeces (see Fig. 11.7). Serology may be helpful in ectopic infections.
- **Management**—praziquantel 25mg/kg tds for 2 days

Ectoparasites

Introduction

An ectoparasite is an organism that survives through interaction with the cutaneous surface of the host (e.g. obtaining a blood meal or living in the skin). Most ectoparasites belong to the phylum *Arthropoda*. Two classes are important in human disease: *Hexapoda* (six-legged insects, e.g. lice, bugs, flies, mosquitoes) and *Arachnida* (eight-legged mites, spiders, and ticks). Ectoparasitic diseases are a common health problem in non-industrialized tropical countries, but outbreaks of lice and scabies commonly occur in institutional settings around the world.

Hexapoda

Lice (pediculosis)

Aetiology

Three species of sucking lice affect humans: *Pediculus humanus capitis* (head louse), *Pediculus humanus humanus* (also known as *P.h. corporis*, or body louse), and *Phthirus pubis* (pubic or crab louse). The first two species are morphologically similar, with small, flat, elongated bodies and pointed heads. The pubic louse is shorter and wider, and resembles a crab. Small ovoid eggs (nits) are laid by the adult female and adhere to hair and clothing; 7–10 days later, the nymphs emerge, and after three successive moults, the adult lice develop and mate. The females produce up to 300 eggs per day for 3–4 weeks until they die. Lice pierce the skin, inject saliva, and defecate while feeding.

Epidemiology

Lice infestations (otherwise known as pediculosis) occur worldwide, are transmitted by direct contact, and are associated with poor hygiene and overcrowding. Lice cause skin disease and, in the case of *P.h. humanus*, can also act as vectors for other infectious diseases such as epidemic typhus (*Rickettsia prowazekii*), trench fever (*Bartonella quintana*), and relapsing fever (*Borrelia recurrentis*).

Clinical features

- *P.h. capitis* affects the scalp and causes pruritus, predominantly in school-aged children. Complications include secondary bacterial infection and regional adenopathy.
- *P.h. corporis* is usually found in the seams of clothing. Symptoms include pruritus, erythematous macules, papules, and excoriations, usually on the trunk. Complications include impetigo, hyperpigmentation, and hyperkeratosis, alongside acting as a vector of the pathogens described above.
- *P. pubis* resides in the pubic hair but may also be found in eyebrows, eyelashes, and axillary and chest hair. Symptoms include pruritus, erythematous macules, papules, and excoriations, but are usually less severe than with other species. Small greyish-blue macules (maculae ceruleae), caused by injection of an anticoagulant, may be seen. Eyelash infestation may be associated with nits at the base of the eyelashes and crusting of the eyelids.

Diagnosis

Diagnosis is usually clinical but may be confirmed by microscopic examination of the organism after detection via systematic combing of hair with a fine-toothed comb.

Management

- *P.h. capitis*—nits can be removed by combing wet hair with a fine-toothed head louse comb. Dimethicone 4% (interferes with water excretion on the surface of lice) is the first-line treatment in the UK for those aged 6 months or older. Two doses are given a week apart. Malathion 0.5% (requires prolonged application, is malodorous, and may be irritant to the eyes) is second line and resistance has been reported. Topical ivermectin or benzyl alcohol 5% are alternatives. Systemic treatment (e.g. ivermectin, co-trimoxazole) is reserved for those who fail topical therapy, under advice from an infection specialist.
- Children with a diagnosis of head lice should not be excluded from school. All affected family members should be treated on the same day, and detection combing should be performed after therapy to confirm treatment success.
- *P.h. corporis*—body lice can be eradicated by washing clothes in a hot cycle (60°C), alongside bedding and towels. Occasionally, a topical pediculicide (e.g. permethrin 5% cream or benzyl alcohol 5%) may be required.
- *P. pubis* may be treated with topical pyrethroids such as permethrin 1% or malathion 0.5%. Eyelid infestation may be treated by applying topical pyrethroids or a thick layer of petrolatum bd for 8 days.
- Pruritus is treated symptomatically with antihistamines and topical corticosteroids. Secondary bacterial infection should be treated with a PO antistaphylococcal agent (e.g. flucloxacillin).

Further reading

National Institute for Health and Care Excellence (NICE) Clinical Knowledge Summaries (CKS) (2021). *Head lice*. Available at: ℘ https://cks.nice.org.uk/topics/head-lice/

Scabies

Aetiology

Sarcoptes scabiei var. *hominis* is an eight-legged mite that resides in human skin. The adult ♀ lays 2–3 eggs per day, which burrow into the skin. After 72–84h, the larvae emerge and, after several moults develop into adults and mate. The ♂ die shortly afterwards, but the gravid ♀ lives for 4–6 weeks.

Epidemiology

Scabies occurs worldwide, and epidemics are associated with poverty, malnutrition, overcrowding, and poor hygiene. Scabies is transmitted by direct contact or by fomites.

Clinical features

- Human scabies—symptoms include intense pruritus (more severe at night). Signs include linear burrows (classically in the web spaces of the hands, arms, and feet), with associated excoriations, but can occasionally present as erythematous papules and vesicles. Complications include secondary bacterial infection and hypersensitivity reactions (e.g. eczematous eruption, nodular scabies).

- Crusted scabies, or 'Norwegian scabies', is a severe variant which may occur in institutionalized, debilitated, or immunosuppressed patients. Cutaneous lesions are hyperkeratotic, crusted nodules or plaques, and nail involvement may occur. Complications include secondary bacterial infection, septicaemia, and even death.
- Animal scabies—humans may occasionally be infected by *S. scabiei* var. *canis* from their pet dog. Skin lesions are pruritic, papular, or urticarial.

Diagnosis

Diagnosis is usually clinical but may be confirmed by microscopic examination of skin scrapings for the organism, egg, or faeces.

Management

- Permethrin 5% cream applied for 8–10h is the most effective treatment and suggested first-line therapy by the National Institute for Health and Care Excellence (NICE) for patients over 2 months old. A second application is required 1 week after the first.
- PO ivermectin is an alternative—two doses are as effective as permethrin. Its use is favoured in institutional outbreak settings or in severe disease. It should not be used in pregnant women or children.
- Other agents include malathion aqueous lotion 0.5%, benzyl benzoate lotion 10–25%, and sulfur 6–33% ointment or lotion.
- Permethrin and malathion can be used in pregnancy and breastfeeding.
- It should be advised that itching can continue for up to 2 weeks after successful treatment.
- Secondary bacterial infection should be treated with an antistaphylococcal agent (e.g. PO flucloxacillin).
- Household members and close contacts should be treated simultaneously, even if asymptomatic. Potentially infected clothing, towels, and bed linen should be washed and dried on a hot cycle (at least 60°C).

Further reading

National Institute for Health and Care Excellence (NICE) Clinical Knowledge Summaries (CKS) (2023). *Scabies*. Available at: ⌕ https://cks.nice.org.uk/topics/scabies/

Myiasis

Epidemiology

Myiasis is an infestation caused by the larvae (maggots) of dipterous (two-winged) flies. It occurs more commonly in tropical climates and is an important veterinary problem. Human disease occurs as a result of travel to an endemic area or exposure to infected animals.

Aetiology

A number of species may cause myiasis:
- *Dermatobia hominis* (human or tropical botfly);
- *Cordylobia anthropophaga* (tumbu fly);

- *Cordylobia rodhaini*;
- *Oestrus ovis* (sheep botfly);
- *Gasterophilus* spp. (horse botfly);
- *Hypoderma bovis* (cattle botfly);
- *Cuterebra* spp. (North American botfly);
- *Cochliomyia hominivorax* (New World screwworm);
- *Chrysomya bezziana* (Old World screwworm).

Clinical features

- Furunculoid myiasis is usually caused by *D. hominis* (Central and South America), *C. anthropophaga*, or *C. rodhaini* (sub-Saharan Africa), and occurs in travellers returning from those areas. It is characterized by single or multiple cutaneous nodules, each containing a larva. A central punctum develops and may exude serosanguineous or purulent fluid. *D. hominis* deposits its eggs directly onto the skin, so infestations occur over exposed surfaces, such as the scalp, face, and extremities, and may be associated with local pain. *C. anthropophaga* usually affects the trunk, buttocks, and thighs, as it tends to lay its larvae on damp clothing. *C. rodhaini* is similar, but lesions are larger and more painful.
- Subcutaneous infestation is caused by *Gastrophilus* spp. and characterized by migratory integumomiasis (creeping eruption), which is due to migration of larvae through the skin. *H. bovis* may cause similar lesions, which become furunculoid as the larvae mature.
- Wound myiasis may be caused by the screwworm flies *C. hominivorax* (Central America) or *C. bezziana* (Asia, Africa), and is characterized by local tissue destruction and secondary bacterial infection.
- Ophthalmomyiasis is caused by *O. ovis* (widely distributed) and may be superficial (ophthalmomyiasis externa) with conjunctivitis, lid oedema, and punctate keratopathy, or deep (ophthalmomyiasis interna) with invasion of the globe.

Management

- Cutaneous myiasis—removal of the larvae from the affected tissue may be achieved by occlusion of the punctum (e.g. with white soft paraffin or cling film), which encourages the larva to partially emerge from the punctum to avoid asphyxiation. It can then be removed with forceps. Surgical excision may be required.
- Wound myiasis—treatment requires removal of larvae and wound debridement.
- Ophthalmomyiasis—external infection is managed by removal of larvae under local anaesthesia, using forceps and slit-lamp examination. With internal infection, dead larvae (without associated inflammation) may be left *in situ*. Inflammation requires topical corticosteroids and mydriatics. Surgical intervention is indicated for live larvae or involvement of critical structures.

Arachnida

Mites

Aetiology

Mites belong to the class *Arachnida*. They occur worldwide and may be free-living or parasitize plants, insects, animals, and humans. Mites that infect humans include:

- chiggers (harvest mite, red bug, trombiculid mite);
- animal mites (e.g. *S. scabiei* var. *canis*, *Cheyletiella* spp., *Liponyssoides sanguineus*, *Ornithonyssus bacoti*);
- bird mites (e.g. *Dermanyssus gallinae*);
- food, grain, and straw mites;
- follicle mites (e.g. *Demodex folliculorum*, *Demodex brevis*);
- house dust mites (e.g. *Dermatophagoides pteronyssinus*, *Dermatophagoides farinae*);
- scabies (➡ see Scabies, pp. 627–8).

Clinical features

Mites may cause cutaneous disease in humans or act as vectors for infectious diseases—for example, rickettsial diseases (➡ see Rickettsial diseases, pp. 380–2), Q fever (➡ see *Coxiella burnetii*, pp. 382–4), tularaemia (➡ see *Francisella*, pp. 352–3), and plague (➡ see *Yersinia pestis*, pp. 349–50).

Management

Treatment of mite bites is symptomatic, with PO antihistamines or topical corticosteroids. Most lesions resolve within a week. Secondary bacterial infection should be treated with an antistaphylococcal antibiotic.

Ticks

Ticks are bloodsucking arthropods of the class *Arachnida*. There are three classes: *Ixodidae* (hard ticks), *Argasidae* (soft ticks), and *Nuttalliellidae* (with characteristics of both).

Epidemiology

Ticks occur worldwide and are important vectors of infectious diseases—for example, Lyme disease (➡ see Lyme disease, pp. 374–6), babesiosis (➡ see *Babesia*, pp. 560–2), erlichiosis, rickettsial diseases (➡ see Rickettsial diseases, pp. 380–2), Q fever (➡ see *Coxiella burnetii*, pp. 382–4), tularaemia (➡ see *Francisella*, pp. 352–3), and relapsing fever (➡ see *Borrelia* species, pp. 372–4).

Clinical features and management

- Tick bites—most bites are asymptomatic. Attached ticks should be removed with forceps to prevent disease transmission. After removal, a pruritic, erythematous papule or plaque may persist for 1–2 weeks. Sometimes a tick bite granuloma may develop.
- Tick paralysis is a rare complication of prolonged attachment of certain tick species. Clinical features are of an ascending paralysis caused by a neurotoxin in the tick salivary gland. Symptoms usually resolve with removal of the tick. A hyperimmune globulin against *Ixodes holocyclus* is effective against tick paralysis caused by this species.

Part 4

Clinical syndromes

Fever

Fever: introduction

Fever has been recognized as a clinical syndrome since the sixth century BC. Several centuries later, Hippocratic physicians proposed that body temperature was a balance between the four corporal humours: blood, phlegm, black bile, and yellow bile. Devices to measure body temperature have been around since the first century BC. Thermometry became a part of clinical practice in 1868, when Wunderlich declared 37.4°C (98.6°F) to be the normal body temperature and described the diurnal variation of body temperature.

Definitions

The definitions of sepsis are constantly evolving. 'Sepsis-3',[1] published in February 2016, moved away from the use of systemic inflammatory respiratory syndrome (SIRS) in the identification of sepsis, focusing instead on life-threatening organ dysfunction.

- **Fever**—defined as 'a state of elevated core temperature which is often, but not necessarily, part of the defensive responses of a multicellular organism (the host) to the invasion of live (microorganisms) or inanimate matter recognized as pathogenic or alien to the host'.
- **Infection**—the presence of organisms in a normally sterile site, usually accompanied by a host inflammatory response.
- **Bacteraemia**—the presence of viable bacteria in the blood; may be transient.
- **SIRS**—response to a wide variety of clinical insults, which include infectious and non-infectious causes.
- **Sepsis**—a clinical syndrome defined as life-threatening organ dysfunction caused by a dysregulated immune response to infection.
- **Septic shock**—sepsis that has circulatory, cellular, and metabolic abnormalities that are associated with a greater risk of mortality than sepsis alone.

Sepsis

Sepsis is a clinical syndrome characterized by systemic inflammation caused by infection. There is a continuum of severity, ranging from sepsis to septic shock. Worldwide the mortality of sepsis and septic shock is between 15% and 30%.

Clinical features

- **Sepsis**—symptoms and signs that are non-specific but include: (1) physiological variables (e.g. temperature >38.3°C or <36°C, pulse >90 bpm, systolic blood pressure <90mmHg, respiratory rate >20 breaths/min, altered mental state, significant oedema or positive fluid balance, hyperglycaemia), (2) inflammatory variables (e.g. leucocytosis >12 000 cells/microlitre, leucopenia <4000 cells/microlitre, CRP >2 standard deviations above normal, plasma procalcitonin >2 standard deviations above normal value, (3) organ dysfunction (e.g. arterial hypoxaemia, acute oliguria, creatinine increase >44.2 micromoles/L, coagulation abnormalities, ileus, thrombocytopenia, hyperbilirubinaemia, and (4) tissue perfusion variables (e.g. decreased capillary refill, hyperlactataemia).

- **Septic shock**—sepsis-induced tissue hypoperfusion or organ dysfunction, with any of the following thought to be due to infection: (1) requiring vasopressors to maintain a mean arterial pressure of ≥65mmHg, (2) lactate >2mmol/L (18mg/dL), (3) urine output <0.5mL/kg/h for 2h, despite adequate fluid resuscitation, (4) acute lung injury with FaO_2/FiO_2 ratio <250 in the absence of pneumonia as the infection source, (5) acute lung injury with PaO_2/FiO_2 ratio <200 in the presence of pneumonia as the infection source, (6) serum creatinine >176.8 micromoles/L, (7) serum bilirubin >34.2 micromoles/L, (8) platelet count <100 000/microlitre, and (9) coagulopathy—international normalized ratio (INR) >1.5.
- **Scoring systems**—the international 2021 guidelines for management of sepsis and septic shock recommend against using the Sequential (sepsis-related) Organ Failure Assessment (SOFA) score as a single screening tool, compared to SIRS, National Early Warning Score (NEWS), or Modified Early Warning Score (MEWS).[2]

Laboratory diagnosis

- Routine investigations may show a number of abnormalities, as described in the clinical features above. Adults with suspected sepsis should have the blood lactate level measured.
- Blood cultures (BCs) and samples from suspected sites of infection (e.g. sputum, urine, faeces, pus) should be taken for culture, ideally prior to administration of antimicrobial therapy.
- The role of procalcitonin is unclear, with its utility varying greatly with the pre-test probability of infection. It appears to be no better than CRP at predicting bacterial infection as a cause of sepsis (as opposed to other causes of SIRS). Sensitivity for predicting a positive BC in medical intensive care patients has been reported as 75%, equating to a positive predictive value (PPV) of 20% and a negative predictive value (NPV) of 97% (using a cut-off of 3.61ng/mL). Studies during the coronavirus disease 2019 (Covid-19) pandemic suggested it may have a role in ruling out bacterial co-infection in patients with Covid-19 but again had a poor PPV. It has a more established place in supporting decisions to stop antibiotic therapy once started empirically.[3]

Management

Sepsis and septic shock are medical emergencies, and treatment and resuscitation should begin immediately.[2]

- **Therapeutic priorities**—these include early initiation of supportive care to correct physiological abnormalities and institution of appropriate therapy for sepsis.
- **Stabilizing respiration**—supplemental oxygen should be given to all patients with sepsis, and oxygen saturations monitored. Intubation and mechanical ventilation may be required. A CXR and an arterial blood gas (ABG) should be obtained.
- **Assessing perfusion**—blood pressure should be assessed early and often. An arterial line may be required in patients who are shut down or have labile blood pressures.

- **Establishing venous access**—a central venous catheter (CVC) may be required in those with shock.
- **Initial resuscitation**—goals during the first 6h, as suggested by the Surviving Sepsis Campaign Guidelines, include: (1) central venous pressure of 8–12mmHg, (2) central venous (superior vena cava) or mixed venous oxygen saturation of 70% or 65%, respectively, and (3) mean arterial pressure of ≥65mmHg; and (4) urine output of ≥0.5mL/kg/h.
- **Restoration of perfusion**—at least 30mL/kg of IV crystalloid fluid within the first 3h of resuscitation. Careful monitoring is required, as patients may develop non-cardiogenic pulmonary oedema. Vasopressors (e.g. noradrenaline) may be required in patients who remain hypotensive, despite adequate fluid resuscitation. Guiding resuscitation is performed to decrease the serum lactate level in those with elevated levels. Additional therapies, such as inotropic therapy (e.g. dobutamine) or red cell transfusions, are sometimes given.
- **Identification of septic focus**—prompt identification and treatment of the focus of infection are essential.
- **Antimicrobial therapy**—this should be instigated promptly, ideally within 1h of recognition; the empirical regimen will depend on the likely source of infection, local antibiotic policies, and antibiotic resistance profiles. Poor outcome is associated with delayed or inappropriate therapy.
- **Additional therapies**—in adults with septic shock and an ongoing requirement for vasopressor therapy, IV corticosteroids should be used. Nutritional support improves nutritional outcomes in critically ill patients, but its impact on clinical outcomes from sepsis is uncertain. Insulin therapy should be initiated at a glucose level of ≥180mg/dL (10mmol/L). One study has suggested that external cooling may be helpful in patients with severe sepsis. Sepsis treatment protocols also appear to improve outcome.

References

1 Singer M, Deutschman C, Seymour C, et al.; The Third International Consensus Definitions for Sepsis and Septic Shock (Sepsis-3). *JAMA*. 2016;**315**:801–10.

2 Evans L, Rhodes A, Alhazzani W, et al.; Surviving Sepsis Campaign Guidelines Committee including the Pediatric Subgroup (2021). *Surviving Sepsis Campaign: international guidelines for management of severe sepsis and septic shock 2021*. Available at: ℛ http://www.survivingsepsis.org/Guidelines/Pages/default.aspx

3 Azzini AM, Dorizzi RM, Sette P, et al. A 2020 review on the role of procalcitonin in different clinical settings: an update conducted with the tools of the Evidence Based Laboratory Medicine. *Ann Transl Med*. 2020;**8**:610.

Pyrexia of unknown origin

Definition

The first definition of pyrexia of unknown origin (PUO) was proposed by Petersdorf and Beeson in 1961: 'fever of >38.3°C (101°F) on several occasions persisting without diagnosis for at least 3 weeks despite at least 1 week's investigation in hospital'.

Since then, the definition has been modified to reflect changes in medical practice, and there are now four different subtypes:

- classic PUO (>38°C for >3 weeks, >2 visits, or 3 days in hospital);
- nosocomial PUO (>38°C for 3 days, not present or incubating on admission);
- immune-deficient PUO (>38°C for >3 days, negative cultures after 48h);
- HIV-related PUO (>38°C for >3 weeks for outpatients or >3 days for inpatients).

Causes of pyrexia of unknown origin

(See Durack, 1997.)[4]

- **Classic PUO**—although a wide variety of conditions can cause classic PUO, most fall into five categories:
  - infections (27–50%; e.g. abscesses, endocarditis, TB, complicated urinary tract infection (UTIs), prosthetic joint infections, *Mycobacterium* chimera in patients post-cardiac surgery). Some causes show distinct geographical variation (e.g. visceral leishmaniasis (Spain), melioidosis (South East Asia));
  - neoplasms (13–25%; e.g. lymphoma);
  - connective tissue disorders (9–17% e.g. Still's disease, systemic lupus erythematosus (SLE), granulomatous processes (sarcoidosis), rheumatoid arthritis, temporal arteritis, polymyalgia rheumatica, polyarteritis nodosa (PAN));
  - miscellaneous disorders (15–21%; e.g. drug fever, factitious fever, inflammatory bowel disease, hyperthyroidism, hypoadrenalism, hypothalamic dysfunction);
  - undiagnosed conditions (5–23%).

The relative frequency of disorders within these five categories varies according to the era in which the study was conducted, geographical region, age of the patient, and type of hospital.

- **Nosocomial PUO** presents as fever after hospitalization for at least 24h. Risk factors include intravascular devices, urinary or respiratory tract instrumentation, surgical procedures, immobility, and drug therapy. However, knowledge is limited due to lack of published data.
- **Immune-deficient PUO** occurs in patients receiving cytotoxic therapy or with haematological malignancies. Because of impaired immune function, signs of inflammation may be modest, leading to atypical presentations. During episodes of neutropenia, infections caused by pyogenic bacteria are commonest. In patients with impaired cell-mediated immunity (CMI), viral infections are commoner.
- **HIV-related PUO** may occur with primary infection or in advanced disease where it is due to opportunistic infections (e.g. mycobacteria, visceral leishmaniasis, *Pneumocystis jirovecii*, bacterial infections, cytomegalovirus (CMV), toxoplasmosis, cryptococcosis) or malignancies.

Evaluation of pyrexia of unknown origin

- **History and examination**—a comprehensive history should include details of recent travel, contact with persons who have a similar illness, exposure to animals, work environment, past medical history, drug history (including over-the-counter, alternative herbal, or traditional medications, and recreational drugs), recent vaccinations, sexual history, and family history for hereditary causes of fever. History should be revisited at regular intervals. A careful physical examination may reveal clues as to the aetiology (e.g. stigmata of endocarditis, spinal tenderness), paying close attention to any implant which can be examined. The presence of fever should be verified, although fever patterns are neither sensitive nor specific enough to be diagnostically reliable.

- **Laboratory investigations** include simple blood tests (e.g. FBC, CRP, ESR, biochemical profile, including LFTs, creatine phosphokinase (CPK)) and urinalysis. BCs (at least three sets drawn from different sites at different times) should be taken prior to initiation of antimicrobial therapy. Mycobacterial blood cultures should be considered, especially if previous cardiac surgery has occurred. Serology may be helpful for viral infections (e.g. hepatitis A, B, and C, Epstein–Barr virus (EBV), CMV, and HIV) and autoimmune disorders (e.g. antinuclear antibody (ANA), antineutrophil cytoplasmic antibody (ANCA), rheumatoid factor). Serum protein electrophoresis may be helpful.
- **Imaging studies**—all patients should have a chest radiograph and abdominal ultrasound. Further radiological imaging should be guided by the clinical presentation. Positron emission tomography–computed tomography (PET-CT) scans have become more widely available and can identify metabolically active foci of infection, inflammation, or cancer. Venous duplex scans of the lower extremities may reveal deep vein thromboses.
- **Invasive procedures**—directed diagnostic biopsies may be helpful (e.g. liver, lymph node, temporal artery, pleural, pericardial, or bone marrow biopsies). Muscle biopsy may be helpful in suspected PAN.
- **Therapeutic trials**—these may confound or delay the diagnosis of PUO. Thus, therapeutic trials should be reserved for those few patients in whom all other approaches have failed or for the occasional patient who is too ill for therapy to be withheld.

Management

A fundamental principle of management of classic PUO is that therapy should be delayed, until the cause has been identified, so that it can be targeted appropriately. However, this ideal is frequently ignored in clinical practice and may confound or delay the diagnosis of PUO. In contrast, for neutropenic sepsis, which carries a high risk of serious bacterial infections, empirical broad-spectrum antibiotic therapy should be started immediately after appropriate cultures are taken.

Prognosis

Nine to 51% of cases of PUO defy diagnosis. Prognosis depends on the cause of the fever and the underlying disease. Elderly patients and those with malignant disease have the poorest prognosis. Diagnostic delay adversely affects outcome in intra-abdominal infections, disseminated TB and fungal infections, and recurrent pulmonary embolism (PE). Patients who have undiagnosed PUO after extensive evaluation generally have a favourable outcome (5-year mortality rate of 3.2%).

References

4 Durack DT. Fever of unknown origin. In: Mackowiak PA (ed). *Fever. Basic Mechanisms and Management*, second edition. Philadelphia, PA: Lippincott-Raven, 1997: pp. 237–49.

Imported fever

Fever in returning travellers is estimated to affect 22–64% of the 50 million people who travel from industrialized countries to the developing world each year. Although most illnesses are mild, up to 8% of people are ill enough to seek medical attention; 0.1% require medical evacuation, and 1 in 100 000 dies. An increased risk of travel-associated infections is seen in people who visit family and friends abroad and in adventure travellers.

Clinical features

The top diagnoses in 32 136 travellers presenting in Europe between 2008 and 2012, ranked by proportionate morbidity, were: malaria, acute diarrhoea, dengue, giardiasis, and insect bites. Patients may present with a wide spectrum of disease,[5] ranging from asymptomatic carriage to fulminant disease (see Table 13.1).

Viral haemorrhagic fever (VHF) risk assessment should be completed for all febrile returning travellers.

Table 13.1 Causes of imported fever

Incubation	Syndrome	Causes
<14 days	Undifferentiated fever	Malaria, dengue, rickettsial spotted fevers, scrub typhus, leptospirosis, bacterial gastroenteritis, typhoid, acute HIV, Covid-19
	Fever with respiratory symptoms	Influenza, legionellosis, Q fever, acute histoplasmosis, acute coccidioidomycosis
	Fever with CNS symptoms	Bacterial meningitis, viral meningitis, encephalitis, cerebral malaria, typhoid, typhus, rabies, arboviral encephalitis, *Angiostrongylus cantonensis* eosinophilic meningitis, polio, East African trypanosomiasis
	Fever with haemorrhage	Meningococcaemia, leptospirosis, *Streptococcus suis*, malaria, VHF
14 days to 6 weeks		Malaria, typhoid, hepatitis A, hepatitis E, acute schistosomiasis, amoebic liver abscess, leptospirosis, acute HIV infection, East African trypanosomiasis, VHF, Q fever, brucellosis, ascariasis, Chagas' disease
>6 weeks		Malaria, TB, hepatitis B, hepatitis E, visceral leishmaniasis, lymphatic filariasis, schistosomiasis, amoebic liver abscess, chronic mycosis, rabies, African trypanosomiasis, HIV, brucellosis

Covid-19, coronavirus disease 2019; VHF, viral haemorrhagic fever

History and examination
The following are essential in the assessment of a returning traveller:
- geography—countries visited or passed through, urban or rural, dates of travel and duration of stay in each place, means of transportation, accommodation;
- activities and exposures—sexual or other intimate contact, animal contact, insect bites, exposure to blood or needles, food and beverages, soil and water contact;
- host factors—age, gender, past medical history, past surgery, past infections and vaccines, current medications including immunosuppressive/immunomodulatory drugs, pre-travel immunizations, antimalarial chemoprophylaxis;
- symptoms—nature and duration of symptoms;
- physical findings—fever, rash, eschar, lymphadenopathy, splenomegaly, genital lesions, retinal or conjunctival haemorrhages, neurological signs. Findings that require urgent intervention are confusion, lethargy, meningism, hypotension, respiratory distress, and haemorrhagic manifestations.

Laboratory investigations
- FBC, WCC and differential, thick and thin films for malaria.
- Urea, creatinine, electrolytes, LFTs, CRP.
- Urinalysis, microscopy and culture.
- Faeces for microscopy (ova, cyst, parasites) and culture.
- Skin scrapings or biopsy of lesions.
- Sputum microscopy and culture.
- BCs—two sets.
- Serum to save for sending away later.
- Serology—HIV, others (e.g. arboviral, *Brucella* if indicated).
- Imaging (e.g. CXR, abdominal USS).
- Bone marrow examination may be helpful in certain conditions.

Treatment
- Supportive treatment (mild infections or those with no treatment).
- Specific treatment according to the causative organism.

Prevention
- Pre-travel consultation is associated with significantly lower morbidity rates for *Plasmodium falciparum* malaria, acute hepatitis, and HIV.
- Vaccination and antimalarial prophylaxis, if indicated.
- Advice regarding risk avoidance (e.g. water purification, avoiding uncooked food, barrier contraception).

References
5 Ryan ET, Wilson ME, Kain KC. Illness after international travel. *N Engl J Med.* 2002;**347**:505–16.

Eosinophilia in travellers

Eosinophilia in returning travellers and migrants is common. Helminth infection accounts for most in which a cause is identified, and many patients experience little in the way of significant symptoms. However, some helminths have the potential for causing significant health problems. The pattern of disease tends to differ between migrants from, and travellers making short trips to, the regions in which infection is acquired. The former are more likely to experience a larger burden of infection or present with complications of chronic infection (e.g. bladder cancer or portal hypertension due to chronic schistosomiasis); the latter are more likely to present with features of acute infection (e.g. Löeffler's syndrome) and higher eosinophil counts.

General points when assessing a patient

- History—a detailed travel history is important. Some organisms can be acquired worldwide (e.g. *Strongyloides*), others in specific regions (e.g. *Taenia solium*), and still others are more geographically restricted (e.g. schistosomiasis). Establish dates of symptom onset, timings of water exposure, foods eaten, specific regions visited within a country, and any activities undertaken.
- The asymptomatic patient with eosinophilia—it is worthwhile performing faeces microscopy and *Strongyloides* serology on such patients. Other screening tests may be appropriate, depending on the region visited (e.g. terminal urine microscopy, filarial serology and day/ night blood films in those returning from relevant regions of Africa). Some authorities recommend empirical albendazole as treatment for undiagnosed ascariasis/hookworm infection in patients with a suitable travel history and transient eosinophilia. Those with the necessary expertise should make such decisions.
- Timing of investigations—eosinophilia can occur briefly in association with the tissue migration phase of infection, and eggs/larvae may not yet be detectable. Faeces microscopy then becomes positive after eosinophilia resolves. Serological tests are likely to become positive only 4–12 weeks after infection, and many of these tests cross-react between helminth species. Filarial blood films are most likely to be positive at specific times of the day (e.g. *Loa loa* from 10 a.m. to 2 p.m., lymphatic filariasis from 10 p.m. to 2 a.m.).
- Those with sustained eosinophilia in whom no diagnosis is reached or with symptoms that are not in keeping with a parasitic infection should be investigated for other infectious causes (e.g. fungi, HIV) and non-infectious causes such as allergy, malignancy (especially leukaemia and lymphoma), and connective tissue disease.

Eosinophilia with specific symptoms

- Fever with or without respiratory symptoms—Katayama fever (➋ see *Schistosoma* species, pp. 618–20), Löeffler's syndrome (➋ see *Strongyloides stercoralis*, pp. 595–7), acute toxocariasis (➋ see Toxocariasis, pp. 601–2), tropical pulmonary eosinophilia due to filarial infection (➋ see Filariasis, pp. 604–6), pulmonary hydatid disease (➋ see Echinococcosis, pp. 615–16), paragonimiasis (➋ see Paragonimiasis, pp. 622–3). Also consider endemic fungi (e.g. coccidioidomycosis; ➋ see *Coccidioides immitis*, pp. 547–50) and non-infectious causes (drugs, connective tissue diseases).

- Gastrointestinal symptoms—*Strongyloides* (➔ see *Strongyloides stercoralis*, pp. 595–7), schistosomiasis (➔ see Trematodes (flukes), pp. 616–17), ascariasis (➔ see *Ascaris lumbricoides*, pp. 589–91), tapeworm (➔ see Cestodes, pp. 611–12), hookworm (➔ see *Ancylostoma duodenale* and *Necator americanus* (hookworm), pp. 593–5), whipworm (➔ see *Trichuris trichiura*, pp. 592–3), *Enterobius vermicularis* (➔ see *Enterobius vermicularis*, pp. 597–600), trichinellosis (➔ see *Trichinella* species, pp. 602–3).
- Right upper quadrant pain, with or without jaundice—hydatid disease of the liver (➔ see Echinococcosis, pp. 615–17), fasciola hepatica (➔ see Fascioliasis, p. 621), schistosomiasis (➔ see Trematodes (flukes), pp. 616–17).
- Neurological symptoms—ask the laboratory to specifically examine the CSF for eosinophils. Causes include gnathostomiasis, neurocysticercosis meningitis (➔ see Cysticercosis, pp. 613–14), neurological schistosomiasis (➔ see *Schistosoma* species, pp. 618–20), toxocariasis (➔ see Toxocariasis, pp. 601–2), and endemic fungi (➔ see *Histoplasma capsulatum*, pp. 540–4). Also consider non-infectious causes such as lymphoma and vasculitis.
- Rash, itch, urticaria—onchocerciasis (➔ see *Onchocerca volvulus*, pp. 607–9), larva currens due to *Strongyloides* (➔ see *Strongyloides stercoralis*, pp. 607–9), lymphatic filariasis (➔ see Filariasis, pp. 604–6), loiasis (calabar swellings; ➔ see *Loa loa*, pp. 606–7), gnathostomiasis, trichinellosis (➔ see *Trichinella* species, pp. 602–3), swimmer's itch due to exposure to avian schistosomiasis.
- Urinary symptoms—schistosomiasis.

Further reading

Checkley AM, Chiodini PL, Dockrell DH, *et al.*; British Infection Society and Hospital for Tropical Diseases. Eosinophilia in returning travellers and migrants from the tropics: UK recommendations for investigation and initial management. *J Infect*. 2010;**60**:1–20.

Respiratory, head, and neck infections

Acute bronchitis

A syndrome of tracheal and bronchial inflammation not associated with evidence of pneumonia on chest radiograph. Usually of viral aetiology. Diagnosis peaks in winter months and is made most frequently in children <5 years of age.

Aetiology

- Usually viral—influenza A and B, parainfluenza, coronavirus (types 1–3), rhinovirus, respiratory syncytial virus (RSV), and human metapneumovirus.
- Around 10% of cases are bacterial—*Mycoplasma pneumoniae*, *Chlamydia pneumoniae* (also known as *Chlamydophila pneumoniae*), and *Bordetella pertussis*.
- Relative proportion varies according to age and season.

Pathogenesis

- The exact nature of pathogenesis depends on the pathogen involved and the host response. Some (e.g. influenza) invade the lower respiratory tract. Others (e.g. rhinovirus) do not, and symptoms may be secondary to inflammatory mediators. Either way, the outcome is an inflamed, oedematous tracheobronchial tree, with increased secretions.
- Attack severity may be increased by exposure to irritants, such as cigarette smoke, and may lead to long-term airway damage. Patients with acute bronchitis are more likely to have a history of atopic disease, which may be associated with airway hyper-reactivity. Some progress to develop adult-onset asthma.

Clinical features

- Disease severity and symptoms vary according to the underlying pathogen. Nasal congestion, rhinitis, sore throat, malaise, and low-grade fever typical of respiratory viral pathogens are first noted, followed by onset of cough, which becomes the predominant symptom.
- Dyspnoea and more severe respiratory symptoms are seen only in those with underlying chest disease. Fever is seen in some cases—most frequently with agents such as influenza or *M. pneumoniae*.
- Cough caused by bacterial causes, especially *B. pertussis*, may persist for several months.

Diagnosis

- Bronchitis is a diagnosis of exclusion, and a complete history and examination should be performed, seeking any more serious cause of cough.
- Respiratory viral PCR may identify viral causes of acute bronchitis.
- Cultures of respiratory secretions may be useful in looking for specific agents such as *B. pertussis*. Serological tests or PCR may be used to confirm infection with *M. pneumoniae* and *C. pneumoniae*.
- Those in whom cough persists beyond a reasonable duration of illness should be investigated for other causes (e.g. foreign body, TB, malignancy).

Treatment

- The National Institute for Health and Care Excellence (NICE) guidance for adults advises self-care strategies, adequate fluid intake, simple analgesia, and over-the-counter cough medicine containing expectorants or suppressants (but not codeine).
- Antibiotics are not usually indicated unless systemically very unwell or at risk of complications (e.g. heart, lung, renal, liver, neuromuscular disease, immunosuppression, cystic fibrosis (CF)). The recommended first-line antibiotic for adults (non-pregnant) is doxycycline; the first-line antibiotic in young people (aged 12–17 years) is amoxicillin. Antibiotic duration is 5 days.
- Routine follow-up is not usually indicated unless symptoms significantly worsen, in which case the person should be reassessed for other diagnoses such as pneumonia.[1]
- Smoking cessation advised.

References

1 National Institute for Health and Care Excellence (2019). *Cough (acute): antimicrobial prescribing.* NICE guideline [NG120]. Available at: 🔗 https://www.nice.org.uk/guidance/ng120

Chronic bronchitis

Defined as a cough productive of sputum on most days during at least 3 months of two successive years, which cannot be attributed to other specific diseases (e.g. TB, bronchiectasis). Chronic obstructive pulmonary disease (COPD) includes both emphysema and chronic bronchitis.

Epidemiology

- Common, affecting 10–25% of the adult population. Men > women, commoner in those >40 years of age
- Associations—cigarette smoking (although only 15% of smokers develop chronic bronchitis), pollution, and exposure to allergens.

Pathogenesis

- Inflammation and oedema seen in patients with chronic bronchitis result from the interaction between exogenous irritants (mostly cigarette smoking) and the pathological response: an increase in bronchial mucus-secreting cells, granulocytic infiltration in response to chemokines produced by epithelial cells, increased airway secretions, and production of neuropeptides promoting bronchospasm.
- Airways are frequently colonized with bacteria, making interpretation of sputum culture difficult, although higher bacterial loads are associated with exacerbations. *Haemophilus influenzae*, *Streptococcus pneumoniae*, and *Moraxella catarrhalis* are the most frequently isolated pathogens. Increased severity of airway disease, recent antibiotic use, and steroid therapy are associated with increased rates of Gram-negative infection (e.g. *Pseudomonas aeruginosa*, *Stenotrophomonas maltophilia*).
- One-third of acute exacerbations are thought due to viral infections.

Clinical features

- Frequent productive cough, most severe in the morning when patients may produce large amounts of sputum, which may be mucoid and white or obviously purulent in appearance.
- COPD exists as a spectrum of clinical disease, with emphysema predominant at one end (breathlessness, less sputum, fewer infections, barrel chest with hyperexpanded, clear lungs) and bronchitis predominant at the other (productive cough, frequent infections, wheeze, widespread crepitations, right heart failure in severe cases).

Diagnosis

- An exacerbation is an acute worsening of the patient's symptoms from their usual state. Common symptoms are worsening breathlessness, cough, increased sputum, and change in sputum colour.
- CXR, electrocardiogram (ECG) (to exclude differentials), FBC, urea and electrolytes (U&Es), sputum culture, and (if pyrexial) blood cultures (BCs) in those presenting to hospital.
- About half of exacerbations are caused by bacterial infections (with the remainder secondary to viral infections and environmental factors, e.g. smoking).

Treatment

General measures

- Exclude other causes of recurrent chest infections, and have a high index of suspicion for lung malignancy.
- Smoking cessation, weight control, avoidance of environmental irritants, and assessment for allergic disease.
- Record of baseline spirometry, arterial blood gas (ABG), and oxygen saturations.
- Pneumococcal and influenza vaccinations.
- Pulmonary rehabilitation programmes and postural drainage where appropriate.

Maintenance therapy to improve airflow obstruction symptoms

- For example, regular inhaled steroids, β2-agonists, anticholinergic agents. PO steroids as required.
- Prophylactic azithromycin (usually 250mg, three times a week) may be considered in patients who, despite optimized inhaled therapies, smoking cessation, vaccinations, and pulmonary rehabilitation, have frequent (typically four or more per year) prolonged exacerbations or require hospitalization. Prior to commencement, ensure sputum culture (including mycobacterial) has been sent and CT thorax performed, to identify an alternative pathology. Do ECG to rule out prolonged QT interval, and baseline LFTs. Advise patients to be alert to hearing loss and tinnitus and to inform a health professional if these occur. Review for benefit at 3 months and then 6-monthly.

Intensive therapy for acute exacerbations

- Intensification of normal therapy (e.g. short-acting bronchodilators, systemic steroids).

- Antibiotic therapy[2]—only about half of exacerbations are caused by bacterial infections. Consider an antibiotic after taking into account the severity of symptoms, sputum changes, and previous cultures. Empirical first-line antibiotics—amoxicillin, doxycycline or clarithromycin. Alternatives in those at higher risk of treatment failure (multiple antibiotic exposure, history of resistant bacteria) include co-amoxiclav and co-trimoxazole. Rationalize with culture results.

References

2 National Institute for Health and Care Excellence (2018). *Chronic obstructive pulmonary disease (acute exacerbation): antimicrobial prescribing*. Available at: ℛ https://www.nice.org.uk/guidance/ng114/chapter/Recommendations#treatment

Bronchiolitis

An acute infection of the lower respiratory tract, characterized by acute onset of wheeze and associated with cough, nasal discharge, breathlessness, and respiratory distress.

Aetiology

- RSV is the commonest cause (60–75%), followed by rhinovirus. Less common causes include parainfluenza virus, human metapneumovirus, influenza virus, adenovirus, coronavirus, and parainfluenza virus. Viral co-infection occurs in up to one-third of infants.
- Rarely caused by *M. pneumoniae*.

Epidemiology

- In the UK, RSV is a winter virus, with peak cases occurring between October and March.
- Most children have evidence of previous RSV infection by their second birthday.
- Previous infection confers only partial immunity, so individuals may be repeatedly infected by the same or different strains. Modelling indicates RSV burden in UK children exceeds that of flu.
- Risk factors for severe disease—age <12 weeks, prematurity, underlying cardiopulmonary disease or immunodeficiency.

Pathogenesis

- Virus infects the upper respiratory mucosa and spreads to the lower airways. Bronchial and bronchiolar inflammation and necrosis follow, with oedema and peribronchiolar mononuclear cell infiltration. In severe cases, interstitial pneumonitis may develop.
- Inflammation and oedema reduce the airway calibre. Necrotic material may block small airways. Distally trapped air is later absorbed, resulting in multiple areas of atelectasis and a low ventilation/perfusion ratio.

Clinical features

- Coryzal prodrome over 1–3 days, followed by persistent cough, tachypnoea, and wheeze or crackles on chest auscultation. Fever usually <39°C.

- Severe cases develop tachypnoea, tachycardia, and signs of increased breathing work (nasal flaring, chest wall retraction, grunting). Cyanosis is rare, even in the presence of hypoxia. Apnoea is relatively common in young infants hospitalized with RSV infection.
- Otitis media may occur.
- Symptoms begin to settle after 2–3 days, with recovery taking 2 weeks or more.

Diagnosis

- Largely clinical, but general features include: elevated WCC in severe cases, and CXR showing hyperinflation, hyperlucent parenchyma, and multiple areas of atelectasis. Pneumonia may be present. Findings do not correlate well with clinical severity.
- Differentials—pneumonia (fever usually >39°C ± persistently focal crackles), viral-induced wheeze, early-onset asthma.
- Viral agents may be identified from respiratory secretions (preferably a nasopharyngeal aspirate (NPA)) by respiratory virus PCR.

Treatment

- Give oxygen supplementation to babies and children with bronchiolitis if their oxygen saturation is persistently less than:
  - 90% for children aged 6 weeks and over;
  - 92% for babies aged under 6 weeks or children of any age with underlying health conditions.
- Bronchodilators and steroids are not recommended.
- No role for antibiotics unless concomitant bacterial infection.
- Ribavirin is not recommended routinely due to lack of evidence. Its use is reserved for immunocompromised patients with severe bronchiolitis due to RSV infection.
- Monoclonal therapies used in prevention (e.g. palivizumab) have no role in acute treatment, based on current evidence.

Prevention

Passive immunization with palivizumab, a humanized monoclonal antibody against the RSV F glycoprotein, decreases the risk of hospitalization due to RSV amongst high-risk children. Recommended as a monthly IM injection during the RSV season for children with bronchopulmonary dysplasia, congenital heart disease, and severe combined immunodeficiency disease (SCID).

Complications

- Children who have RSV bronchiolitis in early life may be at increased risk of developing recurrent wheeze in later childhood.
- Most at risk of severe, or fatal, disease are premature infants, chronic lung disease, congenital heart disease immunodeficiency.

Further reading

National Institute for Health and Care Excellence (2015, updated 2021). *Bronchiolitis in children: diagnosis and management.* NICE guideline [NG9]. Available at: ℘ https://www.nice.org.uk/guidance/ng9/chapter/1-Recommendations

Ralston SL, Lieberthal AS, Meissner C, *et al.* Clinical practice guideline: the diagnosis, management and prevention of bronchiolitis. *Pediatrics.* 2014;**134**:e1474–502. Available at: ℘ https://publicati

ons.aap.org/pediatrics/article/134/5/e1474/75848/Clinical-Practice-Guideline-The-Diagnosis?autologincheck=redirected?nfToken=00000000-0000-0000-0000-000000000000

UK Health Security Agency (2013). *Respiratory syncytial virus: the green book, chapter 27a*. Available at: ℛ https://www.gov.uk/government/publications/respiratory-syncytial-virus-the-green-book-chapter-27a

Community-acquired pneumonia

Epidemiology

- Incidence >1 per 100 people per year; 20–40% of cases require hospital admission. Mortality varies with the patient group (overall 5–10%, 50% in those requiring admission to the intensive care unit (ICU)).
- Peak age 50–70 years, and onset in mid winter and early spring; 58–89% have an underlying disease (e.g. COPD, diabetes, cardiovascular disease, immunosuppression).
- Some organisms are acquired by person-to-person spread or are existing commensals (*S. pneumoniae*, *H. influenzae*). Others are acquired from the environment (*Legionella pneumophila*) or animals (*Chlamydophila psittaci*).
- Seventy per cent to 80% of community-acquired pneumonia (CAP) is managed in primary care—viruses, *S. pneumoniae*, and *M. pneumoniae* are the commonest causes.

Aetiology

- Organisms vary with country, study, age, and patient group (e.g. *Moraxella* and *H. influenzae* are commoner in COPD).
- Pneumonia in childhood is usually viral.
- Common bacterial isolates vary with age:
  - 0–1 month—*Escherichia coli*, group B *Streptococcus* (GBS), *Listeria monocytogenes*;
  - 1–6 months—*Chlamydia trachomatis*, *Staphylococcus aureus*, RSV;
  - 6 months to 5 years—RSV, parainfluenza viruses;
  - 5–15 years—*M. pneumoniae*, influenza;
  - 16–30 years—*M. pneumoniae*, *S. pneumoniae*;
  - older adults—*S. pneumoniae*, *H. influenzae*.
- Some infections (e.g. *M. pneumoniae*) are associated with epidemics.
- *S. pneumoniae* infection is associated with viral illness (e.g. influenza).
- Mixed infections are commoner in the elderly—*S. aureus* and Gram-negatives are seen more frequently amongst those in residential care.
- Severe disease occurs with *S. pneumoniae*, meticillin-resistant *S. aureus* (MRSA), *L. pneumophila*, and Gram-negative organisms. Mortality is 20–53%.
- Rare causes of pneumonia include anthrax, plague, and melioidosis.
- *Pneumocystis jirovecii* (➔ see *Pneumocystis jirovecii*, pp. 522–4) is an important cause in HIV-infected patients, who are also at increased risk of infection with mycobacteria, *Cryptococcus neoformans*, and viruses (e.g. cytomegalovirus (CMV)).

Clinical features

- History—most patients present with sudden-onset chills, fever, cough, mucopurulent sputum, pleuritic chest pain, fatigue, anorexia, sweats,

and nausea. Cough is noted in >80% of cases, and productive in >60%. Ask about predisposing conditions, travel, and exposure to animals.
- Symptoms and signs—sputum; often purulent, fever, tachypnoea, tachycardia, crepitations on chest examination indicating consolidation. Signs of respiratory distress in severe cases. Classic findings may be absent in the elderly, and the main presenting features may be non-respiratory (e.g. confusion, abdominal pain). Other findings—herpes labialis (40% of pneumococcal pneumonia patients), bullous myringitis (rare in *Mycoplasma* pneumonia).

Investigations
- Blood tests—FBC, most commonly neutrophilia. Leucopenia is a poor prognostic sign. Biochemical abnormalities include raised urea level, hyponatraemia (especially in the elderly due to syndrome of inappropriate antidiuretic hormone (SIADH)), abnormal LFTs (especially *Legionella*), raised CRP level.
- CXR—all patients admitted to hospital with suspected CAP require CXR. An infiltrate pattern may indicate the aetiology but can be non-specific:
  - lobar consolidation, cavitation, and effusions suggest a bacterial cause, most often pneumococcal;
  - CXR worse than examination findings suggest mycoplasmal or viral pneumonia;
  - diffuse bilateral involvement may suggest *Pneumocystis* pneumonia (PCP), *Legionella* infection, or primary viral pneumonia;
  - thin-walled cavities (pneumatoceles) classically seen in *S. aureus*, but also *Klebsiella pneumoniae*, *H. influenzae*, and *S. pneumoniae*, infections;
  - *S. aureus* producing Panton–Valentine leucocidin (PVL) is associated with necrotizing pneumonia with multilobar cavities.
- CT has little role in the usual management of CAP. Helpful in recurrent pneumonias or those unresponsive to therapy (e.g. to identify a tumour, foreign body, empyema, or lung abscess). In immunocompromised patients, with a broad differential of potential pathogens, CT may indicate a particular aetiology (e.g. *Aspergillus* infection) and identify an area amenable to diagnostic biopsy.

Microbiological investigations
Microbiological tests are not routinely recommended for patients managed in the community—consider in those who do not respond to empirical antibiotic therapy or in whom unusual pathogens are suspected. The following are advisable in those unwell enough for hospital admission:
- BCs—all patients with moderate/high-severity CAP, preferably before starting antibiotics;
- sputum culture and sensitivity—all moderate/high-severity CAP or those who fail to improve;
- antigen testing—*Legionella* antigen testing should be performed on all patients with moderate or severe disease, in the presence of specific epidemiological risk factors, and during outbreaks. Commercial tests

detect only serogroup 1, responsible for around 85% of reported cases of legionellosis. Pneumococcal urinary antigen may be reassuring if positive, but some laboratories have abandoned it as the result rarely changes management;

- PCR—where PCR is available for respiratory viruses and atypical pathogens (M. pneumoniae, Chlamydophila pneumoniae), this is preferable to serological investigation;
- Serology—consider paired serology tests (M. pneumoniae, C. pneumoniae) for patients with severe CAP in whom no particular microbiological diagnosis has been made by other means (e.g. culture, urine antigen, PCR) and who fail to improve and/or where there are particular epidemiological risk factors
- Bronchoalveolar lavage (BAL)—a bronchoscope is used to instil sterile fluid into a segment of the lung, and the fluid examined microscopically and cultured. A threshold of 10^4 cfu/mL is used to define significant isolates. It is particularly useful in the diagnosis of Mycobacterium tuberculosis (MTB), P. jirovecii, CMV, and ventilator-associated pneumonia (VAP) infections. Legionella cultures should be performed on invasive samples in patients with CAP, especially if a non-serogroup 1 infection is suspected.
- Pleural fluid sampling—where positive, pleural fluid cultures are specific for the organism causing the underlying pneumonia. Fluid analysis helps differentiate other causes of lung disease (e.g. TB, tumour).
- Other tests—cold agglutinins for M. pneumoniae (<25% positive), lung biopsy (e.g. immunosuppressed patients with no diagnosis).

Severity assessment

- The CURB-65 score (**C**onfusion, **U**rea, **R**espiratory rate, **B**lood pressure, age **65** or over) enables rapid assessment of severity and guides initial management (see Fig. 14.1).
- Additional adverse features—hypoxia regardless of oxygen therapy (arterial oxygen saturation (SaO_2) <92% or partial pressure of arterial oxygen (PaO_2) <8kPa), bilateral or multilobar involvement on CXR, positive BCs, WCC $<4 \times 10^9$/L or $>20 \times 10^9$/L.
- Severity should be reassessed regularly during the course of the illness.

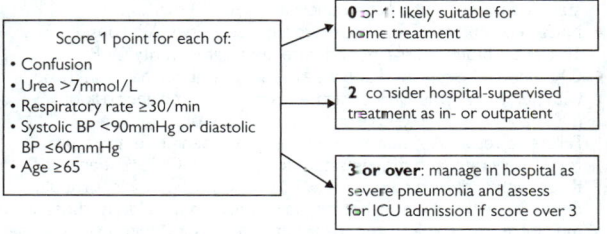

Score 1 point for each of:
- Confusion
- Urea >7mmol/L
- Respiratory rate ≥30/min
- Systolic BP <90mmHg or diastolic BP ≤60mmHg
- Age ≥65

0 or **1**: likely suitable for home treatment

2: consider hospital-supervised treatment as in- or outpatient

3 or over: manage in hospital as severe pneumonia and assess for ICU admission if score over 3

Fig. 14.1 The CURB-65 severity assessment tool.

Management

See British Thoracic Society (BTS) guidelines for CAP (2009) and annotated 2015 update.[3]

- General—IV fluids, appropriate oxygen therapy (with repeated ABG for those at risk of hypercapnic respiratory failure), fluids, frequent reassessment of progress and severity, particularly aimed at early identification of those who may require ICU support.
- Antibiotics—empirical therapy should be started as soon as possible:
  - CURB-65 score 0 or 1—amoxicillin 500mg tds PO. Alternative: doxycycline 200mg loading, then 100mg od;
  - CURB-65 score 2—amoxicillin 500mg tds PO and clarithromycin 500mg bd. Monotherapy with a macrolide may be appropriate if failure to respond to an adequate course of amoxicillin prior to admission. Alternative: doxycycline 200mg loading, then 100mg od;
  - CURB-65 score ≥3—IV β-lactamase-stable antibiotic (e.g. co-amoxiclav) plus macrolide (e.g. clarithromycin 500mg bd; or if *Legionella* strongly suspected, consider adding levofloxacin).
  - older fluoroquinolones (e.g. ciprofloxacin) are not recommended for empirical treatment due to poor activity against *S. pneumoniae*. Newer agents (e.g. levofloxacin and moxifloxacin) may be used.
- Antibiotic therapy should be tailored to the causative organism in the light of microbiological data:
  - *S. pneumoniae*—amoxicillin; alternative: clarithromycin;
  - *M. pneumoniae*—clarithromycin; alternative: doxycycline;
  - *C. pneumoniae*—clarithromycin; alternative: doxycycline;
  - *C. psittaci*—doxycycline;
  - *Coxiella burnetii*—doxycycline;
  - *Legionella* spp.—levofloxacin; alternative: clarithromycin;
  - *H. influenzae*—amoxicillin (non-β-lactamase producer) or co-amoxiclav (β-lactamase producer);
  - Gram-negative enteric bacilli—cefuroxime, cefotaxime, or ceftriaxone;
  - *P. aeruginosa*—ceftazidime and gentamicin or tobramycin;
  - *S. aureus* (meticillin-sensitive)—flucloxacillin ± rifampicin;
  - MRSA—vancomycin.
- IV antibiotics—convert to PO route when clinical improvement (e.g. afebrile for 24h) and no contraindications to PO therapy.
- NICE recommends 5-day course for low-severity CAP; consider 7- to 10-day antibiotic course in moderate- and high-severity CAP.
- CXR should be repeated at 6 weeks if initially abnormal or in those with persisting symptoms or signs—especially if at higher risk of malignancy (e.g. smokers or those aged >50 years).
- Failure to respond—median time to improvement in temperature, respiratory rate, and oxygen saturation is 3 days. Older patients and those with underlying disease may take longer. CXR findings should normalize within 4 weeks but may take longer in the elderly, those with multilobar involvement, and those with pre-existing pulmonary disease. In those failing to improve, consider an incorrect diagnosis (pulmonary embolism (PE), carcinoma, eosinophilic pneumonia), atypical pathogen or resistant organism, antibiotic hypersensitivity, poor absorption or

inadequate dose of antibiotic, impaired immunity, or development of complication (see below).

Complications

- Parapneumonic effusion.
- Empyema (➔ see Pleural infection and empyema, pp. 658–61).
- Lung abscess.
- Acute respiratory distress syndrome (ARDS).
- Sepsis syndrome.
- Metastatic infection (meningitis, arthritis, endocarditis).
- End-organ sequelae of septicaemia (e.g. renal failure).
- Rare neurological sequelae may follow *M. pneumoniae* infection (e.g. meningoencephalitis, cranial nerve palsies, and GBS).

Prevention

UKHSA guidelines in relation to influenza and pneumococcal immunization of at-risk individuals should be followed.

All patients aged >65 years or at risk of invasive pneumococcal disease who are admitted with CAP and who have not previously received the pneumococcal vaccine should receive the 23-valent pneumococcal polysaccharide vaccine (23-PPV) at convalescence.

References

3 British Thoracic Society; Community Acquired Pneumonia in Adults Guideline Group (2009). *BTS guidelines for the management of community acquired pneumonia in adults: update 2009.* Available at: ✎ www.brit-thoracic.org.uk/quality-improvement/guidelines/pneumonia-adults/

Atypical pneumonias

A term coined in the 1930s to describe a clinical presentation that did not follow the 'typical' pneumococcal-like pattern, being, for example, non-responsive to penicillin, with less classic CXR appearances, and causing dyspnoea/cough without sputum. It is now known that this syndrome is seen with various pathogens including *M. pneumoniae*, *C. pneumoniae*, *L. pneumophila*, and respiratory viruses. Clinical signs tend to be milder than what the CXR would suggest, with infiltration usually of the lower lobes, either bilateral or unilateral. The clinical course is usually benign, although certain organisms may cause extrapulmonary symptoms (e.g. mycoplasmal infection and neurological sequelae) or severe disease (e.g. *Legionella*). The CXR tends to improve faster than in typical pneumonia. It is good practice to avoid the term 'atypical pneumonia', although it is still useful to refer to 'atypical organisms', as they have certain features in common—they tend not to be respiratory tract colonizers; they affect healthy individuals of all age groups; they occur in epidemics, and they do not respond to penicillin.

Mycoplasma pneumoniae

(➔ See *Mycoplasma*, pp. 386–8.)

- Causes 10–30% of CAP, mostly mild disease treated as outpatient.
- Typically autumn epidemics every 4–8 years (more frequently within closed populations such as in prisons, military bases, and boarding schools). Majority of cases under 40 years of age.

- Protracted clinical course with constitutional and upper respiratory tract symptoms for up to 10 days prior to development of non-productive cough, which may persist for weeks. Mostly mild disease, but occasionally severe and requiring intensive care.
- Difficult to culture—diagnosis is usually by PCR or paired serology.
- Serum cold agglutination is a non-specific test (positive in 50–70% of patients after 7–10 days of infection).
- CXR appearance is of unilateral or bilateral patchy infiltrates, usually in the lower lobes. Sometimes a nodular infiltration resembling that associated with other diseases with granulomatous pathology such as TB, mycoses, and sarcoidosis.
- Treatment—clarithromycin or doxycycline.
- Rare extrapulmonary manifestations—pericarditis, arthritis, bullous myringitis, Stevens–Johnson syndrome, haemolytic anaemia, thrombocytopenia, CNS infections, GBS, peripheral neuropathy, other neurological manifestations, and ocular complications.

Legionella pneumophila

(➔ See *Legionella*, pp. 353–5.)
- Legionnaire's disease (first described as an epidemic involving attendees at an American Legion convention) is an acute pneumonic illness caused by *Legionella* spp., with over 80% of cases due to *L. pneumophila* serogroup 1. *Legionella* is also responsible for Pontiac fever, which is a febrile, non-pneumonic illness.
- Accounts for 1–20% of CAP cases. Commoner in summer.
- The organism colonizes water piping systems, and outbreaks are associated with acquisition from contaminated water sources, including cooling systems, showers, decorative fountains, humidifiers, respiratory therapy equipment, and whirlpool spas.
- Risk factors—smoking, chronic lung disease, diabetes, malignancy, uncontrolled HIV, end-stage renal disease, alcohol abuse.
- Clinical features—1- to 2-day prodrome (mild headache and myalgias) is followed by high fever (often >40°C), chills and rigors, cough (non-productive, becoming productive as the disease progresses), dyspnoea, pleuritic chest pain, haemoptysis, nausea, vomiting, diarrhoea, abdominal pain, altered mental status, arthralgias, and myalgias. Consider it in those with high fever, multilobar involvement, a need for ICU admission, and rapidly evolving GI, neurological, and radiographic abnormalities. Laboratory abnormalities include disseminated intravascular coagulopathy (DIC), SIADH, abnormal LFTs, and renal impairment.
- Diagnosis—urine antigen testing is most commonly used but has poor sensitivity for non-*L. pneumophila* serotype 1 subtypes. Culture or PCR testing of sputum or deep respiratory samples can be performed.
- Treatment—levofloxacin. Alternative clarithromycin.
- Mortality rate of 25% (may be related to comorbidities).

Chlamydophila pneumoniae

(➔ See *Chlamydophila pneumoniae*, p. 391.)
- Accounts for 3–10% of CAP cases in adults.
- Usually occurs sporadically, but epidemics are well documented.

- Upper respiratory tract symptoms (hoarseness, sore throat) precede a typically mild pneumonia. May be more severe in the elderly.
- Cough and malaise can persist for weeks to months.
- Extrapulmonary manifestations include otitis, sinusitis, pericarditis, myocarditis, and endocarditis.
- Treatment—clarithromycin or doxycycline.

Chlamydophila psittaci

(➋ See Chlamydophila psittaci, pp. 390–1.)
- Usually associated with exposure to birds—pet shop employees and poultry industry workers are at risk.
- Clinical spectrum ranges from asymptomatic infection to fulminant toxicity.
- Consider in those patients with pneumonia splenomegaly, and a history of bird exposure (especially sick birds).
- May develop rash, hepatitis, haemolytic anaemia, DIC, meningoencephalitis, or reactive arthritis.
- Treatment—tetracycline.
- Mortality rate <1%.

Coxiella burnetii

(➋ See Coxiella burnetii, pp. 382–4.)
- An intracellular pathogen found worldwide, with the exception of New Zealand. Highly prevalent in parts of Spain and France (second commonest cause of CAP in some regions).
- Reservoir primarily are farm animals (e.g. cattle, goats, sheep). Excreted in urine, milk, and faeces, and attains high concentrations in birth products.
- Persists in environment.
- Acquisition is mainly inhalational via contaminated aerosolized dust/soil.
- Rare human-to-human transmission from exposure to the placenta of an infected woman and from blood transfusions.
- Acute Q fever may cause a febrile illness, pneumonia, or hepatitis. Disease is more severe in pregnancy (also associated with miscarriage and intrauterine growth restriction (IUGR)).
- Diagnosis—paired serum samples (response to phase II antigen is associated with acute disease, with a shift to phase I in chronic disease). PCR may be performed on whole blood or serum.
- Most cases of acute Q fever resolve spontaneously within 2 weeks, but progression to chronic Q fever occurs in <5% of cases.
- Treatment—doxycycline and hydroxychloroquine combination. Prolonged duration in chronic disease.

Aspiration pneumonia

Elderly patients, those with neurological impairment (e.g. acute phase of stroke), and others with altered consciousness (e.g. alcoholics) and abnormal swallow/gag reflexes are at risk of aspiration. Acid aspiration results in the release of proinflammatory cytokines that recruit neutrophils into the lung. These are thought to be the key mediators of acute lung injury. This chemical pneumonitis, along with acute obstruction (secondary to aspirated matter), results in acute symptoms, with bacterial pneumonia developing several days later. Abscess and empyema are not uncommon complications. The organisms involved in aspiration pneumonia reflect the microbiota of the oropharynx. Subsequently, anaerobes, either alone or mixed with oral aerobes or facultative anaerobes, are the predominant causative organisms (e.g. *Bacteroides* spp., *Porphyromonas* spp., *Fusobacterium*). Gram-negative aerobes, including *P. aeruginosa*, occur at higher frequency in hospital- or ventilator-related aspiration. Bronchoscopy may be indicated to provide material for culture and exclude foreign bodies. BTS guidelines recommend co-amoxiclav as first-line treatment.[4]

References

4 www.brit-thoracic.org.uk/quality-improvement/guidelines/pneumonia-adults/

Hospital-acquired pneumonia

- Hospital-acquired pneumonia (HAP) is the leading cause of infection-related deaths in hospital. Defined as pneumonia developing >48h after admission.
- Sixty per cent of cases are caused by aerobic Gram-negatives, the majority being *Enterobacterales* (*K. pneumoniae*, *E. coli*, *Serratia marcescens*, *Acinetobacter*) and *Pseudomonas* spp. Other causes include *S. aureus*, *S. pneumoniae*, and anaerobes. Nosocomial outbreaks of viral pneumonia are not uncommon.
- Risk factors include:
  - patient-related—age >70 years, severe underlying disease, malnutrition, coma, metabolic acidosis, and possibly sinusitis;
  - infection control-related—poor healthcare worker (HCW) hand hygiene, contaminated respiratory equipment;
  - intervention-related—sedatives, corticosteroids, cytotoxic drugs, prolonged antibiotic use, ventilation (risk of acquiring pneumonia 20 times that in unventilated patients).
- Send sample (sputum sample, nasopharyngeal swab, or tracheal aspirate) for microbiological testing.
- Treatment[5]—should reflect severity of symptoms (based on clinical assessment), length of inpatient stay, recent antibiotic use, local antimicrobial resistance data, patient microbiological results (colonization, multidrug resistance), and risk of adverse effects with antimicrobial therapy (including *Clostridioides difficile* infection). Empirical PO therapy for non-severe HAP is co-amoxiclav (alternatives: doxycycline, co-trimoxazole). IV options for severe disease or higher risk of resistance include piperacillin–tazobactam, levofloxacin, or ceftazidime. Antibiotic choice should be altered (ideally to a narrow-spectrum agent) once microbiological results are available. Review IV therapy at 48h, and switch to a PO agent if clinically improving. Review antibiotic treatment at total 5 days' therapy, and consider stopping if stable.

References

8 National Institute for Health and Care Excellence (2019). *Pneumonia (hospital-acquired): antimicrobial prescribing*. NICE guideline [NG139]. Available at: ℞ https://www.nice.org.uk/guidance/ng139

Ventilator-associated pneumonia

Defined as a type of HAP that develops after >48h of mechanical ventilation. Complicates the clinical course of around 10% of intubated patients.

- Causes—predominant organisms are *P. aeruginosa*, *S. aureus*, *Enterobacterales*, *Haemophilus* spp., and *Acinetobacter* spp., but aetiology varies according to the ICU, duration of inpatient stay, and prior antibiotic use. Patients hospitalized for prolonged periods and who are antibiotic-exposed are at risk of *S. maltophilia*, *Burkholderia cepacia*, and other difficult-to-treat infections. Polymicrobial infections are common, especially in aspiration pneumonia and ARDS.
- Pathogenesis—factors combine to increase the risk of pneumonia in ventilated patients, including endotracheal tube (ETT) placement compromising the natural barrier between the oropharynx and the trachea, pooling of respiratory secretions above the cuff facilitating entry into the lungs, and rapid formation of biofilm serving as a bacterial reservoir.
- Risk factors—hypoalbuminaemia, age ≥60 years, ARDS, COPD, coma, burns, trauma, organ failure, gastric aspiration, gastric colonization and pH, upper respiratory tract colonization, sinusitis, H2 receptor antagonists, paralytic agents, prior antibiotics, continuous sedation, mechanical ventilation >2 days, reintubation, tracheostomy, nasogastric tube, supine position.
- Clinical features—can be non-specific. A diagnosis of VAP is based on new or worsening pulmonary infiltrates, with clinical evidence of infection (e.g. fever, purulent sputum, leucocytosis, decline in oxygenation), together with a significant pathogen identified in respiratory samples. Differentials—aspiration pneumonitis, PE, ARDS, pulmonary haemorrhage, lung contusion, vasculitis.
- Diagnosis—there is no gold standard for diagnosis. Most experts agree that cultures of the lower respiratory tract should be sent, but there is disagreement on the method of sampling (invasive versus non-invasive) and whether cultures should be quantitative or not.[5,6] European guidelines state a preference for invasive sampling (e.g. BAL, protective specimen brush), with quantitative cultures.[6] Practice varies across institutions.
- Treatment[5]—once respiratory samples have been obtained, empirical therapy targeting likely organisms and susceptibility patterns should be commenced. In early-onset VAP (≤5 days after hospital admission), the organisms are community-acquired and unlikely to be multidrug-resistant (MDR). Treatment options include piperacillin–tazobactam or levofloxacin. In cases of late-onset VAP (>5 days after hospital admission), recent IV antibiotic use (within 90 days), or septic shock, there is an increased risk of MDR organisms. Infectious Diseases Society of America (IDSA)/American Thoracic Society (ATS) guidelines

recommend treatment with an antipseudomonal agent (cephalosporin, piperacillin–tazobactam, or carbapenem) plus a fluoroquinolone or an aminoglycoside. Vancomycin or linezolid should be added if there is a possibility of MRSA. Refer to local guidelines and resistance rates.
- Prognosis—mortality ranges from 24% to 76%.

References

5 Kalil AC, Metersky ML, Klompas M, *et al.* Management of adults with hospital-acquired and ventilator-associated pneumonia: 2016 clinical practice guidelines by the Infectious Diseases Society of America and the American Thoracic Society. *Clin Infect Dis.* 2016;**63**:e61–111.

6 Torres A, Niederman MS, Chastre J, *et al.* International ERS/ESICM/ESCMID/ALAT guidelines for the management of hospital-acquired pneumonia and ventilator-associated pneumonia. *Eur Respir J.* 2017;**50**:1700582.

Pulmonary infiltrates with eosinophilia

Pulmonary infiltrates with eosinophilia (PIE), or eosinophilic pneumonia, is a syndrome caused by a range of aetiologies, some of which are infection-related. These include:
- tropical pulmonary eosinophilia, most cases being secondary to microfilarial infection with *Wuchereria bancrofti* or *Brugia malayi*;
- Löffler's syndrome (pulmonary eosinophilia with transient pulmonary infiltrates) is associated with *Ascaris* (most commonly), *Strongyloides*, and hookworm infection;
- TB;
- brucellosis;
- psittacosis;
- coccidioidomycosis;
- histoplasmosis;
- bronchopulmonary mycosis (e.g. *Aspergillus*);
- PCP.

Non-infectious causes include:
- drug effect (e.g. NSAIDs, sulfasalazine) and toxin ingestion (e.g. particulate metals, inhalation of heroin);
- idiopathic acute eosinophilic pneumonia (associated with vaping and heavy exposure to smoke or fine sand);
- chronic eosinophilic pneumonia;
- sarcoidosis;
- eosinophilic granulomatosis with polyangiitis (Churg–Strauss syndrome);
- eosinophilic leukaemia;
- paraneoplastic syndromes;
- hypersensitivity pneumonitis.

Pleural infection and empyema

Pleural infection is bacterial entry and replication in the pleural space. Empyema refers to pleural fluid that is purulent or has positive microbial culture. The BTS guidelines use the term 'pleural infection' to include both empyema and 'complicated' parapneumonic effusion (CPPE).

Aetiology

- Usually secondary to pneumonia. Cases may occur with no evidence of pneumonia (primary empyema). Other precipitants: surgery, trauma, oesophageal perforation, chest drains.
- Pathogens differ between community and hospital settings. Community-acquired: *S. pneumoniae*, *Streptococcus milleri* group, *S. aureus*, *Streptococcus pyogenes*, anaerobes, and *Enterobacterales*. Hospital-acquired: MRSA and Gram-negative organisms are becoming commoner. TB is a common cause where the disease is prevalent.
- Cases associated with aspiration or arising from GI sites are more likely to be due to anaerobic organisms. Those associated with subdiaphragmatic disease are often polymicrobial. Aerobic Gram-negative organisms are common in cases complicating trauma or surgery and those associated with serous effusions.
- The immunocompromised have higher rates of Gram-negative and fungal empyema generally in the context of disseminated disease.
- Rare: parasites, including *Echinococcus* spp. (hydatid disease) and *Entamoeba histolytica* (amoebiasis).

Clinical features

- Chest pain, breathlessness, weight loss, night sweats, fever. Examination reveals only signs of effusion in most cases
- Consider an oesophageal rupture in those who develop a pleural effusion soon after significant retching or vomiting.
- Features of ongoing sepsis and raised CRP after >3 days in patients with pneumonia may indicate progression to pleural infection.

Diagnosis

See BTS guidelines for management of pleural infection.[7] A new BTS guideline is currently out for public consultation.[8]

- BCs—should be performed in all cases of suspected pleural infection.
- Radiology—CXR shows pleural effusion. USS permits diagnostic aspiration and identification of loculated effusions. Contrast CT distinguishes empyema from most lung abscesses and is used to monitor treatment.
- Diagnostic sampling—should be performed in all patients with a pleural effusion of >10mm in depth in the context of pneumonia or sepsis. Samples should be kept tightly sealed on ice to prevent changes in pH and glucose. The presence of frank pus is diagnostic of an empyema and indicates the need for prompt chest tube drainage. Cultures may be negative in patients receiving antibiotics.
- Pleural fluid biochemistry—pH should be measured immediately (see Table 14.1).[7,8] Low pH values (6–6.7) should raise suspicion of oesophageal rupture or chronic empyema. Remember low pH/glucose may occur in TB, malignancy, etc. Where immediate pH measurement is not possible, glucose levels of <4.0mmol/L indicate moderate to high risk of CPPE.

Table 14.1 Pleural fluid characteristics in pleural infection

Stage	Pleural fluid findings	Comments
Very low risk of CPPE	pH >7.4	No indication for immediate ICD
		Monitor clinical progress; reassess need for repeated aspiration if not improving.
Intermediate risk of CPPE	pH >7.2 and <7.4 LDH >900IU/L Glucose <4.0mmol/L	Chest tube drainage should be considered, particularly if febrile, high pleural fluid volume, pleural enhancement on CT, or septation on USS
High risk of CCPE	Clear or cloudy fluid; pH <7.2; may be Gram stain- or culture-positive	Requires chest tube drainage
Empyema	Purulent fluid; may be Gram stain- or culture-positive	Requires chest tube drainage

CPPE, complicated parapneumonic effusion; ICD, intercostal drainage; LDH, lactate dehydrogenase.

- Pleural fluid Gram staining and culture—positive Gram staining and/or culture indicates progression to complicated effusion and the need for chest tube drainage.
- Culture-negative cases—consider BCs, urine antigen testing for *Legionella* or histoplasmosis, pleural biopsy in suspected TB (95% positive on histology, compared to 23% on pleural fluid culture/ microscopy), serology for *E. histolytica* (positive in 98% of patients with pleural amoebiasis), microscopy/culture of empyema pus for acid-fast bacilli (AFB) in those at risk of nocardiosis, and examination of faecal/ sputum samples for eggs in cases with pleural or blood eosinophilia suggestive of paragonimiasis.

Management

- Drainage—adequate drainage of infected fluid from the pleural space is the cornerstone of pleural infection management. Empyema requires prompt ICD insertion. Where diagnostic aspiration does not yield frank pus, pH analysis should be performed (see Table 14.1).[7,8] If pH is <7.2 indicating a high risk of CPPE, an ICD should be inserted. If pH >7.2 and <7.4 indicating an immediate risk of CCPE, then ICD should be considered, particularly if the presence of other factors (pleural fluid biochemistry, clinical and radiological features) indicates progression to a complicated clinical course. Involve respiratory physicians.

- Antibiotics—should be guided by culture results where available. Culture-negative cases should receive antibiotics covering community-acquired and anaerobic organisms (e.g. co-amoxiclav). Broader-spectrum cover should be initiated in hospital-acquired empyema. Consider adding a macrolide in known/suspected *Legionella* infections. Once fever has settled, convert to PO antibiotics and continue treatment for a total of 2–6 weeks, with the total duration based on the clinical, biochemical, and radiological response.
- New in 2022 guideline: intrapleural fibrinolytics (combination of tissue plasminogen activator and DNAse) should be considered for treatment of pleural infection where initial chest tube drainage has ceased and leaves a residual pleural collection.[1]
- Consider bronchoscopy if there is a high index of suspicion of bronchial obstruction.
- In patients with persistent sepsis and/or residual pleural effusion, review the diagnosis and perform a CT chest to confirm chest tube position and effusion anatomy, and look for obstructing lesions, etc.
- Surgery—patients should be considered for surgery if they have ongoing sepsis with a persistent pleural collection by day 7, despite chest tube drainage and antibiotics. Modalities include video-assisted thoracoscopic surgery (VATS), open thoracic drainage, or thoracotomy and decortication.

References

7 British Thoracic Society; *BTS pleural disease guideline 2022*. Available at: ⅍ https://www.brit-thoracic.org.uk/quality-improvement/guidelines/pleural-disease/

Lung abscess

Lung abscess is defined as necrosis of the pulmonary parenchyma caused by microbial infection, resulting in a pus-filled fluid cavity.

Pathogenesis

- Most lung abscesses are polymicrobial infections involving bacteria from the oropharynx.
- Primary abscesses (comprising 80%) follow aspiration in the context of states of altered consciousness (e.g. alcoholism, stroke) or dysphagia (e.g. neurological disease). Strongly associated with periodontal disease.
- In secondary abscesses, the inciting factor is underlying disease or surgery—tumour, infectious mass, septic embolization, bronchiectasis, immunosuppression, and pharyngeal instrumentation (e.g. endotracheal intubation). Up to 5% of PEs may become secondarily infected.
- Most patients present with a single abscess. Location reflects that of aspiration pneumonia—the posterior segment of the right upper lobe and apical segments of the lower lobes.
- Lung bases may be affected in cases of subdiaphragmatic extension (e.g. amoebic liver abscess).
- Multiple abscesses follow septic embolization (e.g. *S. aureus* right heart endocarditis) or bacteraemia (enteric Gram-negatives and anaerobes).

Microbiology

- Most frequently caused by oral anaerobes (e.g. *Peptostreptococcus*, *Prevotella*, *Bacteroides* (usually not *Bacteroides fragilis*), and *Fusobacterium*).
- Common non-anaerobes—*S. milleri* group.
- Other bacterial include *S. aureus*, *K. pneumoniae*, other Gram-negative bacilli, group A *Streptococcus* (GAS), *Burkholderia pseudomallei*, *H. influenzae* type b, *Actinomyces*, mycobacteria (TB and non-tuberculous).
- Immunocompromised hosts—*Legionella*, *Nocardia*, *Rhodococcus*, and moulds such as *Aspergillus*.
- Rare—*E. histolytica* (amoebiasis).

Clinical features

- Cases diagnosed late may present with several weeks or months of cough, low-grade fever, weight loss, anaemia, and clubbing. Sputum is copious and may be foul-smelling. Findings are those of severe pneumonia, with or without effusion.
- In cases of secondary lung abscess, the primary lesion may also be apparent (endocarditis, subphrenic infection, etc.), and lung lesions multiple (e.g. *S. aureus* in people who inject drugs).
- Necrotizing pneumonia—seen in severe cases of anaerobic infection and may affect a single segment or extend to involve one or both lungs, with associated empyema. Disease rapidly spreads, destroying large volumes of parenchyma. Patients appear ill, with pronounced leucocytosis. Pulmonary actinomycosis may present similarly.
- Amoebic lung abscesses—features of coexisting liver abscess and presents with cough productive of brown-red (anchovy sauce) sputum.
- Complications—empyema (one-third of cases), brain abscess, localized bronchiectasis. TB should be considered.

Diagnosis

- Radiology—CXR may reveal a cavity with an air–fluid level. CT facilitates detection of smaller lesions.
- Microbiology—sputum culture typically yields polymicrobial respiratory flora. Quantitative culture of bronchoscopic sampling can provide good results. It is essential samples are placed in anaerobic conditions for transport to the laboratory. BCs may be positive but may not reveal the entire infecting flora. Culture of empyema fluid or percutaneous transtracheal aspiration (CT-guided) may be useful if poor clinical response or secondary abscess; consider mycobacteria, fungi, and parasites in appropriate clinical contexts.

Treatment

- Empirical therapy while awaiting culture—community-acquired cases (e.g. co-amoxiclav); nosocomially acquired infection may require broader cover. Vancomycin should be considered if local rates of MRSA warrant it.
- Limited data on duration, minimum 3–4 weeks with clinical monitoring. Longer for large abscesses or immunocompromise.
- Bronchoscopy and postural physiotherapy may facilitate drainage.

- Medical management is sufficient for most cases. Risk factors for failure include malignancy, large abscess, and resistant organisms. Surgical resection (segmentectomy) has been employed in the past, but percutaneous and endoscopic drainage is increasingly used, with success.

Prognosis
- Overall mortality is <5–10% for primary lung abscesses, and higher for secondary abscesses, depending on the cause.
- Mortality is higher in acute pneumonias caused by resistant or virulent organisms such as *P. aeruginosa* and *S. aureus*.

Cystic fibrosis

CF is the commonest life-limiting autosomal recessive disease in the UK, affecting approximately 10 500 people (1 in 2000–3000 live births). CF usually presents with respiratory infections and pancreatic insufficiency.

Pathogenesis

CF is caused by mutations in the CF transmembrane conductance regulator (CFTR) protein, which is found in all exocrine tissues. Defective transport of chloride and other ions leads to thick, viscous secretions in the lungs, pancreas, liver, intestine, and reproductive tract, and to increased sweat chloride levels.

Microbiology

- *S. aureus*—most prevalent organism in childhood, persists in adulthood.
- *H. influenzae*—affects 20–30% of children, less prevalent in adults.
- *P. aeruginosa*—colonizes in childhood or early adolescence; >80% are infected by adulthood. Early non-mucoid isolates can be eradicated. Later isolates produce large amounts of mucoid polysaccharide (alginate), are difficult to eradicate, and are associated with higher mortality than non-mucoid strains. Chronic infection is associated with rapid decline in lung function and increased mortality.
- *B. cepacia* complex—an important and highly transmissible group of pathogens, intrinsically resistant to aminoglycosides and polymyxins. May be difficult to identify, requiring specific isolation media ± referral to reference laboratory. Colonized patients should be separated from non-colonized patients. Infection with *Burkholderic cenocepacia* can lead to rapid deterioration in pulmonary function bacteraemia, and even death amongst adolescents and young adults (cepacia syndrome).
- Other pathogens—non-typeable *H. influenzae*, *S. maltophilia*, *Achromobacter* (formerly *Alcaligenes*) *xylosoxidans*, non-tuberculous mycobacteria (NTM) (e.g. *Mycobacterium abscessus* complex, *Mycobacterium avium* complex (MAC)), *Aspergillus* spp.

Clinical features

- Reflect obstruction of organs by viscous secretions and the presence of chronic bacterial lung infection.
- General features—chronic cough, wheeze, recurrent pneumonia, sinusitis, clubbing, haemoptysis, pneumothorax, signs of respiratory

impairment. Hypoxia and carbon dioxide retention are uncommon. CXR may show airway thickening, retained secretions, and bronchiectasis.

- Acute respiratory infections—patients often produce a large amount of purulent sputum, even when well. Episodes of deterioration are associated with increased volume and purulence of sputum, dyspnoea, wheeze, chest ache, anorexia, and malaise. High fever or sepsis is unusual, despite the large number of organisms in secretions (10^8 organisms/mL of sputum). CXR may be unchanged from the patient's normal film. Forced expiratory volume in 1s (FEV_1) falls, returning to pre-infection levels with successful antibiotic therapy.
- Other clinical features include meconium ileus, distal ileal obstruction, rectal prolapse, biliary disease, infertility, musculoskeletal disorders, recurrent venous thrombosis, nephrolithiasis, and nephrocalcinosis.

Management

The aims are to slow lung damage by removing viscous airway secretions, control bacterial infection, and monitor the appearance of highly transmissible or antibiotic-resistant organisms. Antibiotics need to be given to CF patients for longer and at frequent, higher doses than to non-CF patients. Outpatient IV antibiotic therapy may be given via a long line. Those requiring very frequent antibiotics may require insertion of a Port-a-cath.

- General measures—postural drainage, deep breathing, coughing, exercise, aerosolized dornase alfa (reduces mucus viscosity, clears airway secretions), inhaled steroids, bronchodilators (helpful in some patients). Pneumococcal and annual influenza vaccinations are recommended. Lung transplantation should be considered if life expectancy is <2 years and quality of life is severely impaired despite medical therapy.
- CFTR modulator therapy—aims to increase protein expression at the cell surface, or its function, with drug therapy. NHS England-approved modulators (ivacaftor, tezacaftor/ivacaftor, and elexacaftor/tezacaftor/ivacaftor) are available for those with specific *CFTR* genotypes.[9]
- Antimicrobial prophylaxis—controversial. A Cochrane review[10] found that antibiotic prophylaxis against *S. aureus* infection reduced isolation of *S. aureus* from the sputum but had no impact on lung function. Endorsed by guidelines in some countries, including the UK Cystic Fibrosis Trust; recommends PO flucloxacillin from diagnosis until the age of 2 years, and some UK clinics promote lifelong prophylaxis.[11]
- Eradication of *Pseudomonas* colonization—the first isolation of a non-mucoid *Pseudomonas* strain should be treated with the aim of eradication (e.g. an initial treatment protocol combining 3 months with nebulized colistin is widely used). If presenting with respiratory exacerbation, a 2-week course of IV antipseudomonal antibiotic should be considered prior to eradication therapy.
- Long-term management of *Pseudomonas* colonization—a Cochrane review concluded that nebulized antibiotic treatment improves lung function and reduces the frequency of respiratory exacerbations. Colistin achieve low systemic and high local concentrations in the lung, and is the initial treatment of choice. If not tolerated/poor response,

tobramycin is second line.[11,12] Some centres advocate elective courses of IV antipseudomonal therapy every 3 months to reduce the frequency of exacerbations and consequent lung damage. There is no evidence to support this.

- Treatment of acute exacerbations[11,13]—the patient's most recent sputum culture result should be used to guide therapy. However, antibiogram and clinical response may be discordant (presence of small colony variants and biofilm). Broad-spectrum PO agents may be beneficial, despite the presence of resistant *P. ceruginosa*. High doses and prolonged therapy (3–4 weeks) are recommended. Aggressive IV therapy is indicated in those patients who do not respond to PO treatment. Such therapy is usually directed at *P. aeruginosa* (e.g. ceftazidime combined with tobramycin or colistin). *H. influenzae* and *S. aureus* should be treated if isolated, even if the patient is asymptomatic. *B. cepacia* is very resistant and should be treated with a combination of two or three agents such as ceftazidime and an aminoglycoside. Nebulized vancomycin can be used to treat MRSA colonization of sputum, but IV therapy is required for exacerbations. Parenteral therapy may be given on an outpatient basis and should continue for 10–14 days or longer. *Aspergillus* is frequently cultured from sputum. Treatment (steroids ± antifungals) is indicated if allergic bronchopulmonary aspergillosis (ABPA) is present (well-described complication in CF).

References

9 NHS England (2023). *Updated commissioning statement: ivacaftor, tezacaftor/ivacaftor, lumacaftor/ ivacaftor and elexacaftor/tezacaftor/ivacaftor for icensed and off-label use in patients with cystic fibrosis who have named mutations.* Available at: 🔗 https://www.england.nhs.uk/wp-content/ uploads/2021/03/Commissioning-statement-CF-modulator-therapies-for-cystic-fibrosis-vers ion-4.pdf

10 Smyth AR, Walters S. Prophylactic anti-staphylococca. antibiotics for cystic fibrosis. *Cochrane Database Syst Rev.* 2012;**12**:CD001912.

11 UK Cystic Fibrosis Trust Antibiotic Working Group (2009). *Antibiotic treatment for cystic fibrosis,* third edition. Available at: 🔗 https://www.cysticfibrosis.org.uk/sites/default/files/2020-11/ Anitbiotic%20Treatment.pdf

12 Ryan G, Mukhopadhyay S, Singh M. Nebulised anti-pseudomonal antibiotics for cystic fibrosis. *Cochrane Database Syst Rev.* 2003;**3**:CD001021.

13 Smyth A, Bell S, Bojcin L, *et al.* European Cystic Fibrosis Society standards of care: best practice guidelines. *J Cyst Fibros.* 2014;**13**(Suppl 1):S23–42. Available at: 🔗 https://www.cysticfibrosis journal.com/article/S1569-1993%2814%2900085-X/fulltext

Bronchiectasis

Bronchiectasis is a respiratory condition characterized by chronic daily cough, mucopurulent sputum production, and bronchial wall thickening and luminal dilatation on CT chest.

Epidemiology

- UK prevalence of around 500/100 000, commoner in women.

Aetiology and pathogenesis

- Induction of bronchiectasis requires an infectious insult and impaired drainage, airway obstruction (e.g. foreign body, tumour, anatomical abnormality), or a defect in host defence (e.g. ciliary dyskinesia,

α1-antitrypsin (A1AT) deficiency, hypogammaglobulinaemia, immunosuppression).
- Conditions associated with bronchiectasis include COPD, A1AT deficiency, asthma, CF, Young's syndrome, rheumatoid arthritis, Sjögren's syndrome, inflammatory bowel disease (IBD), gastro-oesophageal reflux disease (GORD), and rarely systemic lupus erythematosus (SLE) and Marfan's syndrome.
- A number of pulmonary infections are associated with development of bronchiectasis (e.g. ABPA, pertussis, MTB, NTM infections).
- Often no cause is found despite aetiological testing.
- Organisms isolated during acute exacerbations include *H. influenzae*, *Moraxella catarrhalis*, *S. aureus*, *P. aeruginosa*, and less commonly *S. pneumoniae*.

Clinical features
- The classic feature is chronic cough, productive of mucopurulent sputum for months to years. Other symptoms—dyspnoea, wheezing, rhinosinusitis, fatigue, haemoptysis, and pleuritic chest pain.
- Physical findings include crackles, wheezing, and finger clubbing.

Diagnosis
- Consider investigation for bronchiectasis in patients with persistent mucopurulent sputum production, particularly those with relevant risk factors.
- Imaging—perform a baseline CXR. Diagnosis is confirmed by CT, demonstrating bronchial dilatation. CT can also aid in identification of the aetiology (e.g. ABPA, NTM, primary ciliary dyskinesia (PCD)).
- Aetiological investigations—past medical history to identify possible causative disease, FBC, total immunoglobulin E (IgE), and assessment of sensitization (specific IgE) to *Aspergillus fumigatus*, immunoglobulins (if raised, follow with serum protein electrophoresis); consider pneumococcal antibody titres (and vaccinate if deficient prior to retesting); *CFTR* gene mutation analysis. Test for PCD if supporting clinical features: neonatal distress, symptom onset in childhood, recurrent otitis media, infertility.
- A sputum sample should be sent for smear and culture for pyogenic bacteria, mycobacteria, and fungi.
- Investigate for reflux and aspiration in symptomatic patients.
- In younger patients (usually <50 years), consider rheumatoid factor (RF), anti-cyclic citrullinated peptide (CCP), antinuclear antibody (ANA), antineutrophil cytoplasmic antibody (ANCA), A1AT deficiency testing.
- Lung function tests show an obstructive defect.

Imaging
- CXR findings include linear atelectasis, dilated and thickened airways ('tramline' thickening or ring shadows), and irregular peripheral opacities (mucus plugs).
- CT is the imaging modality of choice—characteristic features include airway dilatation (bronchoarterial ratio >1), lack of tapering, bronchial wall thickening, mucopurulent plugs/debris with distal airway trapping, and cysts of the bronchial wall.

Management

- Airway clearance techniques (e.g. active cyc e of breathing) should be taught to all patients.
- Treatment of underlying disease if possible (e.g. immunodeficiency, ABPA, GORD).
- Annual influenza and pneumococcal vaccines.
- If >3 exacerbations/year despite above measures, consider mucoactive treatment. If no improvement, the next step is consideration of long-term PO or inhaled antibiotic by a respiratory specialist (e.g. inhaled colistin for *Pseudomonas* if colonized or azithromycin).
- Acute exacerbations—should be promptly treated with antibiotics. Empirical antibiotics can be commenced while awaiting sputum culture; antibiotics can then be modified. Antibiotic courses of 14 days are standard, particularly in *P. aeruginosa* infection. Manual airway clearance should be offered.
- Inhaled glucocorticoids are not routinely used, unless other indications (e.g. ABPA, asthma).
- Patients with severe haemoptysis may require interventions to control bleeding (e.g. bronchial artery embolization or surgery).
- Surgical resection of bronchiectatic lung or lung transplantation may be required in some cases.
- Long-term oxygen therapy should be recommended using the same eligibility criteria as those with COPD.
- All patients with bronchiectasis should undergo routine monitoring.

Further reading

Hill AT, Sullivan AL, Chalmers JD, *et al.*; BTS Bronchiectasis in Adults Guideline Development Group. British Thoracic Society guideline for bronchiectasis in adults. https://www.brit-thoracic.org.uk/quality-improvement/guidelines/bronchiectasis-in-adults/

National Institute for Health and Care Excellence (2018). *Bronchiectasis (non-cystic fibrosis), acute exacerbation: antimicrobial prescribing*. NICE guideline [NG117]. Available at: ℘ https://www.nice.org.uk/guidance/ng117

Pulmonary tuberculosis

TB is caused by the MTB complex, which comprises seven closely related species—*M. tuberculosis* (➔ see *Mycobacterium tuberculosis*, pp. 391–5), *Mycobacterium bovis*, *Mycobacterium africanum*, *Mycobacterium microti*, *Mycobacterium canetti*, *Mycobacterium caprae*, and *Mycobacterium pinnipedii*.

Epidemiology

Reduced access to TB services during the coronavirus disease 2019 (Covid-19) pandemic has resulted in a reversal of progress in global TB Milestones. In 2020, there were an estimated 9.8 million new cases of TB worldwide, and 1.3 million TB deaths amongst HIV-negative people (up from 1.2 million in 2019) and an additional 214 000 amongst HIV-positive people (up from 209 000 in 2019). Most TB cases were in the World Health Organization (WHO) regions of South East Asia (43%), Africa (25%), and the Western Pacific (18%). Additionally, there was a 15% worldwide reduction in people with MDR/rifampicin-resistant (RR) TB (box 14.1) receiving treatment in 2020, compared to 2019. This level of enrolment was equivalent to about

Box 14.1 Resistant tuberculosis

- RR—rifampicin resistance
- MDR—combined rifampicin and isoniazid resistance
- XDR—Previously defined as MDR-TB plus resistance to any fluoroquinolone (levofloxacin or moxifloxacin) and to at least one of three second-line injectable drugs (capreomycin, kanamycin, and amikacin). MDR also resistant to at least one fluoroquinolone (levofloxacin or moxifloxacin) and to at least one other Group A drug (bedaquiline or linezolid).

one in three people who develop MDR/RR-TB each year. Modelling projections suggest that the impact of disruptions caused by the pandemic are likely to worsen in the next few years.[14]

Pathogenesis

- Primary disease—TB is transmitted by inhalation of infected droplet nuclei, which results in primary infection in the lungs. If the innate immune system of the host fails to eliminate the infection, bacilli proliferate inside alveolar macrophages, resulting in the formation of a granulomatous tubercle. If bacterial replication is not controlled, the tubercle enlarges and the bacilli enter local draining lymph nodes, causing lymphadenopathy (Ghon focus). Bacteraemia may accompany initial infection. Failure by the host to mount an effective cell-mediated response and tissue repair leads to progressive destruction of the lung. Unchecked bacterial growth may lead to haematogenous spread of bacilli to produce disseminated TB.
- Latent disease—in most individuals (90%), MTB infection is contained initially by host defences and infection remains latent. However, latent infection has the potential to develop into active disease at any time.
- Reactivation disease—results from proliferation of previously dormant bacteria seeded at the time of the primary infection. Reactivation disease occurs in ~10% of cases. Risk factors include increased age, HIV infection, corticosteroid use, inhibitors of tumour necrosis factor (TNF)-α and its receptor, end-stage renal disease, diabetes mellitus, and lymphoma.

Clinical features

- Clinical presentations of pulmonary TB include:
  - primary TB—symptoms include fever, pleuritic chest pain, and less commonly retrosternal pain, fatigue, cough, arthralgia, and pharyngitis. The CXR may be normal or show hilar adenopathy, pleural effusions, and upper or lower lobe pulmonary infiltrates;
  - reactivation TB—symptoms include fever, night sweats, cough, weight loss, fatigue, chest pain, and haemoptysis. The CXR typically shows upper lobe pulmonary infiltrates, but other findings include hilar adenopathy, infiltrates or cavities in the middle or lower lung zones, pleural effusions, and solitary nodules;
  - endobronchial TB—occurs in 10–40% of patients with pulmonary TB and presents acutely with cough, sputum production, wheezing, haemoptysis, and chest pain. The CXR may be normal or show upper lobe infiltrates and cavitation;.

- Other presentations—include laryngeal TB, lower lung field TB, and tuberculoma.
- Complications—include haemoptysis pneumothorax, bronchiectasis, extensive tissue destruction, septic shock, malignancy, venous thromboembolism, and chronic pulmonary aspergillosis.

Diagnosis

(See NICE, 2016.)[15]
- CXR.
- Three respiratory samples for TB microscopy and culture, preferably spontaneously produced deep cough, otherwise induced sputum or BAL.
- Special stains—for example, Ziehl–Neelsen (ZN) or auramine phenol stain shows AFB. Fluorescence microscopy increases sensitivity (for laboratory diagnostics, ⊃ see Mycobacterium tuberculosis in chapter 7, Bacteria, pp. 391–5).
- Mycobacterial culture—this is the diagnostic gold standard but may not be available in resource-limited settings. Automated liquid culture systems (e.g. MGIT) are increasingly used.
- Nucleic acid amplification tests (NAATs)—rapid diagnostic NAATs (e.g. the Xpert® Rif/TB assay) simultaneously detect MTB DNA and rifampicin resistance. NICE recommends NAAT testing of respiratory samples if the person is living with HIV, a rapid diagnosis will alter the person's care, as part of an outbreak investigation, or if risk of MDR-TB (including previous TB treatment, contact of MDR case, birth or residence in country where >5% new cases are MDR).
- Whole genome sequencing (WGS)—provides speciation and antimicrobial susceptibility, and is now routinely used in UK reference laboratories. Currently only available for culture-positive cases (takes around 7 days after culture received in reference laboratory). The UKHSA-NHS England TB Action Plan for England supports the development of direct WGS (performed without the need for culture) from TB specimens.[16]
- Phenotypic drug susceptibility testing (DST)—is currently performed at reference laboratories to confirm sensitivity to first-line agents. In the case of resistance, phenotypic testing against second-line agents is performed.[17]
- Latent TB—Mantoux ± IGRA testing is recommended for close contacts of pulmonary or laryngeal TB and those deemed at risk of latent TB (e.g. new entrants from high-risk countries).

Management

Guided by drug susceptibility. Seek TB specialist advice.
- For drug-susceptible pulmonary TB, the standard short-course regimen is 2-month initiation phase with four drugs (rifampicin (R), isoniazid (H), pyrazinamide (Z), and ethambutol (E)), followed by a 4-month continuation phase with two drugs (rifampicin and isoniazid).
- Rifampicin-susceptible, isoniazid-resistant tuberculosis (Hr-TB)—WHO recommends rifampicin (R), ethambutol (E), pyrazinamide (Z), and levofloxacin for a duration of 6 months.[16] NICE guidance is RZE for

2 months, with RE continuation up to 7 months (>10 months in severe disease).[15]

- RR-TB and MDR-TB (resistant to at least both rifampicin and isoniazid) are grouped together and treated with the same regimens, reflecting the critical role of rifampicin in treatment. The 2022 update to the WHO treatment guidelines now advises a 6-month treatment regimen composed of bedaquiline, pretomanid, linezolid, and moxifloxacin (BPaLM) rather than 9-month or longer regimens in MDR/RR-TB patients in the absence of contra-indications. See WHO guideline for details and longer regimens.[18]
- Extensively drug-resistant (XDR)-TB: see above definition, box 14.1. Such cases may require the construction of individualised regimes – see the above WHO guideline for details.
- Latent TB—treatment choice is based on individual risk of developing active disease versus treatment adverse effects. Options are: 3 months' RH or 6 months' H.[15]

References

14 World Health Organization (2021). *Global tuberculosis report 2021*. Available at: ᯄ http://www.who.int/publications/digital/global-tuberculosis-report-2021

15 National Institute for Health and Care Excellence (2016). *Tuberculosis*. NICE guideline [NG33]. Available at: ᯄ https://www.nice.org.uk/guidance/ng33

16 UK Health Security Agency (2022). *Mycobacterium tuberculosis whole-genome sequencing and cluster investigation handbook*. Available at: ᯄ https://www.gov.uk/government/publications/tb-strain-typing-and-cluster-investigation-handbook/mycobacterium-tuberculosis-whole-genome-sequencing-and-cluster-investigation-handbook

17 Wales Centre for Mycobacteria (2021). *Information for patients and users*. Available at: ᯄ https://phw.nhs.wales/services-and-teams/reference-laboratories-and-specialist-services/wales-centre-for-mycobacteria-wcm/wales-centre-for-mycobacteria-information-for-patients-and-users/

18 World Health Organization (2022). *WHO operational handbook on tuberculosis. Module 4: treatment - drug-resistant tuberculosis treatment, 2022 update* Available at: ᯄ https://www.who.int/publications/i/item/9789240065116

Cardiovascular infections

Infective endocarditis

Infective endocarditis (IE) is characterized by infection of the endocardial surface of the heart. Historically classified as acute, subacute, or chronic, depending on the time course of the infection. Now more commonly classified according to the type of valve (native or prosthetic) and the aetiological agent (e.g. staphylococcal, streptococcal, enterococcal, fungal, culture-negative).

Epidemiology

The incidence of IE is estimated to be 0.16–5.4 cases per 1000 hospital admissions. Most patients are aged over 50 years; ♂ > ♀. The disease is uncommon in children in the absence of a predisposing condition. Risk factors include congenital heart disease, rheumatic heart disease, degenerative heart disease, prosthetic valves, intravascular catheters (IVCs), people who inject drugs (PWID), and mitral valve prolapse.

Pathogenesis

The development of IE requires the simultaneous occurrence of a number of events: alteration of the valvular surface, deposition of platelets and fibrin, colonization by bacteria, bacterial multiplication, and development of a vegetation.

Aetiology

- The commonest causes of native valve endocarditis (NVE) are *Staphylococcus aureus*, coagulase-negative staphylococci, streptococci (especially *Streptococcus sanguinis*, *Streptococcus mitis*, and *Streptococcus gallolyticus*), and enterococci.
- *S. aureus* is associated with healthcare contact, intravascular devices, and PWID.
- *S. gallolyticus* (of the *Streptococcus bovis* group) inhabits the GI tract. Bacteraemia is associated with GI malignancy (particularly *S. gallolyticus* subsp. *gallolyticus)* and should prompt GI investigation (e.g. colonoscopy).
- Enterococcal endocarditis is usually associated with manipulation of the genitourinary (GU) or GI tracts and colonic malignancy. For those with IE and an unknown source of bacteraemia, consider colonoscopy.
- HACEK (*Haemophilus*, *Aggregatibacter*, *Cardiobacterium*, *Eikenella*, *Kingella*) organisms classically present subacutely with large, friable vegetations and frequent emboli. See Box 7.9 (p. 342) for detailed names of HACEK bacteria.
- Other organisms (e.g. corynebacteria, *Listeria*, *Bacillus*, *Salmonella*, *Escherichia coli*, *Enterobacter*, *Citrobacter*, *Pseudomonas*) are uncommon.
- Culture-negative endocarditis (30% of cases) may be caused by *Coxiella burnetii*, *Chlamydia* spp., *Legionella* spp., *Mycoplasma pneumoniae*, *Bartonella* spp., *Brucella* spp., and *Tropheryma whipplei*.
- Early-onset (<2 months) prosthetic valve endocarditis (PVE) is commonly caused by *S. aureus* or coagulase-negative staphylococci. However, less virulent organisms acquired perioperatively may manifest months or years later. *Mycobacterium chimaera* is associated with a specific brand of heater–cooler unit used during cardiac surgery,

particularly valve replacement (1 case per 5000 procedures), and symptoms can develop several years post-operatively.[1]
- Most cases of late PVEs are unrelated to the perioperative period, with microbiology similar to that of NVE.
- Fungi—rare, usually *Candida* or *Aspergillus*, associated with prosthetic valves, PWID, and hospitalization on antibiotics. Poor prognosis.
- Polymicrobial infections occur in 1–2%.

Clinical features

- The incubation period may vary from days to weeks.
- Symptoms are protean and include fever (up to 90% of cases), chills, weakness, dyspnoea, sweats, anorexia, weight loss, malaise, cough, skin lesions, stroke, nausea, vomiting, headache, myalgia, arthralgia, oedema, chest pain, abdominal pain, delirium, coma, haemoptysis, and back pain.
- Physical findings include fever, cardiac murmur (85%), Roth spots, clubbing, splinter haemorrhages, Osler's nodes Janeway lesions, petechiae, peripheral emboli, splenomegaly, and septic complications (pneumonia, meningitis, mycotic aneurysms ➋ see Endovascular infections, pp. 677–9).

Diagnosis

- Blood cultures (BCs) are the most important laboratory test, and positive in approximately two-thirds of cases. Three sets should be obtained in the first 24h, from differing venepuncture sites, prior to antibiotic therapy. Bacteraemia is typically continuous, so BCs do not require timing with fever.
- Mycobacterial BCs required if *M. chimaera* is suspected.
- Blood tests may show elevated ESR (90–100%), anaemia (70–90%), leucocytosis (20–30%), leucopenia (5–15%) and thrombocytopenia (5–15%). Hypergammaglobulinaemia (20–30%) may result in false-positive results for rheumatoid factor and Venereal Disease Research Laboratory (VDRL) test. Renal impairment and hypocomplementaemia occur in 5–15%.
- Urinalysis is frequently abnormal, with proteinuria (50–60%), microscopic haematuria (30–60%), gross haematuria, pyuria, bacteriuria, and red and white cell casts. *S. aureus* in the urine may represent spillover from *S. aureus* bacteraemia/IE.
- Serology, polymerase chain reaction (PCR) on blood, and PCR and histology of surgical material are useful for diagnosis of culture-negative endocarditis.
- Echocardiography—transthoracic echocardiography (TTE) allows visualization of vegetations in 60–75% of cases, compared to >95% of cases with transoesophageal echocardiography (TOE).
- Cardiac CT and fluorodeoxyglucose (FDG)-positron emission tomography (PET)/CT may be useful where a definite diagnosis cannot be established by TTE or TOE. Sensitivity and specificity of FDG-PET/CT are reported as 36% and 99%, respectively, for NVE and as 86% and 84%, respectively, for PVE.
- ECG—lengthening of the PR interval in aortic valve endocarditis indicates aortic root involvement.

Modified Duke criteria

This schema stratifies patients with suspected IE into three categories:
- definite—identified histopathologically or by clinical criteria. Clinical diagnosis requires the presence of two major criteria, one major and two minor criteria, or five minor criteria:
  - major criteria—≥2 positive BCs (or a single positive culture for *C. burnetii*), echocardiographic evidence for endocardial involvement;
  - minor criteria—predisposing condition (heart condition, PWID), temperature >38°C, vascular phenomena, immunological phenomena, microbiological evidence (not satisfying major criteria).
- possible—one major and one minor criteria, or three minor criteria;
- rejected—firm alternative diagnosis, rapid resolution with no or short-course antibiotics, no pathological evidence of IE.

Management

- Antimicrobial therapy is targeted at the causative organism:
  - UK endocarditis guidelines;[2]
  - European Society of Cardiology (ESC) endocarditis guidelines.[3]
  - Following the findings of the 2018 POET trial (N Engl J Med 2019 Jan 31; 380(5):415–424), there is a move toward the use of oral antibiotic treatment for the treatment of endocarditis in those patients with uncomplicated disease . This is recognised in the 2023 ESC guidance above.
- Surgery is indicated in patients with life-threatening congestive cardiac failure (CCF) or cardiogenic shock due to surgically treatable valvular disease if the patient has a reasonable prospect of recovery. Surgery is recommended for annular or aortic abscesses, heart block, recurrent emboli on therapy, antibiotic-resistant infections, and fungal endocarditis.

Prevention

National Institute for Health and Care Excellence (NICE) guidelines do not recommend routine antibiotic prophylaxis for those at increased risk of endocarditis. However, any infections should be treated promptly, and if antibiotics are given for a GI or GU procedure at an infected site, they should cover causative IE organisms.[4]

References

1 Public Health England (2017). *Mycobacterium chimaera* infections: guidance for secondary care. Available at: ℗ https://www.gov.uk/government/publications/mycobacterium-chimaera-infections-guidance-for-secondary-care

2 Gould FK, Denning DW, Elliot TS, *et al.*; Working Party of the British Society for Antimicrobial Chemotherapy. Guidelines for the diagnosis and antibiotic treatment of endocarditis in adults: a report of the Working Party of the British Society for Antimicrobial Chemotherapy. *J Antimicrob Chemother.* 2012;**67**:269–89.

3 Delgado et al; 2023 ESC Guidelines for the management of endocarditis; European Heart Journal, Volume 44, Issue 39, 14 October 2023, Pages 3948–4042. Available at: https://doi.org/10.1093/eurheartj/ehad193

4 National Institute for Health and Care Excellence (2008). *Prophylaxis against infective endocarditis: antimicrobial prophylaxis against infective endocarditis in adults and children undergoing interventional procedures.* Clinical guideline [CG64]. Available at: ℗ http://www.nice.org.uk/guidance/CG64

Intravascular catheter-related infections

Definitions
- **Catheter colonization**—significant growth of organism in quantitative or semi-quantitative culture from catheter tip, subcutaneous segment, or catheter hub.
- **Phlebitis**—induration, erythema, pain, or tenderness around the exit site.
- **Exit site infection**—exudate at exit site yielding microorganism or phlebitis <2cm from the exit site plus signs of infection (fever, pus) ± bloodstream infection (BSI).
- **Tunnel infection**—phlebitis ≥2cm from the exit site, along the subcutaneous tract of the catheter ± BSI.
- **Pocket infection**—infected fluid in subcutaneous pocket of implanted intravascular device, often associated with local erythema, induration, tenderness, rupture and drainage, and necrosis of skin ± BSI.
- **BSI**—bacteraemia or fungaemia in a patient who has an intravascular device and ≥1 positive BC obtained from a peripheral vein and no obvious source (apart from the device).

Epidemiology
In the USA, >200 000 nosocomial BSIs occur per year; most of these are related to intravascular devices. Risk factors for IVC-related infections include type of catheter, site of catheter, duration of placement, and hospital demographics.

Aetiology
- Staphylococci (e.g. CoNS, *S. aureus*).
- Aerobic Gram-negative bacilli (e.g. *E. coli*, *Klebsiella* spp., *Pseudomonas* spp., *Enterobacter* spp., *Serratia* spp., *Acinetobacter* spp.).
- Fungi (e.g. *Candida* spp., *Malassezia furfur*).

Clinical features
Clinical features are unreliable. The most sensitive clinical features (e.g. fever, chills) lack specificity, whereas inflammation and purulence at the catheter site are specific but not sensitive. See the Visual Infusion Phlebitis (VIP) score for peripheral catheters in Table 6.4 (p 163).

Diagnosis
- Cultures of IVC tips—semi-quantitative (roll plate) or quantitative (flush, vortex, or sonication) methods have greater specificity than qualitative methods.
- Paired BCs drawn through the IVC and peripherally—all patients with suspected IVC-related infections should have two sets of BCs drawn, at least one peripherally. A positive culture from a line requires clinical interpretation, whereas a negative line culture virtually excludes catheter-related BSI.
- Quantitative cultures of central venous catheter (CVC) and peripheral blood samples—>3-fold greater colony count between central and peripheral cultures supports a diagnosis of catheter-related BSI.

- Differential time to positivity (DTP) for CVC and peripheral cultures—growth of microbes from a blood sample drawn from a catheter hub at least 2h before microbial growth is detected in a blood sample obtained from a peripheral vein best defines catheter-related BSI.

Management

- See Infectious Diseases Society of America (IDSA) guidelines for management of IVC-related infections.[5]
- Peripheral venous catheters (PVCs)—remove the device; swab the exit site if pus is present, and take two sets of BCs before starting antimicrobial therapy.
- Non-tunnelled CVCs—if there are local or systemic signs or positive BCs, the CVC should be removed, antimicrobial therapy started, and the CVC replaced at a new site:
  - complicated infections (septic thrombosis, endocarditis, osteomyelitis): remove the CVC, and treat with systemic antimicrobials for 4–6 weeks; 6–8 weeks for osteomyelitis;
  - uncomplicated CoNS infection: remove the CVC, and treat with 5–7 days of systemic antibiotics; if the catheter is retained, treat with systemic antibiotic + lock therapy for 10–14 weeks.
  - uncomplicated *S. aureus* bacteraemia: remove the CVC, and treat with 14 days of systemic antibiotics (if negative TOE) or 4–6 weeks of antibiotics (if positive TOE);
  - uncomplicated Gram-negative bacteraemia: remove the CVC, and treat with 10–14 days of systemic antibiotics;
  - uncomplicated candidaemia: remove the CVC, and treat with antifungals for 14 days after the last positive BC.
- Tunnelled CVCs and implanted devices (IDs)—investigations should be performed to establish the CVC or ID as the source of infection:
  - tunnel infection or port abscess: remove the CVC/ID, and treat with systemic antibiotics for 7–10 days;
  - complicated infections (septic thrombosis, endocarditis, osteomyelitis): remove the CVC/ID, and treat with systemic antibiotics for 4–6 weeks; 6–8 weeks for osteomyelitis;
  - uncomplicated CoNS infection: may retain the CVC/ID, and treat with 10–14 days of systemic antibiotics plus antibiotic lock therapy. Remove the CVC/ID if persistent bacteraemia or clinical deterioration;
  - uncomplicated *S. aureus* bacteraemia: remove the CVC/ID, and treat with 14 days of systemic antibiotics (if negative TOE) or 4–6 weeks of antibiotics (if positive TOE). For salvage therapy, see IDSA guidelines;[5]
  - uncomplicated Gram-negative bacteraemia: remove the CVC/ID, and treat with 7–14 days of systemic antibiotics.

Prevention

See IDSA guidelines for the prevention of IVC-related infections.[6]

References

5 Mermel LA, Allon M, Bouza E, *et al*. Clinical practice guidelines for the diagnosis and management of intravascular catheter-related infection: 2009 update by the Infectious Diseases Society of America. *Clin Infect Dis*. 2009;**49**:1–45.

6 O'Grady NP, Alexander M, Burns LA, *et al*.; Healthcare nfection Control Practices Advisory Committee (HICPAC). Guidelines for the prevention of intravascular catheter-related infections. *Clin Infect Dis*. 2011;**52**:e162–93.

Endovascular infections

Persistent bacteraemia (i.e. multiple BCs taken on different occasions which are positive for the same isolate) suggests endovascular infection. These include endocarditis, IVC-related infections, mycotic aneurysms, pacemaker infections, and vascular graft infections.

Mycotic aneurysm

- Definition—localized dilation of an artery due to destruction of the vessel wall by infection.
- Aetiology—in the pre-antibiotic era, mycotic aneurysms were usually associated with IE and caused by streptococci and staphylococci. Today mycotic aneurysms are usually due to haematogenous seeding of atherosclerotic vessels or trauma. Pathogens include *S. aureus*, *Salmonella* spp., aerobic Gram-negative bacilli, *Streptococcus pneumoniae*, *Streptococcus pyogenes*, *Streptococcus dysgalactiae*, *Listeria monocytogenes*, *Bacteroides fragilis*, *Clostridium septicum*, enterococci, and *C. burnetii*.
- Clinical features—symptoms and signs of IE ➲ see Infective endocarditis, pp. 672–4) may be present. Superficial infected aneurysms may present as a painful, pulsatile, and enlarging mass, together with systemic features of infection such as fever. Deeper aneurysms may not be palpable; present with fever, weight loss, and site-dependent features (e.g. back pain—aorta or iliac arteries; headache, stroke, or subarachnoid haemorrhage—intracerebral vessels; mesenteric ischaemia—superior mesenteric artery).
- Diagnosis—BCs may identify the causative organism in 50–85% of cases. Serology, PCR, and histology may aid diagnosis in culture-negative cases. CT angiography is the most useful imaging for diagnosing mycotic aneurysm. Magnetic resonance (MR) angiography is an alternative when IV contrast is contraindicated. FDG-PET/CT is an increasingly used modality.
- Management—there are no randomized control led trials to guide management, which is instead based on clinical experience and case series. Standard treatment is antibiotic therapy ± surgical excision. Empirical choice of antibiotic should be based on likely infecting organisms (e.g. vancomycin plus agent with activity against Gram-negatives, including *Salmonella* and enteric organisms, e.g. ceftriaxone, piperacillin–tazobactam). Seek microbiology advice. Intracranial aneurysms should be treated with antimicrobial therapy, monitored by angiography, and excised if they enlarge or bleed.
- Aortic mycotic aneurysms are generally managed with debridement and reconstruction and extended courses of antibiotics. Peripheral vessel mycotic aneurysms are managed by surgical resection/reconstruction

and antibiotic therapy. However, many may now be managed endovascularly (EVAR: EndoVascular Aneurysm Repair), which, while less invasive, can necessitate long-term empirical antibiotic therapy, often in the absence of culture results.

Pacemaker infections

- Implantable cardiac electronic devices (ICEDs) include implantable cardiac defibrillators (ICDs), cardiac resynchronization therapy devices (CRTDs), and permanent pacemakers (PPMs). Infection is an uncommon (incidence 0.5–2.2%), but serious, complication which can manifest as infection of the generator ('box') pocket and the leads and can also involve endocardial structures.
- Aetiology—CoNS and *S. aureus* are the commonest isolates. Other organisms include *Enterobacterales* spp., *Pseudomonas aeruginosa*, streptococci, enterococci, *Cutibacterium* (formerly known as *Propionibacterium*), and (rarely) *Candida* spp.
- Clinical features—generator pocket infection is characterized by localized cellulitis, swelling, discharge, dehiscence, or pain. Wound inflammation can be an early presentation of generator pocket infection. ICED infection may be associated with pericarditis (➔ see Pericarditis, pp. 681–3), mediastinitis (➔ see Mediastinitis, pp. 683–4), or endocarditis (➔ see Infective endocarditis, pp. 672–4). Non-specific signs and symptoms of systemic infection (including fevers, chills, night sweats, malaise, and anorexia) may be the only clinical features. May present with secondary foci such as spinal or pulmonary infection. The modified Duke criteria (although of unproven benefit in this scenario) may aid diagnosis.
- Sampling—appropriate microbiological samples include: culture of blood (×3 prior to antibiotics), lead fragments (ideally distal and proximal), lead vegetation, generator pocket tissue, and pus from a generator pocket wound.
- Management—complete and early (as soon as possible, but not >2 weeks after diagnosis) removal of an infected ICED system (generator and all leads), combined with appropriate antimicrobial therapy, is the most effective, safe, and efficient treatment option for generator pocket, ICED-LI (lead infection), and ICED-IE. If extraction is considered too risky or is declined, salvage with prolonged antibiotic therapy can be attempted. See guidelines for empirical and targeted antibiotic therapies.[7] Seek local microbiologist advice.

Prosthetic vascular graft infections

- **Epidemiology and pathogenesis**—the incidence of vascular graft infection is 1–5%. Three mechanisms are thought to be responsible for infection: intraoperative contamination (commonest), extension from adjacent infected tissue, and haematogenous seeding.
- **Aetiology**—CoNS and *S. aureus* cause the majority of infections. Less common are *Enterobacterales* spp., enterococci, streptococci, *P. aeruginosa*, *Bacteroides* spp., corynebacteria, and *Candida* spp.
- **Clinical features**—these depend on the site of the graft infection:
  - inguinal graft infections present with an inguinal mass ± pain, erythema, fever, and sinus formation;

- abdominal graft infections present with fever, abdominal pain or mass, retroperitoneal bleeding, lower extremity emboli, and GI bleeding due to erosion into the GI tract.
- **Diagnosis**[9]—superficial graft infections may be readily diagnosed clinically. Deep grafts require radiological imaging (e.g. CT or MRI abdomen) to confirm the infection. PET-CT is increasing utilized and reported as 95% sensitive and 80% specific for aortic graft infection, compared to CT angiography reported as 67% sensitive and 63% specific. BCs are often negative, unless infection involves the graft lumen.[8]
- **Management**—surgical resection of the infected graft, extensive debridement of all infected, devitalized tissues, and revascularization (preferably through an extra-anatomical, uninfected route) are the treatment of choice. Systemic antimicrobial therapy is given for 4–6 weeks post-operatively, based on microbiological identification of the causative organism if possible. Conservative management is associated with high mortality. In cases where complete excision of the infected graft is not feasible, lifelong suppressive therapy is recommended.[9]

References

7 Sandoe J, Barlow G, Chambers J, et al. Guidelines for the diagnosis, prevention and management of implantable cardiac electronic device infection. Report of a joint Working Party project on behalf of the British Society for Antimicrobial Chemotherapy (BSAC, host organization), British Heart Rhythm Society (BHRS), British Cardiovascular Society (BCS), British Heart Valve Society (BHVS) and British Society for Echocardiography (ESE). J Antimicrob Chemother. 2015;**70**:325–59.

8 Nagpul A, Sohail M. Prosthetic graft infections; a contemporary approach to diagnosis and management. Curr Infect Dis Rep. 2011;**13**:317–23.

9 American Heart Association (s016). Scientific statement diagnosis and management of vascular graft infection.

Myocarditis

An inflammatory disease of the myocardium, which may be caused by a variety of infectious and non-infectious causes. May be acute, subacute, or chronic, and focal or diffuse.

Aetiology

- Myocardial injury may be a consequence of direct cell damage by an infectious agent, by a circulating toxin, or by immune reactions following infection. The cause is not identified in most cases.
- Viruses are the most important infectious agent in the developed world, particularly Coxsackie viruses, adenoviruses, parvovirus B19, cytomegalovirus (CMV), Epstein–Barr virus (EBV), influenza, and severe acute respiratory syndrome coronavirus 2 (SARS-CoV-2). Dengue virus is a significant cause in endemic regions.
- Bacterial infections cause myocarditis via three key mechanisms: (1) immune-mediated (e.g. acute rheumatic fever), (2) direct myocardial infection with associated inflammation (e.g. brucellosis, meningococcal, streptococcal, and staphylococcal sepsis, Legionella spp., M. pneumoniae, and Chlamydia psittaci infection), and (3) toxin-mediated damage, seen with Corynebacterium diphtheriae and C. perfringens.

- Parasitic causes include trypanosomal disease; for example, *Trypanosoma cruzi* (Chagas' disease) is a common cause in South America.
- Disseminated infection in the immunocompromised may lead to myocarditis (e.g. *Toxoplasma*, *Aspergillus*, and *Cryptococcus* spp.). HIV infection, particularly in advanced disease, is associated with cardiomyopathy, but the pathogenesis is unclear.
- Rarely, myocarditis occurs after vaccine administration (e.g. Covid mRNA vaccines); however, in this case, note that the risk of myocarditis is higher with natural infection, with the exception of men under 40 years of age.

Pathogenesis

The pathological process varies according to the mechanism of the injury and whether it is acute or chronic. All lead to an inflammatory infiltrate and damage to adjacent myocardial cells. In addition, some agents damage vascular endothelial cells. Routine histology rarely allows a definitive aetiological diagnosis. Where normal cardiac function is regained, histological abnormalities may lag behind clinical improvement. Cases that leave permanent damage are marked by interstitial fibrosis and loss of muscle fibres.

Clinical presentation

- Clinical manifestations are highly variable, ranging from asymptomatic to chest pain, heart failure, arrhythmias, and sudden death.
- Myocarditis should be considered in a young person developing cardiac abnormalities in the context of a recognized systemic illness or in an otherwise well individual developing unexpected heart failure or arrhythmias (e.g. supraventricular tachycardia (SVT) or extrasystoles).
- Fever, malaise, arthralgias, upper respiratory tract symptoms, tachycardia, dyspnoea, and chest pain may precede Coxsackie virus myocarditis.
- On examination, there may be cardiomegaly, murmurs, and signs of cardiac failure.
- Pericarditis may coexist.

Diagnosis[10]

- Requires a high index of suspicion, particularly in the context of fulminant systemic infection.
- ECG is usually abnormal, but changes are non-specific (e.g. sequential ST elevation and T wave inversion).
- Serum troponin levels may be extremely high; ESR and CRP are commonly elevated.
- Echocardiography should be performed in all suspected cases—rules out alternative causes and monitors progression.
- Cardiac MRI scanning can support the diagnosis.
- Endomyocardial biopsy (EMB) is considered the gold standard for diagnosis, and identifies the aetiology and type of inflammation. There are regional variations in the use of EMB, but it has a role in establishing a diagnosis of myocarditis in new-onset heart failure.

- Molecular techniques have been used to identify viruses in cardiac tissue; however, the pathogenic significance remains uncertain, particularly in the absence of histological criteria for myocarditis. Diagnosis is also inferred by serology (e.g. Lyme disease) or detection of the organism in other specimens (e.g. faecal sample or blood).

Treatment

- Therapy should be directed at the causative agent where possible.
- General measures include bed rest (exercise is associated with increased death in mouse models) and management of heart failure and arrhythmias.
- Severe cases may require cardiac assist devices.
- Steroids are of no benefit and are probably deleterious overall.

Prognosis

Acute myocarditis resolves in less than month in about 50% of cases; 25% will develop persistent cardiac dysfunction; 12–25% may either die or progress to end-stage dilated cardiomyopathy.

Differential diagnosis

Pericarditis, idiopathic congestive cardiomyopathy, acute rheumatic fever, non-infectious myocarditis (collagen vascular disease, thyrotoxicosis, drug- or radiation-induced).

References

10 Caforio AL, Pankuweit S, Arbustini E, *et al*. Current state of knowledge on aetiology, diagnosis, management, and therapy of myocarditis: a position statement of the European Society of Cardiology Working Group on Myocardial and Pericardial Diseases. *Eur Heart J*. 2013;**34**:2636.

Pericarditis

Inflammation of the pericardium which may be acute or chronic.

Aetiology

- The result of a wide variety of infectious and non-infectious causes.
- The cause of acute, self-limited pericarditis is undetermined in most cases and is termed 'idiopathic'; most are probably viral.
- Viruses—enteroviruses, especially Coxsackie B virus, adenovirus, hepatitis C, HIV, CMV, echovirus, influenza virus (including H1N1), EBV, parvovirus B19, and human herpesvirus 6 (HHV-6).
- Bacteria—purulent pericarditis occurred fairly commonly in the pre-antibiotic era as a complication of pneumonia (e.g. *S. aureus* and *S. pneumoniae*) but is now uncommon. Gram-negative infections have become more prominent and patients are often older with a predisposing condition (e.g. oesophageal perforation, head/neck infections (usually anaerobes)). Purulent pericarditis may occur as a complication of meningococcal meningitis or septicaemia. Other bacterial causes include *M. pneumoniae*, *Neisseria gonorrhoeae*, *Legionella pneumophila*, and *Haemophilus influenzae*. Tuberculous pericarditis is a major cause of heart failure in sub-Saharan Africa—chronic disease is associated with constrictive pericarditis.

- Fungi—rare; include *Histoplasma capsulatum*, *Coccidioides immitis*, *Aspergillus* spp., *Cryptococcus neoformans*, and *Candida* spp.
- Parasites—include *Toxoplasma gondii*, *Entamoeba histolytica*, and *Toxocara canis*.

Pathogenesis

- Viruses usually reach the pericardium haematogenously, and infection results in inflammation of both the visceral and parietal pericardium, with or without a pericardial effusion. Most patients recover—some may experience episodes of relapse, a phenomenon that is probably related to immune mechanisms, rather than to persistent viral infection. It is rare that viral pericarditis leads to constriction.
- Bacterial infection may occur as a result of direct inoculation (trauma or surgery), contiguous spread (e.g. endocarditis or untreated pneumonia), or bacteraemia. Fluid is usually grossly purulent, and subsequent organization with adhesions may lead to constriction.
- Tuberculous pericarditis may arise from haematogenous spread (during primary infection), lymphatic spread (from regional lymph nodes), or contiguous spread (from the infected lung or pleura). Initial fibrin deposition, granuloma formation, and polymorphonuclear cell infiltration are followed by the development of a serous/serosanguinous effusion with lymphocytes and plasma cells. Later, the pericardium is thickened by fibrin deposition and granulomas. In late disease, the pericardial space is taken up with adhesions and fibrous tissue, leading to constriction.

Clinical presentation

- Depends on the aetiology. Typical manifestations are chest pain, pericardial friction rub, ECG changes, and pericardial effusion.
- Idiopathic or viral pericarditis—retrosternal chest pain, radiating to the shoulder/neck and aggravated by breathing or lying flat. Fever may be present, along with flu-like features.
- Bacterial pericarditis is usually seen in the context of severe systemic infection in an acutely ill patient. Chest pain and pericardial rubs may be reported in less than one-third of patients. Bacterial pericarditis may be recognized late, after the onset of haemodynamic complications.
- Tuberculous pericarditis has an insidious onset with chest pain, weight loss, night sweats, cough, and breathlessness. The classic clinical finding is a pericardial rub. Where the effusion is significant, there may be jugular venous distension and pulsus paradoxus.
- Regardless of the cause, assess for cardiac tamponade.

Diagnosis

- Diagnosis is often made clinically and depends on the history.
- The ECG is abnormal in 90% of cases (due to diffuse subepicardial inflammation), with 50% showing the classic findings of early ST elevation in multiple leads, resolving over a few days, to be replaced with T wave flattening/inversion.
- Echocardiography is useful in diagnosing and assessing effusions and the extent of any compromise.

- Virus isolation from throat swabs or stool sample, or acute and convalescent viral serology, can be attempted but rarely yields a diagnosis.
- Diagnostic sampling may be indicated if the effusion persists for >3 weeks, when tuberculosis, fungal infection, malignancy, or connective tissue disorders should be considered.
- Pericardiotomy with biopsy is preferable to pericardiocentesis, as it has a higher diagnostic yield and fewer complications.

Treatment

- Viral/idiopathic—bed rest, analgesia, and monitoring for haemodynamic complications. Non-steroidal anti-inflammatory drugs (NSAIDs) are often useful for symptomatic relief, continued for a few weeks, then tapered to stop to avoid recurrence. The efficacy of colchicine has been assessed in several systematic reviews and meta-analyses and proved to reduce symptoms and recurrences, usually when prescribed for up to 3 months.
- Purulent bacterial—surgical drainage and appropriate antibiotic therapy are essential. Early pericardiocentesis may be lifesaving, but fluid often reaccumulates. Overall mortality, however, remains at around 30%—particularly in those cases associated with endocarditis or following surgery.
- Tuberculous—antituberculosis therapy should be initiated with prednisolone (60mg once daily in adults, gradually withdrawing 2–3 weeks after starting treatment); see NICE tuberculosis treatment recommendations.

Mediastinitis

Acute mediastinitis is an uncommon, but potentially devastating, infection involving the mediastinal structures.

Epidemiology and pathogenesis

- Primary infection is rare. Almost all cases are secondary to:
  - cardiothoracic surgery, now the commonest cause;
  - oesophageal perforation (e.g. iatrogenic, trauma, spontaneous);
  - head and neck infections (e.g. odontogenic, Ludwig's angina, pharyngitis, tonsillitis, epiglottitis, parotitis);
  - spread from other infections (e.g. pneumonia, empyema, subphrenic abscess, pancreatitis, skin or soft tissue infections of the chest wall, osteomyelitis of the sternum, clavicle, ribs, or vertebrae, haematogenous seeding).

Aetiology

- The spectrum of organisms causing infection varies strikingly according to the underlying cause.
- Post-surgical infections are usually monomicrobial and caused by meticillin-sensitive *S. aureus* (MSSA; 45%), meticillin-resistant *S. aureus* (MRSA; 16%), Gram-negative bacilli (17%), CoNS (13%), and streptococci (5%).

- Oesophageal perforation or head and neck infections are usually polymicrobial and caused by oral streptococci (e.g. viridans streptococci, peptococci, peptostreptococci) and anaerobic Gram-negative bacilli (e.g. *Bacteroides* spp., *Fusobacterium* spp., *Prevotella* spp., *Porphyromonas* spp.).

Clinical features

- Clinical manifestations also depend on the underlying cause.
- Head and neck infections usually present with fever, pain, and swelling of the affected site.
- Oesophageal perforation may be obvious or clinically inapparent. Boerhaave syndrome (transmural perforation of the oesophagus) typically presents with severe anterior chest pain following vomiting/retching.
- Symptoms include chest pain (site depends on the location of infection), respiratory distress, and dysphagia.
- Physical signs include fever, tachycardia, crepitus, and oedema of the head and neck. Hamman's sign (a crunching sound heard over the precordium synchronous with the cardiac rhythm) is due to emphysema of the mediastinum.
- Post-cardiothoracic mediastinitis usually presents within 2 weeks of surgery, with fever, wound erythema/discharge, and chest pain (often pleuritic). Sternal instability, wound dehiscence, and chest wall emphysema may occur.

Diagnosis

- Blood tests show leucocytosis and raised inflammatory markers. BCs may yield the causative organism(s).
- Chest X-ray may show mediastinal widening, air–fluid levels, and subcutaneous or mediastinal emphysema.
- CT thorax is particularly useful in post-operative mediastinitis to distinguish superficial wound infections from deep retrosternal infections.

Management

- Prompt surgical intervention is required with drainage, debridement, and repair (e.g. oesophageal stent in cases due to oesophageal perforation). Post-operative mediastinitis may be managed by the open technique (wound debrided and left open to heal by secondary intention) or the closed technique (debridement, primary closure, and irrigation through drains).
- Appropriate parenteral antibiotic therapy should be initiated promptly. Empirical therapy should cover the most likely organisms (e.g. co-amoxiclav, piperacillin–tazobactam). Local resistance data should be considered (e.g. MRSA rates), and empirical therapy should reflect this. Rationalize therapy once culture results are available. Duration is determined by the extent of infection, effectiveness of drainage/debridement, bone involvement, presence of prosthetic material, and causative pathogen.
- Complications include pericardial effusion/cardiac tamponade, Pleural effusions/empyema, Peritonitis, and Sternal osteomyelitis (post-operative mediastinitis).

Gastrointestinal infections

Oesophagitis

Inflammation of the oesophagus, generally non-infectious (e.g. gastro-oesophageal reflux), but may also be caused by a variety of infectious agents, usually in the context of impaired immunity (HIV, transplant recipients, or those receiving cancer chemotherapy).

Aetiology

- *Candida*—*Candida albicans* is the commonest cause of oesophagitis. Other *Candida* spp. (*Candida glabrata*, now called *Nakaseomyces glabrata*; or *Candida krusei*, now called *Pichia kudriavzevii*) are less commonly isolated. Colonization is seen in up to 75% of the population (particularly those receiving antacid therapy). Seen in both immunosuppressed and immunocompetent hosts (those with dentures or dry mouth or using inhaled corticosteroids). Infection follows when breakdown of local and systemic defences permit invasion to the deeper epithelial layers. Endoscopy reveals yellow-white plaques adhering to a hyperaemic oesophagus (usually the distal third). Removing these reveals an inflamed, friable surface. Perforation occurs rarely. Predisposing factors: acute or advanced HIV infection, diabetes mellitus, haematological malignancy, broad-spectrum antibiotic therapy, inhaled or PO corticosteroid therapy, conditions that impair oesophageal motility (systemic sclerosis, achalasia), reflux oesophagitis.
- Cryptococcosis, blastomycosis, histoplasmosis, and aspergillosis—have occasionally been found to cause oesophagitis.
- Cytomegalovirus (CMV)—seen usually in advanced HIV (the cause in around 30% of such patients reporting oesophageal symptoms) or the severely immunosuppressed. Endoscopy may demonstrate large (10cm²), shallow, 'punched-out' ulcers, usually at the lower oesophageal sphincter, but can be diffuse inflammation. Diagnosis is best made by histopathological examination of biopsies obtained from the ulcer edge and base, which show enlarged endothelial cells with large intranuclear owl's eye inclusions (cytomegalic cells). Isolation of CMV in culture is not reliable due to contamination from blood or saliva. Co-infection with HSV or *Candida* spp. is common. Detection in the blood via PCR is not diagnostic, as 50% of patients with positive PCR and advanced HIV have no symptoms.
- Herpes simplex virus (HSV)—usually seen in those with significant immunosuppression; rare in healthy adults. HSV-1 is commoner than HSV-2. Seen most frequently in solid organ and bone marrow transplant recipients, less common in advanced HIV, causative agent in estimated 5% of patients with advanced HIV and oesophagitis. Presentation may be with odynophagia, chest pain, fever, nausea, and vomiting; <25% may develop clinically significant GI bleeding. Oral/labial or cutaneous HSV infection may be apparent (<38% of cases). Endoscopy reveals multiple small, superficial ulcers in the distal third of the oesophagus. Large confluent ulcers and denuded epithelium may be seen as infection progresses. Viral PCR of brushing or biopsies is the most sensitive means of diagnosis.
- Idiopathic ulceration—extensive ulceration may occur in those with acute or advanced HIV, or in mild form in those otherwise

healthy. These may be attributed to unrecognized infectious agents. Management is based upon limited evidence and includes good oral hygiene, avoiding exacerbating factors, pain control with topical anaesthetic agents, and topical corticosteroids. In complex disease, systemic treatment is often required; prednisolone (40mg a day for 14 days, then tapered to stop) improves symptoms in the majority of HIV-related aphthous ulceration. Second-line treatment includes dapsone and colchicine.

Clinical features

Key feature is odynophagia or dysphagia. Liquids may be better tolerated than solids. Pain may be worse with acidic substances. Severe ulcerative oesophagitis can cause such severe pain that oral intake is limited to the point of weight loss and dehydration. GI bleeding can occur. Oesophagitis can exist in the absence of symptoms <41%. Fever may be seen in those with CMV or mycobacterial infection. Vomiting is commoner with CMV than with other causes. The presence of oral lesions may be indicative of the cause of oesophagitis (e.g. oral thrush, herpetic ulceration).

Diagnosis and treatment

Often a clinical diagnosis based on the presence of visible oral lesions—oral candidiasis, herpetic ulcers. Accurate diagnosis of oesophageal candidiasis requires endoscopic brushing (with a sheathed cytology brush) and biopsy. The gross appearance can mislead—white lesions may be seen with HSV, CMV, and candidal infection. Histopathological examination and viral PCR may identify viral causes. Fungal culture is useful only in the management of refractory cases (e.g. to identify the species and sensitivities).

Management

- Diagnostic endoscopy may not always be feasible (bleeding, severe pain, critical illness), particularly in those patients developing oesophagitis secondary to cancer chemotherapy. Empirical treatment for *Candida* and HSV infection may be appropriate (e.g. IV amphotericin and aciclovir), particularly if symptoms are very severe or oral thrush/HSV stomatitis are apparent.
- Patients receiving immunosuppressant therapy may need drug level monitoring if treated with antifungals such as fluconazole.
- *Candida* spp.—fluconazole 200–400mg PO or IV for 14–21 days.
- HSV—aciclovir 5mg/kg tds IV, followed by PO valaciclovir or famciclovir for a total of 14 days or until healing is complete.
- CMV—ganciclovir 5mg/kg bd IV for 14–21 days or until symptoms/signs have resolved. PO valganciclovir 900mg bd can be substituted for some or all of the duration if swallowing and absorption are unaffected. Maintenance therapy is not indicated unless concomitant ophthalmological disease.

Oesophagitis in advanced HIV

(See British HIV Association, 2022.)[1]
- Oesophageal symptoms are seen in 40–50% of patients with HIV at some point in their illness, and affect nutritional status and morbidity. Prior to widespread use of combination antiretroviral therapy,

oesophageal candidiasis was seen in up to 50% of patients presenting with CD4 count of <350 cells/mm³ and is still the commonest late-presenting feature. Seventy per cent of cases due to *C. albicans*—rates of non-*albicans* spp. continue to rise and are responsible for ~30% in many cohorts.

- Diagnosis is clinical and can be treated empirically with fluconazole in mild cases if oral thrush is observed in a symptomatic patient (70% will have oesophageal involvement). Alternative agents include itraconazole solution, voriconazole, posaconazole, or IV echinocandins (caspofungin, micafungin, or anidulafungin). Amphotericin is now rarely used, as it is more toxic than other agents.
- Microbiological confirmation and susceptibility testing of *Candida* spp. are required when symptoms of candidiasis persist or recur during antifungal therapy, to establish whether ongoing symptoms reflect an azole-resistant strain or an alternative diagnosis.
- Endoscopic diagnosis should be undertaken in patients with oesophageal symptoms without oropharyngeal candidiasis, in those who do not respond to initial treatment, and in the case of relapse.
- CMV and HSV cause one-third of cases (often in association with candidiasis). Three-quarters will have a partial or complete response to induction therapy with antiviral drugs, but relapses are common without maintenance treatment; 70% of HSV oesophagitis responds to aciclovir, but relapse is seen in 15% within 4 months.
- Rarer causes include tuberculosis, *Mycobacterium avium* complex, primary syphilis, Epstein–Barr virus (EBV), *Cryptococcus neoformans*, *Cryptosporidium*, and *Actinomyces*. Idiopathic ulcers are also common.
- Other non-infectious causes of dysphagia include pill-associated ulcers. These have been associated with a number of medications, most commonly in the mid oesophagus. Doxycycline and related antimicrobials, NSAIDs, potassium supplementation, and iron tablets are the commonest causes that are likely to be encountered in people living with HIV.

References

1 British HIV Association (2022). *BHIVA guidelines on the management of opportunistic infection in people living with HIV: the clinical management of gastrointestinal opportunistic infections 2020* (2022 interim update). Available at: ℞ https://www.bhiva.org/OI-guidelines-gastrointestinal

Peptic ulcer disease

Peptic ulcer disease has two main risk factors which cause disease both independently and synergistically: NSAIDs and infection by the Gram-negative organism *Helicobacter pylori*. *H. pylori* is a motile, curved Gram-negative rod (GNR) that lives within the mucus layer overlying the gastric (and occasionally duodenal or oesophageal) mucosa. It is the commonest chronic bacterial infection in humans, present in most people with peptic ulcer disease and increasing the risk of several inflammatory and neoplastic processes. All clinical isolates of *H. pylori* produce urease. It has been isolated from people in all parts of the world—humans appear to be the major reservoir, with the route of transmission unknown, but likely faeco-oral, and possibly oral–oral, routes. Rates of colonization are equal between men and women.

Most infections are acquired during childhood. Carriage is near universal by the age of 20 years in developing countries, with a prevalence of over 50% by the age of 50 in the UK. One to 3% of those who remain free of the organism by adulthood acquire the bacteria each year.

Clinical features

- Acute acquisition—may cause an acute upper GI illness with nausea and abdominal discomfort, with vomiting, burping, and fever lasting 3–14 days. However, infection is clinically silent in most individuals. There have been some documented cases of acute self-limiting infection.
- Persistent colonization—*H. pylori* persists for decades in most people. Acute symptoms do not usually recur, although the incidence of non-ulcer dyspepsia is slightly higher in colonized individuals.
- Duodenal ulceration—70% have *H. pylori* infection. Prevalence is falling in the USA and parts of Europe. The organism is found only in areas of metaplastic gastric-type epithelium, and its presence is associated with an over 50 times greater risk of duodenal ulceration.
- Gastric ulceration—50–80% are colorized with *H. pylori*. A greater proportion of gastric ulcers are associated with NSAIDs or aspirin.
- Gastric carcinoma—the presence of *H. pylori* has been identified as a risk factor for gastric carcinoma. Pathogenesis is incompletely understood but is thought to be related to the strain of bacteria, host immune response, and environmental factors such as diet (high salt intake), obesity, and high glycated haemoglobin (HbA1c). Although only a small proportion of those infected with *H. pylori* will develop gastric cancer, eradication appears to reduce the risk of cancer development.
- Gastric lymphoma—*H. pylori* colonization is strongly associated with mucosa-associated lymphoid tissue (MALT) tumours (lymphomas arising from B lymphocytes). The mechanism is thought to be related to specific strains expressing cytotoxin-associated gene A (CagA). Initial treatment for stage 1 and 2 disease is eradication therapy and surveillance rather than radiotherapy. Around 80% achieve cure with this treatment.
- Oesophageal disease—as the incidence of *H. pylori* colonization falls, it appears the incidence of gastro-oesophageal reflux disease (GORD), Barrett's oesophagus, and oesophageal adenocarcinoma are on the rise. Certain *H. pylori* strains may have an inverse association with Barrett's oesophagus. It has been shown that eradication of *H. pylori* in those with duodenal ulceration doubles the rate of GORD development and patients with GORD are less likely to be colonized with *H. pylori* than controls.

Diagnosis

- Endoscopy with biopsy—*H. pylori* infection is diagnosed by one of three methods: biopsy urease test, histology or less commonly bacterial culture. Antral biopsies can be tested for urease activity by using commercial tests (e.g. CLO test), which detect the production of ammonia from urea that results in a colour change. Sensitivity and specificity are 90 and 95%, respectively, and results are available in 1h. False negatives can occur in the presence of GI bleeding, use of proton pump inhibitors (PPIs), bismuth-containing compounds, and antibiotics.

Gastric biopsy histology may demonstrate *H. pylori* and also provides information about the presence of gastritis, intestinal metaplasia, or MALT. Bacterial culture and sensitivity testing of *H. pylori* are difficult and rarely performed.

- Urea breath tests (UBTs) and stool antigen tests (SATs) are the preferred methods of diagnosis in primary care.
- UBT is based on the ability of *H. pylori* to convert urea to ammonia and carbon dioxide (CO_2). Urea labelled with a carbon isotope is swallowed, and detection of isotope-labelled CO_2 in exhaled breath after 30 minutes indicates the presence of urease; 88–95% sensitive and 95–100% specific; PPIs can cause false negatives.
- SAT—detection of bacterial antigen in faecal samples. Most cost-effective test in areas of low to moderate prevalence. Can be used to confirm eradication 4 weeks after treatment.
- Serology—enzyme-linked immunoassay (EIA) tests detect immunoglobulin G (IgG), which is positive in nearly all colonized patients (sensitivity 90–100%, specificity 76–96%). Not recommended first line due to accuracy concerns. Good negative predictive value in areas of low prevalence. Most useful in patients on PPIs or with acute GI bleeds when UBTs or SATs cannot be used. Retesting is indicated in areas of high antibiotic resistance rates, and in cases of severe, persistent symptoms or with associated ulcer or malignancy.

Treatment

- Treatment involves a triple therapy regimen of a PPI and two antibiotics. Choice of antibiotics should take into consideration the patient's treatment history, as each additional course of macrolide, metronidazole, or quinolone increases the risk of resistance.
- Various treatment regimens for the treatment of *H. pylori* have been evaluated in clinical trials, but the optimal therapy has not been defined. See National Institute for Health and Care Excellence (NICE) guidelines for details.
- Consider referral to a specialist if the patient remains *H. pylori* positive after second-line eradication therapy. Patients should be referred for an endoscopy, culture, and susceptibility testing if the choice of antibacterial treatment is reduced due to allergy or known high local resistance rates, or if they previously received treatment with clarithromycin, metronidazole, and a quinolone.
- Triple therapy—this is used in areas with low levels of clarithromycin resistance (<15%). The commonest regimen is a PPI plus amoxicillin and either clarithromycin or metronidazole for 7 days, depending on previous treatments used. In penicillin allergy, the first line is PPI plus clarithromycin and metronidazole. If previously treated with metronidazole, tetracyclines or levofloxacin can be used.
- Quadruple therapy—this is indicated in areas with high levels of resistance to clarithromycin or metronidazole, or in patients who have recent or repeated exposure to either drug. It consists of a PPI (combined with bismuth subsalicylate) and two antibiotics (e.g. amoxicillin, metronidazole, tetracycline, or levofloxacin) for 10–14 days. Either rifabutin or furazolidone (both unlicensed) may also be used.

Infectious diarrhoea

Definitions

- Gastroenteritis is inflammation of the stomach and intestinal epithelium.
- Diarrhoea is passage of ≥3 loose/liquid faeces within 24h.
- Food poisoning is vomiting and/or diarrhoea caused by eating food contaminated with microorganisms or toxins (bacterial or otherwise, e.g. poisonous mushrooms).
- Dysentery is bloody diarrhoea with mucus, tenesmus, pain, and fever, usually caused by bacterial, parasitic, or protozoan infection.

Aetiology

- Most cases of infectious aetiology in the UK are self-limiting, with 50% lasting <24h.
- One of the leading causes of childhood death in resource-limited settings.
- Transmission of GI infection from person to person may occur through one or more of a variety of different pathways, including faeco-oral, food-borne, environmental, and airborne routes.
- Risk factors in the UK include immunosuppression, nursing home residence, recent hospital stays, and certain sexual practices. Recent antibiotic use predisposes to antibiotic-associated diarrhoea. Bacterial infections are commoner in the tropics. In the UK, causes of gastroenteritis include:
  - general patients—viruses (50–70% of cases, e.g. rotavirus, norovirus), Campylobacter, Shigella, Salmonella, Clostridium perfringens, Staphylococcus aureus, Bacillus cereus, Escherichia coli, Clostridioides difficile, parasites (10–15%, e.g. Giardia, Cryptosporidium);
  - immunosuppressed patients—general causes plus increased E. coli, Cryptosporidium, mycobacteria, microsporidia, CMV, and HSV (especially HIV patients with CD4 count <200/mm^3);
  - returning travellers—enterotoxigenic E. coli (30–70%), Shigella spp. (5–20%), Salmonella spp. (5%), Campylobacter (5–20%), Vibrio parahaemolyticus (shellfish), viral (10–20%), protozoal (5–10%).

Clinical features

- History:
  - nature of diarrhoea—blood, mucus, or pus? Painful? Frequency?
  - associated systemic symptoms (e.g. fever, rash);
  - onset—acute onset <14 days—usually viral, but if severe, may be bacterial; can also be protozoal. Persistent (14–29 days)—differential diagnosis depends on exposures and travel history: protozoal, C. difficile, parasitic, viral. Chronic (>29 days)—often non-infectious or seen in immunocompromised;
  - food history—specific restaurant, reheated food, unusual diets, fish;
  - are other people affected—is it an outbreak and, if so, what was the source?
  - recent antibiotic use (in community or hospital);
  - foreign travel—country, city, or rural, with reference to timing of possible exposures (e.g. food from a street vendor);
  - risk factors for immunosuppression.

- Examination:
  - look for signs of fever and volume depletion; is the patient systemically unwell or hypovolaemic?
  - examine for an acute abdomen; surgical cause for presentation?
  - wasting implies a longer-standing problem (e.g. small bowel malabsorption, immunosuppression, malignancy);
  - rectal examination—blood, mucus, faecal occult blood, impacted faeces causing overflow diarrhoea, rectal carcinoma.
- When GI symptoms are followed by neurological signs, think of *Clostridium botulinum* (nausea, dry mouth, cranial nerve palsies, and descending weakness with respiratory and autonomic dysfunction) or *Campylobacter jejuni* infection-associated Guillain–Barré syndrome (GBS) (occurs 1–3 weeks after GI symptoms).
- Differential diagnosis—non-infectious causes of food poisoning include mushrooms and metal poisoning. Non-infectious causes of diarrhoea include perforation, appendicitis, diverticulosis, inflammatory bowel disease (IBD), colonic malignancy, ischaemic colitis, malabsorption, irritable bowel syndrome, constipation with overflow, thyrotoxicosis, drugs, and autonomic neuropathy.

Investigations

- Not routinely indicated in most cases, unless systemically unwell and hospitalized or immunocompromised.
- Blood tests—anaemia or macrocytosis may be due to malabsorption. Renal failure may occur with dehydration or haemolytic uraemic syndrome (HUS). Blood film shows red cell fragmentation in HUS.
- Sigmoidoscopy may show inflamed colonic mucosa ± pseudomembrane (*C. difficile* colitis). Biopsies may be taken to exclude IBD.
- Abdominal X-ray or CT abdomen may exclude surgical causes.
- Faecal samples should be sent to the laboratory for:
  - microscopy—blood and pus cells indicate infectious diarrhoea (e.g. *Salmonella*, *Shigella*, or *Campylobacter* spp.) or IBD. Ova, cysts, and parasites are only reported if requested and may be diagnostic in patients with a history of foreign travel. Modified Ziehl–Neelsen (ZN) stain for *Cryptosporidium* (preschool children and the immunocompromised);
  - culture—detects specific pathogens such as *Salmonella* spp., *Shigella* spp., *C. jejuni*, *E. coli* O157, *Yersinia* spp., and *Vibrio* spp.; special media are required;
  - toxin detection—either the toxin itself within faecal samples (e.g. *C. difficile*) or the toxin gene in isolated organisms (e.g. *E. coli* O157).

Management

- Oral rehydration is sufficient in mild cases. Oral rehydration salts (ORS) are commercially available. Patients with moderate or severe dehydration require IV replacement of fluid and electrolytes.
- Antibiotics are not usually recommended for adults with diarrhoea of unknown pathology. Empirical antibiotic therapy is only indicated if severe diarrhoea: >6 unformed faeces/day, pyrexia, tenesmus, or high WCC. Use ciprofloxacin or azithromycin for 3 days. Alternative regimens include co-trimoxazole.

- If pathogen identified, most do not require specific treatment. Exceptions are: early *C. jejuni* enteritis (within 3 days of onset), *C. difficile*, *Yersinia enterocolitica* (children and the immunocompromised), *Shigella dysenteriae*, severe *Salmonella enteritidis* and *Salmonella typhimurium* (e.g. bacteraemia), *Giardia lamblia*, and *Entamoeba histolytica*.
- Antispasmodic agents—useful in mild diarrhoea without blood. Do not use if there is a suggestion of dysentery or *C. difficile* infection (CDI).
- Refer to secondary care all previously healthy children with acute painful, bloody diarrhoea or confirmed cases of verocytotoxigenic (VTEC) *E. coli* O157. Avoid antibiotics, as they may increase the risk of HUS.
- Cases and all household contacts should be provided with advice on minimizing spread of infection, including hand hygiene, safe preparation of food, and avoiding towel sharing.
- Repeat faecal sampling is unnecessary, unless specifically advised by public health guidelines or if parasitic infection is suspected.

Public health aspects

All persons with gastroenteritis should be excluded from work, school, or other institutional and social settings until a minimum of 48h symptom-free/no loose faeces.

All cases of suspected food poisoning or dysentery should be notified to public health. UK Health Security Agency (UKHSA) has issued guidelines for public health management of GI infections in 2019.[2]

References

2 Public Health England, Chartered Institute of Environmental Health (2020). *Recommendations for the public health management of gastrointestinal infections 2019: principles and practice.* Available at: https://assets.publishing.service.gov.uk/media/5e3027c7ed915d1f28fe88ff/manage-ment_of_gastrointestinal_infections.pdf

Enteric fever

The clinical and pathological features of typhoid fever were first described in the nineteenth century by Louis (1829) and then by Jenner (1850). The term enteric fever was proposed by Wilson in 1869. Typhoid Mary (Mary Mallon) worked as a cook in New York in early 1900s and infected 49 people with typhoid, three of whom died. She was forcibly quarantined and died after almost 30 years in isolation. The species that cause enteric fever are the Gram-negative bacterium *Salmonella enterica* serotype Typhi and *S. enterica* serotype Paratyphi A, B, or C. Please see chapter 7 (bacteria) p. 323 Salmonella.

Epidemiology

Enteric fever is a global health problem, affecting an estimated 12–33 million people per year, and predominantly a disease in countries with inadequate sanitation and poor standards of hygiene. Regions with a high incidence (>100 cases per 100 000 person-years) include south-central Asia, South East Asia, the Pacific, and Southern Africa. The organisms are spread by ingestion of faecally contaminated food or water. Direct person-to-person spread is rare, and laboratory transmission has been reported. Outbreaks in developing countries may result in high morbidity and mortality. In developed countries, infection is usually associated with international travel, although food-borne outbreaks do occur.

Pathogenesis

Inoculum size and decreased gastric acidity are important determinants of disease severity. The ability of the organisms to survive within macrophages is essential to disease pathogenesis and spread. Organisms multiply in Peyer's patches, then enter the bloodstream and reinvade the small bowel, causing bleeding and peritonitis. The Vi antigen of *S.* Typhi prevents antibody-mediated opsonization, increases resistance to peroxide, and confers resistance to complement-mediated lysis.

Clinical features

- The incubation period averages from 7 to 20 days, depending on the inoculum size, age, gastric acidity, and host immune status. Diarrhoea may be absent.
- Fever is present in 98–100% of cases, often gradually rising to >39±C over the first week, then becoming sustained.
- Non-specific symptoms include abdominal pain, constipation, malaise, and headaches. Can also present with sore throat, delirium, or psychosis.
- On examination, patients are acutely ill with fever, rash (macular rose-coloured spots—occur in 2–40% of cases), abdominal tenderness, and hepatosplenomegaly. Cervical lymphadenopathy, respiratory crepitations, cholecystitis, pancreatitis, seizures, or coma may also occur. May have relative bradycardia (Faget's sign).
- Complications occur in the third or fourth week of illness and include intestinal perforation or haemorrhage, endocarditis, pericarditis, hepatic or splenic abscesses, and orchitis. Usually occur in delayed or untreated patients.
- Mortality rates are <1% in developed countries but may be as high as 10–30% in developing countries, as a result of delayed treatment or multidrug-resistant (MDR) strains.
- Long-term carriage (presence of salmonellae in faeces or urine for >1 year) occurs in 1–4% of patients with *S.* Typhi. It is associated with biliary abnormalities, concurrent infection with *Schistosoma haematobium*, and an increased risk of developing cholangiocarcinoma.

Diagnosis

Culture—definitive diagnosis requires isolation of the organism from cultures of blood (40–80% positive,), faecal samples (30–40% positive), or bone marrow (50–90% positive). Other diagnostic samples include urine, rose spots, or duodenal contents. A combination of specimens increases the likelihood of diagnosis. Antibiotic susceptibility testing is vital. Serological tests (e.g. Widal) detect antibodies to *S.* Typhi but are of limited clinical utility in endemic areas, because they do not distinguish recent from past infection. Newer EIAs for antibodies to the polysaccharide Vi antigen are useful for diagnosing carriers, but not in acute illness. PCR-based diagnostics have limited sensitivity and there are newer approaches in development—antibody tests to detect serum immunoglobulin A against haemolysin E.

Management

- High levels of MDR strains (resistant to previous first-line treatment—ampicillin, co-trimoxazole, and chloramphenicol) and increasing resistance to fluoroquinolones have made treatment challenging. There have also been outbreaks of extensively drug-resistant (XDR) strains resistant to ceftriaxone, as well as to ciprofloxacin, amoxicillin, chloramphenicol, and co-trimoxazole, in Pakistan and Iraq. Currently, the XDR strain remains susceptible to azithromycin and carbapenems.
- Antibiotic selection depends on local resistance patterns, patient age, whether PO medications are feasible, and the clinical setting.
- In uncomplicated enteric fever of unknown susceptibility, known quinolone resistance, or XDR strain, azithromycin for 7 days is the first-line treatment. If fully susceptible or MDR strain, ciprofloxacin for 7 days is first line.
- In severe disease requiring parenteral treatment, ceftriaxone (2–3g daily IV) for 10–14 days, or if susceptibility known, ciprofloxacin. In XDR disease, meropenem should be used.
- Alternative agents include chloramphenicol, amoxicillin, co-trimoxazole, or cefixime, depending on susceptibility.
- Surgery—this is indicated in patients with ileal perforation.

Relapse

This may occur 2–3 weeks after treatment in 1–6% of patients. These are treated with an additional course of therapy to which the organism is susceptible.

Chronic carriage

Chronic carriage with excretion of organisms in the faeces occurs in 1–6% of patients—rates are higher in patients with biliary tract abnormalities. Carriers do not develop recurrent disease but pose a risk to others, particularly if they are food handlers. Eradication therapy is recommended, using susceptibility profiles to guide. Duration of 4–12 weeks. Either ciprofloxacin for a minimum of 4 weeks, or amoxicillin or co-trimoxazole for a minimum of 6 weeks. Cholecystectomy may be required.

Prevention

- There are two vaccines available for protection against S. Typhi—neither is completely effective nor do they provide protection against S. Paratyphi.
- The live oral vaccine Ty21a has an efficacy of 35% and 58% at years 1 and 2, respectively.
- The parenteral Vi polysaccharide vaccine has an efficacy of 69% and 59% at years 1 and 2, respectively. Protective antibodies fall over time, and revaccination is necessary when continuing protection is required.
- Immunization is recommended for travellers to typhoid-endemic areas or laboratory personnel who handle S. Typhi in their course of work.

Cholera

Cholera is an acute diarrhoeal disease caused by toxigenic strains of *Vibrio cholerae*, a highly motile, halophilic, curved GNR. *V. cholerae* is classified on the basis of the O-antigen. Over 200 serotypes exist, but only *V. cholerae* O1 and O139 cause epidemics. *V. cholerae* O1 is the predominant cause of cholera worldwide, and has two major serotypes (Inaba and Ogawa) and two biotypes (El Tor and classical). Please see chapter 7 (bacteria) p. 356 Cholera for further details.

Epidemiology

- Cholera has the ability to either cause epidemics with pandemic potential or remain endemic in affected areas.
- Predominantly occurs in areas with poor access to clean water.
- Epidemic cholera affects non-immune individuals of all ages, occurs after a single introduction, spreads by the faeco-oral route, and has high secondary spread.
- Endemic cholera affects children aged 2–15 years, has an aquatic or asymptomatic human reservoir, and is spread by water or food or faeco-orally. Immunity increases with age, and secondary spread is variable. Cases show seasonal variation.
- Six pandemics occurred between 1817 and 1923 caused by *V. cholerae* O1 classic biotype originating from the Indian subcontinent. The seventh originated in Indonesia in 1961 caused by *V. cholerae* O1 El Tor biotype. Following the 2010 Haiti earthquake, there was a huge O1 outbreak—the worst in recent history and thought to be introduced from South Asia.
- In 1992, a new epidemic caused by *V. cholerae* O139 occurred in India and Bangladesh. This has subsequently subsided.
- Worldwide cases are increasing since 2015, mainly in Africa and the Eastern Mediterranean.

Pathogenesis

The infectious dose varies from 10^2 to 10^8 organisms. Reduced gastric acidity is associated with an increased severity of disease. Pathogenic strains have two virulence factors—cholera toxin and toxin co-regulated pilus. The latter is a pilus that aggregates organisms on the surface of the small intestine and allows bacteria to resist killing by bile. The cholera toxin is the main virulence factor and primary cause of the profuse watery diarrhoea. It has a B subunit that binds to gangliosides on the epithelial surface and allows the A subunit to enter the cell. Once inside the cell, the A subunit increases cyclic adenosine monophosphate (cAMP) activity, resulting in chloride secretion at the apical surface and concurrent losses of sodium and water.

Clinical features

- Infection with *V. cholerae* results in a spectrum of disease, from asymptomatic to severe diarrhoea. Incubation period is usually 18–40h.
- Abdominal pain, vomiting, and borborygmi (abdominal rumbling) are common early symptoms.
- Fever is uncommon, occurring in <5% of cases.
- Severe disease is characterized by profuse watery diarrhoea ('rice water stool') and can result in hypovolaemia and electrolyte loss. Patients

may be anxious, restless, or obtunded with sunken eyes, dry mucous membranes, and loss of skin elasticity. Severe disease is commoner in pregnancy and associated with fetal loss in up to 50%.

- Complications—hypoglycaemia, coma, acute kidney injury, pneumonia, bacteraemia (rare), 'cholera sicca' (fluid accumulation in the intestinal lumen without diarrhoea).

Laboratory diagnosis

- Most cases are diagnosed on clinical suspicion, with management initiated presumptively.
- Faecal sample culture is the definitive test—on selective media (thiosulfate–citrate–bile salts–sucrose agar, or tellurite taurocholate gelatin agar), followed by identification using biochemical tests or matrix-assisted laser desorption/ionization (MALDI). Serogroup and serotype are determined by specific antibodies. Please see chapter 7 (bacteria) p. 357 Cholera and Table 7.15.
- Dark-field microscopy of fresh rice water stool shows large numbers of motile vibrios whose movement can be blocked by specific antisera. Lacks sensitivity.
- Rapid tests—these include commercial immunochromatographic lateral flow devices (e.g. Crystal VC™ dipstick).

Management

As per World Health Organization (WHO) treatment guidelines for cholera.[3]

- The goal of therapy is to restore fluid losses rapidly and safely.
- Evaluate the patient for the degree of dehydration:
  - mild (<5% fluid loss);
  - moderate (5–10% fluid loss)—sunken eyes, dry mouth, slow return of skin pinch;
  - severe (>10% fluid loss)—absent radial pulse, low blood pressure.
- Rehydrate the patient in two phases: intensive phase (2–4h); maintenance phase (until diarrhoea resolves).
- Giver ORS if the patient can drink, while a drip is being set up, and continue in addition to IV fluids.
- Use IV fluids only for—severely dehydrated patients in intensive phase (30mL/kg within 30 minutes and 70mL/kg in next 2h), moderately dehydrated patients who cannot tolerate oral fluids, and high faecal volumes (>10mL/kg/h) in the maintenance phase.
- Monitor the patient after 3h and assess hydration status. If the pulse remains weak, continue IV fluids. If moderate dehydration, use ORS 2200–4000mL over 4h. Reassess after 4h. If mild dehydration, continue to the maintenance phase.
- Most patients absorb enough ORS to achieve rehydration.
- Use oral hydration salts (OHS) for patients in the maintenance phase (800–1000mL/h), matching input with output.
- Discharge patients when all the following criteria are fulfilled—PO intake ≥1000mL/h, urine volume ≥400mL/h, and faecal volume ≤400mL/h.
- Antimicrobial agents play a secondary role in treatment and have been shown to reduce the duration and volume of diarrhoea. Only used in those with severe dehydration; start after vomiting has stopped.

Preferred is doxycycline 300mg stat dose. Alternatives include tetracycline (500mg four times daily (qds) PO for 3 days), furazolidone if pregnant (100mg qds PO for 3 days), co-trimoxazole (960mg bd PO for 3 days), ciprofloxacin (20mg/kg stat), or azithromycin (20mg/kg stat).

Prevention

- Clean water supply and good sanitation are the cornerstones of prevention.
- Vaccines—two oral cholera vaccines (OCVs) are available: (1) WC-rBS, a killed whole-cell vaccine of *V. cholerae* O1 and recombinant cholera toxin B subunit, and (2) bivalent killed whole-cell vaccine containing *V. cholerae* O1 and O139. The WHO recommends these vaccines should be used in areas with endemic cholera, in humanitarian crises with a high risk of cholera, and during cholera outbreaks. OCVs should be considered for travellers and emergency and relief workers at high risk.[4]

References

3 World Health Organization. WHO treatment guidelines for cholera. https://www.paho.org/en/resurgence-cholera-hispaniola/cholera-technical-guidelines-and-resources
4 World Health Organization. Cholera vaccines: WHO position paper, August 2017. *Wkly Epidemiol Rec.* 2017;**92**:477–500.

Clostridioides difficile diarrhoea

Diarrhoea is the commonest complication of antibiotic therapy, occuring in up to 15% of those receiving β-lactam antibiotics and 25% of those receiving clindamycin. *C. difficile* is the most frequent cause (20–30% of antibiotic-associated diarrhoea, 50–75% of antibiotic-associated colitis). See Infection prevention and control chapter 6, p. 196.

Epidemiology

- Antibiotic-associated diarrhoea and colitis were reported soon after the widespread use of antibiotics. In 1978, *C. difficile* was identified as the main causative agent and largely attributed to clindamycin. Since then, it has been associated with a range of antibiotics, including penicillins, cephalosporins, and fluoroquinolones.
- Between 1989 and 1992, the 'J strain', a strain of *C. difficile* resistant to clindamycin, was implicated in large outbreaks in the USA.
- From 2003 to 2006, CDIs became more frequent, severe, and resistant to treatment in North America and Europe. These were attributed to a new strain designated B1, NAP1, or ribotype 027. This strain occurred in older hospitalized patients, and was associated with fluoroquinolones and high rates of colectomy/death.
- Since 2005, *C. difficile* ribotype 078 has emerged in the Netherlands. It caused severe disease but was community-acquired, occurred in a younger population, and is genetically similar to porcine isolates.
- Transmission—patients with *C. difficile* carriage, whether symptomatic or not, are a reservoir for environmental contamination. *C. difficile* is highly transmissible via fomites, as well as via the hands, clothing, and stethoscopes of healthcare workers (HCWs).

- Risk factors—age >65 years, antibiotic use, hospitalization, chronic kidney disease (CKD), diabetes, cancer, gastric acid suppression, enteral feeding, GI surgery, obesity, cancer chemotherapy, haematopoietic stem cell transplantation, previous CDI.

Microbiology

- *C. difficile* is an anaerobic, Gram-positive, spore-forming, toxin-producing bacillus, which is difficult to culture in conventional media. It exists in spore form in the environment and converts to its vegetative form in the colon where it produces toxins.
- *C. difficile* produces two potent exotoxins—toxin A (enterotoxin) and toxin B (cytotoxin). Toxin A activates neutrophils and causes mucosal injury, fluid secretion, and inflammation. Toxin B is essential for virulence and 10 times more potent than toxin A. Non-toxigenic strains do not cause infection.

Clinical features

- Infection with toxigenic *C. difficile* may be asymptomatic (particularly in neonates) or symptomatic, or cause fulminant colitis. Carrier state—about 20% of hospitalized adults carry *C. difficile* and shed it in their faeces but do not have diarrhoea.
- *C. difficile* diarrhoea—symptoms commonly start 5–10 days after antibiotic therapy (<10 weeks after therapy has finished). Features include fever, abdominal pain, and leucocytosis.
- Severe disease—temperature >38.5°C, WCC >15 × 10^9/L, acutely rising creatinine level, and evidence of severe colitis.
- Pseudomembranous colitis—patients present with symptoms of colitis and have yellow/white pseudomembrane visible on sigmoidoscopy/colonoscopy.
- Fulminant colitis—severe abdominal pain and distension, fever, hypovolaemia, marked leucocytosis, and lactic acidosis. Toxic megacolon is a clinical diagnosis based on systemic symptoms plus colonic dilatation of >7cm on abdominal X-ray. Bowel perforation leads to peritonitis.
- Other presentations—protein-losing enteropathy with ascites, *C. difficile*-associated diarrhoea (CDAD) in IBD, appendicitis, skin and soft tissue infection, splenic abscess, osteomyelitis, reactive arthritis (previously known as Reiter's syndrome) (all rare).
- Differential diagnosis—other infectious causes of diarrhoea, adverse drug reaction, ischaemic colitis, IBD.

Diagnosis

- Requires the presence of diarrhoea and either a faecal test positive for *C. difficile* toxins or toxigenic *C. difficile* or endoscopic/histological evidence of pseudomembranous colitis.
- Testing protocols generally use a sensitive first assay (nucleic acid amplification test (NAAT) or glutamate dehydrogenase (GDH) EIA) and a more specific second assay (e.g. toxin EIA).
- NAATs (PCR) detect one or more genes specific to toxigenic strains, do not test for active toxin production, and can detect asymptomatic carriers, so they should only be used if clinically indicated,

- EIA for *C. difficile* GDH—useful as a screening test, as GDH is produced by all *C. difficile* isolates, but its detection does not distinguish between toxigenic and non-toxigenic strains.
- EIA for *C. difficile* toxins A and B—sensitivity is about 75%, and specificity is up to 99%.
- Cell culture cytotoxicity assay—the gold standard test that detects the cytopathic effects of *C. difficile* toxins on fibroblast monolayers. Highly sensitive, but labour-intensive and slow (2 days).
- Cepheid Xpert® *C. difficile* PCR assay—97% sensitivity and 93% specificity, compared with cytotoxicity assay.
- Culture—culture on selective anaerobic plates is highly sensitive, but slow. Does not distinguish toxigenic from non-toxigenic strains.
- Endoscopy—colonoscopy or sigmoidoscopy and biopsy are a useful adjunct in the following situations: (1) high clinical suspicion of CDAD, with negative laboratory tests, (2) prompt diagnosis before laboratory tests are available, (3) failure to respond to therapy, and (4) atypical presentation with ileus or minimal diarrhoea.

Management

(See NICE, 2021. See Infection prevention and control chapter 6, pp. 199–201 and table 6.5.)[5]

- General measures—isolate the patient; implement infection control measures; discontinue the precipitating drug; replace fluid/electrolyte losses, and avoid antimotility agents.
- Mild/moderate/severe disease—vancomycin 125mg qds PO for 10 days. Second-line antibiotic for first episode—fidaxomicin 200mg bd for 10 days.
- Antibiotics if first- and second-line antibiotics are ineffective— vancomycin 500mg qds PO for 10 days, with or without metronidazole 500mg tds IV for 10 days.
- Life-threatening infection—vancomycin 500mg qds PO for 10 days, with metronidazole 500mg tds IV for 10 days.
- Relapse (further episode of CDI within 12 weeks of symptom resolution)—fidaxomicin 200mg bd PO for 10 days.
- Recurrent disease—occurs in 20–30% of patients, further episode of infection >12 weeks after symptom resolution. Options for treatment of initial recurrence are vancomycin or fidaxomicin. Second relapses can be treated with tapering doses of vancomycin (125mg qds for 7–14 days, then slowly reducing over 5 weeks). Alternatives—fidaxomicin (200mg bd for 10 days) or vancomycin (125mg qds for 14 days), followed by rifaximin (400mg bd for 14 days).
- Alternative antibiotics include teicoplanin and nitazoxanide, and studies are ongoing on comparing their efficacy.
- Consider a faecal microbiota transplant (FMT) for recurrent infections after two or more previous episodes that have not responded to antibiotics. FMT consists of instillation of processed faeces collected from one or more healthy donors into the intestinal tract of a patient with recurrent CDI. Efficacy is thought to be around 50%, rising to 75% following a second FMT and to 90% for >2 FMTs.
- Surgery is rarely necessary but is lifesaving in cases of toxic megacolon or perforation. Mortality in such cases is around 35%.

Prevention

Limit the use of inciting agents (e.g. antibiotics, PPIs). Infection control measures, such as handwashing, universal precautions, and phenolic disinfectants for environmental cleaning, are of proven benefit in reducing *C. difficile* transmission in healthcare settings. Do not offer antibiotics to prevent CDI. Do not advise people taking antibiotics to take prebiotics or probiotics to prevent infection.

References

5 National Institute for Health and Care Excellence (2021). *Clostridioides difficile infection: antimicrobial prescribing*. NICE guideline [NG199]. Available at $\Re$ https://www.nice.org.uk/guidance/ng199

Cholecystitis

Inflammation of the gall bladder, which may develop acutely or gradually over time. Acute cholecystitis presents with fever and right upper quadrant (RUQ) pain, and is usually related to gallstone disease. Usually inflammatory and non-infectious. Acalculous cholecystitis (without gallstones) presents in a similar fashion, usually in critically ill patients. Chronic cholecystitis is characterized by chronic inflammation of the gall bladder and is usually asymptomatic or minimally symptomatic.

Pathogenesis

Ninety per cent of patients have gallstones impacted in the cystic duct. The consequent increase in intraductal pressure impairs blood supply and lymphatic drainage. Tissue necrosis and bacterial proliferation follow within the gall bladder. Complications occur in 10–15% of cases: gall bladder empyema, emphysematous cholecystitis (elderly diabetic men), gall bladder perforation and peritonitis, pericholecystic abscess, intraperitoneal abscess, cholangitis, liver abscess, pancreatitis, and bacteraemia. Differential diagnosis includes: myocardial infarction, ulcer perforation, intestinal obstruction, and right lower lobe pneumonia.

Clinical features

Early obstruction may cause only mild epigastric pain and nausea. Transient cases may settle in 1–2h. Persistent obstruction sees the symptoms localize to the RUQ and increase in severity, with signs of peritoneal irritation (shoulder tip pain). The gall bladder may be palpable in 30–40% of cases. Patients with acute cholecystitis often have a positive 'Murphy's sign'—pain on inspiration as the gall bladder descends towards, and presses against, the examining fingers. Fever may occur. Most patients settle within 4 days, with 25% requiring surgery or developing complications. Complications include: (1) gall bladder gangrene. (2) gall bladder perforation, (3) cholecystoenteric fistula, (4) gallstone ileus, and (5) emphysematous cholecystitis.

Diagnosis

- Blood tests—WCC is usually raised; 50% of patients have mild elevations in bilirubin level; 40% have raised aspartate aminotransferase (AST) level, 25% raised alkaline phosphatase (ALP) level.

- Microbiology—bacteria may be isolated from bile, even in asymptomatic cases of cholecystitis. Rates of bile infection rise with duration of symptoms and age of the patient, and in jaundiced patients (particularly those with common bile duct (CBD) obstruction). Organisms isolated are those of the intestinal flora: enteric Gram-negative bacilli (*E. coli*, *Klebsiella*, *Enterobacter*, *Proteus* spp.), enterococci, and anaerobes (*Bacteroides*, clostridia, *Fusobacterium* spp.). Anaerobic organisms may be found in polymicrobial infection and are often isolated following biliary tract procedures.
- Radiology—CXR is of limited use. Gas in the gall bladder wall or lumen is diagnostic of emphysematous cholecystitis. USS is the diagnostic study of choice, showing a sensitivity of around 90% (presence of stones, thickened gall bladder wall, dilated gall bladder lumen, pericholecystic collection). Cholescintigraphy (hepatobiliary iminodiacetic acid (HIDA) scan) may be indicated if the diagnosis remains unclear after ultrasonography. Magnetic resonance cholangiopancreatography (MRCP) is used to examine the intra- and extrahepatic bile ducts—its role in the diagnosis of acute cholecystitis is limited. Abdominal CT is usually unnecessary but may show gall bladder wall oedema, pericholecystic stranding, and high attenuation bile.

Treatment

- Supportive therapy—IV fluids, analgesia, fasting, nasogastric (NG) tube if vomiting.
- Antibiotic therapy—acute cholecystitis is primarily an inflammatory process, and the role of antibiotics is not clear, apart from in patients with sepsis (fever and raised WCC). Nevertheless, antibiotics are often given because of the risk of gall bladder empyema and pericholecystic abscesses. The empirical choice should be active against the most likely organisms (e.g. *E. coli*, enterococci, *Klebsiella* spp., *Enterobacter* spp.). Commonly used regimens include amoxicillin/metronidazole/gentamicin, ceftriaxone and metronidazole, or ciprofloxacin. Therapy should be tailored in the light of positive cultures. Antibiotics may be discontinued if no evidence of infection outside the gall bladder.
- Surgery—immediate cholecystectomy may be preferred amongst patients who are hospitalized with acute cholecystitis and good candidates for surgery, as it has been associated with reduced perioperative morbidity and mortality and shorter lengths of hospital stay. Some surgeons prefer to treat with antibiotics and delay surgery (>7 days after admission). Laparoscopic cholecystectomy is the preferred option.

Acute cholangitis

Clinical syndrome characterized by fever, jaundice, and abdominal pain. Usually caused by bacterial infection in patients with biliary obstruction (e.g. gallstones, benign stenosis, malignancy).
- Aetiology—similar to acute cholecystitis (i.e. *E. coli*, *Klebsiella*, *Enterobacter* spp., enterococci, anaerobes).

- Clinical features—onset is acute with fever, jaundice, and RUQ pain (Charcot's triad—seen in 50–75% of cases). The presence of confusion and hypotension (Reynolds' pentad) suggests suppurative cholangitis and is associated with significant morbidity and mortality. Septic shock may lead to multi-organ failure.
- Diagnosis—the 2013 Tokyo guidelines proposed the diagnosis should be suspected if the patient has fever/shaking or has evidence of inflammation (abnormal WCC, raised CRP, etc.), and either jaundice or abnormal liver enzymes (ALP, gamma glutamyltransferase (GGT), alanine aminotransferase (ALT), AST). The diagnosis can be considered definitive if, in addition, the patient has biliary dilatation on imaging or evidence of a cause (e.g. stone).
- Differential diagnosis—acute cholecystitis, liver abscess, infected choledochal cyst, Mirizzi syndrome, biliary leak, acute pancreatitis, appendicitis, acute diverticulitis, intestinal perforation, right lower lobe pneumonia.
- Treatment—management of sepsis (e.g. oxygen, fluid resuscitation, monitoring). Antibiotic therapy—initial broad-spectrum therapy based on likely organisms and local resistance patterns. Biliary drainage—usually endoscopic retrograde cholangiopancreatography (ERCP). If endoscopic drainage is not feasible/successful, either percutaneous transhepatic cholangiography (PTC) or open surgical drainage may be required.
- Prognosis—reported mortality rates range from 2% to 65%.

Pancreatitis

Pancreatitis is inflammation of the pancreas, which may be acute or chronic (>4 weeks' symptoms) in nature.

Causes of acute pancreatitis

- Gallstones, biliary sludge.
- Alcohol.
- Smoking.
- Hypertriglyceridaemia.
- Post-ERCP.
- Hypercalcaemia.
- Genetic mutations (e.g. *PRSSI*, *CFTR*, *SPINK1*, *CTRC* genes).
- Drugs (e.g. diuretics, sulfonamides, aminosalicylic acid, 6-mercaptopurine, valproic acid, didanosine, pentamidine, tetracycline, azathioprine, oestrogens).
- Viruses (e.g. mumps, Coxsackie virus, hepatitis B, CMV, varicella-zoster virus (VZV), HSV, HIV, severe acute respiratory syndrome coronavirus 2 (SARS Cov-2)).
- Bacteria (e.g. *Mycoplasma*, *Legionella*, *Leptospira*, *Salmonella*).
- Fungi (e.g. *Aspergillus*, *Cryptococcus* (HIV patients), *Pneumocystis* pneumonia (PCP)).
- Parasites (e.g. *Toxoplasma*, *Cryptosporidium Ascaris*, *Strongyloides*).
- Toxins (e.g. venom of the brown recluse spider, some scorpions, Gila monster lizard).

- Trauma.
- Pancreas divisum.
- Vascular disease (e.g. vasculitis, atheroembolism, hypotension).
- Pregnancy.
- Idiopathic.

Clinical features

- Symptoms—patients usually present with acute-onset, severe abdominal pain, which is usually epigastric (or RUQ) and radiates through to the back. It may be associated with nausea and vomiting (>90%), dyspnoea (acute respiratory distress syndrome (ARDS), pleural effusions), or hypotension.
- Examination findings—epigastric tenderness, generalized abdominal tenderness, abdominal distension, hypoactive bowel sounds, jaundice (if biliary obstruction). Patients with severe pancreatitis may have fever, tachypnoea, hypoxia, and hypotension. Three per cent of patients may have discoloration around the umbilicus (Cullen sign) or in the flanks (Grey Turner sign), indicating retroperitoneal haemorrhage. Rarely, patients may have panniculitis (subcutaneous fat necrosis). There may also be signs related to the cause (e.g. alcoholic liver disease, hyperlipidaemia, mumps parotitis).

Laboratory diagnosis

- Serum amylase level rises within 6–12h of onset and returns to normal after 3–5 days. It is usually >3 times the upper limit of normal (ULN) but may not rise to this level in patients with alcoholic pancreatitis or hypertriglyceridaemia-related pancreatitis. It has a sensitivity of 67–83% for the diagnosis of acute pancreatitis.
- Serum lipase level rises within 4–8h of onset, peaks at 24h, and returns to normal within 8–14 days. It has a sensitivity of 82–100% for the diagnosis of acute pancreatitis.
- Blood tests—FBC, electrolytes, ALT, AST, bilirubin, calcium, and albumin may rule out other causes of acute abdominal pain.
- Pregnancy test in all women of childbearing age.

Imaging

- Plain radiographs—abdominal X-ray may be unremarkable or show a sentinel loop (localized ileus of the small bowel) or a colon cut-off sign (lack of air in the distal colon, caused by colonic spasm secondary to pancreatic inflammation) in severe disease. CXR may show a raised hemidiaphragm, pleural effusions, basal atelectasis, pulmonary infiltrates, or ARDS.
- USS—the pancreas is diffusely enlarged and hypoechoic, and there may be gallstones, peripancreatic fluid, or evidence of pancreatic necrosis. However, in 25–35% of cases, the pancreas may not be visible because of small bowel ileus.
- CT—this may show focal or diffuse enlargement of the pancreas, with heterogeneous enhancement with IV contrast, necrotizing pancreatitis (best identified 5–7 days after symptoms develop), or gallstones.

- MRI—has a higher sensitivity for the diagnosis of early acute pancreatitis, compared to CT, and can better characterize the pancreatic and bile ducts and complications of acute pancreatitis.
- Urgent ERCP indicated if cholangitis suspected (elevated bilirubin and ALP levels).

Management

- The severity of acute pancreatitis should be assessed for fluid losses and organ failure by using SIRS (systemic inflammatory response syndrome)/APACHE (acute physiology and chronic health evaluation) scores.
- Patients with adverse features of severe acute pancreatitis should be admitted to the intensive care unit (ICU) for management.
- Fluid replacement—aggressive fluid resuscitation (5–10mL/kg/h) may be required initially, and fluid requirements should be reassessed at frequent intervals during the first 24–48h.
- Pain control.
- Nutrition—patients with mild pancreatitis can be managed with fluids, until they are able to tolerate oral nutrition. Those with moderate to severe pancreatitis may require enteral nutrition.
- Antibiotics—prophylactic antibiotics are not recommended, but antibiotics should be commenced if the patient develops an extrapancreatic infection (25% of cases), which is associated with increased mortality.
- Antifungal prophylaxis in severe acute pancreatitis remains controversial. Fluconazole may be given if evidence of pancreatic necrosis. Randomized controlled trials are needed.

Primary peritonitis

Defined as infection of the peritoneal cavity not related to a surgically treatable intra-abdominal source. It can occur in any age group and is most commonly associated with cirrhosis of the liver.

Aetiology

- Children—associated with post-necrotic cirrhosis, nephrotic syndrome, and urinary tract infection (UTI) but can occur in those with no predisposing condition. Its incidence has fallen in children with the use of antibiotics.
- Adults—at-risk groups: hepatic cirrhosis with ascites, chronic active hepatitis, congestive cardiac failure (CCF), metastatic malignancy, systemic lupus erythematosus (SLE), advanced HIV. May cause decompensation in those with previously stable chronic liver disease.

Pathogenesis

- Infection is acquired via the lymph and blood (particularly in those with portosystemic shunting in association with cirrhosis, which may increase the rates and duration of bacteraemia), by bacterial transmural migration from the gut lumen, or via the fallopian tubes in women (e.g. gonococcal or chlamydial perihepatitis).

- Enteric organisms account for nearly 70% of infections in cirrhotic patients (*E. coli*, *Klebsiella pneumoniae*, enterococci, other streptococci). *S. aureus* and anaerobes are less commonly isolated. Bacteraemia may occur in up to 75% of those with aerobic organisms. Unusual causes of peritonitis include *Mycobacterium tuberculosis* (MTB) and *Coccidioides immitis*—such organisms are usually found in disseminated infection. *Streptococcus pneumoniae* is the commonest cause in HIV-infected patients.

Clinical features

- An acute febrile illness, with fever, diffuse abdominal pain, nausea/vomiting, diarrhoea, and rebound tenderness on examination. Resembles acute appendicitis. Onset may be insidious, and patients can present with signs of infection/sepsis and no localizing features.
- Cirrhotic patients may have other features of chronic liver disease and develop hepatic encephalopathy.
- Paralytic ileus, hypotension, and hypothermia are signs of severe disease and associated with poor survival.
- Tuberculous peritonitis is gradual in onset, with fever, weight loss, night sweats, and abdominal distension.
- Gonococcal or chlamydial perihepatitis is usually seen in women. Presents with pain, guarding, and tenderness in the RUQ.

Diagnosis

- Abdominal paracentesis is indicated in all cirrhotic patients with ascites. Ascitic fluid should be sent for cell count, Gram staining, culture, and protein concentration. Culture yield is improved by direct inoculation of 10mL of fluid into blood culture (BC) bottles at the bedside. Positive Gram stain is diagnostic but is negative in 60% of cirrhotics with infection. Ascitic fluid neutrophil count of >500/microlitre is the best single predictor of peritonitis (86% sensitive, 98% specific)—generally a threshold of 250/microlitre is used (93% sensitive, 94% specific). Improved diagnostic accuracy is achieved by combining cell counts and the ascitic fluid pH (neutrophil count >500/microlitre, together with ascitic fluid pH <7.35, gives 100% sensitivity and 96% specificity).
- BCs may be positive in approximately one-third of patients. A diagnosis of primary peritonitis can be made only after other potential primary sources of infection have been excluded.
- Contrast-enhanced CT can help identify intra-abdominal sources of infection.
- Some surgeons will exclude appendicitis in children only at operation. Tuberculous peritonitis may be confirmed at operation or on histology/culture of peritoneal biopsies.

Treatment

- Treat those patients with positive cultures or Gram stain, regardless of the cell count (nearly 40% of those with positive cultures and normal cell counts go on to develop peritonitis), and all culture-negative patients with raised cell counts.
- Initial treatment is empirical, while culture results are awaited—piperacillin–tazobactam, ampicillin in combination with an

aminoglycoside, or a third-generation cephalosporin (avoids the risks of nephrotoxicity). Patients with primary peritonitis respond within 48h to appropriate antibiotic therapy. Antibiotics are usually given for 10–14 days.
- Follow-up peritoneal fluid cell counts are useful, but not essential.
- In those who do not respond, another primary source of infection should be considered (e.g. perforation, intra-abdominal abscess).

Prevention

In patients with known cirrhosis, secondary prophylaxis in patients who have recovered from an episode of spontaneous bacterial peritonitis (SBP) should be considered for treatment with norfloxacin (400mg od), ciprofloxacin (500mg od PO), or co-trimoxazole (960mg od) to prevent further episodes of SBP. Primary prophylaxis should be offered to patients considered at high risk, as defined by an ascitic protein count of <1.5g/day, but risks and benefits of this should be explained prior to use.[6]

References

6 Aithal GP, Palaniyappan N, China L, et al. Guidelines on the management of ascites in cirrhosis. *Gut*. 2020. https://pubmed.ncbi.nlm.nih.gov/33067334/

Secondary peritonitis

Secondary peritonitis occurs as a result of a breach in the mucosal barrier, resulting in spillage of organisms from the GI or genitourinary (GU) tract into the peritoneal cavity. This normally occurs in the context of intra-abdominal infections (e.g. appendicitis, diverticulitis) or surgery (abdominal, gynaecological, or obstetric).

Aetiology
- Most cases are due to infection by commensa flora of the mucous membranes within the abdominal cavity. Peritonitis also complicates an exogenously acquired visceral infection (e.g. S. aureus, MTB).
- Infection is usually polymicrobial. The commonest isolates are *E. coli*, *Bacteroides fragilis*, enterococci, other *Bacteroides* spp., *Fusobacterium*, *C. perfringens*, *Peptococcus*, and *Peptostreptococcus*. Antibiotic-resistant organisms are more likely to be found in patients who acquire peritonitis while receiving antibiotics in hospital (e.g. *Candida*, enterococci, *Enterobacter*, *Serratia*, *Acinetobacter* spp.). Vaginal flora (e.g. *Streptococcus agalactiae*) may be present after vaginal surgery or labour.

Pathogenesis
- Many anaerobic infections are synergistic (e.g. facultative anaerobes providing a sufficiently reduced environment for the establishment of obligate anaerobic organisms).
- Leaking bile or acid may cause chemical peritonitis that leads to inflammation, necrosis, and further intra-abdominal damage, facilitating the establishment of bacterial infection.
- Local response—local inflammatory response of the peritoneum leads to fluid production and granulocyte entry into the peritoneal cavity. The exudate contains fibrinogen, which forms plaques around inflamed

surfaces, aimed at localizing infection, and may later lead to adhesions. Some instances of infection may be contained and resolve. Others may lead to local abscess formation. If localization fails completely, diffuse peritonitis may result.

Clinical features

- Symptoms—initial features are those of the primary disease process (e.g. appendicitis). Moderate abdominal pain, aggravated by movement, becomes more severe and diffuse, as infection spreads throughout the abdomen. Pain may reduce in intensity and become more focal if localization strategies are effective. Other: vomiting, fever, distension, anorexia, inability to pass flatus, thirst.
- Signs—patient lying still, alert, and restless at first, later becoming listless. Fever is usually present. Hypothermia may be noted in early chemical peritonitis and is a severe sign late in the course of patients presenting with sepsis. Tachycardia, hypotension, tachypnoea, abdominal tenderness (maximal over primarily affected organ) with rebound and guarding, and bowel sounds present initially but later disappear. Some of these features may be masked in patients receiving glucocorticoids or whose abscess has been localized away from the anterior abdominal wall (e.g. subphrenic).

Diagnosis

- Laboratory tests—peripheral WCC 17 000–25 000 cells/mL, with a left shift (in some situations, massive peritoneal inflammation may lead to low peripheral WCC, with an extreme shift to immature forms), haemoconcentration, elevated amylase levels, acidosis in late disease, features of underlying condition (diabetic ketoacidosis (DKA), haematuria, pyuria, pancreatitis).
- Radiology—contrast CT is preferred initially; plain erect chest and abdominal X-ray: signs of inflammation, free air, distended loops of adynamic bowel, signs of the underlying condition (obstruction, volvulus, intussusception, gall bladder calcification); USS may be limited by the presence of air-filled loops of bowel.
- BCs.
- Peritoneal lavage or aspiration may be appropriate
- Differential diagnosis—pneumonia, sickle-cell anaemia, herpes zoster, DKA, porphyria, familial Mediterranean fever, SLE, uraemia.

Treatment

- General measures—fluid resuscitation, circulatory and respiratory support, appropriate surgical interventions. Exclude pregnancy.
- Operative management is usually indicated to eliminate the source of contamination, reduce bacterial load, and prevent recurrence.
- Antimicrobial therapy—empirical antibiotic therapy should cover Gram-negative aerobes, enteric streptococci, and anaerobes. Broad-spectrum antimicrobial therapy should be started immediately after taking BCs (e.g. IV ampicillin, metronidazole ± gentamicin, or IV piperacillin–tazobactam). Detailed culture and sensitivity results may take several days, as cultures are often mixed and some organisms are slow-growing. Antibiotics may not need to be active against every organism

isolated—elimination of the majority may allow host defences to eliminate the remainder. Antifungal therapy (e.g. amphotericin) should be used if *Candida* spp. are isolated; 5–7 days of treatment should be sufficient after adequate surgical intervention, depending on the severity of infection and clinical response. Conversion to PO therapy may be indicated in those patients with a good response.

Prognosis

- Survival depends on age, comorbid conditions, duration of peritoneal contamination, primary process, and microorganisms involved.
- Mortality ranges from 3.5% in those with early infection caused by penetrating trauma to 60% in those with established infection and secondary organ failure. Death is thought to follow uncontrolled cytokine release.

Prevention

Pre-/perioperative antibiotics reduce infections in clean-contaminated surgery (e.g. appendectomy for appendicitis without rupture, penetrating wounds of the abdomen, vaginal hysterectomy in premenopausal women). Post-operative infection rates fall from 20–30% to 4–8% with prophylactic antibiotic use in such infections.

Peritoneal dialysis peritonitis

Peritonitis was a common complication of peritoneal dialysis (PD), until Tenckhoff introduced his improved catheter in 1968. Rates fell further, as techniques and bag adapters improved. However, it still occurs at around one episode per patient year, with up to 70% of patients experiencing an episode of infection in their first year of dialysis. Recurrent infection is one of the commonest reasons for discontinuing continuous ambulatory peritoneal dialysis (CAPD) (20–30% of patients). Prognosis is good—mortality is <1%.

Pathogenesis

Infection is commonly acquired by contamination of the catheter by skin organisms. Enteric organisms may be cultured from the skin of some CAPD patients. Organisms can also enter via the catheter exit site and through contamination of the dialysate delivery system, as well as transmurally, as seen in some cases of primary peritonitis.

Microbiology

Gram-positive organisms account for 50% of isolates (coagulase-negative staphylococci (CoNS), *S. aureus*, streptococci, enterococci, and diphtheroids); Gram-negative infections account for 15% (*E. coli*, *Klebsiella*, *Enterobacter*, and *Pseudomonas*), and polymicrobial infections for 4%. Anaerobes and yeasts are uncommon isolates. ~20% of cases are culture-negative. *Pseudomonas* and fungal peritonitis are difficult to eradicate and require catheter removal. TB peritonitis should be suspected in patients from TB-endemic areas with lymphocytic peritoneal fluid and culture-negative peritonitis. Non-tuberculous mycobacteria (NTM) may also cause PD peritonitis.

Clinical features

Patients are often unaware of an antecedent event (e.g. possible contamination or breaks in sterile technique). There may be a history of a recent exit site or tunnel infection. Commonest symptoms are abdominal pain and cloudy peritoneal fluid. Other symptoms include fever, abdominal tenderness, nausea, diarrhoea, and hypotension.

Diagnosis

PD patients presenting with cloudy fluid should be presumed to have peritonitis and treated as such until the diagnosis is confirmed or excluded. Peritoneal fluid should be taken from the catheter by using a sterile technique. PD peritonitis should be diagnosed if at least two of the following are present: clinical features consistent with peritonitis (cloudy dialysis fluid and/or abdominal pain), PD WCC >100 cells/mL (>50% neutrophils), positive PD fluid culture. Eosinophilia may be seen after tube placement (an allergic reaction to the tubing) and in some cases of fungal infection. A predominance of lymphocytes may be seen in mycobacterial infection. Gram stain is positive in less than half of the cases. BCs are rarely positive. Fluid should be inoculated into BC bottles. Yield can be improved by culturing the sediment of 50mL of the centrifuged fluid.

Differential diagnosis

Other causes of cloudy peritoneal fluid include chemical peritonitis, eosinophilia of the effluent, haemoperitoneum, malignancy, chylous effluent, and specimen taken from a 'dry' abdomen.

Treatment

- General measures—heparin (500U/L of dialysate) may be used to help lyse or prevent fibrin clots. Analgesia for abdominal pain.
- Bacterial—intraperitoneal antibiotics are preferred and can be given with each exchange (continuous dosing) or od (intermittent dosing). Empirical therapy should cover both Gram-positive and Gram-negative organisms, according to local antibiotic policies and then guided by Gram staining and culture results. Treatment should continue for between 10 and 21 days, or for 1 week after catheter removal. Most patients improve within 2–4 days. Those who do not should be re-evaluated, and unusual (e.g. fungi) or resistant organisms considered, as well as alternative diagnoses.
- Fungal—most cases can be treated with amphotericin, which can be given intraperitoneally but may cause abdominal pain. Most patients with fungal infections will require catheter removal and IV therapy. Flucytosine may be used, but levels must be carefully monitored. Some *Fusarium* spp. are resistant to amphotericin.
- Catheter removal—up to 20% of patients require catheter removal. Indications include: refractory peritonitis, relapsing peritonitis, refractory exit site/tunnel infection, *Pseudomonas* peritonitis with concomitant exit site and tunnel infection, fungal peritonitis, mycobacterial peritonitis, and multiple enteric organisms.

Prevention

Good technique helps to reduce infection rates (e.g. exit site care, connection methods, patient training). Antibiotic prophylaxis may be of some benefit in those patients undergoing extensive dental procedures or lower GI endoscopy. Further details are available in the guidelines produced by the International Society for Peritoneal Dialysis.[7]

References

7 Li et al ISPD peritonitis guideline recommendations: 2022 update on prevention and treatment. Peritoneal Dialysis International. 2022;42(2):110-153. doi:10.1177/08968608221080586

Diverticulitis

Pathogenesis

Diverticulae are sac-like protrusions of the colonic wall. They are associated with a low-fibre diet, constipation, and obesity. Diverticulosis is the presence of diverticulae and affects >10% of those over 45 years of age, and 80% of those over 85 years. Acute (uncomplicated) diverticulitis is defined as inflammation of the diverticulae—it occurs in 20% of patients with diverticulae and is commoner in the elderly and those with extensive disease. Complicated diverticulitis is defined as acute diverticulitis with one of the following complications: abscess, colovesical or colovaginal fistula, perforation, or obstruction.

Presentation

Abdominal pain is the commonest symptom and usually affects the left lower quadrant (sigmoid colon). However, it may occur in the right lower quadrant (mimicking appendicitis) or suprapubically. The pain is usually constant and lasts for several days. Fifty per cent of patients report previous episodes. Other symptoms include nausea, vomiting, fever, a palpable mass, localized peritoneal signs, altered bowel habit (constipation or diarrhoea), or urinary symptoms (bladder irritation).

Diagnosis

Acute diverticulitis should be suspected in a patient with lower abdominal pain/tenderness and is usually confirmed by abdominal CT scan or USS. Blood WCC is often elevated, but this is neither sensitive nor specific. Differential diagnosis includes acute appendicitis, IBD, ischaemic colitis, infectious colitis, and colorectal cancer.

Management

- Uncomplicated diverticulitis—only offer antibiotics if systemically unwell, immunosuppressed, or significant comorbidities. A 5-day PO course is sufficient.
- Complicated disease (abscess formation, perforation, fistula, or obstruction)—often requires surgical or radiological intervention, alongside broad-spectrum IV antibiotic therapy (e.g. piperacillin–tazobactam) for 10–14 days.
- Drainage of diverticular abscesses should be considered if >3cm—this can be performed percutaneously under radiological guidance or

surgically. Surgery is indicated in patients who present with sepsis or diffuse peritonitis, or who fail medical therapy or percutaneous drainage of abscesses.
- After recovery—6 weeks after recovery from acute diverticulitis, selected patients should undergo colonoscopy to exclude other pathologies (e.g. colonic carcinoma) and evaluate the extent of the disease.

Intra-abdominal abscess

Intra-abdominal abscesses may complicate peritonitis of any cause. Primary abscesses develop following primary peritonitis. Secondary abscesses may follow appendicitis, diverticulitis, biliary tract lesions, pancreatitis, IBD, perforated peptic ulcers, trauma, and surgery.

Pathogenesis

Infections are usually polymicrobial, with anaerobes isolated in up to 70% of cases. Other organisms include *Enterobacterales*, *Streptococcus milleri*, enterococci, *Pseudomonas aeruginosa*, and *S. aureus*. Abscess location is related to that of the primary disease and the direction of peritoneal drainage; for example, most appendicitis-related abscesses occur in the right lower quadrant or pelvis.

Clinical features

These include high/fluctuating fever, rigors, abdominal pain, and tenderness over the affected area. Specific features will vary with the location; for example, subphrenic abscesses may cause costal tenderness and chest signs on examination. Presentation can be acute or chronic (particularly subphrenic abscesses where the patient has been receiving antibiotics), and may follow primary abdominal disease (e.g. pancreatitis) or abdominal surgery with prolonged recuperation.

Diagnosis

CT most helpful, occasionally USS or MRI. A pleural effusion on CXR may indicate a subphrenic abscess. The diagnosis is confirmed by radiologically guided diagnostic aspiration. Send BC and abscess material (ideally aspirate/fluid rather than swabs) for microscopy and culture.

Treatment

- Drainage is key—percutaneous drainage (radiologically guided) is suitable for unilocular collections that are readily accessible, are not vascular, and are likely to drain easily by simple dependent drainage. Repeat scanning should be used to confirm resolution, following adequate drainage. Surgical drainage is usually required for multiple or loculated abscesses, or those with very viscous pus.
- Antibiotics—agents should be directed against the most likely organisms (e.g. *Enterobacterales*, anaerobes). Therapy should be started immediately after BCs have been taken. The antimicrobial regimen should be tailored to culture results. Repeat samples may be required in patients with prolonged antimicrobial therapy.

Retroperitoneal abscess

- Abscesses may form in the retroperitoneal space, following direct extension of infection from a retroperitoneal structure (e.g. pyelonephritis, spinal osteomyelitis), intra-abdominal sepsis, traumatic haemorrhage, or bacteraemia.
- Common organisms include S. aureus and coliforms. Anaerobes and polymicrobial infections are less common. MTB may be seen in endemic areas.
- Clinical features—fever, abdominal/flank/lumbar pain, and a palpable mass. If the psoas sheath is involved, there may be pain on hip flexion.
- Diagnosis is made by CT or MRI. BCs and aspirated pus should be sent to the laboratory for culture.
- Management is by surgical drainage and with empirical broad-spectrum IV antibiotic therapy, while awaiting results of cultures. Treatment should be tailored to culture results.

Pancreatic abscess

- Up to 9% of patients with acute pancreatitis develop a pancreatic abscess. Abscesses may also develop following penetration by a peptic ulcer or secondary infection of a pancreatic pseudocyst. Up to 50% of abscesses are polymicrobial. Haematogenous seeding of bacteria may explain those abscesses caused by single organisms.
- Clinical features—presents with failure to improve or abrupt deterioration following initial recovery from acute pancreatitis. Most patients experience abdominal pain radiating to the back, with fever and vomiting. Rarer manifestations include jaundice, distension, peritonitis, and abdominal mass.
- Diagnosis—USS and CT demonstrate an abscess in the majority of cases, but distinguishing the abscess from a pseudocyst may require guided diagnostic needle aspiration. Gas is seen in ~50% of abscesses. Serum amylase may be elevated.
- Treatment—surgical drainage/debridement are essential (53–86% survival). Percutaneous drainage may be helpful in some patients requiring stabilization prior to surgery but is rarely sufficient. Initial antibiotic therapy needs to be broad and can later be adjusted according to sensitivity testing.
- Complications—retroperitoneal extension of infection; fistula formation between the abscess and the stomach, duodenum, or colon; erosion of major blood vessels causing intra-abdominal haemorrhage.

Splenic abscess

- Uncommon and may be due to bacteraemic seeding of infection (e.g. bacterial endocarditis, people who inject drugs (PWID)), splenic infarction (e.g. blunt trauma, sickle-cell disease), or direct extension of intra-abdominal infection. They are usually multiple.
- Aetiology—causes include S. aureus, streptococci, Enterobacterales, anaerobes, and Candida spp. (neutropenic or chronic corticosteroid use). Around a quarter are polymicrobial.
- Clinical features—left upper quadrant pain, with shoulder tip discomfort and fever. Multiple small abscesses may not cause spleen enlargement.

- Diagnosis—CXR may demonstrate an elevated hemidiaphragm, basal pulmonary infiltrates, or pleural effusion. USS, CT, or MRI confirm the diagnosis.
- Treatment—initial antibiotic therapy must be broad-spectrum and modified following culture results. Multiple or large single abscesses may necessitate splenectomy. Incision and drainage may be preferred in cases where the spleen is held by extensive adhesions.

Psoas abscess

- A psoas (or iliopsoas) abscess is a collection of pus in the iliopsoas muscle compartment. It may arise by haematogenous or lymphatic spread from a distant site (primary abscess) or from contiguous spread from adjacent structures (secondary abscess) (e.g. vertebrae, hip arthroplasty, GI or GU tract, aorta).
- Aetiology—primary psoas abscesses are usually monomicrobial (e.g. *S. aureus*, streptococci, *E. coli*, MTB). Secondary psoas abscesses may be monomicrobial or polymicrobial (21–55%, often enteric organisms).
- Clinical features—fever, back or flank pain, inguinal mass, limp, anorexia, weight loss. On examination, patients may have lumbar lordosis and a flexed hip—pain is exacerbated by extending the hip (psoas sign).
- Diagnosis—this may be suspected clinically and confirmed by CT. Identification of the causative organism requires aspiration/drainage and culture of pus. BCs are positive in 41–68% of cases.
- Treatment—drainage may be performed percutaneously (under USS or CT guidance) or by an open surgical procedure. Empirical antibiotic therapy should cover the most likely organisms (*S. aureus* and enteric organisms) and be tailored in light of culture results. The optimal duration of therapy is uncertain—usually 3–6 weeks after drainage.
- Outcome—mortality rates vary from 2.4% (primary abscesses) to 19% (secondary abscesses). Risk factors include advanced aged, delayed or inadequate treatment, bacteraemia, and *E. coli* infections. Relapse may occur in 15–36% of cases.

Liver abscess

Liver abscesses account for 48% of visceral abscesses and 13% of intra-abdominal abscesses. The estimated incidence is 2.3 cases per 100 000 population, and they occur more frequently in women than in men. Risk factors include diabetes mellitus, underlying hepatobiliary or pancreatic disease, and liver transplantation.

Aetiology

- Most pyogenic liver abscesses are polymicrobial, with mixed enteric organisms and anaerobes.
- *S. milleri* (*Streptococcus anginosus*) group are important causes.
- *S. aureus*, *Streptococcus pyogenes*, and other Gram-positive cocci are recognized pathogens in certain circumstances.
- *K. pneumoniae* is an important emerging pathogen, especially in Asia where it has been associated with underlying colorectal cancer.

- *Candida* spp. have also been implicated in up to 22% of cases.
- Tuberculous abscesses should be considered in endemic areas and in cases with sterile cultures.
- *Burkholderia pseudomallei* (melioidosis) is an important pathogen in South East Asia and other endemic areas.
- *E. histolytica* (amoebic liver abscess) should be considered in those who come from/have travelled to an endemic area.
- *Echinococcus granulosus*—commonest cause of hydatid cysts.

Presentation

- Pyogenic liver abscess—presents with fever and abdominal pain, over days or weeks. Other symptoms include nausea, vomiting, anorexia, and weight loss. About 50% of patients have hepatomegaly, RUQ tenderness, or jaundice.
- Amoebic liver abscess—usually presents with 1–2 weeks of RUQ pain and fever 8–20 weeks after returning from an endemic area. Other symptoms include sweating, anorexia, malaise, weight loss, cough, and hiccough. There may be a history of previous dysentery, although diarrhoea is present in <30% of cases. Examination may reveal tender hepatomegaly (50%) and jaundice (10%).
- Hydatid cysts are usually asymptomatic, unless leakage, rupture, or enlarging cyst.

Diagnosis

- Radiology—plain CXR may reveal elevation of the right hemidiaphragm, with right pleural effusion or gas in the abscess cavity. USS or CT is most useful and may be used to guide diagnostic aspiration.
- Blood tests—WCC, CRP, and LFTs may be raised.
- BCs—positive in 50% of patients with pyogenic liver abscesses.
- Aspirates—should be examined by microscopy for *E. histolytica* trophozoites, and cultured aerobically and anaerobically. Pus from amoebic liver abscesses is brown, foul-smelling (anchovy pus), and culture-negative.
- Serology and antigen detection—99% of patients with amoebic liver abscess develop antibodies, which are detectable after 7 days, but do not distinguish recent from past infection. More recent tests based on *E. histolytica* antigens, which wane over time, may be more useful in endemic areas.

Treatment

- Pyogenic liver abscesses—the mainstay of treatment is drainage and antibiotic therapy. For single abscesses, percutaneous aspiration or catheter drainage is appropriate. Repeat aspiration may be required in up to 50% of cases. The drain should be kept in, until drainage is minimal. Indications for surgical drainage include: (1) large (>5cm), multiple, loculated, or viscous abscesses, (2) failure to respond to percutaneous drainage within 7 days, and (3) underlying disease requiring surgical management. Empirical broad-spectrum IV antibiotic therapy should be started as soon as the diagnosis is suspected and tailored in light of culture results. The optimal duration of treatment is unknown, but antibiotics are usually continued for 4–6 weeks.

- Amoebic liver abscesses—metronidazole (➔ see *Entamoeba histolytica*, pp. 582–4) is the treatment of choice and has a >90% cure rate. Alternatives include tinidazole, diloxanide furoate, and nitazoxanide. Following this treatment, a luminal agent (e.g. paromomycin) is required to eliminate intraluminal cysts. Aspiration is probably not necessary, unless the lesion is very large, threatens to rupture, or fails to respond to medical therapy. The mortality rate of uncomplicated amoebic abscesses is under 1%. Higher mortalities are associated with those abscesses that rupture into the peritoneum (18%), pericardium (30%), or pleura/bronchi (6%).
- Hydatid (echinococcal) cyst—surgical resection is the standard intervention. Uncomplicated cysts—PAIR (Percutaneous puncture with CT or USS guidance, followed by Aspiration, Injection of a protoscolicidal agent, such as hypertonic saline or ethanol, and Re-aspiration 15 minutes later). Combine with albendazole treatment.

Acute hepatitis

Acute inflammation of the liver characterized by hepatocyte damage and elevations in serum AST and AST levels. May be caused by a variety of infectious and non-infectious agents.

Aetiology

- Hepatitis viruses—hepatitis A virus (HAV) (➔ see Hepatitis A virus, pp. 463–5), hepatitis B virus (HBV) (➔ see Hepatitis B virus, pp. 465–70), hepatitis C virus (HCV) (➔ see Hepatitis C virus, pp. 471–3), hepatitis D virus (HDV) (➔ see Hepatitis D virus, pp. 470–1), hepatitis E virus (HEV) (➔ see Hepatitis E virus, pp. 473–4).
- Other viruses—EBV (➔ see Epstein–Barr virus, pp. 445–8), CMV (➔ Cytomegalovirus, pp. 448–50), HSV (➔ see Herpes simplex, pp. 438–41), VZV (➔ see Varicella-zoster virus, pp. 441–5), measles (➔ see Measles, pp. 421–3), rubella (➔ see Rubella, pp. 425–7), adenovirus (➔ see Adenovirus, pp. 429–30), Coxsackie B virus, enterovirus, and yellow fever virus (➔ see Yellow fever, pp. 496–8).
- Non-viral infectious diseases—syphilis (➔ see Syphilis, pp. 760–2), leptospirosis (➔ see *Leptospira* species, pp. 376–8), Q fever (➔ see *Coxiella burnetii*, pp. 382–4), sepsis, legionellosis (➔ see *Legionella*, pp. 353–5), TB (➔ see *Mycobacterium tuberculosis*, pp. 391–5), brucellosis (➔ see *Brucella*, pp. 347–9), tularaemia (➔ see *Francisella*, pp. 352–3), and plague (➔ see *Yersinia pestis*, pp. 349–50).
- Drug-induced hepatitis (e.g. paracetamol, isoniazid, rifampicin, pyrazinamide, phenytoin, halothane).
- Toxins (e.g. mushrooms, herbal medicines).
- Alcoholic hepatitis.
- Sepsis.
- Ischaemic hepatitis.
- Heat stroke.
- Muscle disorders (e.g. polymyositis), seizures, heavy exercise.

- Autoimmune hepatitis.
- Wilson's disease.
- Budd–Chiari syndrome.
- Sinusoidal obstruction syndrome (veno-occlusive disease).
- HELLP (haemolysis, elevated liver enzymes, low platelets) syndrome.

Clinical features

- There are no clinical features that distinguish the various causes.
- Acute viral hepatitis can be divided into four clinical stages: incubation period, pre-icteric phase, icteric phase, and convalescence.
- Clinical features may range from asymptomatic disease to anorexia, malaise, abdominal pain, and jaundice to fulminant hepatic failure.
- Hepatitis B and C may cause immune complex-mediated diseases (e.g. serum sickness, polyarteritis nodosa (HBV), glomerulonephritis, mixed cryoglobulinaemia).
- Fulminant viral hepatitis, characterized by liver failure and hepatic encephalopathy, occurs within 8 weeks after onset of symptoms.

Diagnosis

- Routine blood tests—AST and ALT levels are usually dramatically elevated, and bilirubin may be variably elevated. A prolonged prothrombin time (PT) is rare and suggests severe hepatic necrosis.
- Serology—anti-HAV IgM, HBsAg, and anti-HBc IgM, and anti-HCV should be performed initially. If these are negative, other diagnoses should be considered. Discuss with an infection expert.
- Liver USS is usually normal in acute viral hepatitis. Abnormalities (e.g. hepatic lesions, cirrhosis, portal hypertension, ascites) suggest alternative diagnoses.
- Liver biopsy may be performed to establish the diagnosis in acute hepatitis with negative serology.

Management

- Supportive care—most patients with acute viral hepatitis do not require hospitalization, unless they are at risk of dehydration, have clinical evidence of liver failure, or have a rising bilirubin level or PT. Bed rest and alcohol avoidance are recommended, while patients are symptomatic. Most medications should be avoided, but symptomatic therapy for nausea or pain may be required. Vitamin K may be given if the PT is prolonged.
- Treatment—there is no specific treatment for acute viral hepatitis. Corticosteroids have been recommended for cholestatic hepatitis and fulminant hepatic failure, although clinical trials have failed to show benefit. α Interferon alfa has also been used in fulminant HBV infection, but the evidence is poor. There is some evidence that treatment of acute HCV infection with β interferon beta may prevent chronic infection.
- Monitoring—inpatients should be monitored regularly for signs of liver failure and with blood tests (bilirubin, AST, ALT, and PT). Hepatitis serology should be rechecked after 6 months to determine chronicity.

- Liver biopsy may be performed for various reasons (e.g. diagnostic uncertainty, if >1 cause is a possibility, or if specific treatment is being considered).
- Liver transplantation is the only available treatment for fulminant hepatic failure, and patients should be promptly referred for consideration of transplantation.

Chronic hepatitis

This is used to describe chronic inflammation of the liver (lasting >6 months) and may be caused by a variety of infectious and non-infectious agents.

Causes

- Chronic viral hepatitis: HBV (❯ see Hepatitis B virus, pp. 465–70), HCV (❯ see Hepatitis C virus, pp. 471–3), HDV (❯ see Hepatitis D virus, pp. 470–1), HEV (❯ see Hepatitis E virus, pp. 473–4).
- Autoimmune hepatitis.
- Hereditary haemochromatosis.
- Wilson's disease.
- α1-antitrypsin deficiency.
- Fatty liver and non-alcoholic steatohepatitis (NASH).
- Alcoholic liver disease.
- Drug-induced liver disease.
- Hepatic granulomas—infectious, drug-induced, neoplastic, idiopathic.

Clinical features

There are no specific clinical features, and many patients remain asymptomatic until they develop end-stage liver disease. Non-specific features (e.g. fatigue, RUQ discomfort) are common. Symptoms, such as jaundice, weight loss, abdominal distension, or confusion, suggest decompensation. Examination may show signs of chronic liver disease (e.g. palmar erythema, Dupuytren's contractures, jaundice, spider naevi, hepatosplenomegaly, caput medusae, ascites). Clinical features of hepatic encephalopathy include confusion, drowsiness, asterixis, ophthalmoplegia, and ataxia.

Diagnosis

- Routine blood tests—AST and ALT levels are usually elevated, and bilirubin levels may be variably elevated. A prolonged PT suggests hepatic failure. A low albumin level occurs in cirrhosis.
- Serology—HBsAg and anti-HCV should be performed in patients with suspected chronic viral hepatitis. If these are negative, other diagnoses should be considered. Discuss with an infection expert.
- Liver USS may show hepatomegaly or cirrhosis, portal hypertension, or ascites. Hepatic lesions may be due to hepatocellular carcinoma.
- Liver biopsy may be performed to establish the diagnosis in chronic hepatitis with negative serology or to determine the degree of fibrosis in patients with suspected cirrhosis. In patients with deranged clotting, this may be performed by the transjugular route.

Management

- Chronic HBV infection is usually treated with antiviral agents (⊃ see Antivirals for hepatitis B, pp. 101–3) (e.g. interferon alfa α, lamivudine, tenofovir disoproxil, tenofovir alafenamide, entecavir). Liver transplantation may be performed for patients with end-stage liver disease. However, the risk of reinfection is 20%, even with prophylaxis (lamivudine and polyclonal anti-hepatitis B immunoglobulin (HBIG)). For full details, ⊃ see Treatment, p. 101.
- Chronic hepatitis C—all patients should be offered treatment with direct-acting antivirals for 8–12 weeks, with the aim of achieving a sustained virological response and cure.[8] For more details, ⊃ see Treatment, p. 104.
- Liver transplantation—end-stage liver disease secondary to chronic HCV infection is the leading indication for hepatic transplantation. Patients with decompensated cirrhosis without hepatocellular carcinoma awaiting liver transplantation should be transplanted first, and the HCV infection treated after transplant. If the waiting time on the transplant list exceeds 6 months, then treatment should be given.

References

8 European Association for the Study of the Liver. EASL recommendations on treatment of hepatitis C: final update of the series. *J Hepatol.* 2020;73:1170–218

Other gastrointestinal infections

Mesenteric adenitis

- Inflammation of the mesenteric lymph nodes—may be acute or chronic, depending on the infecting agent. Organisms are thought to pass through intestinal lymphatics to the lymph nodes where they produce inflammation and sometimes suppuration. Commonest in children <15 years of age.
- Causes—these include *Yersinia* spp., *Staphylococcus* spp., *E. coli*, *Streptococcus* spp., MTB, *G. lamblia*, non-typhoidal salmonellae, and viruses (e.g. Coxsackie virus, adenovirus).
- Clinical features—fever, abdominal pain, and tenderness. It may be difficult to distinguish clinically from appendicitis.
- Diagnosis—USS or CT may demonstrate enlarged mesenteric lymph nodes. The key feature in diagnosis is to recognize appendicitis and other problems requiring surgical intervention; <20% of appendectomies may reveal evidence of non-specific mesenteric adenitis. BCs may be positive in those bacterial cases that progress to sepsis. Serological tests may demonstrate evidence of *Y. enterocolitica* infection.
- Treatment—patients with mild symptoms need only supportive care. Ill patients with more obvious evidence of infection require antibiotic treatment.
- Complications—abscess formation, sepsis, peritonitis.

Typhlitis

- Inflammation of the caecum. May occur in patients with HIV or severe neutropenia. It is thought that bacteria from the lumen invade ulcerations in the bowel wall during periods of neutropenia, proliferate, and produce exotoxins, causing damage to the gut wall.
- Clinical features—resembles acute appendicitis, with fever, pain, and rebound tenderness in the right iliac fossa. Rapid progression to an acute abdomen may occur.
- Treatment—broad-spectrum IV antibiotic therapy (aerobic and anaerobic cover), with surgical resection of necrotic bowel recommended, as the mortality rate of severe cases of neutropenic enterocolitis is >50%.

Tropical sprue/enteropathy

- A syndrome of acute or chronic diarrhoea, weight loss, and malabsorption of at least two nutrients, which is believed to follow an intestinal microbial infection that causes enterocyte injury and bacterial overgrowth. Villous destruction and demonstrable nutrient malabsorption occur in varying degrees. It has been described in tropical climates throughout the world, but primarily in South East Asia and the Caribbean.
- Clinical features—symptoms develop over months, after several years resident in an affected area. It presents with weight loss, fatigue, and features of loss of specific nutrients—commonly folate, vitamin B_{12}, and iron.
- Diagnosis—there are no specific tests. Laboratory studies reveal features of specific nutritional deficiencies (e.g. megaloblastic anaemia). Faecal studies may demonstrate fat malabsorption, and small bowel biopsy may show villous atrophy. The diagnosis is one of exclusion.
- Treatment—management is with nutritional support and antibiotic therapy (e.g. tetracycline or metronidazole for 6–12 months).

Whipple's disease

- A rare chronic and systemic infectious disorder, caused by the Gram-positive bacterium *Tropheryma whipplei*. Clinical manifestations probably follow a disordered host response to the organism's infiltration of various body tissues. The organism is taken up into tissue macrophages, which may be seen on periodic acid–Schiff (PAS) staining.
- Predominantly affects middle-aged Caucasian men. Patients with HIV infection do not develop the disease, and one small study found *T. whipplei* DNA in 35% of healthy volunteers.
- Clinical features—arthritis, fever, diarrhoea, abdominal pain, and weight loss (90%). Malabsorption follows disruption of the villous architecture. Cardiovascular (endocarditis), respiratory, and CNS (supranuclear ophthalmoplegia, cerebellar ataxia, disinhibition, meningoencephalitis, dementia) involvement may occur.
- Diagnosis—PCR or immunohistochemistry now available. Traditionally, biopsy of affected organs (small bowel, synovium, brain, endocardium) to demonstrate the typical histopathology. PAS-positive, large foamy macrophages (not pathognomonic and may be seen with *Mycobacterium*

avium intracellulare (MAI), cryptococcal, or other parasitic infections, usually observed in patients who are immunosuppressed with HIV disease). Serology has low specificity.

- Treatment—prolonged course of antibiotics (e.g. 2 weeks of IV ceftriaxone, followed by 1 year of co-trimoxazole or doxycycline plus hydroxychloroquine). PCR may be the best way to demonstrate remission—therapy should be continued if patients remain positive, perhaps with an alternative regimen. Malnourished patients will need nutritional support and vitamin supplementation.
- Prognosis—almost universally fatal within 12 months, if untreated. Most treated patients do well, apart from those who have CNS disease or those who relapse (17–35%).

Urinary tract infections

Introduction

Definitions

- The term 'urinary tract infection' (UTI) covers the whole spectrum of infection, from cystitis to catheter-associated UTI (CAUTI) to pyelonephritis. The term 'asymptomatic bacteriuria' (ASB) refers to the presence of bacteria in the urine without symptoms of a UTI.
- Uncomplicated UTI is considered to be infection of a structurally and functionally normal urinary tract (e.g. acute cystitis in women).
- A complicated UTI is associated with an underlying factor that increases the risk of failing therapy (e.g. diabetes mellitus, hospital-acquired infection (HAI), urinary tract obstruction, renal failure, presence of urinary catheter/stent/nephrostomy tube, recent urinary tract instrumentation, anatomical or functional abnormality of the urinary tract, renal transplantation, immunosuppression).
- All UTIs in men, pregnant women, and children are considered complicated. Patients with a complicated UTI may need referral to a specialist for assessment and follow-up.

Epidemiology

- Asymptomatic bacteriuria occurs in all age groups and does not necessarily result in clinical infection.
- Infants—incidence of UTI 1–2%, commoner in $\male$.
- Children—ASB and UTI commoner in girls. UTI is rare in boys and suggests a structural abnormality.
- Women—asymptomatic bacteriuria occurs in 1–5% of healthy, non-pregnant women and in 2–9.5% of pregnant women. Ten to 20% of women experience symptomatic UTI during their life. Risk factors: frequent sexual intercourse, diaphragm use, spermicide use, lack of urination after intercourse, and history of recurrent infections. Twenty to 30% of pregnant women with untreated ASB go on to develop acute pyelonephritis.
- Men—ASB <0.1%. Circumcision is associated with a decreased risk of UTI.
- Elderly—10% of men and 20% of women aged >65 years have bacteriuria. Risk factors: prostatic disease, poor bladder emptying, perineal soiling, and urinary tract instrumentation.
- Hospitalized patients—high rates of bacteriuria; 10% of catheterized patients develop UTI. Other risk factors: $\female$, diabetes, pregnancy, sickle-cell trait, patients with interstitial renal disease, and renal transplant recipients.
- Renal transplant patients—ASB is associated with a high incidence of pyelonephritis and a higher risk of graft loss, although guidelines advise against screening in those who had the transplant surgery >1 month prior (insufficient evidence to make a recommendation in those within 1 month of transplant).

Aetiology

- Seventy-five to 95% of acute community infections are due to *Escherichia coli*. Other organisms include *Proteus mirabilis*, *Klebsiella pneumoniae*, and *Staphylococcus saprophyticus*.

- The microbial spectrum for complicated UTIs is broader and includes the above, as well as *Serratia*, *Pseudomonas*, *Enterobacter*, *Providencia*, enterococci, staphylococci, and fungi.
- Polymicrobial infections are common in those with structural abnormalities, as are antibiotic-resistant organisms (secondary to antibiotic exposure and instrumentation).
- Fungi (particularly *Candida*) occur in patients with indwelling catheters who receive antimicrobial therapy.
- *Staphylococcus aureus* infection is usually haematogenous and can be associated with renal/perinephric abscesses.
- Adenoviruses (especially type 11) and BK virus are implicated in acute haemorrhagic cystitis in allogeneic bone marrow transplant (BMT) recipients.

Diagnosis

- Specimen collection—urine may be collected by midstream clean-catch (to reduce the number of urethral organisms collected), by catheterization, or by suprapubic aspiration of the bladder.
- Urine dipstick analysis—pyuria (>10 white cells/mm³ of urine) is non-specific and does not necessarily indicate infection, but most patients with UTI have pyuria. *Proteus* rarely produces pyuria due to urease causing alkalinity and white cell lysis.
- The dipstick leucocyte esterase test is sensitive (75–96%) and specific (94–98%) for detecting >10 white cells/mm³ of urine. Haematuria may be seen in certain infections, but calculi, tumour, vasculitis, glomerulonephritis, and renal TB should be considered. Proteinuria is common in UTI and should be <2g/24h. The dipstick nitrite test detects the products of bacterial nitrate reduction. It may be falsely negative in the presence of diuretic use, low dietary nitrate, or organisms that do not produce nitrate reductase (e.g. *Enterococcus*, *Pseudomonas*, *Staphylococcus*). A negative leucocyte esterase test plus a negative nitrite test has a high negative predictive value for a positive urine culture.
- **Urine dipsticks become more unreliable with increasing age (i.e. over 65 years) and should not be performed in this patient group.**
- Urine culture—patients with UTI usually have ≥10⁵ organisms/mL of urine in properly collected specimens. Patients without infection will have counts of <10⁴ organisms/mL of urine. However, symptomatic infections can result with counts of 10⁴–10⁵ organisms/mL of urine.
- Blood cultures (BCs)—if systemic infection or symptoms of upper UTI.
- Urological assessment—consider for exclusion of anatomical abnormalities, stones, or tumours in patients with recurrent or complicated UTIs.

Cystitis

An infection of the bladder characterized by dysuria, frequency, and urgency. These symptoms may also be related to urethritis or inflammation without infection. Non-bacterial causes of cystitis include infectious agents (viral, mycobacterial, chlamydial, and fungal species) and non-infectious pre-cipitants (radiation, chemical, autoimmune, hypersensitivity, and interstitial cystitis). Consider these non-bacterial causes in cases of cystitis that are culture-negative and fail to respond to antibiotic therapy.

Clinical features
- These include dysuria, urgency, hesitancy, polyuria, incomplete voiding, urinary incontinence, haematuria, and suprapubic or low back pain.
- Elderly patients may present with confusion and no localizing features.
- Constitutional symptoms, such as fever, are mild or absent.

Management
(See NICE, 2018.)[1]
- General measures—these include hydration, management of diabetes, and investigation and management of obstruction or structural abnormalities.
- Antibiotic therapy—empirical regimens based on local resistance data. The resolution of bacteriuria is related to the concentration of the antimicrobial agent achieved in the urine—dosage modifications are necessary in patients with renal insufficiency for agents excreted primarily by the kidney:
  - cystitis in non-pregnant women—backup prescription or immediate prescription. Appropriate empirical agents include nitrofurantoin (100mg bd for 3 days), trimethoprim (200mg bd for 3 days), fosfomycin (3g stat), or pivmecillinam (400mg stat, then 200mg tds for a total of 3 days);
  - cystitis in pregnant women—appropriate regimens include amoxicillin (500mg tds for 7 days) or cefalexin 500mg bd for 7 days. Nitrofurantoin (7 days) is best avoided in the third trimester;
  - cystitis in men—appropriate agents include nitrofurantoin (7 days) or trimethoprim (7 days);
  - cystitis in children—antibiotic treatment will depend on the age of the child. If <3 months, refer to a paediatric specialist. If >3 months, appropriate agents would include trimethoprim, nitrofurantoin, or cefalexin.

Recurrent infection
May be due to relapse (bacteriuria with the same organism that was present when treatment was started) or reinfection (bacteriuria with a different or-ganism from that before treatment). Reinfection with the same organism may occur due to persistence in nearby areas (e.g. vagina).[2]
- Relapse—consider renal involvement (necessitating a longer course of therapy), a structural abnormality (e.g. calculi, obstruction—consider urological investigation), or chronic prostatitis (➔ see Prostatitis, pp. 734–5). Certain patients experiencing repeated relapses in whom surgical correction is not advised or is not feasible may be appropriate for long-term antibiotic therapy. Such patients should have regular urine cultures (looking for antibiotic resistance), assessment of renal function, and renal imaging. There is no consensus on how long prophylaxis should last; it should be reviewed at least every 6 months. Rates of

infection return to pre-treatment levels once therapy is stopped. Evidence of benefit for the use of cranberry products is limited.

- Reinfection—certain patients experience repeated reinfections (with successful clearance following appropriate therapy between each episode). Those cases related to sexual intercourse may benefit from a single dose of antibiotic taken immediately after sexual intercourse. Where no associated precipitating event can be identified, long-term chemoprophylaxis may be appropriate, particularly in children who may be at risk of renal damage.

Prognosis

- Children—those without obstruction (e.g. urethral valves) or vesico-ureteric reflux (VUR) have a good prognosis. Obstruction can lead to severe destruction of the renal parenchyma. VUR is seen in 30–50% of children with bacteriuria and can lead to renal scarring. Infants and preschool children are at greatest risk. Severe reflux may lead to repeated infection and renal impairment. Reflux alone, particularly intrarenal reflux, may be capable of causing renal scarring, even in the absence of infection. Infection exacerbates reflux, which reduces with elimination of bacteriuria.
- Adults—once a woman has had a UTI, she is more likely to go on to have further episodes.

Urethral syndrome

Seen in women with acute onset of urinary symptoms (e.g. dysuria), but with <10^5 bacteria/mL. Studies have shown that the majority of these patients have genuine infection, with a low number of organisms confined to the lower urinary tract. Others may represent patients with sterile pyuria and urethritis secondary to infection with *Chlamydia trachomatis* or *Neisseria gonorrhoeae*. However, some patients with the syndrome have no pyuria and have persistently sterile cultures—vaginitis and genital herpes should be excluded.

References

1 National Institute for Health and Care Excellence (2018). *Urinary tract infection (lower): antimicrobial prescribing*. NICE guideline [NG109]. Available at: ⌖ https://www.nice.org.uk/guidance/ng109/resources/urinary-tract-infection-lower-antimicrobial-prescribing-pdf-66141546350533
2 National Institute for Health and Care Excellence (2013). *Urinary tract infection (recurrent): antimicrobial prescribing*. NICE guideline [NG112]. Available at: ⌖ https://www.nice.org.uk/guidance/ng112/resources/urinary-tract-infection-recurrent-antimicrobial-prescribing-pdf-66141595059397

Acute pyelonephritis

Infection of the kidney, which may be caused by ascending infection from the bladder or by seeding of the kidneys during bacteraemia. Uncomplicated pyelonephritis occurs in non-pregnant women, and the annual incidence of pyelonephritis is 1.2–1.3 cases per 100 000 women. Complicated pyelonephritis is progression of disease to emphysematous pyelonephritis, renal corticomedullary abscess, perinephric abscess, or papillary necrosis.

Clinical features

Clinical symptoms of pyelonephritis include symptoms of cystitis, plus fever, chills, nausea, vomiting, flank pain, and tenderness. May rarely present with sepsis, shock, acute kidney injury (AKI), and multi-organ failure.

Microbiology

- *E. coli* is the commonest isolate in uncomplicated pyelonephritis. Other species include *Proteus*, *Klebsiella*, *Enterobacter*, and *Pseudomonas* spp.

Diagnosis

- Usually easily diagnosed in women, but may be less obvious in men, the elderly, and hospitalized patients in whom infection may develop insidiously. (For general points on the diagnosis of UTI, ⭢ see Introduction, pp. 724–5.)
- Urinalysis—pyuria is present in most cases; haematuria is unusual and suggests another pathology.
- Urine culture—all patients with presumed pyelonephritis should be tested because of the possibility of antibiotic resistance.
- BCs—up to 20% are positive.
- Imaging—indicated for patients who fail to respond to 48–72h of therapy or who are severely ill with pyelonephritis. Other indications include a history of renal stones, symptoms of renal colic, diabetes mellitus, previous urological surgery, immunosuppression, and repeated episodes of urosepsis. USS or CT is useful to demonstrate renal tract abnormalities—the latter may be contraindicated in those with renal impairment if IV contrast is required.

Management

(See NICE, 2018.)[3]

- General—rehydration, antipyretics, analgesics.
- Antibiotic therapy—start empirically, as guided by local resistance patterns, while awaiting culture and sensitivity testing.
- Uncomplicated pyelonephritis in non-hospitalized patients—empirical options include cefalexin for 7–10 days or ciprofloxacin for 7 days.
- Hospitalized patients should usually treated with IV antibiotics, based on local antibiotic susceptibility data. Possible regimens include: extended-spectrum cephalosporin, ciprofloxacin, or gentamicin.
- Drainage or surgery may be required in some patients with predisposing conditions who fail to respond to therapy and in those developing certain complications (e.g. renal cortical abscess, corticomedullary abscess, emphysematous pyelonephritis).

Prevention

- Cases with an obvious precipitant—changes in practice (e.g. different means of contraception, administration of prophylactic antibiotics, early identification and treatment of lower UTIs) may help.
- Long-term catheter-related infections—ensure a closed catheter system; consider intermittent or suprapubic catheterization. Renal transplant recipients—most centres advise recipients receive 3–6 months of post-operative prophylaxis (e.g. co-trimoxazole 480mg od).

Prognosis

- AKI is rare outside the context of hypovolaemia, obstruction, or sepsis. It may follow papillary necrosis, which may be seen in those with diabetes mellitus, sickle-cell disease, or urinary tract obstruction.
- Renal scarring: adults—a single episode of acute pyelonephritis in an adult woman leads to renal scarring in 46%, as demonstrated by Tc-99m-labelled DMSA (dimercaptosuccinic acid) scanning 10 years later. Acute pyelonephritis in pregnancy may lead to acute renal impairment, AKI, acute respiratory distress syndrome (ARDS), low-birthweight children, preterm delivery, and sepsis. Renal scarring is four times more likely after pyelonephritis in pregnant women than in non-pregnant women. Renal impairment is seen particularly in infections causing severe papillary necrosis.
- Pyelonephritis becomes potentially fatal when secondary conditions develop such as emphysematous pyelonephritis (20–80% mortality rate), perinephric abscess (<15% mortality rate), or sepsis.
- Acute renal transplant pyelonephritis occurring in the first 3 months after transplant has a significant association with graft loss (>40%) by 96 months, compared to all renal transplant cases, with or without the occurrence of pyelonephritis at any time after the transplant up to 96 months (25–30%).

References

3 National Institute for Health and Care Excellence (2018). *Pyelonephritis: antimicrobial prescribing*. NICE guideline [NG111]. Available at: ℅ https://www.nice.org.uk/guidance/ng111/resources/pyelonephritis-acute-antimicrobial-prescribing-pcf-66141393279781

Complications of pyelonephritis

Chronic pyelonephritis secondary to vesico-ureteric reflux

VUR is congenital incompetence of the ureterovesical valve due to an abnormally short intramural segment of the ureter. The condition is present in 30–40% of young children with symptomatic UTIs and in almost all children with renal scars. VUR may also be acquired by patients with a flaccid bladder due to spinal cord injury. This may lead to reflux nephropathy. Sometimes this diagnosis is established, based on radiological evidence obtained during an evaluation for recurrent UTI in young children. Infection without reflux is less likely to produce injury.

- Symptoms—patients with chronic pyelonephritis present with fever, lethargy, nausea and vomiting, flank pain, and dysuria, and children may fail to thrive. Hypertension may be noted
- Investigations—pyuria, proteinuria (poor prognostic feature), urine cultures (negative cultures do not exclude the diagnosis), demonstration of renal stones/dilatation (IV urography, renal USS), reflux (voiding cystourethrography, cystoscopy), and renal scarring (radioisotopic scanning with technetium-labelled DMSA).
- Management—infection should be treated, and underlying structural abnormalities corrected (e.g. ureteric reimplantation).
- Complications—proteinuria, focal glomerulosclerosis, renal impairment secondary to scarring (rate of progress of scars can be slowed by

speedy institution of appropriate antibiotic therapy), pyonephrosis (if obstructed), nephrosis (may occur in cases of obstruction), hypertension (increases the rate of decline in renal function), and xanthogranulomatous pyelonephritis (see below).

Emphysematous pyelonephritis

- Severe, necrotizing, acute, multifocal bacterial nephritis, with extension of the infection through the renal capsule. Gas is found in the renal substance and perinephric space. More common in patients with diabetes.
- Eighty-five to 100% of cases are seen in patients with diabetes mellitus.
- Most cases due to *Enterobacterales*.
- Patients present with fever, chills, pain, flank mass (50%), crepitation (over thigh or flank), and urinary symptoms.
- Diagnosis is confirmed by CT.
- Treatment—antibiotics, percutaneous drainage, nephrectomy.
- Mortality—depends on the extent of gas production and therapeutic approach used. Ranges from 20% to 80%.

Xanthogranulomatous pyelonephritis

- A rare, serious, debilitating illness characterized by a chronic inflammatory mass originating in the renal parenchyma. Gross appearance: mass of yellow tissue composed of lipid-laden macrophages and inflammatory cells (perhaps with an abscess cavity), regional necrosis, and haemorrhage.
- Causes—often associated with infection by *Proteus*, *E. coli*, or *Pseudomonas* spp. in the context of chronic obstruction (stones are seen in 75% of patients, e.g. staghorn calculus).
- Patients are often immunocompromised or diabetic, and it is four times commoner in women than in men.
- Clinical features—patients appear chronically ill, with dull, persistent flank pain, fever, weight loss, and fistulae (pyelocutaneous and ureterocutaneous fistulae have been described). Can present acutely with fever and flank pain. Renal function is usually reduced.
- Diagnosis—CT scan helps diagnosis. Resembles a neoplastic lesion in its radiographic appearance, and tendency to involve adjacent structures, including the psoas muscle and perirenal space. The renal pelvis is dilated. Urine culture may be negative, with the diagnosis confirmed only on histology at operation.
- Treatment—appropriate antibiotic therapy may be important in initial stabilization, but definitive therapy is always surgical, usually by nephrectomy. Other factors complicating response to therapy: obstructing calculus, renal papillary necrosis.

Renal abscess

Perinephric abscess

- Follows chronic or recurrent pyelonephritis, rupture or extension of suppuration within the kidney (usually due to Gram-negative enteric bacilli or a polymicrobial infection), or haematogenous dissemination from another site (mostly due to *S. aureus*). Located between the renal capsule and surrounding fascia, and may extend to involve the GI tract, groin, lung (pleuritic pain, raised hemidiaphragm, pleural effusion), and psoas (may be signs of psoas irritation, e.g scoliosis, pain on hip flexion). Risk factors include urinary tract calculi and diabetes mellitus.

- Clinical features—presentation is insidious, with fever, chills, unilateral flank pain (70%), dysuria (40%), nausea, vomiting, weight loss (25%), flank tenderness, abdominal tenderness (60%), referred pain (i.e. hip, thigh, or knee), flank or abdominal mass (<30%), pyuria (70%), sterile urine (40%), and bacteraemia (40%).
- Diagnosis is often not apparent—one-third of patients are diagnosed at autopsy. CT scan confirms the diagnosis. USS may be falsely negative. Microbiology—midstream urine (MSU) (often normal as abscess does not communicate with the collecting system), BCs, culture of pus obtained by percutaneous drainage.
- Treatment—choice of empirical antibiotic agent depends on suspected pathogenesis of abscess. Percutaneous drainage is often performed. Small abscesses (<3cm) may respond to antibiotic therapy alone. Nephrectomy may be necessary.
- Mortality—<15% with early diagnosis and prompt treatment.

Renal corticomedullary abscess

- Occurs in the setting of pyelonephritis. Usually associated with urinary tract abnormalities and commonly caused by *Enterobacterales*. Disease starts with acute focal bacterial nephritis, which progresses to tissue necrosis and abscess formation.
- Clinical features—fever, chills, flank pain, nausea, vomiting (usually absent in cortical abscesses), flank mass, hepatomegaly. Urinary symptoms may be absent (but seen more frequently than with cortical abscesses), and urinalysis is normal in 30%.
- Diagnosis is best confirmed by CT. Microbiology: MSU, BCs, culture of pus obtained by CT/USS-guided aspiration or drainage.
- Treatment is with empirical antibiotic therapy and drainage. Small abscesses may respond to antibiotic therapy alone. Structural abnormalities should be corrected (e.g. obstruction relieved).

Renal cortical abscess

- Uncommon and usually due to haematogenous spread of *S. aureus*, most commonly from a skin infection. Risk factors include PWID, diabetes mellitus, and haemodialysis. Microabscesses forming in the cortex coalesce to form a circumscribed abscess over days to months. Commoner in men than in women.
- Clinical features—the onset is often insidious. Symptoms include fever, chills, back pain, abdominal pain, flank mass, and rarely urinary symptoms (if the abscess communicates with, and involves, the collecting system).
- Diagnosis best confirmed by CT, and this or USS may be used to guide aspiration or drainage. Microbiology—MSU (often negative), BCs (often negative), culture of aspirated pus.
- Treatment—IV antibiotics (e.g. high-dose flucloxacillin for 4 weeks) and drainage (for all but the smallest abscesses), which may be successfully achieved percutaneously. Nephrectomy is rarely required.

Catheter-associated urinary tract infections

UTIs associated with urinary catheters are the leading cause of secondary healthcare-associated bacteraemia, accounting for around 20% of cases.

Pathogenesis of urinary tract infections

- Catheterization thwarts a number of defence mechanisms that reduce the incidence of UTI in healthy individuals.
- Organisms may be introduced from the perineum or urethra at the time of catheter insertion, contaminate the collecting device, or enter via the space between the catheter and the urethral mucosa.
- Once in the urinary tract, organisms are not eliminated as efficiently as usual, and can reach large numbers within a couple of days. Some are capable of producing biofilms which facilitate their growth. An inflammatory response may result in cystitis and pyuria. Organisms may ascend and cause upper UTI.
- Risk factors associated with catheter-associated bacteriuria include duration of catheterization, ♀ sex, older age, diabetes mellitus, bacterial colonization of the drainage bag, and errors in catheter care.

Short-term catheterization

Up to 25% of patients have a catheter in at some point during a hospital stay. The rate of bacteriuria is 3–10% per day of catheterization. Common organisms: *E. coli* (24%), *Candida* spp. (26%), *Pseudomonas aeruginosa*, *K. pneumoniae*, *P. mirabilis*, enterococci, and coagulase-negative staphylococci (CoNS). Most bacteriuric episodes in this group are caused by a single organism. Organisms isolated from the catheter itself may not be found in the urine. Most episodes of bacteriuria are asymptomatic, but 10–25% develop symptoms of UTI. Bacteraemia occurs at higher rates in bacteriuric patients undergoing instrumentation (e.g. prostatectomy).

Long-term catheterization

The two most frequent indications are urinary incontinence (women) and outflow obstruction (men). Such patients may be catheterized for months to years. All develop bacteriuria at some point, and certain species possess adhesins that enable them to persist in the catheterized urinary tract. Polymicrobial bacteriuria is seen in 95% of long-term catheterized patients. Mildly symptomatic UTIs occur fairly regularly, most lasting only a day and resolving without treatment. Bacteraemia occurs in 4–10% of institutionalized patients undergoing catheter removals or replacements, often following the development of acute pyelonephritis. Other complications of long-term catheterization: symptomatic UTI, catheter obstruction (by bacteria, crystals, protein, and glycocalyx), urinary stones, chronic renal inflammation, peri-urinary infection, bladder metaplasia, and malignancy (in very long-term patients). Some of the complications of long-term catheterization once seen in spinal injury patients are now seen much less frequently, as such individuals manage themselves with intermittent catheterization.

Prevention

- Patients should be catheterized for clear indications only. Incontinence, in particular, may be more appropriately managed by other means.
- When urethral catheterization cannot be avoided, carers should be meticulous in maintaining a closed collection system and the catheter should be used for as short a period as possible.
- Alternatives to indwelling urethral catheterization: conveens (lower incidence of bacteriuria, but have infection risks and complications of their own), intermittent catheterization, and suprapubic catheterization (cleaner skin region is associated with lower rate of infection).
- A single dose of gentamicin at insertion may reduce infection.

Treatment

- Asymptomatic bacteriuria—no evidence that treating catheterized patients with bacteriuria in the absence of symptoms significantly reduces the number of people who go on to develop symptoms. Long-term catheterized patients treated with antibiotics for bacteriuria, regardless of symptoms, showed no difference in the number of febrile episodes. Certain situations may warrant treatment (e.g. patients undergoing urological surgery).
- Symptomatic CAUTI—cultures of blood and urine should be taken. Patients are treated with empirical antibiotics, based on local antibiotic susceptibility patterns and previous infections. Empirical oral options include nitrofurantoin, trimethoprim, and pivmecillinam. Empirical IV options include an extended-spectrum cephalosporin, ciprofloxacin, gentamicin, or amikacin. Therapy can be modified in light of culture results. Treatment duration is usually 7 days. Bacteria may persist in the catheter biofilm, and it is sensible to remove or replace the catheter, if possible.
- Candiduria—seen in many catheterized patients and particularly related to hospitalization and previous antibiotic exposure. It is usually asymptomatic, in which case treatment is only required for neutropenic patients or those undergoing a urological procedure. Catheter removal resolves it in 40% of cases; changing the catheter resolves it in 20% of cases. Patients who must remain catheterized and continue to have symptomatic candiduria may benefit from a course of fluconazole if they have *Candida albicans*, or amphotericin B or flucytosine for fluconazole-resistant *Candida*. Note that treatment failures have been reported with echinocandins, due to low urine concentration. Complications: perinephric abscess, fungus balls in the bladder and renal pelvis, prostatic abscess, dissemination.

Further reading

National Institute for Health and Care Excellence (2018). *Urinary tract infection (catheter-associated): antimicrobial prescribing*. NICE guideline [NG113]. Available at: ℞ https://www.nice.org.uk/guidance/ng113/resources/urinary-tract-infection-catheterassociated-antimicrobial-prescribing-pdf-66141596739013

Prostatitis

Up to 50% of men will experience symptoms of prostatitis at some time in their lives.

Acute bacterial prostatitis

- Usually caused by bacteria entering the prostate from the urinary tract. Occurs spontaneously or after urological procedures (e.g. prostate biopsy).
- Clinical features—symptoms are those of lower UTI (dysuria, frequency) and possibly obstruction (due to prostatic oedema) and fever. On examination: lower abdominal/suprapubic discomfort, a firm and exquisitely tender prostate on PR examination.
- Investigations—urinalysis shows pyuria, and cultures are positive. The usual pathogens are *E. coli*, *Proteus* spp., other *Enterobacterales* (*Klebsiella*, *Enterobacter*, *Serratia* spp.), and *P. aeruginosa*. BCs may be positive either spontaneously or following vigorous PR.
- Management—response to antimicrobial therapy is usually rapid; empirical PO agents include ciprofloxacin and co-trimoxazole. Empirical IV agents include cefuroxime, ceftriaxone, gentamicin, and ciprofloxacin. Treatment duration is usually 14–28 days. Urinary retention is best managed by suprapubic catheterization to avoid obstructing the drainage of prostatic secretions.
- Complications—prostatic abscess, prostatic infarction, chronic prostatitis, metastatic infection (e.g. spinal or sacroiliac infection).

Chronic bacterial prostatitis

- Chronic/recurrent bacterial infections of the prostate which occur in young and middle-aged men. Risk factors include previous acute prostatitis, a history of prior manipulation of the urinary tract, voiding symptoms, diabetes, smoking, and higher prostate volumes.
- Patients often experience repeated infections with the same organism (with symptoms of lower UTI) and are asymptomatic between episodes, with a normal prostate on examination.
- *E. coli* causes 75–80% of episodes. *K. pneumoniae*, *P. mirabilis*, *P. aeruginosa*, and other Gram-negative rods (GNRs) are the next most commonly reported organisms. *S. aureus*, *Enterococcus faecalis*, and streptococcal species are occasional pathogens.
- Diagnosis is usually clinical, as obtaining prostatic fluid or a urine sample post-prostatic massage requires specialist input.
- Treatment is usually with a fluoroquinolone for 6 weeks. Co-trimoxazole is an alternative. Long treatment courses fail in one-third, cure one-third, and bring about resolution (while on treatment) with subsequent relapse in one-third of patients. These poor results may be a consequence of poor drug penetration into the prostatic parenchyma or perhaps due to infected calculi serving as persistent foci for infection. Those not cured may remain asymptomatic on long-term low-dose suppressive antibiotic therapy, despite persistence of prostatic bacteria.

Chronic prostatitis/chronic pelvic pain syndrome

- The largest subset of patients with symptoms of prostatitis. This is a syndrome defined by pain in the pelvic region ± urological symptoms and sexual dysfunction.
- Symptoms—difficulty voiding, erectile dysfunction, and a dull, aching pain, which may be pelvic, perineal, suprapubic scrotal, or inguinal and is exacerbated by ejaculation. Examination is unremarkable.
- There is no history of bacteriuria or evidence of bacterial infection of prostatic secretions. Diagnosis is one of exclusion. It has been proposed by experts that this syndrome is not an infectious disease.

Asymptomatic inflammatory prostatitis

Prostate inflammation with no symptoms. Such patients may be identified in working up the cause of a raised prostate-specific antigen (PSA) level, with prostate biopsy showing a simple inflammatory process.

Granulomatous prostatitis

A histological reaction that may follow acute bacterial prostatitis, tuberculous prostatitis (and that following Bacillus Calmette–Guérin (BCG) therapy for transitional cell carcinoma of the bladder), and systemic mycoses. It may cause an indurated, firm, or nodular prostate, clinically indistinguishable from that caused by malignancy.

Prostatic abscess

- A rare complication of acute bacteria prostatitis. Patients most commonly affected: those with urinary tract obstruction or foreign bodies, those with diabetes, the immunocompromised, and those not adequately treated for their acute episode.
- Most cases are caused by the common uropathogens acquired by the ascending route. *S. aureus* is associated with haematogenous spread. Rare causes include *Nocardia*, *Blastomyces*, *Cryptococcus*, and *Burkholderia pseudomallei*.
- Symptoms resemble those of acute bacterial prostatitis: fever, dysuria, and signs of urinary sepsis. A fluctuant area of the prostate may be apparent on PR examination.
- Definitive diagnosis can be made by USS, CT, or MRI of the pelvis.
- Treatment—drainage (perineal or transurethral) and appropriate antibiotics for 4–6 weeks.

Further reading

National Institute for Health and Care Excellence (2018). *Prostatitis (acute): antimicrobial prescribing*. NICE guideline [NG110]. Available at: ℞ https://www.nice.org.uk/guidance/ng110/resources/prostatitis-acute-antimicrobial-prescribing-pdf-66141591700165

Epididymitis

An inflammatory reaction of the epididymis caused by infection or trauma. There are two distinct patterns of infective epididymitis: sexually transmitted and non-specific (non-sexually transmitted) bacterial epididymitis. Underlying genitourinary (GU) tract abnormalities are common only in the latter group.

General features
- Symptoms—painful swelling of the scrotum which may be acute (over 1–2 days) or more gradual in onset, dysuria with or without urethral discharge. Fever may be present, particularly in hospitalized patients who develop the condition following urinary tract manipulation.
- Examination—tender swelling and erythema of the scrotum, usually unilateral. Early in disease, swelling may be localized to one portion of the epididymis. Consequent involvement of the associated testis is common, producing epididymo-orchitis. Secretion of inflammatory fluid can lead to the development of a hydrocele.

Non-specific bacterial epididymitis
- The commonest pathogens in men aged >35 years are *Enterobacterales* and *Pseudomonas* spp. Other infectious agents: *Mycobacterium tuberculosis* (MTB) (tuberculous epididymitis is the commonest form of ♂ genital TB), systemic mycoses (e.g. *Blastomyces*), *Brucella*.
- Patients often have an underlying urinary tract pathology or a history of recent GU tract manipulation (cases may occur weeks or months after the intervention), particularly if bacteriuric at the time. Bacterial prostatitis or long-term urethral catheters are other important predisposing factors.
- Management—empirical antibiotics aimed at covering Gram negative rods and Gram-positive cocci, while awaiting urinary cultures. Bed rest, scrotal elevation, analgesics. Some complications may require surgical intervention.
- Complications—scrotal abscess, testicular infarction, pyocele, scrotal sinus, infertility, chronic epididymitis.

Sexually transmitted epididymitis
- The commonest form in young men.
- Major pathogens—*C. trachomatis*, *N. gonorrhoeae*.
- Many patients do not complain of discharge. *Chlamydia* spp. may be carried for prolonged periods (≥1 month) before developing symptoms.
- Diagnosis requires a high index of clinical suspicion and appropriate testing, including nucleic acid amplification tests (NAATs). The patient should be evaluated for the presence of other sexually transmitted infections (STIs), and sexual partners followed up. Underlying GU abnormalities are uncommon in this group.
- Treatment—specific therapy covering both chlamydial and gonococcal infections (e.g. ceftriaxone 1g IM single dose plus doxycycline 100mg bd PO for 10–14 days).
- Complications—abscess, testicular infarction, infertility, chronic epididymitis.

Orchitis
Less common than epididymitis or prostatitis. Blood-borne dissemination is the major route of infection.

Viral orchitis

Viruses are by far the commonest cause (e.g. mumps, Coxsackie B virus). Mumps rarely causes orchitis in pre-pubescent ♂, but orchitis is seen in 20% of post-pubertal patients. Testicular pain and swelling follow 4–6 days after parotitis and may be seen even in the absence of parotid involvement. Seventy per cent of cases are unilateral, but contralateral testicular involvement may occur after a few days. Symptoms range from mild discomfort to severe pain, with nausea, vomiting, prostration fever, and constitutional symptoms. Mild cases resolve within 4–5 days; severe ones may take 3–4 weeks. Fifty per cent of patients experience some degree of testicular atrophy. Testicular atrophy has been documented in 30–50% of cases after mumps orchitis—impaired fertility occurs in 13% of cases, but sterility is rare.

Bacterial orchitis

Isolated bacterial orchitis is extremely rare. It usually follows from contiguous spread from an infected epididymis. Most cases of pyogenic orchitis are caused by *E. coli*, *K. pneumoniae*, *P. aeruginosa*, staphylococci, and streptococci. Patients are acutely ill with high fever, marked discomfort, testicular swelling, and nausea and vomiting. Pain radiates to the inguinal canal. There is usually an acute hydrocele, and the testis is swollen and tender. Overlying skin may be erythematous and oedematous. Treatment is as for bacterial epididymitis. Complications (e.g. infarction, abscess, pyocele) may require surgery.

Sexually transmitted infections

Introduction

Sexually transmitted infections (STIs) have been on the rise in the UK and many other Western countries in recent years, fuelled by a decline in the practice of 'safer sex'. The most severely affected groups are younger women and homosexual men. The number of new STI diagnoses made in England continues to rise.

Risk factors

Risk factors that influence an individual's chance of acquiring a particular STI are broadly the same for all STIs. This means that patients with one STI should be assessed for the presence of others, including syphilis and HIV. Risk factors include: number of sexual partners an individual has, failure to use barrier contraception, frequency of partner change, lower socio-economic status, age <25 years, residence in an inner city, symptomatic partner, sexual orientation (syphilis, gonorrhoea, HIV, and hepatitis B are more prevalent amongst men who have sex with men (MSM) in the UK), and sexual practices (orogenital and anogenital contact).

Contact tracing

During the Second World War, fears of a UK STI epidemic led to laws enabling compulsory treatment of a sexual contact named by >1 person with a diagnosed STI. These laws were repealed after the war and led to the concept of partner notification. Partner notification aims to prevent reinfection of treated persons and break any chain of onward STI transmission. Patients are encouraged to notify their sexual partners of any infection risk, with the help and advice of trained health advisers. This process should be carried out by a genitourinary medicine (GUM) clinic, and it is essential that individuals experiencing such infections are referred. It may be appropriate to treat asymptomatic contacts presumptively. Partner notification is voluntary in the UK, but a legal requirement in some states of the USA and Sweden.

Patient assessment

- History—last intercourse, contraceptive method, nature of sexual contacts and number, frequency of partner change, sexual orientation, sexual practices, previous history of STI, previous treatments received, menstrual history, drug use, foreign travel.
- Examination—skin (rashes, lesions), lymphadenopathy, hair loss, jaundice, mucosal lesions, conjunctivitis, urethritis, arthritis, detailed examination of the genitalia, including a speculum examination in women and the subpreputial space and men urethra in men. A rectal examination and proctoscopy may be indicated.
- Tests—should be adapted to the patient's clinical history. Tests include serology (HIV, syphilis, hepatitis A/B) and swabs as indicated (urethral, rectal, vaginal, endocervical, any ulcers or vesicles) for nucleic acid amplification tests (NAATs) (*Chlamydia*, *Neisseria gonorrhoeae*, *Mycoplasma genitalium*, *Trichomonas*), microscopy (*N. gonorrhoeae*, bacterial vaginosis (BV), *Candida*), culture (*N. gonorrhoeae*), and PCR (herpes simplex virus (HSV)).

Differential diagnoses

- Men with urethritis—*N. gonorrhoeae*, non-gonococcal urethritis (*Chlamydia*, trichomoniasis, *M. genitalium*, urinary tract infection (UTI)).
- Balanitis—if associated with ulcers or blisters, consider causes of genital ulceration. If associated with erythema or excoriation, consider *Chlamydia*, causes of urethritis, trichomoniasis, *Candida*, and bacterial infection. Non-STI causes—consider dermatological causes such as dermatitis, lichen simplex, lichen planus, etc.
- Vulval irritation/pain—if associated with ulcers/blisters, consider causes of genital ulceration. Otherwise, consider candidiasis (especially in pregnancy, diabetes, discharge, or recent use of antibiotics), trichomoniasis, and BV. Non-STI causes: dermatological conditions, especially atopic vulvitis, and consider vulval intraepithelial neoplasia.
- Abnormal vaginal discharge—watery, white/grey with fishy smell, consider BV; white, curdy discharge with vulval rash, consider candidiasis; malodorous green/yellow discharge, consider trichomoniasis. Other: gonorrhoea, *Chlamydia*, cervical herpes simplex. Non-STI causes: retained foreign body (e.g. tampon).
- Anogenital ulceration—herpes (preceded by vesicles), syphilis, chancroid, lymphogranuloma venereum (LGV), donovanosis. Non-STI causes: neoplasia, drug reactions, Behçet's disease, trauma.
- Genital lumps—genital warts, molluscum contagiosum, condylomata lata. Non-STI causes: folliculitis, lichen planus, keratoacanthoma, carcinoma.
- Infestations that may be transmitted sexually include pubic lice and scabies.

Bacterial vaginosis

BV is the commonest cause of abnormal discharge in women of child-bearing age. Rather than being due to a single organism, BV is caused by complex changes in the balance of the microbiological flora.

Epidemiology

- Worldwide prevalence ranges from 5% to 50% in women of childbearing age.
- Risk factors for acquisition—new or multiple sexual partners, vaginal douching, smoking, receptive cunnilingus, presence of an STI. It can occur in women who have never had vaginal intercourse.

Pathology

- Lactobacilli produce hydrogen peroxide (H_2O_2), which lowers the pH—the loss of these organisms permits an increase in pH and overgrowth of vaginal anaerobes. These produce proteolytic enzymes, which degrade vaginal peptides into offensive-smelling products and promote discharge and exfoliation of the epithelial layers.
- A reduction in the normally dominant lactobacilli and an increase in other organisms such as *Gardnerella vaginalis*, *Prevotella* spp., *Porphyromonas* spp., *Bacteroides* spp., *Peptostreptococcus* spp., *Mycoplasma hominis*, *Ureaplasma urealyticum*, and *Mobiluncus* spp.

Clinical features
- Fifty per cent of cases are asymptomatic.
- Thin, white/grey, fishy-smelling discharge, most noticeable after intercourse.
- May be associated with cervicitis, which may or may not occur in the presence of simultaneous chlamydial or gonococcal infection.
- Vaginal pain or vulval irritation is uncommon.
- Complications—pregnant women with BV have a higher rate of late miscarriage, preterm delivery, premature rupture of membranes, and post-partum endometritis; BV is a risk factor for HIV acquisition and transmission, and acquisition of HSV-2, *Chlamydia*, trichomoniasis, and gonorrhoea.

Diagnosis
- The Amsel criteria—sensitivity is 90%, and specificity 77% if three of the four criteria are present. Remember that trichomonal infection may cause the first three findings:
  - homogeneous, watery, white discharge coating the vaginal walls;
  - vaginal pH >4.5;
  - positive amine test—add 10% potassium hydroxide (KOH) to a sample of discharge—positive if produces a fishy odour;
  - the presence of 'clue cells' (vaginal epithelial cells studded with adherent coccobacilli) on a saline wet mount—the single best predictor of BV. At least 20% of epithelial cells should be clue cells in those women with BV.
- Gram-stained vaginal smear to determine the relative concentration of different bacteria—gold standard laboratory method, but impractical in standard clinical practice.
- Commercial tests (e.g. a DNA probe test which detects high concentrations of *G. vaginalis*, and a chromogenic test which detects vaginal fluid sialidase activity).
- No bacteria are specific for BV, and bacterial culture is not useful.

Differential diagnosis
Trichomoniasis, candidiasis, atrophic vaginitis (dyspareunia and inflammation are present in these cases), gynaecological malignancy. Up to 10% of infections are mixed (e.g. BV together with trichomoniasis or candidiasis).

Management
(See Clinical Effectiveness Group and British Association for Sexual Health and HIV, 2012.)[1]
- Infection resolves spontaneously in one-third of cases.
- Treatment may reduce the risk of acquiring other STIs.
- Reduce exposure to contributing factors (e.g. vaginal douching).
- Who to treat:
  - symptomatic women—PO treatment is safe in pregnancy and not associated with adverse fetal effects;
  - asymptomatic women proceeding to abortion or hysterectomy—reduces the risk of post-operative infection;
  - asymptomatic pregnant women with previous preterm delivery—may also benefit from treatment. BV is associated with a higher rate

of preterm birth (perhaps due to chorioamnionitis), but studies have not demonstrated that treating it brings about a significant reduction. However, treating BV in those women with a history of preterm delivery is associated with reduced rates of preterm pre-labour rupture of membranes and low-birthweight babies. Consider screening those women with a history of preterm labour for BV.

- Regimens:
  - metronidazole—500mg bd PO for 5–7 days (single 2g dose has lower efficacy and is no longer recommended) or 5g od PV of 0.75% metronidazole gel for 5 days. Early cure rates >90%; 80% at 4 weeks;
  - clindamycin—300mg bd PO for 7 days or 5g od PV of 2% clindamycin cream for 7 days. Use of clindamycin may be associated with acquisition of clindamycin-resistant anaerobes;
  - no resistance to metronidazole has been demonstrated;
  - other agents—tinidazole;
  - no evidence yet to support use of intravaginal *Lactobacillus* formulations or probiotics.
- Test of cure not required if symptoms resolve.
- Thirty per cent of patients experience recurrence within 3 months. A prolonged (e.g. 14 days) or alternative treatment course should be used in such patients. Those who experience multiple relapses may benefit from a long-term maintenance regimen of twice-weekly PV metronidazole gel. Clindamycin should not be used for this purpose.
- Treating partners does not appear to reduce recurrence. Sexual intercourse appears to play a role in disease activity. Some studies have reported reduced rates of recurrence when $\male$ sexual partners used condoms routinely during coitus or when women remained abstinent.

References

1 Clinical Effectiveness Group, British Association for Sexual Health and HIV (2012). *UK national guideline for the management of bacterial vaginosis 2012*. Available at: ℞ https://www.bashhguidelines.org/media/1041/bv-2012.pdf

Vulvovaginal candidiasis

Vulvovaginal candidiasis (VVC) accounts for one-third of cases of vaginitis. See candida in fungal chapter.

Epidemiology

- *Candida* spp. may be found in the lower genital tract of 10–20% of asymptomatic women.
- It is common, with 75% of women reporting at least one episode. It is less common in post-menopausal women.
- Candidal infection is uncommon in prepubertal women but does occur in children who have had recent antibiotic therapy, wear nappies, or are immunosuppressed.
- There is an increase in incidence at the time at which most women begin regular sexual activity.

Pathology

- *Candida albicans* is the cause of 80–89% of cases, but the incidence of other *Candida* spp., such as *Candida glabrata* (now called *Nakaseomyces*

glabrata) and *Candida krusei* (now called *Pichia kudriavzevii*), may be increasing as a result of increasing use of over-the-counter drugs.
- Sporadic episodes usually occur with no identifiable predisposing factor. Risk factors include: diabetes mellitus, immunosuppression, recent antibiotic use, oral contraceptive use, and oestrogen therapy.

Clinical features
- Vulval itch, dysuria, dyspareunia, soreness.
- There may be discharge which may be white and clumpy, or thin and watery, but it is often absent, with only vulvar and vaginal erythema on examination.
- Recurrent infection—defined as ≥4 episodes a year and seen in 5–8% of women. Predisposing factors, such as diabetes, are seen in a minority, and susceptibility seems to be largely determined genetically. Behavioural factors seem to play a part—a 2-fold increase in risk has been associated with the consumption of cranberry juice, use of sanitary towels, and sexual lubricants.

Diagnosis
(See Fig. 18.1.)
- Self-diagnosis unreliable—one study demonstrated that only 34% of those women self-diagnosing candidal infection actually had it.
- Acute VVC: microscopy (high vaginal swab (HVS) for Gram staining and/or phase contrast wet film microscopy). Culture not necessary.

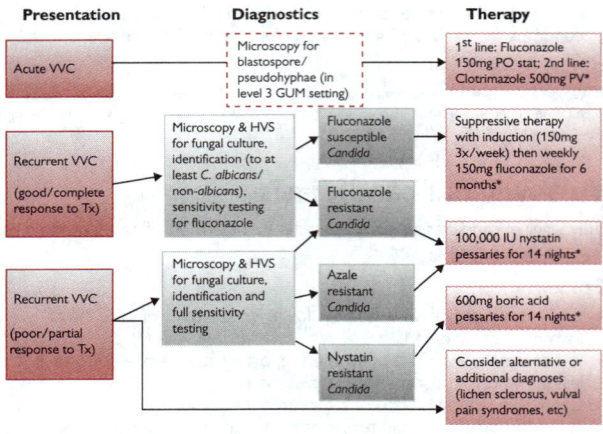

*See relevant section for more details and other treatment options

Fig. 18.1 Summary of the diagnostic and management pathway for vulvovaginal candidiasis. GUM, genitourinary medicine; HVS, high vaginal swab; PO, per oral; PV, per vagina; Tx, treatment; VVC, vulvovaginal candidiasis.

Reproduced from Saxon C et al (2020) 'British Association for Sexual Health and HIV national guideline for the management of vulvovaginal candidiasis (2019)' *International Journal of STD & AIDS* **31**(12) 1124–1144 with permission from SAGE.

- Recurrent VVC: microscopy, culture, and sensitivity testing.
- Vaginal pH is around 4–4.5 (unlike trichomonal infection or BV).
- Limited evidence to recommend molecular and point-of-care testing.
- Differential diagnosis: dermatitis/eczema, lichen sclerosis, vulvodynia, aerobic vaginitis, cytolytic vaginosis, other infective causes.

Management

(See Fig. 18.1.)

- Treatment is indicated for symptoms. Asymptomatic carriage does not require therapy.[2]
- Avoid local irritants; use emollient as soap substitute.
- For severe VVC—first line: PO fluconazole (150mg) on days 1 and 4. Second line: PV clotrimazole 500mg on days 1 and 4.
- Pregnancy—treat only for symptoms using a topical imidazole for 7 days (e.g. PV clotrimazole 500mg). PO azoles are contraindicated in pregnancy. Vaginal candidiasis is not associated with adverse outcomes in pregnancy.
- Recurrent infection (four or more episodes per year)—aim to eliminate risk factors (e.g. screen for diabetes mellitus and iron deficiency anaemia, lower oestrogen-containing contraceptives, behavioural changes where appropriate).
- Most experts do not recommend treatment of asymptomatic sexual partners.
- Treatments with insufficient or no evidence of benefit: probiotics, tea tree oil, PV yoghurt, and honey mix.

References

2 British Association for Sexual Health and HIV (2019). *British Association for Sexual Health and HIV national guideline for the management of vulvovaginal candidiasis (2019)*. Available at: ℅ https://www.bashhguidelines.org/media/1249/vvc-ijsa-pdf.pdf

Genital warts

Anogenital warts are one of the commonest viral STIs. They are caused by human papillomavirus (HPV), a highly infectious double-stranded (ds)DNA virus, of which there are over 70 distinct subtypes. Ninety per cent of cases are related to subtypes 6 and 11. Subtypes 16 and 18 are associated with squamous cell carcinoma.

Epidemiology

- Exposure is usually sexual, and the incubation period ranges from a few weeks to several months. The risk of disease increases with the number of sexual partners. Women tend to be affected more than men in most settings.
- Anal disease can occur in women as a result of extension of perineal infection or receptive anal intercourse. Men usually experience lesions on the shaft of the penis or the preputial cavity. Anal lesions are commoner amongst MSM but also occur among heterosexual men.
- The prevalence of anogenital warts is higher amongst those who are HIV-positive or have other STI. The risk increases with lower CD4 counts.

- Most infections are cleared within 2 years, but persistent infections can occur and are associated with the development of squamous cell carcinoma.

Clinical features

- Those with a small number of lesions may experience no symptoms.
- A larger number of lesions may be associated with pruritus, bleeding, dysuria, PV discharge, pain, and tenderness.
- Rarely, warts may form larger exophytic masses that can interfere mechanically with intercourse, defecation, and even childbirth.
- Anal disease may cause strictures.

Diagnosis

- Usually made visually. Lesions can take the form of flattened papules or the more classic verrucous papilliform warts. Application of 5% acetic acid causes lesions to turn white. This is not specific for anogenital warts, however.
- Anoscopy/colposcopy allows the extent of disease to be assessed.
- Biopsy should be performed where the diagnosis is in doubt, in immunocompromised patients (higher risk of malignancy), and in cases that do not respond to therapy.
- The differential includes: condyloma lata (flat, velvety lesions of secondary syphilis), anogenital squamous cell carcinoma (may coexist with genital warts), vulvar intraepithelial neoplasia, skin tags, and molluscum contagiosum.

Management

Spontaneous regression is seen in up to 30% of immunocompetent cases by 3 months. The choice of therapy, where indicated, is governed by the number and extent of the lesions. All modalities have high rates of recurrence. Women should have a Pap smear. Small external lesions can be managed by the application of a topical treatment, either in clinic or by the patient where appropriate. Large, multiple, or internal lesions should be referred to a surgeon or gynaecologist, and pathological studies undertaken where indicated.[3]

- Chemical agents:
  - podophyllotoxin is a purified extract of the cytotoxic agent podophyllin and can be self-administered to external warts. A treatment cycle is typically bd application for 3 days followed by 4 days' rest, for 4–5 cycles. It should be avoided in pregnancy;
  - trichloroacetic acid acts by protein coagulation and has similar rates of success to podophyllotoxin. It can be used on internal lesions and during pregnancy. Neighbouring skin can be protected from its caustic effects by application of petroleum jelly prior to use;
  - Catephen® 10% ointment—extract of the leaf of the green tea plant *Camellia sinensis*, mechanism of action uncertain. Avoid in pregnancy;
  - fluorouracil/adrenaline gel injected intralesionally.
- Immuno-modulatory agents:
  - imiquimod is applied topically as a cream to external lesions only and acts by cytokine induction. Not approved for use in pregnancy.

- Physical ablation:
  - excision—used for pedunculated, large, or keratinized lesions. Patients may develop strictures. Excised lesions should be sent for histology to look for malignancy;
  - cryotherapy—uses liquid nitrogen or a cryoprobe, usually repeated at weekly intervals. Safe in pregnancy;
  - electrosurgery—places the operator at risk of developing warts;
  - laser treatment—especially suitable for large-volume warts and difficult anatomical sites. Expensive. Places the operator at risk of developing warts.

References

3 Clinical Effectiveness Group, British Association for Sexual Health and HIV (2015). *UK national guidelines on the management of anogenital warts 2015*. Available at: ℘ https://www.bashhguideli nes.org/media/1075/uk-national-guideline-on-warts-2015 final .pdf

Tropical genital ulceration

Genital ulceration is much commoner in patients presenting with STI in the developing world and is an important factor in the spread of HIV. The common causes of genital ulcers in the developed world (HSV and syphilis) remain common in developing regions (e.g. HSV remains the top cause in Jamaica and South Africa) but may be pushed out of the top place by certain other infections (e.g. chancroid in Rwanda). Diagnosing lesions clinically can be difficult—syphilis classically causes a single painless ulcer, but so may HSV and LGV. Where facilities allow, investigations should include: serological testing for syphilis, a diagnostic evaluation for herpes, and, where appropriate, culture on selective media or NAATs (for *Haemophilus ducreyi*).

Chancroid

- Caused by *H. ducreyi*, a fastidious Gram-negative rod (GNR). See chapter 7, p. 341.
- It produces a potent 'cytolethal distending toxin', which is likely to contribute to both the formation of ulcers and their slow healing.
- Incubation after infection is around 1 week, following which painful, erythematous papules develop on the external genitalia (prepuce, corona, or glans in men; the labia, vagina, and perianal areas in women), progress into pustules, and then erode into sloughy, non-indurated haemorrhagic ulcers. Lesions are usually multiple, often developing on adjacent skin surfaces (thigh and scrotum). Unilateral, painful, suppurative inguinal lymphadenopathy is common (sometimes forming fluctuant buboes). Co-infection with HIV may result in atypical presentations with multiple lesions, extragenital involvement, and delayed response to treatment.
- Diagnosis is by clinical appearance, culture (sample is taken from an undermined edge of the ulcer; enriched culture media are required), or NAATs (more sensitive). Microscopy is not recommended due to poor sensitivity (organisms clump in a 'school of fish' appearance). First-line treatment is with azithromycin 1g PO stat or ceftriaxone 250mg IM stat. Second-line treatment is ciprofloxacin 500mg bd PO for 3 days or erythromycin 500mg qds PO for 7 days (second-line treatments are recommended for HIV-infected patients).[4]

- Partners who had sexual contact with the patient in the 10 days preceding the patient's onset of symptoms should also be treated, regardless of whether symptoms are present.

Lymphogranuloma venereum

- Genital ulcer disease caused by the L1, L2, and L3 serovars of *Chlamydia trachomatis*. Endemic in areas of East and West Africa, India, South East Asia, and Caribbean. In the UK, 95% of cases occur amongst MSM.
- Asymptomatic infection in women is common and may serve as a reservoir. Incubation is 3–30 days. Primary infection is characterized by a transient, painless genital ulcer. Haemorrhagic proctitis is the primary manifestation of infection seen in MSM. Direct local extension leads to a secondary lesion 2–6 weeks later—an inflammatory reaction in the inguinal lymph nodes, with fever, headache, weight loss ± pneumonia, meningoencephalitis, and arthritis. Lymphadenopathy may be so severe as to bulge on each side of the inguinal ligament ('groove sign'). An inflammatory mass may form in the rectum, leading to pain, constipation, tenesmus, and rectal discharge. LGV proctitis may be confused with inflammatory bowel disease (IBD). Late disease may lead to fibrosis and strictures in the anogenital tract, genital elephantiasis, anal fistulae, frozen pelvis, and infertility.
- Diagnosis is clinical and by NAATs, followed by detection of LGV DNA. Culture of material from suspected lesions is possible but has increasingly restricted availability. Chlamydial serology is useful, but not specific for serovars.
- Treatment is with doxycycline 100mg bd PO or erythromycin 500mg qds PO for 21 days.[5] All patients should be followed clinically until signs and symptoms have resolved.

Granuloma inguinale (donovanosis)

- Caused by *Klebsiella granulomatis*.
- Endemic in Papua New Guinea, South Africa, parts of India and Brazil; granuloma inguinale (or donovanosis) is primarily an STI, but infection may be acquired faecally and by passage through an infected birth canal.
- Incubation is 1–3 months. The first sign of infection is usually a firm papule or a subcutaneous nodule that then ulcerates (beefy red, painless, non-purulent ulcers that bleed readily are commonest). Auto-inoculation may see ulcers forming on adjacent skin. Local extension and fibrosis occur, and late lesions may cause elephantiasis-like swelling of the external genitalia. Regional lymphadenopathy is rare, but metastatic spread to the bones, joints, and liver has been reported.
- Diagnosis is clinical and by microscopy of Giemsa-stained material from ulcers, which may demonstrate bipolar intracellular bacteria ('Donovan bodies'—a characteristic safety-pin appearance). Culture is extremely difficult and rarely performed. Serology is unreliable.
- Treatment should be given for a minimum of 3 weeks or until the lesions have healed. Options include azithromycin 1g weekly or 500mg daily, co-trimoxazole 960mg bd, doxycycline 100mg bd, or erythromycin 500mg qds (recommended in pregnancy). An aminoglycoside (e.g. gentamicin 1mg/kg tds IV) may be added if there is no initial response (which may be seen in HIV-positive patients).[6]

References

4 Lautenschlager S, Kemp M, Christensen JJ, et al. (2017). *2017 European guideline for the management of chancroid.* Available at: ℘ https://www.bashhguidelines.org/media/1251/chancroid-iusti-2017.pdf

5 Clinical Effectiveness Group, British Association for Sexual Health and HIV (2013). *2013 UK national guideline on the management of lymphogranuloma venereum.* Available at: ℘ https://www.bashh.org/resources/26/lgv_2013

6 CDC (US) Guidelines for the treatment of Granuloma Inguinale (Donovanosis) 2021, www.cdc.gov/std/treatment-guidelines/donovanosis.htm

Genital herpes

Genital herpes simplex infections are a major public health problem across the world. Like all herpesviruses, herpes simplex establishes a latent state, following primary infection, and may reactivate, causing episodic local disease.

Epidemiology

- HSV-2 is the commonest cause of genital herpes, but an increasing number of cases are due to HSV-1 infection.
- Asymptomatic HSV-2 infection is more likely in those previously infected with HSV-1, and vice versa.
- The incidence of genital herpes has been increasing in the UK, and the presence of HSV-related ulcers is associated with an increased risk of HIV transmission.

Clinical features

- Incubation is usually 3–7 days. Primary infection is characterized by local burning, followed by a painful genital vesicular eruption. These vesicles then rupture, forming ulcers. Other symptoms: fever, dysuria, tender inguinal lymphadenopathy, headache, herpetic proctitis. New lesions appear for around a week. Resolution over 1–3 weeks. Up to 60% of primary cases are asymptomatic; thus, the first clinical attack may actually represent the first reactivation.
- Recurrent attacks tend to be less severe with a shorter duration of symptoms and infrequent systemic features. Up to half of patients with reactivation experience prodromal symptoms (local tingling, shooting pains). The majority of patients developing primary infection will experience a recurrence within the first year. Prolonged first episodes are associated with earlier and more frequent relapses. Recurrence rates are much higher with HSV-2 infection and in immunosuppressed patients.
- Rare extragenital features of primary infection include: meningitis, urinary retention due to autonomic dysfunction, and distant skin lesions.
- Subclinical viral shedding can occur in the absence of lesions. This is of importance, as it leads to unrecognized transmission to neonates and sexual partners. It is commoner with HSV-2.

Diagnosis

- PCR-based viral detection is rapid and specific, and allows recognition of asymptomatic viral shedding.

- Type-specific antibodies to HSV develop in the first few weeks of infection and are maintained indefinitely. A positive test does not allow one to distinguish present from previous infection.
- Viral culture from lesions allows definitive diagnosis—it is more likely to be positive if the fluid is taken from vesicles that have not yet ruptured. Less sensitive than PCR.

Management

- Symptomatic treatment—saline bathing, analgesia, and topical local anaesthetic agents (e.g. 5% lidocaine) as ointment for painful micturition. Hospitalization may be required for urinary retention, meningism, or severe constitutional symptoms. If catheterization is required (e.g. autonomic disturbance or pain), the suprapubic route may be better to reduce pain, aid recognition of return of normal micturition, and reduce the risk of ascending infection.
- Antiviral treatment—this is indicated within 5 days of onset or while new lesions are forming. Recommended regimens include: (1) aciclovir 200mg five times a day for 5 days, (2) aciclovir 400mg tds for 5 days, (3) valaciclovir 500mg bd for 5 days, and (4) famciclovir 250mg tds for 5 days. Antivirals reduce the severity and duration of episodes but do not alter the natural history of the disease. Topical agents are less effective. IV aciclovir is indicated if patients are unable to take PO therapy.
- Recurrent disease—episodic antiviral therapy reduces the duration and severity of recurrent episodes. Recommended regimens include: aciclovir 200mg five times a day for 5 days or 400mg tds for 5 days, valaciclovir 500mg bd for 5 days, or famciclovir 125mg bd for 5 days. Alternative short-course regimens include: aciclovir 800mg tds for 2 days, famciclovir 1g bd for 1 day, or valaciclovir 500mg bd for 3 days.
- Suppressive antiviral therapy—patients with frequent recurrences (>4 per year) may benefit from suppressive antiviral therapy. Recommended regimens include: aciclovir 400mg bd, famciclovir 250mg bd, or valaciclovir 500mg od for up to 1 year.
- Consider giving HIV-infected patients who develop severe genital herpes secondary prophylaxis with antivirals if their CD4 count is under 100 cells/mm³.[7]

References

7 Clinical Effectiveness Group, British Association for Sexual Health and HIV (2014). *2014 UK national guideline for the management of anogenital herpes.* Available at: ℞ https://www.bashhguidelines.org/media/1019/hsv_2014-ijstda.pdf

Pelvic inflammatory disease

An acute infection of the ♀ upper genital tract which may involve the uterus, Fallopian tubes, ovaries, and even adjacent pelvic structures.

Epidemiology

- The majority of cases present within 1 week of menses, which is thought to enhance the ascent of vaginal organisms.

- Those at greatest risk of pelvic inflammatory disease (PID) are those with multiple sexual partners. It is rarely seen in celibate women and those in long-standing monogamous relationships.
- Other risk factors include: age (highest incidence in those aged 15–25 years), the presence of symptomatic STI in the partner, previous PID, and possibly vaginal douching.

Microbiology

- *C. trachomatis* and *N. gonorrhoeae* are commonly identified pathogens. The National Chlamydia Screening Programme has reduced the incidence of PID.
- Other organisms include *M. genitalium*, *Escherichia coli*, and anaerobes (including *Prevotella* and *Leptotrichia*). Rarely, *Mycobacterium tuberculosis*, *Haemophilus influenzae*, *Streptococcus pyogenes*, and *Streptococcus agalactiae* have been identified.
- Pathogen-negative PID is common.

Clinical features

- Infection of the upper genital structures may precipitate any or all of endometritis, salpingitis, parametritis, oophoritis, tubo-ovarian abscess, peritonitis, and perihepatitis.
- Symptoms—lower abdominal pain (typically bilateral), vaginal discharge, abnormal uterine bleeding, deep dyspareunia. Signs—lower abdominal tenderness, adnexal and cervical motion tenderness on pelvic examination, fever. Those with perihepatitis may also develop upper abdominal pain (Fitz-Hugh–Curtis syndrome).
- PID can be a subclinical disease and a cause of infertility—one-third of women with no history of PID were found to have *C. trachomatis* in the upper genital tract, with no clinical findings, except infertility.

Diagnosis

- Consider the diagnosis in patients with abdominal pain and one of: cervical or uterine/adnexal tenderness, fever >38°C, raised WCC, abnormal cervical or vaginal discharge, or raised inflammatory markers.
- Investigations include:
  - NAATs for *N. gonorrhoeae*, *C. trachomatis*, and *M. genitalium*;
  - microscopy of vaginal discharge—the absence of pus cells on Gram staining has a good negative predictive value (NPV) (85%), but their presence is non-specific (positive predictive value (PPV) ~17%);
  - imaging—USS can be helpful if an abscess or a hydrosalpinx is suspected. CT or MRI may be helpful but are not routinely indicated;
  - laparoscopy—although specificity approaches 100%, laparoscopy has been found to be only around 50% sensitive in the diagnosis of PID. It should be considered in patients who do not respond to empirical therapy within 72h (less if acutely ill) and those in whom there is high suspicion of an alternative diagnosis (e.g. appendicitis);
  - endometrial biopsy—the demonstration of plasma cell endometritis is a common finding in cases of clinical PID, but it is also found in asymptomatic women with no other evidence of PID.
- Confirmed cases are considered to be those with pelvic pain/tenderness and one of: endometritis/salpingitis on biopsy, *N.*

gonorrhoeae, *C. trachomatis*, or *M. genitalium* in the genital tract, salpingitis seen on laparoscopy or laparotomy, isolation of pathogenic bacteria from the upper genital tract, or inflammatory pelvic peritoneal fluid with no other cause.
- All patients should have a pregnancy test and urinalysis.
- Differential diagnosis—appendicitis, cholecystitis, IBD, UTI, dysmenorrhoea, ectopic pregnancy, ovarian cyst/torsion/tumour.[8]

Treatment

- Most people can be treated as outpatients. Consider admitting pregnant women, those failing to respond to PO medications, those with severe clinical features (high fever, vomiting, severe pain), and those with tubo-ovarian abscesses or likely to require surgery. Selected antibiotics should cover *N. gonorrhoeae*, *C. trachomatis*, *S. pyogenes*, and *S. agalactiae*, anaerobes, and the common Gram-negative enterics. Suitable regimens include:
  - outpatient therapy—ceftriaxone 1g IM stat, followed by doxycycline 100mg bd PO for 14 days and metronidazole 400mg bd PO for 14 days. Alternative regimens: ofloxacin 400mg bd PO plus metronidazole 400mg tds PO for 14 days; ceftriaxone 500mg IM stat plus azithromycin 1g PO weekly for 2 weeks; moxifloxacin 400mg od PO for 14 days. Fluoroquinolones are recommended as second-line therapy, except for the treatment of *M. genitalium*-associated PID;
  - inpatient therapy—IV therapy should be given until 24h after clinical improvement and then changed to a PO regimen to complete a 14-day course. Regimens include: ceftriaxone 2g od IV plus doxycycline 100mg bd PO, followed by doxycycline 100mg bd PO plus metronidazole 400mg bd PO; clindamycin 900mg tds IV plus gentamicin 5–7mg/kg od IV, followed by clindamycin 450mg qds PO (or metronidazole 400mg bd PO) plus doxycycline 100mg bd PO).
- As with all STIs, contacts should be contacted and screened.

References

8 Ross J, Cole M, Evans C, et al. (2019). *United Kingdom national guideline for the management of pelvic inflammatory disease (2019 interim update)*. Available at: ℞ https://www.bashhguidelines.org/media/1217/pid-update-2019.pdf

Toxic shock syndrome

Although not technically an STI, toxic shock syndrome (TSS) is a syndrome of fever, skin rash, and shock due to toxins produced by certain organisms—for example, *Staphylococcus aureus* (➡ see *Staphylococcus aureus*, pp. 261–4), group A *Streptococcus* (GAS)/*S. pyogenes* (➡ see Group A *Streptococcus*, pp. 280–3), and *Clostridium sordellii* (➡ see Other clostridia, pp. 304–5).

Epidemiology

- Staphylococcal TSS—classically associated with tampon use, although non-menstrual TSS (e.g. surgical and post-partum wound infections, mastitis, septo-rhinoplasty, sinusitis, osteomyelitis, arthritis, burns, skin and soft tissue infections, respiratory infections following influenza, enterocolitis) is commoner.

- Streptococcal TSS—associated with severe invasive GAS infections (e.g. necrotizing skin and soft tissue infections, bacteraemia, pneumonia). Risk factors for development of severe GAS include minor trauma, non-steroidal anti-inflammatory drugs (NSAIDs), recent surgery, viral infections (e.g. influenza, varicella), and post-partum state.
- *C. sordellii* TSS—this is associated with gynaecological procedures, childbirth, abortion, and people who inject drugs (PWID).

Pathogenesis

- Staphylococcal TSS—TSS toxin-1 (TSST-1) was the initial exotoxin isolated from cases reported in 1981. It is found in 90–100% of *S. aureus* strains associated with menstrual TSS and in 40–60% of non-menstrual cases. The staphylococcal enterotoxins A, B, C, D, E, and H have also been implicated in TSS. They act as superantigens, activating large numbers of T cells and massive cytokine production.
- Streptococcal TSS—streptococcal pyogenic exotoxins A, B, and C (SPEA, SPEB, and SPEC, respectively) act as superantigens, resulting in T-cell proliferation and production of cytokines that mediate shock and tissue injury.
- *C. sordellii* TSS—the production of two cytotoxins, lethal toxin (LT) and haemorrhagic toxin (HT), causes diffuse capillary leak, oedema, and shock. Another toxin *C. sordellii* neuraminidase modifies vascular adhesion molecules and stimulates promyelocytic proliferation.

Clinical features

- Staphylococcal TSS—symptoms develop rapidly, 2–3 days after the onset of menstruation or surgery, in otherwise healthy individuals. Clinical features include fever, hypotension, and skin lesions (erythroderma, diffuse macular rash, mucosal hyperaemia, ulceration, desquamation of the palms and soles 1–2 weeks after illness onset). Myalgia, weakness, and raised creatine kinase (CK) levels are common. Diarrhoea is common, and renal failure and CNS symptoms (confusion, seizures) may occur. Recurrent TSS may occur days to months after the initial episode, usually in patients who have not been treated adequately or who fail to develop an appropriate antibody response.
- Streptococcal TSS—typically presents with pain prior to developing symptoms of infection. Clinical features include localized swelling and erythema, followed by bruising, sloughing of the skin, and progression to necrotizing fasciitis or myositis. Twenty per cent of patients develop an influenza-like illness with fever, chills, myalgia, nausea, vomiting, and diarrhoea. Fever is common, but hypothermia may occur. Patients may be normotensive at presentation but rapidly become hypotensive. Altered mental status occurs in 50% of patients. Complications include bacteraemia, renal failure, acute respiratory distress syndrome (ARDS), disseminated intravascular coagulopathy (DIC), and rarely Waterhouse–Friderichsen syndrome.
- *C. sordellii* TSS—characterized by rapid or set of severe illness/septic shock in previously healthy individuals. Early symptoms include nausea, vomiting, lethargy, 'flu-like' symptoms, and abdominal pain/tenderness.

This is followed by development of massive generalized tissue oedema, pleural, pericardial, and peritoneal effusions, refractory hypotension, and absence of fever. Laboratory tests show profound leucocytosis and haemoconcentration.

Diagnosis

- Staphylococcal TSS—the US Centers for Disease Control and Prevention (CDC) clinical criteria[9] include: (1) fever, (2) hypotension, (3) rash, (4) desquamation, (5) involvement of three or more systems (e.g. GI, muscular, mucous membranes, renal, hepatic, haematological, CNS), and (6) negative tests (e.g. blood, throat, and CSF cultures for other pathogens; negative serology for measles, leptospirosis, Rocky Mountain spotted fever).
- Streptococcal TSS—the US CDC clinical criteria[10] include: (1) isolation of GAS from a normally sterile site AND (2) hypotension PLUS (3) two or more of the following: renal dysfunction, coagulopathy, liver dysfunction, ARDS, erythematous macular rash, and soft tissue necrosis (e.g. necrotizing fasciitis, myositis, gangrene).
- *C. sordellii* TSS—the diagnosis should be suspected in young women with rapid clinical deterioration following a gynaecological procedure, abortion, or delivery, and in PWID. Blood cultures (BCs) are positive in 20% of cases. Vaginal and/or wound specimens should be cultured.

Management

- Supportive therapy—patients may require extensive fluid replacement (10–20L/day) to maintain tissue perfusion. Vasopressors may be required.
- Surgery—for menstrual TSS, foreign bodies should be removed and surgical drainage/debridement may be required for post-surgical cases. Extensive surgical debridement is required for necrotizing fasciitis cases.
- Empirical antibiotic therapy may need to be broad if the diagnosis of TSS is not yet established and Gram-negative or anaerobic cover indicated.
- Staphylococcal TSS—no randomized studies have evaluated antibiotic regimens. Antibiotic therapy should include an active drug, such as a β-lactam or vancomycin, plus a drug that suppresses protein synthesis (and therefore potentially toxin production) such as clindamycin. In the absence of bacteraemia or a distinct focus of infection, aim for 10–14 days of treatment.
- Streptococcal TSS—empirical treatment for streptococcal TSS would be the same as for staphylococcal TSS. Once the diagnosis is confirmed, treatment should be changed to benzylpenicillin 4 million units every 4h plus clindamycin 900mg tds IV. The duration of therapy is 14 days after the last surgical debridement.
- *C. sordellii* TSS—empirical treatment is with clindamycin 900mg tds IV plus piperacillin–tazobactam 4.5g tds IV. Once the diagnosis is confirmed, treatment should be changed to benzylpenicillin 4 million units every 4h plus clindamycin 900mg tds IV.
- Adjunctive therapies—more evidence is needed to assess the effectiveness of these. They include: (1) IVIG (staphylococcal and streptococcal TSS are listed as 'blue' indications by the Department

of Health, meaning approval by the local IVIG lead is required), (2) corticosteroids, (3) hyperbaric oxygen, (4) *C. sordellii* anti-toxin, and (5) anti-tumour necrosis factor (TNF) antibody.

Prognosis

- Staphylococcal TSS—death usually occurs within a few of days of presentation but can occur up to 2 weeks later. Causes of death include cardiac arrhythmias, respiratory failure, and bleeding. Mortality in menstrual cases is around 1.8%, and in non-menstrual cases 6%.
- Streptococcal TSS—the mortality rate is 30–70% in adults, and 18% in children.
- *C. sordellii* TSS—mortality is high and ranges from 50% to 100%.

References

9 Centers for Disease Control and Prevention. *Toxic shock syndrome (other than streptococcal) (TSS). 2011 case definition.* Available at: https://ndc.services.cdc.gov/case-definitions/toxic-shock-syndrome-2011/

10 Centers for Disease Control and Prevention. *Streptococcal toxic shock syndrome (STSS) (Streptococcus pyogenes). 2010 case definition.* Available at: https://ndc.services.cdc.gov/case-definitions/streptococcal-toxic-shock-syndrome-2010/

Gonorrhoea

A purulent infection of mucous membranes (e.g. urethra, rectum, cervix, conjunctiva, pharynx) caused by *N. gonorrhoeae*. See chapter 7, pp. 311–13.

Epidemiology

- Infection is common across the world. In the developing world, perinatal transmission and neonatal eye infections remain a significant problem.
- It is the second commonest STI in the UK, affecting predominantly young people (peaking in ♂ aged 20–24 years and in ♀ aged 16–19 years), with the highest rates in deprived urban areas. Infection is concentrated amongst MSM and black ethnic minority populations. Since 2015, gonorrhoea diagnoses in the UK have risen by 71%.
- The recent increase in incidence and growing prevalence of antimicrobial resistance have made it a major public health concern.
- Resistance to first-line antibiotic treatment is related to an increased risk of treatment failure (with consequent disease complications) and onward transmission within a community. In 2017, 36% of isolates in the UK were resistant to ciprofloxacin.

Clinical features

- Incubation is 2–5 days. Lower genital tract infection may be asymptomatic or cause urethritis, with purulent discharge and dysuria in men and endocervicitis with PV discharge, itch, and dysuria in women. Although infection of the ♀ urethra, pharynx, and rectum (common in MSM, uncommon otherwise and causing discharge and tenesmus) is probably common, they are usually asymptomatic.
- Retrograde spread may occur, causing salpingitis/endometritis, PID (➔ see Pelvic inflammatory disease, pp. 750–2), and tubo-ovarian abscesses in up to 20% of women with cervicitis. In rare cases,

frank peritonitis or perihepatitis (Fitz-Hugh–Curtis syndrome) is seen. Men with gonococcal urethritis can develop epididymitis or epididymo-orchitis.

- Disseminated gonococcal infection may follow around 1% of genital infection; 75% of such cases occur in women who are at increased risk if mucosal infection occurs during menstruation or pregnancy. Features include: rash, fever, arthralgias, migratory polyarthritis, septic arthritis, endocarditis, and meningitis.
- Neonates acquiring infection intrapartum present with ophthalmia neonatorum and disseminated infection. Conjunctivitis can also occur in adults, following direct inoculation of organisms, and may lead to blindness.[11]

Diagnosis

- NAATs—the screening test of choice for asymptomatic individuals with urethral and endocervical infection, and for rectal and pharyngeal infection in MSM. They are highly sensitive (>95%). In low-prevalence populations (<1% prevalence), a positive NAAT result may have a PPV of <90% and confirmatory supplementary testing is required.
- Microscopy—provides rapid, near-patient diagnosis in symptomatic patients and shows Gram-negative diplococci within polymorphonuclear cells. Sensitivity is high in men with urethral discharge (90–95% sensitive) and lower in asymptomatic men (50–75% sensitive) and in women with endocervical discharge (37–50% sensitive). It should not be performed on pharyngeal or rectal specimens.
- Culture—all infected areas should be swabbed and plated onto selective media, both to confirm diagnosis and to provide antibiotic susceptibility data. Culture has a sensitivity of 85–95% for urethral and endocervical infection.
- Disseminated infection—joint effusions, blood, and CSF should be sent for culture and Gram staining, where appropriate. Negative cultures do not rule out disseminated infection.

Management

- Indications for treatment—these include: (1) identification of Gram-negative intracellular diplococci on microscopy of a genital tract smear, (2) a positive culture of *N. gonorrhoeae* from any site, (3) a positive NAAT from any site, and (4) consideration on epidemiological grounds in sexual assault cases.
- Antibiotics for uncomplicated anogenital or pharyngeal infection—first-line therapy is ceftriaxone 1g IM single dose. Alternative regimens include azithromycin 2g PO as a single dose PLUS: (1) cefixime 400mg PO single dose, (2) spectinomycin 2g IM single dose, or (3) gentamicin 240mg IM single dose. If the isolate is ciprofloxacin-susceptible, use ciprofloxacin 500mg PO single dose.[12]
- Test of cure (TOC)—this is recommended following treatment of gonococcal infections, because of treatment failures and increasing antimicrobial resistance. Where a universal TOC is not feasible, it is recommended for the following groups: persisting symptoms/signs, pharyngeal infection, treatment with a second-line regimen or acquired in the Asia-Pacific region when antimicrobial susceptibility is unknown.

- Partner notification and treatment of contacts—if presenting after 14 days of exposure, treat only following a positive test for gonorrhoea. If presenting within 14 days of exposure, consider epidemiological treatment.

References

11 Public Health England (2014, updated 2021). *Detection of gonorrhoea in England*. Available at: ℘ https://www.gov.uk/government/publications/guidance-for-the-detection-of-gonorrhoea-in-england

12 Fifer H, Saunders J, Soni S, et al. (2018). *2018 UK national guideline for the management of infection with Neisseria gonorrhoeae*. Available at: ℘ https://www.bashhguidelines.org/media/1238/gc-2018.pdf

Chlamydia

Epidemiology

The commonest STI in the UK, with rates highest in the under 25s. A significant number of cases are asymptomatic, and 10–40% of untreated infected women develop PID, making it an important reproductive health issue. The number of cases in the UK has been rising steadily since the mid 1990s, prompting the establishment of the National Chlamydia Screening Programme (NCSP) in 2003. The responsible organisms are *C. trachomatis* serovars D–K (➔ see *Chlamydia*, p. 388).

Clinical features

- Incubation period is 1–3 weeks.
- Around 50% of infected ♂ and 80% of infected ♀ are asymptomatic—such infection may persist for many years, if untreated.
- Symptoms—mucopurulent cervicitis in ♀ and urethritis with dysuria and discharge in ♂. Ascending genital tract infection may lead to PID in women and is the commonest cause of epididymitis in men aged under 35 years. Proctitis and pharyngitis occur in men and women.
- Other presentations—LGV (the cause of 10% of genital ulcers in tropical countries; ➔ see Tropical genital ulceration, pp. 747–9), neonatal conjunctivitis, and neonatal pneumonia may occur in children born to infected mothers.
- Complications—PID (➔ see Pelvic inflammatory disease, pp. 750–2), reactive arthritis (formerly known as Reiter's disease: urethritis, conjunctivitis, reactive arthritis), perihepatitis, conjunctivitis.
- Co-infection of *Chlamydia* and gonorrhoea is common (40% of women and 20% of men with *Chlamydia* also have gonorrhoea).

Diagnosis

- NAATs—these have become the diagnostic test of choice, as they are highly sensitive (90–95%). A vulvovaginal swab is the specimen of choice in women. Appropriate samples in men include a first-catch urine sample or a urethral swab. Pharyngeal and rectal swabs are recommended in MSM.
- Enzyme-linked immunoassays (EIAs), direct fluorescent antibody (DFA) tests, and cell culture are no longer recommended.[13]

Management
- General measures—patients should be advised to avoid sexual intercourse until treatment has finished (or for 7 days after azithromycin treatment). Patients should be offered screening for other STIs, including HIV and hepatitis B virus (HBV) screening, and vaccination. All contacts should be offered the same tests.
- Antibiotics—first-line treatment is doxycycline 100mg bd PO for 7 days. Single-dose azithromycin is no longer recommended. Alternative regimens are azithromycin 1g single dose, followed by 500mg daily for 2 days, erythromycin 500mg bd for 10–14 days, or ofloxacin 200mg bd or 400mg od for 7 days. First-time cure rates of over 95%.
- Pregnancy—doxycycline and ofloxacin are contraindicated. Treat with azithromycin 1g single dose, followed by 500mg daily for 2 days (*British National Formulary* (*BNF*) caution), erythromycin 500mg qds PO for 7 days, erythromycin 500mg bd for 14 days, or amoxicillin 500mg tds PO for 7 days.
- TOC recommended in pregnancy where poor compliance is suspected and where symptoms persist (perform at least 3 weeks after treatment is completed).
- The NCSP recommends that people <25 years old with a positive test should be offered a repeat test 3 months after treatment of the initial infection.[13]

References
13 Nwokolo NC, Dragovic B, Patel S, *et al.* (2015). *2015 UK national guideline for the management of infection with Chlamydia trachomatis.* Available at: 🔗 https://www.bashhguidelines.org/media/1192/ct-2015.pdf

Mycoplasma genitalium

A fastidious bacterium that is an increasingly recognized cause of non-gonococcal urethritis in men and cervicitis in women. See chapter 7, p. 387.

Epidemiology
- Prevalence in the general population of 1–2%.
- Risk factors include: younger age, increasing number of sexual partners, non-white ethnicity, smoking.

Clinical features
- The majority of infections are asymptomatic.
- Signs and symptoms—urethral discharge, dysuria, and urethritis in men; and dysuria, abnormal bleeding, cervicitis, and lower abdominal pain in women.
- Complications—reactive arthritis, epididymo-orchitis in men; PID and preterm delivery in women.

Diagnosis
- NAATs are the diagnostic test of choice. All positive specimens should be tested for macrolide resistance. A first-void urine is the most sensitive specimen in men, and a vulvovaginal swab is the specimen of choice in women.
- Culture not appropriate, as organism is fastidious and slow-growing.

Management

- Uncomplicated urogenital infection—doxycycline 100mg bd PO for 7 days. If macrolide-sensitive or resistance unknown, follow with azithromycin 1g PO as a single dose, then 500mg od PO for 2 days. If macrolide-resistant or treatment with azithromycin has failed, give moxifloxacin 400mg od PO for 10 days.
- Treatment of PID/epididymo-orchitis—moxifloxacin 400mg od PO for 14 days.
- Pregnancy—the 3-day azithromycin regimen can be used for uncomplicated infection. Options limited in those with macrolide-resistance or upper genital tract infection. Where possible, treatment should be delayed until after pregnancy.
- TOC should be performed in all patients 5 weeks after the start of treatment.

Further reading

Soni S, Horner P, Rayment M, et al. (2018). British Association for Sexual Health and HIV national guideline for the management of infection with Mycoplasma genitalium (2018). Available at: ℘ https://www.bashhguidelines.org/media/1228/mg-ijstdaids.pdf

Trichomoniasis

An infection caused by the flagellated protozoan *Trichomonas vaginalis* (➔ see *Trichomonas vaginalis*, pp. 581–2).

Epidemiology

- Transmission is by sexual contact, and its incidence is highest in women with multiple sexual partners and those with other STIs, including HIV. Vertical transmission may take place during delivery.
- Non-sexual transmission (e.g. by contact with contaminated linen in institutions) occurs but is very rare.

Clinical features

- Incubation is 5–28 days.
- Infection is asymptomatic in up to 50% of people.
- Symptoms tend to develop during menstruation or pregnancy (higher vaginal pH provides a favourable environment for parasite replication) and include: frothy, yellow vaginal discharge (may be itchy and smelly), dyspareunia, dysuria, and lower abdominal pain.
- On examination, the vulva may be erythematous, with obvious discharge, vaginal inflammation, and punctate haemorrhages on the cervix ('strawberry cervix').
- Symptomatic men experience urethritis indistinguishable from other causes of non-gonococcal urethritis.
- Complications—vaginitis emphysematosa (gas-filled blebs in the vaginal wall), vaginal cuff cellulitis after hysterectomy premature labour, low-birthweight infants.

Diagnosis

- Microscopy—light-field microscopy of wet preparation of genital specimens will demonstrate motile flagellated protozoans. Highly specific, but not sensitive. Culture is more sensitive than microscopy but requires specialist media (e.g. InPouch™ TV media or Diamond's media).
- Point-of-care tests (e.g. OSOM® *Trichomonas* rapid test) has a sensitivity of 80–94% and a specificity of >95%.
- NAATs offer the highest sensitivity and are becoming the gold standard.

Management

- Metronidazole 2g stat dose, metronidazole 400–500mg bd for 5–7 days, or tinidazole 2g stat dose. Partners and asymptomatic individuals should be treated.
- TOC recommended if the patient remains symptomatic following treatment or if symptoms recur.[14]

References

14 British Association for Sexual Health and HIV (BASHH) United Kingdom national guideline on the management of Trichomonas vaginalis 2021, www.bashh.org/resources/20/trichomonas_vaginalis_2021

Syphilis

Caused by *Treponema pallidum* subspecies *pallidum* (◗ see *Treponema* species, pp. 369–72).

Epidemiology

- Generally transmitted by sexual contact; can also be transmitted vertically and via blood transfusions. Highest rates are seen in adults.
- Cases of syphilis have risen dramatically in the UK since the late 1990s. A reduction in cases at the peak of the coronavirus pandemic was followed by a rapid rise, with cases of syphilis in England reaching their highest levels for 75 years in 2023.
- HIV infection is associated with treatment failures and more frequent, earlier neurological disease.

Clinical features

- **Primary syphilis**—after an incubation period of 14 days to 3 months, a painless, erythematous papule develops. This ulcerates, forming a painless, 'punched-out' chancre on the genitalia (rarely on the mouth, hands, and anus). Associated with regional lymphadenopathy. Multiple chancres can occur, particularly in HIV-infected patients. They are highly infectious and heal spontaneously after 1–2 months.
- **Secondary syphilis**—organisms disseminate from the chancre, causing symptoms 1–6 months later:
  - rash—localized or diffuse mucocutaneous rash may be macular, papular, pustular, or mixed. Involves the trunk, limbs, palms, and soles. Mucosal ulcers may occur. Condylomata lata occur in warm, moist areas (e.g. skinfolds) and are highly infectious;
  - early neurosyphilis (commoner in HIV)—may be asymptomatic (CSF findings: pleocytosis, raised protein level, decreased glucose

level, reactive CSF Venereal Disease Research Laboratory (VDRL) test), presents with syphilitic meningitis (chronic basal meningitis with headache and cranial nerve palsies—fever is usually absent), or causes meningovascular syphilis (headache, fits, limb paralysis). May also present with stroke, cervical myelopathy, and hemiplegia;

- other features—fever, sore throat, 'snail-track ulcers' in the mouth, lymphadenopathy, malaise, hepatitis, periostitis, iritis, arthritis, glomerulonephritis.

- **Latent syphilis**—spontaneous resolution of secondary syphilis occurs after 3–12 weeks. During the latent period, patients are asymptomatic and infectivity is low, but up to one-quarter of patients experience recrudescence of disease. Early latent syphilis is the period up to 2 years after primary infection, and late latent syphilis occurs after 2 years.

- **Late/tertiary syphilis**—rare, follows a latent period of 2–20 years; characterized by chronic inflammation:
  - gummatous syphilis—granulomatous lesions usually affecting the skin, mucous membranes, and bone or organs, causing local destruction (e.g. saddle nose). Gummata may be indurated, nodular, or ulcerated and can be painful;
  - cardiovascular syphilis—endarteritis of the aorta leads to aortic regurgitation (may present with angina and left ventricular failure (LVF)) and aneurysm formation (ascending aorta)). Other large arteries may be affected. VDRL can be negative;
  - late neurosyphilis—two forms: (1) general paresis of the insane (presents with gradual confusion, hallucinations, delusions, fits, cognitive impairment, tremor of the lips and tongue, brisk reflexes, extensor plantars, Argyll Robertson pupils), and (2) tabes dorsalis (atrophy of the dorsal columns of the spinal cord with autonomic neuropathy and cranial nerve lesions). Presents with ataxia, sensory loss, sphincter disturbance, shooting pains, sensory loss, and areflexia.

- **Congenital syphilis**—there are two forms:
  - early congenital syphilis occurs within 2 years of birth and presents with rash, condylomata lata, vesiculobullous lesions, snuffles, haemorrhagic rhinitis, osteochondritis, periostitis, pseudoparalysis, mucous patches, perioral fissures, hepatosplenomegaly, generalized lymphadenopathy, non-immune hydrops, glomerulonephritis, neurological or ocular involvement, haemolysis, and thrombocytopenia;
  - late congenital syphilis presents after 2 years with interstitial keratitis, Clutton's joints, Hutchinson's incisors, mulberry molars, high palatal arch, rhagades, deafness, frontal bossing, short maxilla, protuberance of the mandible, saddle nose deformity, sternoclavicular thickening, paroxysmal cold haemoglobinuria, and neurological or gummatous involvement.

Diagnosis

- Microscopy—detection of organisms on dark-field microscopy.
- PCR-based tests should be used in suspected early primary syphilis and are part of the diagnostic algorithm for congenital syphilis.

- Serology[15]—there are two types of serological tests; may be negative in HIV-infected persons (◑ see *Treponema* species, pp. 369–72):
  - specific treponemal tests (e.g. treponemal EIA to detect IgM and IgG, *T. pallidum* haemagglutination assay (TPHA), *T. pallidum* particle assay (TPPA), and fluorescent treponemal antibody absorption (FTA-ABS) test. Once infected, treponemal tests typically remain positive, even with successful treatment. They cannot differentiate syphilis from endemic treponematoses;
  - non-treponemal/cardiolipin tests (e.g. VDRL test and rapid plasma reagin (RPR)). These are quantitative tests used to detect infection and track response to therapy. A positive treponemal test and an RPR titre >16 indicate the need for treatment. A false-negative RPR test can occur in secondary or early latent syphilis due to the prozone effect. The VDRL/RPR tests may be negative in late syphilis.
- CSF findings in neurosyphilis—raised protein level, CSF pleocytosis (lymphocytic); although CSF is acellular in 10% of cases of tabes dorsalis, positive RPR (highly specific, but only 50% sensitive in CSF), TPPA >1:320 (sensitive but lacks specificity).

Management

- All patients should be tested for other STIs and HIV infection.
- Early syphilis (primary, secondary, and early latent)—benzathine benzylpenicillin 2.4 million IU IM stat as two injections (each of 1.2 million IU) into separate sites, or doxycycline 100mg bd for 14 days. Penicillin treatment may be complicated by the Jarisch–Herxheimer reaction (◑ see *Borrelia* species, Treatment, pp. 373–4).
- Late syphilis (late latent, cardiovascular, and gummatous)—benzathine benzylpenicillin 2.4 million IU IM as two injections (each of 1.2 million IU) into separate sites weekly for 3 weeks, or doxycycline 100mg bd PO for 28 days.
- Neurosyphilis—benzylpenicillin 1.8–2.4g IV 4-hourly for 14 days, or procaine benzylpenicillin 1.8–2.4 million IU IM daily with probenecid 500mg qds PO for 14 days
- Steroids should be given with all anti-treponemal antibiotics for cardiovascular syphilis and neurosyphilis—40–60mg prednisolone od for 3 days, starting 24 hours before antibiotics.
- Recommended clinical and serological (VDRL/RPR) follow-up at 3, 6, and 12 months and then, if indicated, 6-monthly until VDRL/RPR negative or serofast. In neurosyphilis, if VDRL/RPR titres do not decrease 4-fold within 1 year of therapy, CSF examination and retreatment are indicated.[16]

References

15 Public Health England (2014, updated 2016). *SMI V 44: syphilis serology. UK standards for microbiology investigations (SMIs) V 44: syphilis serology*. Available at: ℘ https://www.gov.uk/government/publications/smi-v-44-serological-diagnosis-of-syphilis

16 Kingston M, French P, Higgins S, *et al*. (2015). *UK national guidelines on the management of syphilis 2015*. Available at: ℘ https://www.bashhguidelines.org/media/1148/uk-syphilis-guidelines-2015.pdf

Neurological infections

Acute meningitis

Definition

Acute meningitis is defined as a syndrome characterized by the onset of meningeal symptoms (headache, neck stiffness, vomiting, photophobia), fever, and cerebral dysfunction over hours to days. It is identified by an abnormal number of white blood cells in the CSF. Table 19.1 summarizes the causes.

Table 19.1 Causes of acute meningitis

Category	Causes
Bacteria	*Streptococcus pneumoniae, Neisseria meningitidis, Haemophilus influenzae, Listeria monocytogenes, Streptococcus agalactiae, Escherichia coli, Klebsiella pneumoniae, Klebsiella spp., Salmonella spp., Serratia marcescens, Pseudomonas aeruginosa, Enterobacter spp., Staphylococcus aureus, Staphylococcus epidermidis, Cutibacterium acnes*
Viruses	Enteroviruses, mumps virus, measles virus, herpesviruses, influenza and parainfluenza viruses, HIV, arboviruses, lymphocytic choriomeningitis virus
Rickettsia	*Rickettsia rickettsii, Rickettsia conorii, Rickettsia prowazekii, Rickettsia typhi, Rickettsia tsutsugamushi, Erlichia spp.*
Protozoa	*Naegleria fowleri, Acanthamoeba spp.*
Helminths	*Strongyloides stercoralis, Angiostrongylus cantonensis*
Other infectious diseases	IE, parameningeal foci of infection, viral post-infectious syndromes, post-vaccination
Medications	Antimicrobials, non-steroidals, azathioprine, OKT-3, carbamazepine, immune globulin, ranitidine
Systemic diseases	SLE, sarcoidosis
Procedure-related	Post-neurosurgery, spinal anaesthesia, intrathecal injections
Miscellaneous	Seizures, migraine, Mollaret's meningitis

IE, infective endocarditis; SLE, systemic lupus erythematosus.

Bacterial meningitis

The cause of acute bacterial meningitis depends on age, immune status, and whether there has been recent head trauma or neurosurgery (see Table 19.2). The initiation of infection usually begins with nasopharyngeal colonization by a new organism, followed by systemic invasion. Important bacterial virulence factors include fimbriae, bacterial capsule, and production of immunoglobulin A (IgA) proteases. Host factors that predispose to meningitis include splenectomy and complement deficiencies.

Table 19.2 Causes of bacterial meningitis

Age/condition	Common organisms
0–4 weeks	*Streptococcus agalactiae, Escherichia coli, Listeria monocytogenes, Klebsiella pneumoniae, Enterococcus spp., Salmonella spp.*
4–12 weeks	S. agalactiae, E. coli, L. monocytogenes, K. pneumoniae, Haemophilus influenzae, Streptococcus pneumoniae, Neisseria meningitidis
3 months to 18 years	H. influenzae, N. meningitidis S. pneumoniae
18–50 years	N. meningitidis, S. pneumoniae, Streptococcus suis
>50 years	S. pneumoniae, N. meningitidis, L. monocytogenes, aerobic Gram-negative bacilli, S. suis
Immunocompromised	S. pneumoniae, N. meningitidis, L. monocytogenes, aerobic Gram-negative bacilli (e.g. E. coli, Klebsiella spp., Salmonella spp., Serratia marcescens, Pseudomonas aeruginosa)
Basal skull fracture	S. pneumoniae, H. influenzae, Streptococcus pyogenes
Head trauma, post-neurosurgery	Staphylococcus aureus, Staphylococcus epidermidis, aerobic Gram-negative bacilli
CSF shunt	S. aureus, S. epidermidis, Cutibacterium acnes, aerobic Gram-negative bacilli

Clinical features

- Classical features include fever, headache, meningism (neck stiffness, photophobia, positive Kernig's sign, Brudzinski's sign), and cerebral dysfunction (confusion and/or reduced conscious level).
- Seizures occur in 30% of patients. Cranial nerve palsies (especially III, IV, VI, and VII) and focal signs are seen in 10–20% of cases. Hemiparesis may be due to a subdural effusion.
- Papilloedema is rare (<1%).
- Skin rash (initially macular, then petechial) occurs in patients with meningococcal septicaemia but can occur in pneumococcal, *Haemophilus influenzae*, or *Streptococcus suis* septicaemia.
- Rhinorrhoea or otorrhoea suggests basal skull fracture.
- Patients with *Listeria monocytogenes* have an increased risk of seizures and focal signs; some patients present with ataxia, cranial nerve palsies, and nystagmus caused by rhomboencephalitis.
- Neonates may present with non-specific symptoms (e.g. temperature instability, listlessness, poor feeding, irritability, vomiting, diarrhoea, jaundice, respiratory distress). Seizures occur in 40% of cases, and a bulging fontanelle is a late sign.
- Elderly patients may present insidiously with confusion, lethargy, obtundation, no fever, and variable signs of meningeal inflammation.

Diagnosis

The diagnosis is confirmed by examination and culture of the CSF (⤴ see tables on the inside of the back cover). In bacterial meningitis, the following are typically seen:

- opening pressure >18mm of CSF;
- CSF WCC 1000–5000 cells/mL (but 40% of cases have less than this; range 100–10 000);
- CSF neutrophils ≥80%;
- CSF protein 0.1–0.5g/dL;
- CSF glucose ≤40mg/dL or ≤2.2mmol/L;
- Gram stain positive in 60–90%;
- Culture positive in 70–85%;
- bacterial PCR: sensitivity 87–100%, specificity 98–100%.

Management

- For acute management, ⤴ see flow chart in back cover.[3]
- Appropriate empirical antimicrobial therapy should be commenced immediately, pending investigations (see Table 19.3). If CSF Gram stain or culture is positive, treatment should be tailored to the infecting organism (see Table 19.4).
- Adjunctive corticosteroids have been recommended for the treatment of acute bacterial meningitis.[1] The recommended regimen is dexamethasone 10mg qds for 4 days, administered before or with the first dose of antibiotic. A systematic review only recommends their use in high income-countries.[2] Benefit is proven only for pneumococcal infection; thus, steroids can be stopped before 4 days if an alternative causative agent is identified.
- Reduction of raised intracranial pressure (ICP) may be achieved by various methods: elevating the head of the bed to 30° to maximize

Table 19.3 Examples of empirical antibiotic therapy

Age/condition	Empirical therapy
Age 0–4 weeks	Cefotaxime + amoxicillin
Age 4–12 weeks	Cefotaxime or ceftriaxone + amoxicillin
Age 3 months to 18 years	Cefotaxime or ceftriaxone
Age 18–49 years	Ceftriaxone or cefotaxime ± vancomycin
Age ≥50 years	Ceftriaxone or cefotaxime + amoxicillin
Immunocompromised	Ceftriaxone or cefotaxime + amoxicillin
Healthcare-associated meningitis	Ceftazidime or meropenem + vancomycin
Basal skull fracture	Cefotaxime or ceftriaxone
Head trauma/ neurosurgery	Vancomycin + ceftazidime
CSF shunt	Ceftazidime or meropenem + vancomycin

Table 19.4 Examples of specific antibiotic therapy

Organism	Antimicrobial therapy
Streptococcus pneumoniae	Penicillin MIC ≤0.06mg/L: benzylpenicillin or cefotaxime or ceftriaxone Penicillin MIC >0.06mg/L, but cephalosporin sensitive: cefotaxime or ceftriaxone Penicillin MIC >0.06mg/L and cephalosporin-resistant: (cefotaxime or ceftriaxone) plus vancomycin or rifampicin Sensitivities unknown: cefotaxime or ceftriaxone
Neisseria meningitidis	Cefotaxime or ceftriaxone
Listeria monocytogenes	Amoxicillin +/– gentamicin
Streptococcus agalactiae	Amoxicillin or benzylpenicillin
Escherichia coli	Ceftriaxone or cefotaxime
Pseudomonas aeruginosa	Ceftazidime or meropenem
Haemophilus influenzae	Cefotaxime or ceftriaxone
Staphylococcus aureus	Meticillin-susceptible: flucloxacillin Meticillin-resistant: vancomycin

MIC, minimum inhibitory concentration.

venous drainage, hyperventilation to cause cerebral vasoconstriction, and use of hyperosmolar agents (e.g. mannitol).
- Neurosurgery may be required in certain circumstances: persistent CSF leak after basal skull fracture, congenital defects leading to recurrent meningitis, and subdural empyema.

Prevention
- Vaccination—Hib, MenB, MenC, Men ACWY, and pneumococcal conjugate vaccine (PCV) are part of the routine childhood immunization schedule in the UK. They are also recommended for patients with asplenia, splenic dysfunction, or a complement disorder. In addition, Men ACWY is recommended for pilgrims to Saudi Arabia and contacts of cases. The pneumococcal polysaccharide vaccine (PPV23) is recommended in certain high-risk groups (e.g. age >65 years, chronic cardiovascular, pulmonary, renal, or liver disease, diabetes mellitus, immunosuppression, CSF leak, cochlear implants, asplenia and splenic dysfunction).
- Chemoprophylaxis is required for certain bacteria. It should be given within 24h to household contacts, kissing contacts, and medical personnel involved in resuscitation of the index case. Rifampicin is the agent of choice for H. influenzae type b meningitis. For N. meningitidis, ciprofloxacin (500mg stat) is first-line, but rifampicin (600mg bd for

2 days) is a suitable alternative. NB Rifampicin interacts with the oral contraceptive pill (OCP) and may reduce its efficacy. Penicillin is not routinely recommended to prevent secondary cases of *Streptococcus pneumoniae* meningitis. IV ampicillin, penicillin, clindamycin, or erythromycin is recommended for pregnant women colonized with group B *Streptococcus* (GBS) or with obstetric risk factors for invasive disease.

References

1 De Gans J, van de Beek D. Dexamethasone in adults with bacterial meningitis. *N Engl J Med.* 2002;**347**:1549–56.
2 Brouwer MC, McIntyre P, Prasad K, *et al.* Corticosteroids for acute bacterial meningitis. *Cochrane Database Syst Rev.* 2013;**6**:CD004405.
3. McGill F, Heyderman RS, Michael BD, *et al.* The UK joint specialist societies guideline on the diagnosis and management of acute meningitis and meningococcal sepsis in immunocompetent adults. *J Infect.* 2016;**72**:405–38

Viral meningitis

Viruses are the major cause of the aseptic meningitis syndrome. This is usually characterized by lymphocytic pleocytosis in the CSF and sterile bacterial cultures.

Causes

- Enteroviruses are the leading cause of viral meningitis (e.g. echoviruses, Coxsackie viruses, enteroviruses 70 and 71).
- Arboviruses (e.g. West Nile virus, St Louis encephalitis virus, California encephalitis group viruses, Colorado tick fever, and Toscana virus).
- Mumps virus is a common cause in unimmunized populations.
- Herpesviruses include herpes simplex virus (HSV)-1 and -2, varicella-zoster virus (VZV), cytomegalovirus (CMV), Epstein–Barr virus (EBV), and human herpesvirus 6 (HHV-6). Although all of these can cause meningitis, HSV is the commonest cause and often associated with primary genital HSV-2 infection.
- HIV may cause meningitis as part of primary infection.
- Adenovirus.
- Lymphocytic choriomeningitis virus (LCMV) is a rare cause of aseptic meningitis. It usually occurs in laboratory personnel, pet owners, or persons living in unsanitary conditions.

Pathogenesis

After colonization of mucosal surfaces, the virus invades and replicates prior to haematogenous dissemination. CNS invasion may occur by several mechanisms: via the cerebral microvascular endothelial cells, via the choroid plexus epithelium, or by spread along the olfactory nerve. Once CNS invasion occurs, inflammatory cells accumulate, leading to the release of inflammatory cytokines (e.g. interleukin-6, interferon-γ, interleukin-1β), and synthesis of immunoglobulins (e.g. oligoclonal immunoglobulin G (IgG)).

Clinical features

- Enterovirus—in neonates, fever is accompanied by vomiting, anorexia, rash, and upper respiratory tract symptoms. Meningeal signs (nuchal

rigidity, bulging anterior fontanelle) may be present or absent, and focal signs are uncommon. A severe form may occur in the early neonatal period with hepatic necrosis, myocarditis, necrotizing enterocolitis, and encephalitis. In older children and adults, symptoms are milder, with fever, headache, neck stiffness, and photophobia. There may be non-specific symptoms (e.g. anorexia, vomiting, rash, diarrhoea, cough, pharyngitis, myalgia). Other clues include community enteroviral epidemics, maculopapular or pustular rashes conjunctivitis, pleurodynia, pericarditis, and herpangina.
- Mumps virus—CNS symptoms usually occur 5 days after the onset of parotitis but can occur in the absence of parotitis.
- Herpesviruses—HSV-2 meningitis presents with classical symptoms. Complications include urinary retention, dysaesthesia, paraesthesiae, neuralgia, motor weakness, paraparesis, difficulties in concentration, and impaired hearing; these usually resolve within 3–6 months. EBV meningitis is associated with pharyngitis, lymphadenopathy, and splenomegaly. VZV meningitis is associated with a characteristic diffuse vesicular rash.
- HIV—HIV-infected patients may present with a typical aseptic meningitis syndrome, associated with acute primary HIV infection.
- LCMV—this is usually a biphasic illness that starts with non-specific viral symptoms, followed by improvement; 15% of patients develop severe headache, photophobia, light-headedness, myalgia, and pharyngitis. Occasionally, arthritis, orchitis, myopericarditis, and alopecia may occur.

Diagnosis

- CSF examination—CSF pleocytosis (100–1000 cells/mL) usually occurs. This may show a neutrophil predominance initially but becomes lymphocytic over 6–48h. CSF protein level may be normal or mildly elevated. CSF glucose level is normal or mildly reduced.
- Molecular methods—PCR-based assays are the diagnostic test of choice for enterovirus and herpesvirus infections. HIV RNA may be isolated from the CSF of patients with acute HIV meningitis.
- Serology—a 4-fold rise in mumps antibody titres confirms the diagnosis of mumps meningitis. HIV, LCMV, and arboviral infections are usually diagnosed serologically.
- Viral culture—not routinely used in clinical practice.

Differential diagnosis

The following may mimic viral meningitis:
- syphilitic meningitis (➋ see Syphilis, pp. 750–2);
- Lyme disease (➋ see Lyme disease, pp. 374–6);
- Rocky Mountain spotted fever (RMSF) (➋ see Rickettsia, p. 380);
- erlichiosis;
- cryptococcal meningitis (➋ see Cryptococcus, pp. 520–2); coccidioidomycosis (➋ see Coccidioides immitis, pp. 547–50);
- tuberculous meningitis (➋ see Mycobacterium tuberculosis, pp. 391–5);
- parameningeal bacterial infections (e.g. epidural/subdural abscess, otitis media, sinusitis);
- Angiostrongylus cantonensis meningitis;
- leptomeningeal neoplasm;

- drug-induced meningitis (e.g. NSAIDs, co-trimoxazole, IV immunoglobulin (IVIG), rofecoxib, cetuximab, anti-epileptics, OKT-3).

Management

- Treatment of viral meningitis is mainly supportive (e.g. analgesics, antipyretics).
- There is little evidence for the use of IV aciclovir in the treatment of HSV meningitis, but some authorities suggest its use in those unwell enough to require hospitalization—but any benefit may be restricted to immunocompromised patients. Pleconaril may have a role in the treatment of enteroviral meningitis.
- No specific antiviral therapy exists for arboviruses, mumps virus, or LCMV meningitis.

Chronic meningitis

Chronic meningitis is a syndrome characterized by a subacute onset of meningoencephalitic symptoms (fever, headache, nausea, vomiting, neck stiffness, lethargy, and confusion) and CSF abnormalities which persist for at least 4 weeks There are a large number of infectious and non-infectious causes (see Table 19.5).

Table 19.5 Causes of chronic meningitis/meningoencephalitis

	Syndrome	Causes
Infectious	Meningitis	*Mycobacterium tuberculosis, Treponema pallidum, Borrelia burgdorferi, Tropheryma whipplei, Brucella, Listeria, Leptospira, Ehrlichia chaffeensis, Candida, Cryptococcus, Histoplasma, Coccidioides, Sporothrix, Acanthamoeba, Balamuthia, Taenia solium*
	Focal lesions	*Actinomyces, Blastomyces, T. solium, Aspergillus, Nocardia, Schistosoma, Toxoplasma, M. tuberculosis*
	Encephalitis	*Trypanosoma brucei*, CMV, enterovirus (hypogammaglobulinaemia), EBV, HIV, HTLV, HSV, measles, SSPE, rabies, VZV
Non-infectious	Meningitis	Drugs (NSAIDs, IVIG, intrathecal agents), Behçet's disease, benign lymphocytic meningitis, CNS vasculitis, Fabry's disease, granulomatous angiitis, malignancy, sarcoidosis, SLE, granulomatosis with polyangiitis (previously known as Wegener's granulomatosis), Vogt–Koyanagi–Harada disease

CMV, cytomegalovirus; EBV, Epstein–Barr virus; HSV, herpes simplex virus; HTLV, human T-cell lymphotropic virus; SLE, systemic lupus erythematosus; SSPE, subacute sclerosing panencephalitis; VZV, varicella-zoster virus.

Clinical features

- History—an exposure history may suggest certain infections (e.g. TB, brucellosis, cysticercosis, coccidioidomycosis, histoplasmosis, Lyme disease, syphilis, HIV infection). In non-infectious cases, there may be a history of pre-existing systemic disease.
- Examination—diagnostic physical findings are rare. Skin lesions may be found in cryptococcosis, sarcoidosis, *Acanthamoeba* infection, coccidioidomycosis, blastomycosis, and secondary syphilis. Subcutaneous nodules may be found in cysticercosis and metastatic carcinoma. Lymphadenopathy and hepatomegaly suggest systemic disease. Eye examination may show choroidal tubercles, sarcoid granulomas, papilloedema, iritis, or uveitis. Neurological examination is non-discriminatory—focal signs indicate a cerebral mass lesion; hydrocephalus and cranial nerve palsies indicate basal meningitis; and peripheral neuropathy suggests sarcoidosis or Lyme disease.

Laboratory diagnosis

- Blood tests—in addition to routine blood tests (FBC, ESR, CRP, creatinine, LFTs), the following may be indicated: blood culture (BC) for fungi and mycobacteria, serology for HIV and syphilis, serum cryptococcal antigen, antinuclear antibody (ANA), and antineutrophil cytoplasmic antibody (ANCA). Depending on the patient's exposure history, the following tests may be indicated: serology for *Brucella*, *Borrelia burgdorferi*, *Histoplasma*, and *Coccidioides*.
- Radiology—a CXR and CT or MRI brain scan should be performed in all cases. Meningeal enhancement and hydrocephalus are common findings.
- CSF examination should be performed in all cases (unless contraindicated by scan findings). The CSF should be analysed for cell count and differential, protein, and glucose (see Table 19.6). Diagnostic tests include Gram staining and culture, Ziehl–Neelsen (ZN) staining for mycobacteria and mycobacterial culture, India ink and cryptococcal antigen, and syphilis serology. Further tests may be indicated, depending on the patient's exposure history (e.g. fungal antigens, 16S/18S PCR, fungal antibodies, parasite serology)

In cases where the diagnosis remains obscure, a biopsy of the brain or other tissues may be indicated. Metagenomic pathogen detection may have a role.

Management

- Specific therapy is tailored according to the cause of chronic meningitis.
- Therapeutic trials may be indicated when a specific cause is not found, despite comprehensive evaluation. Response to treatment may be slow, making interpretation difficult. Attempts to establish a diagnosis should be continued during therapeutic trial. In areas where TB is endemic, tuberculous meningitis (➲ see Tuberculous meningitis, pp. 772–3) is the commonest cause of chronic meningitis, and empirical therapy is often initiated if the clinical presentation and CSF indices are compatible. Positive cultures or a clinical response to treatment are indications for continuing therapy. In areas where TB is not endemic, chronic meningitis is usually not infectious.

Table 19.6 CSF findings in chronic meningitis

CSF characteristic	Causes
Lymphocytic pleocytosis	Viral causes, TB meningitis
Neutrophilic pleocytosis	*Actinomyces*, *Nocardia*, early *Mycobacterium tuberculosis* infection, *Aspergillus*, *Candida*, HIV-associated CMV
Eosinophilic pleocytosis	*Angiostrongylus cantonensis*, *Coccidioides*, *Taenia solium*, *Schistosoma*, lymphoma, chemical
Pleocytosis <50 cells/microlitre	Behçet's disease, benign lymphocytic meningitis, carcinoma, HIV-associated cryptococcosis, sarcoidosis, vasculitis
Low CSF glucose	*Actinomyces*, *Nocardia*, *T. solium*, *M. tuberculosis*, *Treponema pallidum*, *Toxoplasma*, fungi, chronic enterovirus, HIV-associated CMV, sarcoidosis, carcinoma, subarachnoid haemorrhage

CMV, cytomegalovirus.

Tuberculous meningitis

- Caused by *Mycobacterium tuberculosis* (MTB) (➔ see *Mycobacterium tuberculosis*, pp. 391–5). There are three forms of CNS TB—tuberculous meningitis (TBM), intracranial tuberculoma, and spinal tuberculous arachnoiditis.
- Pathogenesis—primary infection or reactivation of latent infection results in bacillaemia and seeding of the brain and meninges. Rupture of these foci into the subarachnoid space results in proliferative basal arachnoiditis, vasculitis, and communicating hydrocephalus.
- Clinical features of TBM—non-specific, with gradual onset of meningeal symptoms, cranial nerve palsies (III, IV, and VI), hemiplegia or paraplegia, and urinary retention. CXR is abnormal in 50% of cases and may show pulmonary or miliary TB. CT or MRI head may show hydrocephalus, basal meningeal enhancement, infarcts, or tuberculomas. There are three clinical stages, which are prognostically useful: (1) stage 1—Glasgow coma scale (GCS) 15/15 with no focal neurological signs, (2) stage 2—GCS 15 with focal signs or GCS 11–14, and (3) stage 3—GCS ≤10. In areas with high HIV prevalence, TB meningitis may be a primary presentation of HIV infection or present as immune reconstitution inflammatory syndrome (IRIS) after initiation of antiretroviral therapy (ART).
- Laboratory diagnosis—CSF findings include raised opening pressure, lymphocytic pleocytosis (100–500 cells/mL), increased CSF protein levels, and decreased CSF glucose levels. Neutrophils may predominate in early disease and HIV-infected patients. Diagnosis is confirmed by detection of *M. tuberculosis* by CSF ZN smear or culture. Smear positivity rates are generally low (10–22%) but may be increased to >50% if the spun deposit of a large volume of CSF (5–10mL) is examined meticulously. PCR: Xpert® MTB/RIF Ultra assay (often

referred as 'Cepheid', the manufacturer) is recommended by the World Health Organization (WHO) for use on CSF as an initial diagnostic test in all patients with signs and symptoms of TBM. CSF adenosine deaminase (ADA) level can be measured, but the cut-off threshold to distinguish TBM from non-tuberculous meningitis is unclear.
- Management—prompt treatment is important when TBM is suspected. The optimum drug choice and duration of treatment have not been established in clinical trials. The TB treatment guidelines from both the UK and the USA recommend a four-drug initiation phase (rifampicin, isoniazid, pyrazinamide, and ethambutol) for 2 months, followed by a two-drug continuation phase (rifampicin and isoniazid) for 10 months. If patients are unable to take PO medication initially, the initiation regimen could consist of IV rifampicin, isoniazid, fluoroquinolone, and amikacin. As isoniazid and pyrazinamide are the only two drugs that have good CSF penetration, some experts recommend continuing pyrazinamide during the continuation phase. Studies from India and South Africa suggest that 6 months of therapy may be adequate. Adjunctive dexamethasone has been shown to reduce short-term mortality. Although a randomized controlled trial (RCT) has shown that treatment with a higher dose of rifampicin and the addition of a fluoroquinolone do not improve survival, there may be a role for this regimen in those at risk of isoniazid-resistant infection. A clinical trial of early versus deferred (around 8 weeks after initiation of TB treatment) ART in HIV-associated TB meningitis showed no survival benefit with immediate treatment, and an increased frequency of severe adverse effects.

Cryptococcal meningitis

- There are estimated to be 223 100 cases of cryptococcal meningitis globally each year, with 181 100 deaths. The highest incidence is in sub-Saharan Africa, followed by South and South East Asia. Most patients are immunocompromised. Advanced HIV infection (CD4 count <100 cells/mL) is a major risk factor, but others include glucocorticoid therapy, solid organ transplantation, malignancy (especially haematological), sarcoidosis, and liver failure.
- *Cryptococcus neoformans* var. *neoformans* occurs worldwide and tends to cause disease in immunocompromised patients. *C. neoformans* var. *gatii* occurs in tropical and subtropical climates, and tends to affect non-immunocompromised patients.
- Clinical features—subacute presentation with fever, malaise, meningoencephalitis, and focal signs (~6%).
- Laboratory diagnosis—CSF findings include raised CSF pressure, lymphocytic pleocytosis (40–400 cells/mL), low CSF glucose levels (55%), and positive India ink staining (≤50%). CSF findings may be normal in HIV patients. Serum and CSF cryptococcal antigen tests can increase the diagnostic rate to ≥90%. CSF cultures are positive in 75% of patients. Cultures of blood, urine, and sputum may increase the diagnostic rate.
- Management:

- HIV-infected patients—induction therapy with liposomal amphotericin B (4mg/kg/day IV) plus flucytosine (100mg/kg/day in four divided doses) for 2 weeks. If there is clinical improvement after 2 weeks, change to consolidation therapy with fluconazole (400mg/day PO) for 10 weeks, followed by maintenance therapy with fluconazole (200mg/day PO). This may be discontinued in asymptomatic patients with CD4 counts >100 cells/mL, who have an undetectable HIV viral load on ART for >3 months. Repeat lumbar punctures (LPs) to reduce the ICP may be necessary in those with high initial opening pressures or ongoing headaches/neurology. Extension of induction therapy until the CSF cultures are negative might be indicated.
- HIV-negative patients—induction therapy with liposomal amphotericin B (3–4mg/kg/day IV) plus flucytosine (100mg/kg/day in four divided doses) for at least 2 weeks (some patients may need up to 6 weeks). This is followed by consolidation therapy with fluconazole (400–800mg/day PO) for 8 weeks, followed by maintenance therapy with fluconazole (200–400mg/day PO) for 12 months.

Further reading

Infectious Diseases Society of America (2020). *Guidelines for the prevention and treatment of opportunistic infections in adults and adolescents with HIV*. Available at: ⌾ https://www.idsociety.org/practice-guideline/prevention-and-treatment-of-opportunistic-infections-among-adults-and-adolescents/

Coccidioidal meningitis

- Coccidioidomycosis is caused by *Coccidioides* spp. (◑ see *Coccidioides immitis*, pp. 547–50), a dimorphic fungus that is endemic in the desert areas of south-western USA and in Central and South America. Two species cause disease: *Coccidioides immitis* (California) and *Coccidioides posadasii* (Arizona, Texas, Central and South America). The exact incidence of coccidioidal meningitis is unknown, but disseminated coccidioidomycosis occurs in 8% of reported cases, of which 17% involve the CNS. In contrast to non-CNS infections, mortality is high—95% if untreated.
- Clinical features—CNS involvement may be part of generalized coccidioidomycosis or may be the only site of extrapulmonary disease. Meningitis usually occurs within weeks or months of primary infection, although it can present years afterwards. Persistent headache is the main symptom (75% of cases), but the clinical syndrome is indistinguishable from other causes of chronic meningitis. Rarer clinical features include tremor, papilloedema, cranial nerve palsies, cerebral infarction, focal neurological deficits, and gait abnormalities.
- Laboratory diagnosis—the CSF usually has raised WCC, which is predominantly lymphocytic, although CSF neutrophilia or eosinophilia may occur. The CSF glucose level is low, and the CSF protein level is elevated. Rarely, the organisms may be seen on CSF microscopy. CSF cultures are positive in 15–30% of cases. Other tests include CSF

antibodies and PCR on the CSF. Occasionally, meningeal biopsy may be required to establish the diagnosis.
- Imaging—CT or MRI may identify abnormalities such as hydrocephalus, basal meningitis, and cerebral infarction; these are not specific to coccidioidal meningitis.
- Management—fluconazole (400mg/day) is associated with a 70% response rate. Higher fluconazole doses (800–1000mg/day) may be used in patients who do not initially respond. Itraconazole (200mg bd or tds) has been reported to have similar efficacy. Intrathecal amphotericin deoxycholate has been used in patients who do not respond to PO azole therapy. Voriconazole and posaconazole have been used as salvage therapy in patients who develop disease progression on fluconazole. Hydrocephalus may require a ventriculoperitoneal (VP) shunt.

Further reading

Galgiani JN, Ampel NM, Blair JE, et al. 2016 Infectious Diseases Society of America (IDSA) clinical practice guideline for the treatment of coccidiomycocis. *Clin Infect Dis.* 2016;**63**:e112–46.

Histoplasma meningitis

- Caused by *Histoplasma capsulatum* (➔ see *Histoplasma capsulatum*, pp. 540–4), which is found worldwide, but particularly in North America (especially the mid-Western states) and Central America. The commonest presentation is pulmonary disease, but disseminated infection may occur in 1 in 2000 patients with acute infection. Risk factors for disseminated infection include HIV infection, solid organ transplantation, treatment with tumour necrosis factor (TNF)-α inhibitors, and extremes of age. CNS involvement occurs in 5–20% of those with disseminated infection.
- Clinical features—these are non-specific with fever and gradual onset of meningitic symptoms over weeks or months.
- Laboratory diagnosis—CSF examination shows lymphocytic pleocytosis, with low glucose and raised protein levels. CSF microscopy is rarely positive. CSF cultures are positive in 27–65% of cases. Large volumes of CSF (10–20mL) should be cultured, on at least two occasions to improve diagnostic yield. Detection of serum and CSF antibodies is the most sensitive test, but problems occur with cross-reactivity to other fungi. Three sets of BCs should also be taken. Bone marrow culture should be considered in patients with suspected disseminated disease.
- Management—treatment is with liposomal amphotericin B (5mg/kg/day IV for a total of 175mg/kg, given over 4–6 weeks), followed by itraconazole (400–600mg/day) for at least 1 year. LPs should be performed every few months to assess response. Treatment should be monitored with serum and/or urine *Histoplasma* antigen tests during therapy.

Further reading

Wheat LJ, Freifeld AG, Kleiman MB, et al.; Infectious Diseases Society of America. Clinical practice guidelines for the management of patients with histoplasmosis: 2007 update by the Infectious Diseases Society of America. *Clin Infect Dis.* 2007;**45**:807–25.

Neuroborreliosis

- Neuroborreliosis is a manifestation of Lyme disease, a tick-borne illness caused by *Borrelia* spp. (➲ see *Borrelia* species, pp. 372–6). There are three pathogenic species: *B. burgdorferi*, *Borrelia afzelii*, and *Borrelia garinii*. All three species cause disease in Europe; *B. burgdorferi* causes disease in the USA, and *B. afzelii* and *B. garinii* cause disease in Asia.
- Clinical features—early infection is characterized by flu-like symptoms and a characteristic rash (erythema chronicum migrans), which is seen in 80% of patients. Joint involvement occurs more frequently in the USA than in Europe. The nervous system is involved in 10–15% of untreated patients. Many patients develop non-specific symptoms (e.g. headache, fatigue, cognitive slowing, memory difficulty), but these do not constitute CNS infection. Neuroborreliosis is characterized by chronic meningitis, cranial nerve palsies, Lyme encephalomyelitis, and benign intracranial hypertension. CNS involvement may occur weeks or months after the tick bite. Peripheral nerve involvement may also occur (e.g. radiculoneuritis, mononeuritis multiplex).
- Laboratory diagnosis—CSF examination shows a lymphocytic pleocytosis. The CSF protein level is raised, but the CSF glucose level is usually normal. Diagnosis is confirmed by positive serology in the context of an appropriate exposure history. Serology is insensitive in early disease, and false-positive and false-negative results are a considerable problem. The most specific test is detection of *B. burgdorferi* antibodies in the CSF, and comparison of CSF and serum antibody levels by an immunocapture assay. PCR detection of *B. burgdorferi* has poor sensitivity, but high specificity.
- Imaging—MRI may show evidence of encephalomyelitis. Electrophysiological studies—electromyography (EMG) and nerve conduction studies may be useful in patients with peripheral neuropathy.
- Management—IV ceftriaxone 2–4g/day (the lower dose is advised by US/European guidelines, the higher dose by National Institute for Health and Care Excellence (NICE)), or alternatively PO doxycycline 400mg/day for 21 days. There is good evidence that these regimens are equally effective.

Further reading

National Institute for Health and Care Excellence (2018). *Lyme disease.* NICE guideline [NG95]. Available at: ✆ https://www.nice.org.uk/guidance/ng95/resources/lyme-disease-pdf-183775 6839877

Neurocysticercosis

- Caused by *Taenia solium* (➲ see Cestodes, pp. 611–12), the commonest parasitic disease of the CNS. Infection is endemic in Mexico, Central/South America, the Caribbean, sub-Saharan Africa, India, and China.
- Clinical features—depend on whether cysts are localized to the parenchyma or extra-parenchymal tissues. Parenchymal cysts are associated with focal or generalized seizures; if there are large numbers

of cysts associated with oedema, there may also be headache, nausea, vomiting, impaired consciousness, reduced visual acuity, and fever. Extra-parenchymal cysts can occur in the ventricles, subarachnoid space, spinal cord, and eye. Intraventricular cysts are associated with symptoms of hydrocephalus (e.g. headache, nausea, vomiting, altered mental status, reduced visual acuity). Subarachnoid lesions can present as chronic meningitis. Spinal cysticercosis may present with radicular pain, paraesthesiae, and sphincter disturbance. Ocular cysticercosis may present with impaired vision, diplopia, and eye pain.

- Imaging—CT may show calcified lesions. MRI is better for smaller lesions, and intraventricular and subarachnoid lesions. Spinal imaging should be performed in patients with basal subarachnoid neurocysticercosis. Plain X-ray may show skeletal muscle calcification.
- Laboratory diagnosis—CSF examination shows lymphocytic or eosinophilic pleocytosis, normal or low CSF glucose levels (25%), and normal or elevated CSF protein levels. Cysticercosis immunoblot and cysticercosis antigen EIA can be performed on CSF and serum. The antigen EIA detects the presence of viable cysticerci, but not degenerate or calcified cysticerci. Its sensitivity decreases with low numbers of viable cysts. Brain biopsy is only warranted in cases where non-invasive testing is non-diagnostic
- Management—those with parenchymal cysts and seizures should receive anti-epileptic therapy. If hydrocephalus or diffuse cerebral oedema is present, management of these is key and antiparasitic therapy is not appropriate acutely. In patients with viable cysts without these complications, treatment depends on the number of cysts and consists of either albendazole monotherapy or albendazole combined with praziquantel. Potential benefits include decreased risk of seizures or recurrent hydrocephalus. Risks include exacerbation of symptoms due to increased inflammation around degenerating cysts—thus, concomitant corticosteroids should be given. Antiparasitic therapy is not recommended for calcified cysts. Management of extra-parenchymal cysts depends on their location but may require surgical intervention ± adjuvant antiparasitic and corticosteroid therapy.

Further reading

White AC, Coyle CM, Rajshekhar V, et al.; Infectious Diseases Society of America. Diagnosis and treatment of neurocysticercosis: 2017 clinical practice guidelines by the Infectious Diseases Society of America (IDSA) and the American Society of Tropical Medicine and Hygiene (ASTMH). Clin Infect Dis. 2017;68:e49–75.

Encephalitis

- Encephalitis is an inflammatory process in the brain accompanied by cerebral dysfunction.
- It may be caused by infectious agents (mainly viruses) or non-infectious conditions (e.g. vasculitis, autoimmune diseases, paraneoplastic syndromes). In some cases, there may be features of meningitis, and it is referred to as meningoencephalitis.
- The incidence of encephalitis varies according to geography and population; the estimated incidence in industrialized countries is 0.7–13.8 cases per 100 000 population.

- The diagnostic evaluation of a patient with encephalitis should be individualized and guided by epidemiological clues (see Table 19.7),[5,6] clinical presentation (see Table 19.8),[5,6] and laboratory tests (see Table 19.9).[5,6]

Table 19.7 Epidemiological factors and causes of encephalitis

Risk factor	Potential causes
Agammaglobulinaemia	Enterovirus, *Mycoplasma pneumoniae*
Age	
- Neonates	HSV-2, CMV, rubella, *Listeria monocytogenes*, syphilis, *Toxoplasma gondii*
- Infants and children	Eastern equine encephalitis, Japanese encephalitis, Murray Valley encephalitis, influenza, La Crosse virus
- Elderly	Eastern equine encephalitis, St Louis encephalitis, West Nile virus, sporadic CJD, *L. monocytogenes*
Animal contact	
- Bats	Rabies, Nipah virus
- Birds	West Nile virus, Eastern and Western equine encephalitis, St Louis encephalitis, Murray Valley encephalitis, Japanese encephalitis, *Cryptococcus neoformans*
- Cats	Rabies, *Coxiella burnetii*, *Bartonella henselae*, *T. gondii*
- Dogs	Rabies
- Horses	Eastern, Western, and Venezuelan equine encephalitis, Hendra virus
- Old world primates	Herpesvirus B
- Raccoons	Rabies, *Baylisascaris procyonis*
- Rodents	Eastern and Venezuelan equine encephalitis, tick-borne encephalitis, Powassan virus, La Crosse virus, *Bartonella quintana*
- Sheep and goats	*C. burnetii*
- Skunks	Rabies
- Swine	Japanese encephalitis, Nipah virus
- White-tailed deer	*Borrelia burgdorferi*
Immunocompromised persons	CMV, EBV, HHV-6, HIV, JC virus, VZV, West Nile virus, *L. monocytogenes*, MTB, *C. neoformans*, *Coccidioides* spp., *Histoplasma* spp., *T. gondii*
Ingestion of food/drink	
- Raw/partially cooked meat	*T. gondii*
- Raw meat/fish/reptiles	*Gnathostoma* spp.

Table 19.7 (Contd.)

Risk factor	Potential causes
- Unpasteurized milk	Tick-borne encephalitis, *L. monocytogenes*, *C. burnetii*
Insect bites	
- Mosquitoes	Dengue, chikungunya, Eastern, Western, and Venezuelan equine encephalitis, St Louis encephalitis, Murray Valley encephalitis, Japanese encephalitis, West Nile virus, La Crosse virus, *Plasmodium falciparum*
- Sandflies	*Bartonella bacilliformis*
- Ticks	Tick-borne encephalitis, Powassan virus, *Rickettsia rickettsii*, *Erlichia chaffeensis*, *Anaplasma phagocytophilum*, *C. burnetii*, *B. burgdorferi*
- Tsetse flies	*Trypanosoma brucei gambiense*, *T.b rhodesiense*
Occupation	
- Exposure to animals	See above for specific animals
- Laboratory workers	West Nile virus, HIV, *C. burnetii*, *Coccidioides* spp.
- Healthcare workers	VZV, HIV, influenza, measles, MTB
- Veterinarians	Rabies, *Bartonella* spp., *C. burnetii*
Person-to-person transmissions	Influenza, VZV, HSV (neonatal), mumps, measles, rubella, polio, enteroviruses, EBV, HHV-6, HIV, Venezuelan equine encephalitis virus (rare), Nipah virus, *M. pneumoniae*, MTB, syphilis
Recreational activities	
- Camping/hunting	See mosquitoes/ticks above
- Caving	Rabies, *Histoplasma* spp.
- Sexual contact	HIV, syphilis
- Swimming	Enteroviruses, *Naegleria fowleri*
Season	
- Late summer/early autumn	Enteroviruses, see mosquitoes/ticks above
- Winter	Influenza virus
Transfusion and transplantation	CMV, EBV, HIV, West Nile virus, tick-borne encephalitis, rabies, iatrogenic CJD, syphilis, *A. phagocytophilum*, *R. rickettsii*, *C. neoformans*, *Coccidioides* spp., *Histoplasma capsulatum*, *T. gondii*
Travel	
- Africa	Rabies, West Nile virus, *P. falciparum*, *Trypanosoma* spp.

(Continued)

Table 19.7 (Contd.)

Risk factor	Potential causes
- Central America	Rabies, Eastern, Western, and Venezuelan equine encephalitis, St Louis encephalitis, *R. rickettsii, P. falciparum, Taenia solium*
- North America	Eastern and Western equine encephalitis, West Nile virus, *B. burgdorferi, E. chaffeensis, A. phagocytophilum, Coccidioides* spp.
- South America	Rabies, Eastern, Western, and Venezuelan equine encephalitis, St Louis encephalitis, *R. rickettsii, P. falciparum, T. solium*
- Australia	Murray Valley encephalitis, Japanese encephalitis, Hendra virus
- Europe	West Nile virus, tick-borne encephalitis, *A. phagocytophilum, B. burgdorferi*
- India, Nepal	Rabies, Japanese encephalitis
- Middle East	West Nile virus, *P. falciparum*
- Russia	Tick-borne encephalitis
- South East Asia/China/ Pacific Rim	Japanese encephalitis, tick-borne encephalitis, Nipah virus, *P. falciparum, Gnathostoma* spp., *T. solium*
Vaccination status	
- Unvaccinated	VZV, mumps, measles, rubella, polio, Japanese encephalitis
- Recent vaccination	Acute disseminated encephalomyelitis

Clinical features

- Viral encephalitis is characterized by alterations in consciousness, progressing from mild lethargy to confusion, to stupor and coma.
- Some patients may present with features of meningitis.
- Focal neurological signs frequently develop, and seizures are common.
- Motor weakness, attenuation of reflexes, and extensor plantar responses may be seen.
- Some viruses may cause CNS symptoms as part of a post-infectious encephalomyelitis (e.g. mumps, measles, rubella, influenza).
- Certain diseases are associated with characteristic symptoms or signs (see Table 19.8).

Diagnosis

- CSF examination is essential. In viral encephalitis, CSF pleocytosis is variable (10–2000 cells/mL) and lymphocytes usually predominate. In early disease, however, there may be no cells, or neutrophils in the CSF. Red cells may be found in HSV encephalitis. CSF protein levels are usually increased. CSF glucose levels are usually normal or slightly low. All patients should have CSF PCR for HSV, VZV, and enteroviruses performed.

Table 19.8 Clinical features and causes of encephalitis

Clinical presentation	Potential causes
Hepatitis	*Coxiella burnetii*
Lymphadenopathy	HIV, EBV, CMV, measles, rubella, West Nile virus, syphilis, *Bartonella* spp., MTB, *Toxoplasma gondii*, *Trypanosoma brucei gambiense*
Parotitis	Mumps
Rash	VZV, rubella, some enteroviruses, HIV, HHV-6, B virus, West Nile virus, *Rickettsia rickettsii*, *Mycoplasma pneumoniae*, *Borrelia burgdorferi*, syphilis, *Ehrlichia chaffeensis*, *Anaplasma phagocytophilum*
Respiratory	Influenza, adenovirus, Venezuelan equine encephalitis, Nipah virus, Hendra virus, *C. burnetii*, *M. pneumoniae*, MTB, *Histoplasma capsulatum*
Retinitis	CMV, West Nile virus, *Bartonella henselae*, syphilis
Urinary symptoms	St Louis encephalitis (early)
Cerebellar ataxia	VZV (children), EBV, mumps, St Louis encephalitis, *Tropheryma whipplei*, *T. brucei gambiense*
Cranial nerve abnormalities	HSV, EBV, *Listeria monocytogenes*, MTB, syphilis, *B. burgdorferi*, *T. whipplei*, *Cryptococcus neoformans*, *Coccidioides* spp., *H. capsulatum*
Dementia	HIV, sporadic and variant CJD, measles (SSPE), syphilis, *T. whipplei*
Myorhythmia	*T. whipplei* (oculomasticatory)
Parkinsonism	Japanese encephalitis, St Louis encephalitis, West Nile virus, Nipah virus, *T. gondii*, *T. brucei gambiense*
Flaccid paralysis	Japanese encephalitis, West Nile virus, tick-borne encephalitis, enterovirus-71, Coxsackie viruses, polio
Rhomboencephalitis	HSV, West Nile virus, enterovirus-71, *L. monocytogenes*

Additional CSF diagnostic studies should be performed, guided by epidemiological risk factors and clinical findings (see Table 19.9).
- Serology—all patients should have an HIV test performed. Other tests should be guided by epidemiological and clinical features (see Table 19.9).
- Imaging—MRI is more sensitive than CT.
- Electroencephalography (EEG)—not helpful, apart from to identify patients with non-convulsive seizures.
- Brain biopsy—this is occasionally performed for diagnostic reasons. There may be a role for metagenomic analysis for identification of unusual pathogens in some settings.

Table 19.9 Laboratory diagnosis of encephalitis

Class of organism	Diagnostic tests
Viruses	CSF PCR for HSV-1, HSV-2, VZV, enteroviruses, EBV, CMV
	Throat swab/respiratory specimens for respiratory virus PCR
	Blister fluid for HSV, VZV PCR
	Serology for HIV, EBV, mumps, measles, rubella, West Nile virus, Eastern, Western, and Venezuelan equine encephalitis, La Crosse virus
Bacteria	CSF and blood cultures
	Serology for *Coxiella burnetii* and *Mycoplasma pneumoniae*
	PCR for *Bartonella* and *Tropheryma whipplei*
Rickettsiae and *Erlichiae*	Serology for *Rickettsia rickettsii*, *Ehrlichia chaffeensis*, and *Anaplasma phagocytophilum*
	Blood smears for *E. chaffeensis* and *A. phagocytophilum*
Spirochaetes	CSF and serology for syphilis and *Borrelia burgdorferi*
Mycobacteria	Sputum and CSF for microscopy (acid-fast stain), mycobacterial culture, and TB PCR
Fungi	Serum and CSF cryptococcal antigen
	Serum and CSF for *Histoplasma* antibody and PCR
	Serum and CSF for *Coccidioides* antibody and PCR
Protozoa	Blood film for malaria
	Blood, CSF, bone marrow films, and serology for *Trypanosoma brucei gambiense* and *T. brucei rhodesiense*
	Serology for *Toxoplasma gondii*
Helminths	CSF eosinophilia, identification of worm in tissues and serology for *Gnathostoma* spp.
	Serum and CSF for *Taenia solium* antigen and antibody

Treatment

- Treatment of encephalitis is mainly supportive.
- Empirical therapy—all patients should be treated with IV aciclovir to cover HSV (the most frequent cause of encephalitis), pending CSF viral PCR. ➲ See Herpes Simplex Virus in chapter 8, pp. 438–40 for discussion on when treatment can be safely stopped. Other empirical antimicrobial agents should be initiated on the basis of epidemiological and clinical features (e.g. ceftriaxone for presumed bacterial meningitis, doxycycline for rickettsial infections, etc.).
- Specific therapy—this should be tailored to the causative organism. For detailed guidance, see guidelines from the Infectious Diseases Society of America (IDSA) and British Infection Association (BIA).

Prevention

Some diseases may be prevented by vaccination (e.g. mumps, measles, rubella, polio, rabies, Japanese encephalitis).

References

5 Tunkel AR, Glaser CA, Bloch KC, et al.; Infectious Diseases Society of America. The management of encephalitis: clinical practice guidelines by the Infectious Diseases Society of America. Clin Infect Dis. 2008;**47**:303–27.

6 Solomon T, Michael BD, Smith PE, et al.; National Encephalitis Guidelines Development and Stakeholder Groups. Management of suspected viral encephalitis in adults—Association of British Neurologists and British Infection Association National Guidelines. J Infect. 2012;**64**:347–73.

Brain abscess

A focal intracerebral infection that begins as a local area of cerebritis and develops into a collection of pus surrounded by a well-vascularized capsule. Bacteria may enter the brain by direct spread from contiguous areas (e.g. ear, sinus, dental infections, post-neurosurgery) or by haematogenous spread from elsewhere (e.g. endocarditis, or pulmonary, intra-abdominal, or skin infections).

Epidemiology

Brain abscesses are an uncommon, but severe, disease. They tend to occur more frequently in ♂. Case fatality rates range from 0% to 24%.

Aetiology

Brain abscesses may be caused by a broad range of organisms, some of which are associated with predisposing conditions (see Table 19.10).

Table 19.10 Factors predisposing to cerebral abscess

Predisposing condition	Microorganisms
Otitis media/mastoiditis	Streptococcus anginosus group, Enterobacterales, Bacteroides spp., Prevotella spp.
Sinusitis	Streptococcus anginosus group, Staphylococcus aureus, Haemophilus spp., Bacteroides spp., Fusobacterium spp.
Dental sepsis	S. anginosus group, Haemophilus spp., Bacteroides spp., Fusobacterium, Prevotella
Pulmonary/pleural sepsis	S. anginosus group, Fusobacterium, Actinomyces, Bacteroides. Prevotella spp.
Endocarditis	S. aureus, S. anginosus group
Congenital heart disease	S. anginosus group. Haemophilus spp.
Head trauma/ neurosurgical	S. aureus, S. anginosus group, Pseudomonas aeruginosa, Enterobacter spp., Clostridium spp.
Immunocompromised hosts, including HIV infection	Toxoplasma gondii, Listeria monocytogenes, Nocardia spp., Aspergillus, Cryptococcus neoformans, Coccidioides immitis, Candida spp., Mycobacterium spp., Mucorales, Scedosporium spp.

Clinical features

Clinical features of brain abscess are initially non-specific, often resulting in delayed diagnosis. Headache is the commonest symptom (69%) and may be localized to the side of the abscess. Other symptoms/signs include fever (45–53%), focal neurological deficits (50%), seizures (25%), and neck stiffness (15%). Nausea, vomiting, cranial nerve palsies, and papilloedema indicate raised ICP. Changes in mental status (lethargy, coma) are associated with poor outcome.

Diagnosis

- Imaging—CT with contrast should be performed urgently to confirm the diagnosis. Early cerebritis appears as an area of low density, which does not enhance with contrast. As the lesion enlarges, it develops an inflammatory capsule that enhances with contrast. MRI is more sensitive than CT and also visualizes the brainstem better.
- An LP is contraindicated if there are focal symptoms or signs, because of the risk of brainstem herniation. If bacterial meningitis is suspected, BCs should be taken and LP deferred until a mass lesion is excluded by CT/MRI.
- Culture—if single or multiple ring-enhancing lesions are seen, then the patient should be referred for CT-guided, or surgical, aspiration. Samples should be sent for microscopy and culture, including TB and fungal cultures. 16S PCR may be helpful in culture-negative cases. BCs should also be taken.
- Serology—this is helpful in cases of cerebral toxoplasmosis (⊃ see *Toxoplasma gondii*, pp. 562–6) and neurocysticercosis (⊃ see Neurocysticercosis, pp. 776–7).

Treatment

- For a brain abscess arising from dental/sinus/ear infections, empirical therapy with ceftriaxone 2g bd IV and metronidazole 500mg tds IV is appropriate.
- For brain abscesses arising from haematogenous spread (e.g. endocarditis), IV vancomycin can be added to the above regimen for empirical therapy.
- For brain abscesses occurring post-neurosurgery, empirical therapy with IV vancomycin and ceftazidime 2g tds IV or meropenem 2g tds IV is appropriate.
- Once culture results are available, treatment can be rationalized according to antimicrobial sensitivities. Antimicrobial therapy is usually given for 2–4 weeks IV, followed by 2–4 weeks PO. The usual duration of therapy is 6–8 weeks, but patients with multiple lesions or multiloculated lesions or those who are immunocompromised may require longer courses. There is limited evidence to inform decision-making with regard to the optimum choice, route, and duration of antibiotic therapy.
- Adjunctive corticosteroids can be given to patients with significant oedema and mass effect.[7]

Subdural empyema

A collection of pus in the space between the dura and the arachnoid.

Epidemiology

Accounts for 15–20% of localized intracranial infections. Risk factors: sinusitis, otitis media, mastoiditis, skull trauma, neurosurgery, infection of pre-existing subdural haematoma, cranial traction devices, nasal surgery, ethmoidectomy, and polypectomy. Metastatic infection accounts for 5% of cases. A rare complication of meningitis in infants

Aetiology

Causative organisms include streptococci, staphylococci, aerobic Gram-negative bacilli, and anaerobes. Polymicrobial infections are common. Post-operative/traumatic empyemas are usually caused by staphylococci or aerobic Gram-negative bacilli. Unusual causes include *Salmonella* spp., *Cutibacterium acnes*, MTB, and *Candida* spp.

Clinical features

Acute onset of fever, headache (may be localized), vomiting, altered mental state (disorientation, drowsiness, coma), and focal neurological signs (hemiparesis, cranial nerve palsies, dysphasia, homonymous hemianopia, cerebellar signs). About 80% of patients have meningeal symptoms/signs. Seizures occur in 25–80% of cases. There may be rapid neurological deterioration, with signs of raised ICP and cerebral herniation. Complications: septic venous thrombosis, cerebritis, cerebral abscess. In infants with subdural empyema, persistent fever, decline in neurological status, and seizures are seen.

Diagnosis

Consider the diagnosis in any patient with meningism and focal neurological signs. LP is contraindicated. CT or MRI head shows a crescentic or elliptical area of hypodensity with contrast enhancement. MRI is more sensitive than CT.

Management

Subdural empyema is an emergency and requires immediate surgical management. Samples should be sent for urgent microscopy and culture. Commence IV antibiotics immediately after aspiration, based on the likely infecting organisms (e.g. ceftriaxone and metronidazole). Vancomycin should be added for suspected staphylococcal infection. Tailor treatment to culture results, once available. Outcome is related to the conscious level at presentation (>90% in patients who are awake/alert and <50% in patients who are unresponsive to pain); 10–44% of survivors experience permanent neurological sequelae.

Epidural abscess

A localized collection of pus between the dura mater and the overlying skull (cranial epidural abscess) or vertebral column (spinal epidural abscess. Cranial epidural abscess may be complicated by subdural empyema.

Epidemiology

The epidemiology of cranial epidural abscess is similar to that of subdural empyema. Spinal epidural abscess usually occurs following haematogenous spread from another site of infection or by extension of vertebral osteomyelitis. Risk factors: bacteraemia, diabetes mellitus, skin infections, spinal trauma/surgery, decubitus ulcers, LP, epidural anaesthesia/analgesia.

Aetiology

The causes of cranial epidural abscess are similar to those of subdural empyema. *Staphylococcus aureus* is the commonest cause of spinal epidural abscess. Other causes include streptococci, Gram-negative bacilli (e.g. *Escherichia coli*, *Pseudomonas aeruginosa*); 5–10% are polymicrobial. Unusual causes include *Nocardia*, MTB, and fungi.

Clinical features

- The presentation of cranial epidural abscess may be insidious, masked by the primary focus of infection (e.g. sinusitis, otitis media). Headache is common, and focal neurological signs and seizures eventually develop, followed by signs of raised ICP.
- Gradenigo's syndrome, characterized by unilateral facial pain and cranial nerve V and VI palsies, may occur if the abscess is close to the petrous bone.
- Spinal epidural abscess may present acutely (hours to days with haematogenous seeding) or chronically (weeks to months with vertebral osteomyelitis). Pain is the commonest symptom (70–90%), followed by fever (60–70%). There are four clinical stages: (1) back pain and tenderness, (2) nerve root pain, (3) spinal cord symptoms (e.g. motor or sensory deficits, sphincter dysfunction), and (4) paralysis.

Diagnosis

Gadolinium-enhanced MRI is the diagnostic investigation of choice.

Management

Cranial epidural abscess—surgical drainage and antibiotics (usually continued for 3–6 weeks after drainage). Spinal epidural abscess—surgical decompression, drainage, and antibiotics. Empirical therapy should cover staphylococci (e.g. vancomyin) and aerobic, Gram-negative bacilli (e.g. ceftriaxone, ceftazidime, or meropenem). The outcome of spinal epidural abscess depends on the level of neurological deficit before decompression. Complete recovery is possible if neurological signs have been present for <24h.

CNS device infections

Infection is a frequent complication of neurosurgical procedures. Neurosurgical devices can be externalized or internalized. The types of devices that may become infected are:
- external ventricular drain (EVD);
- lumbar–peritoneal or lumbar–pleural shunt;

- ventriculo-atrial (VA), ventriculoperitoneal (VP), or ventriculopleural shunt;
- Ommaya reservoir;
- deep brain stimulator.

Aetiology

Depends on the type of device and timing of the infection in relation to device insertion. Causative organisms include:
- *Staphylococcus epidermidis*;
- *S. aureus*, including meticillin-resistant *S. aureus* (MRSA);
- streptococci, enterococci;
- *C. acnes*;
- Gram-negative organisms, including *P. aeruginosa*, *Klebsiella*, *Proteus*, and *E. coli*;
- mycobacteria;
- fungi.

Pathogenesis

Mechanisms of infection include: (1) contamination (at implantation of the device), (2) introduction of infection through the skin (e.g. through accessing the device or through device externalization), (3) retrograde infection from the distal end of the shunt, and (4) haematogenous (rare).

Clinical features

- Depend on the type of device, mechanism of infection, and whether the proximal or distal part of the device is infected. Clinical features can be very variable, and presentation can be acute or insidious.
- Symptoms include fever, headache, nausea, vomiting, lethargy, neck stiffness, and impaired conscious level.
- VA shunts may present with fever, bacteraemia, and endocarditis.
- VP shunts may present as an acute abdomen, with fever, nausea, and abdominal pain.

Diagnosis

- This depends on the type of device and clinical presentation.
- CSF examination—via shunt aspiration or LP. In patients with a suspected shunt infection, shunt aspiration is preferred over LP, if possible. CSF samples should be taken for urgent microscopy, culture, and protein and glucose levels. Abnormal results should be confirmed by a second sample, unless the clinical condition mandates immediate treatment.
- Blood tests—note normal WCC and CRP levels do not exclude shunt infection.
- BCs—90% positive with VA shunt infections.
- Imaging—CT/MRI head to look for raised ICP, CXR (VA or ventriculopleural shunt), abdominal USS/CT (VP shunt), transthoracic echocardiography (TTE) (VA shunt).

Management

- CSF device infections should be managed by neurosurgeons, with infectious diseases/microbiology input. Management varies across the UK; there are no randomized trials to guide clinical practice.
- Shunt infections—management should include device removal, external drainage, IV antibiotics, and subsequent shunt replacement once the CSF is sterile. An example of an empirical antibiotic regimen would be vancomycin IV and an antipseudomonal β-lactam IV (e.g. ceftazidime or meropenem). Intraventricular antibiotics may be required in those who respond poorly to systemic antibiotics.
- EVD-associated ventriculitis—empirical antibiotics (e.g. intrathecal vancomycin and intrathecal gentamicin). A minority of patients will require systemic antibiotics.
- Specific antibiotic therapy should be tailored in light of culture results and clinical response.

Ophthalmological infections

Periorbital infections

Blepharitis

Inflammation of the eyelids. Clinical features: soreness or stinging, erythema, pruritus, and crusting of lid margins. Bacterial infection is usually secondary to minor trauma and often occurs in association with seborrhoeic dermatitis, acne, rosacea, *Demodex* mites, and pubic lice infestations. Blepharitis is usually a chronic condition.

Anterior blepharitis

Inflammation at the base of the eyelashes. Lid-colonizing bacteria (e.g. *Staphylococcus aureus*, coagulase-negative staphylococci (CoNS)) play a role in some cases.

Posterior blepharitis

Inflammation of the inner portion of the eyelid involving the Meibomian glands. Posterior blepharitis can lead to a chalazion (eyelid cyst).

Treatment

Eyelid hygiene is the mainstay of treatment. Blepharitis thought to be infectious in nature should be treated with a topical antibiotic, and the frequency and duration of treatment determined by the severity. Predisposing conditions should be treated (e.g. lice—malathion; rosacea—PO tetracycline; seborrhoeic dermatitis—topical antifungal/steroid combinations).

Other causes of lid inflammation

Cosmetic contact allergy, molluscum contagiosum, dermatoblepharitis secondary to herpes simplex virus (HSV) infection, or spread of adjacent impetigo.

Infections of the lacrimal apparatus

The lacrimal gland is found at the lateral upper lid margin. It produces around 10mL of tears a day, with the act of blinking serving to smear the tear film from the lateral to the medial edge of the eye surface. Drainage is via the puncta at the inner canthus into the canaliculi, and from here to the lacrimal sac and the nasolacrimal duct, and out into the nose.

Canaliculitis

Low-grade inflammation of the canaliculi. Can be primary or secondary to a punctal plug. Forms gritty casts that obstruct the lacrimal duct, leading to eye-watering, chronic conjunctivitis, and nasal lid swelling. Organisms include *Actinomyces*, *Staphylococcus* spp., *Streptococcus* spp., and *Pseudomonas* spp. Treatment: antibiotic irrigation with canaliculotomy and curettage where necessary.

Dacryocystitis

Inflammation of the lacrimal sac usually in the setting of obstruction of the sac or duct (congenital, secondary to infection, tumour, or trauma). Clinical features of acute dacrocystitis: red and tender swelling over the lacrimal sac, excessive tearing. Bacterial overgrowth or secondary infection can occur, and it may be possible to express purulent material through the lacrimal puncta. Organisms include *Streptococcus pneumoniae*, *S. aureus*, *Haemophilus influenzae*, and *Pseudomonas aeruginosa*. Treatment: systemic antibiotics, may require incision and drainage of lacrimal sac abscess or dacryocystorhinostomy. Orbital cellulitis is a serious complication of acute dacryocystitis.

Dacryoadenitis

Inflammation of the lacrimal gland; infections are rare. Symptoms: localized tenderness/swelling of the outer upper eyelid, with conjunctivitis and periorbital oedema. *S. aureus* and *S. pneumoniae* are commonly implicated. Rarer causes include Epstein–Barr virus (EBV), HSV, mumps, TB, brucellosis, and leprosy. Treatment: systemic antibiotics; drainage if a collection develops. Orbital cellulitis is a serious complication of acute dacryoadenitis.

Orbital infections

The orbital septum is a fibrous sheet lying beneath the orbicularis oculi. It extends from the periosteum of the orbit and fuses to the levator aponeurosis in the upper lids and the orbital retractor in the lower lids. It acts as a physical barrier to infection. Orbital cellulitis (infection within the septum) is an ophthalmic emergency and must be differentiated from the less devastating preseptal cellulitis (see Table 20.1). Early involvement of an ophthalmologist is essential. Children with preseptal infection are at high risk of progressing to orbital cellulitis, due to the undeveloped nature of the orbital septum, and should be managed as orbital cellulitis.

Preseptal (periorbital) cellulitis

An infection of the superficial skin around the eyes, anterior to the orbital septum. It may follow infection of adjacent structures (e.g. dacryocystitis) or trauma.

- Aetiology—*S. aureus, S. pneumoniae*, other streptococci, *H. influenzae* (if unvaccinated), anaerobes. Rare causes include *Acinetobacter* spp., *Nocardia* spp., *Bacillus anthracis, P. aeruginosa, Neisseria gonorrhoeae, Proteus* spp., *Pasteurella multocida, Mycobacterium* tuberculosis (MTB), and *Trichophyton* spp.
- Clinical features—ocular pain, eyelid swelling and erythema, low-grade fever. Proptosis and impairment of eye movements are not seen—their presence suggests orbital cellulitis (➔ see Orbital (post-septal) cellulitis,

Table 20.1 Orbital versus preseptal cellulitis

	Preseptal	Orbital
Proptosis	Absent	Present
Ocular motility	Normal	Painful and restricted
Visual acuity	Normal	Reduced in severe cases
Colour vision	Normal	Reduced in severe cases
Relative afferent pupillary defect	Normal	Present in severe cases

Reproduced from Denniston A and Murray P, *Oxford Handbook of Ophthalmology.* Oxford: Oxford University Press, 2018, with permission from Oxford University Press.

p. 792). Optic nerve function is normal. Complications include progression to orbital cellulitis and CNS infections.
• Investigations—Gram staining and culture of any discharge, CT/MRI scan if any question of orbital involvement.
• Management—outpatient management with PO antibiotics is sufficient in simple cases (e.g. co-amoxiclav 625mg tds for 7 days or clarithromycin 500mg bd with metronidazole 400mg tds for 7 days). Infants should be admitted, as should those in whom the distinction between preseptal and orbital cellulitis is unclear.

Orbital (post-septal) cellulitis

An acute infection involving the contents of the orbit (fat and ocular muscles). This is an ophthalmic emergency because of the risk of visual loss and posterior extension to the cavernous sinus (with possible thrombosis and death). Most cases result from contiguous spread from infected sinuses but can occur as a result of trauma, otitis media, and dental infection.

• Aetiology—*S. aureus*, *Streptococcus anginosus* group, *S. pneumoniae*, group A *Streptococcus* (GAS), anaerobes. Rare causes: *H. influenzae*, *Aeromonas hydrophila*, *P. aeruginosa*, *Eikenella corrodens*, MTB, *Aspergillus* spp., mucormycosis.
• Clinical features—ocular pain, swelling, eyelid erythema (may be absent), painful eye movements, proptosis, ophthalmoplegia, diplopia. Fever is commoner in orbital cellulitis than in preseptal cellulitis. Late signs: increased orbital pressure, reduced corneal sensation, and congestion of retinal veins. Complications include subperiosteal abscess, orbital abscess, loss of vision (3–11%), central retinal artery occlusion, cavernous sinus thrombosis, and brain abscess.
• Investigations—CT scan of the orbits/sinuses is indicated if there are any of the following features: proptosis, pain on eye movement, limitation of eye movements, double vision, loss of vision, oedema extending beyond the eyelid margin, signs/symptoms of CNS involvement, inability to examine the patient fully, and failure to improve within 24–48h of starting antibiotic therapy. Blood cultures (BCs) should be taken prior to antibiotics but are rarely positive. If surgical intervention is performed, the organism may be recovered from material, despite empirical antibiotic therapy.
• Treatment—empirical antibiotics should be started as soon as possible (e.g. ceftriaxone and metronidazole ± vancomycin if meticillin-resistant *S. aureus* (MRSA) is suspected/possible). Urgent ophthalmology opinion and ear, nose, and throat (ENT) review (if sinus surgery may be required). Continuing deterioration on therapy suggests the development of an abscess, and repeat CT should be performed, with a view to surgical drainage if necessary. Management of fungal orbital cellulitis is a complex mix of surgical debridement and antifungal therapy.

Conjunctivitis

Conjunctivitis is the commonest ocular inflammation and may be a primary/local infection or part of a systemic infection (e.g. leptospirosis, measles). Some organisms (e.g. *Chlamydia trachomatis*) cause very specific syndromes, but most cannot be distinguished clinically. Viruses are the commonest cause. Acute conjunctivitis resolves within 4 weeks; chronic conjunctivitis persists for ≥4 weeks. Conjunctivitis is typically self-limiting but can progress to potentially sight-threatening infections.

Aetiology

- Viruses—the commonest cause (e.g. adenovirus, Coxsackie A24, enterovirus 70, HSV, varicella-zoster virus (VZV), rubella, measles, mumps, influenza, EBV).
- Chlamydia—*C. trachomatis*, *Chlamydia pneumoniae*.
- Bacterial—*S. aureus*, *S. pneumoniae*, *H. influenzae*, *Moraxella* spp., *Corynebacterium diphtheriae*, *Neisseria* spp., *Leptospira* spp., enteric Gram-negative rods (GNRs).
- Parasitic—*Leishmania* spp., *Trypanosoma* spp., cryptosporidia, fly larvae, *Loa loa*, *Phthyrus pubis* (pubic lice), *Demodex* (mites).
- Fungal—*Candida* spp., *Blastomyces* spp., *Sporothrix schenkii*, microsporidia.
- Allergic or toxic—allergens, cosmetics, soaps, detergents, medications.

Clinical features

- Irritation and itching are the commonest symptoms. Ocular pain is unusual, unless there is ulceration (e.g. HSV) or corneal involvement.
- Visual acuity is normal or slightly reduced (unless the cornea is involved).
- Skin lesions are seen with HSV, VZV, poxviruses, and immune-mediated diseases (e.g. Stevens–Johnson syndrome).
- Conjunctival hyperaemia is worse in the periphery than in the limbal region.
- Ocular secretion may be due to increased lacrimal flow or impaired drainage.
- Conjunctival oedema (chemosis) may be marked, resulting in an inability to close the eyelids.
- Conjunctival papillae—conjunctival inflammation may result in dilated subepithelial blood vessels that become surrounded by an inflammatory infiltrate to form mounds called papillae. Commoner in bacterial and allergic conjunctivitis.
- Conjunctival follicles—small, elevated clusters of lymphocytes, similar to papillae, but with no central vascular core. Most commonly associated with viral, chlamydial, or toxic conjunctivitis.
- Membrane and pseudomembranes—inflammatory exudate may coalesce, forming a yellow-white membrane overlying the palpebral conjunctiva. Commoner in viral and bacterial conjunctivitis.
- Conjunctival phlyctenules—a phlyctenule is a whitish, nodular collection located at or near the limbus, often in the centre of a hyperaemic area. It is a delayed-type hypersensitivity reaction and is associated with *S. aureus* and MTB.
- Conjunctival granuloma—a granulomatous nodule of inflammatory cells. Seen in Parinaud's oculoglandular conjunctivitis, foreign body, TB, and sarcoidosis, and sometimes in chlamydial or fungal conjunctivitis.

- Corneal involvement—may be mild (superficial epithelial erosions) or severe (ulceration or perforation). Corneal dendritic ulceration is a feature of HSV conjunctivitis. Symptoms include foreign body sensation, pain, decreased visual acuity, and photophobia.
- Lymphadenopathy—preauricular adenopathy is a non-specific finding associated with viral, chlamydial, and gonococcal causes of conjunctivitis. Submandibular and submental adenopathy is uncommon but may be present in Parinaud's oculoglandular conjunctivitis.

Diagnosis

- Laboratory investigations are not usually performed for most cases of conjunctivitis, especially if a viral aetiology is suspected.
- Investigations include swab for Gram staining, culture, nucleic acid amplification tests (NAATs) (*C. trachomatis* and *N. gonorrhoeae*), and PCR (adenovirus, HSV).
- All cases of ophthalmia neonatorum (conjunctivitis occurring within the first month of life) should be investigated. The commonest cause in neonates is *C. trachomatis*.

Management

- Treatment should be directed at the likely cause.
- Acute bacterial conjunctivitis—topical antibiotic eye drops (e.g. chloramphenicol, trimethoprim and polymyxin B, fluoroquinolone, or azithromycin drops) or ointment (e.g. erythromycin, bacitracin, or bacitracin and polymyxin B).
- Viral conjunctivitis usually resolves spontaneously and is usually treated supportively (e.g. artificial tears and cold compresses). There is no role for antivirals or corticosteroids.
- Chlamydial conjunctivitis—adult inclusion conjunctivitis is treated with doxycycline 100mg bd PO for 7 days or azithromycin 1g single dose followed by 500mg daily for 2 days. Patients should be screened for other sexually transmitted infections (STIs). Neonatal infection should be treated with erythromycin 12.5mg/kg qds PO for 14 days.
- *N. gonorrhoeae*—IM ceftriaxone 1g single dose. Patients should be screened for other STIs. Neonatal infection should be treated with a third-generation cephalosporin.
- Chronic bacterial conjunctivitis—treat with appropriate antibiotic therapy (e.g. against *S. aureus*) and aggressive lid hygiene.

Keratitis

Keratitis is an inflammation of the cornea that may be caused by infectious or non-infectious agents. Corneal inflammation is potentially sight-threatening and requires prompt investigation/management, as corneal perforation can occur within 24h with certain organisms. Subsequent endophthalmitis may lead to loss of vision or even loss of the eye.

Aetiology

- Microbial agents do not usually cause keratitis in immunocompetent patients with an intact corneal epithelium. Exceptions include *N. gonorrhoeae*, *Listeria monocytogenes*, *Shigella* spp., and *Corynebacterium* spp.

- Risk factors—trauma, contact lens use, contaminated cleaning fluids, immunological impairment secondary to malnutrition, alcoholism or diabetes, recent or pre-existing eye disease (e.g. sicca syndrome, recent topical steroid use).
- Bacteria—the commonest cause of keratitis. Causes include *Staphylococcus* spp., *Streptococcus* spp., *Corynebacterium* spp., *Bacillus* spp., *Cutibacterium* spp., *Pseudomonas* spp., *Haemophilus* spp., *Moraxella* spp., *N. gonorrhoeae*, *C. trachomatis*, and *Enterobacterales*.
- Mycobacteria—MTB, *Mycobacterium chelonae*, *Mycobacterium gordonae*, *Mycobacterium avium intracellulare* (MAI).
- Spirochaetes—*Treponema pallidum*, *Borrelia burgdorferi*.
- Viruses—HSV, VZV, adenovirus, enterovirus, EBV, Coxsackie virus, measles.
- Fungi—*Fusarium* (commonest), *Aspergillus*, *Curvularia*, *Paecilomyces*, *Phialophora*, *Blastomyces*, *Sporothrix*, *Exophiala*, *Pseudallescheria*, *Scedosporium*, and *Alternaria* spp., microsporidia.
- Parasites—*Acanthamoeba*, *Onchocerca volvulus*, *Leishmania*, and *Trypanosoma* spp.

Clinical features

- Rapid onset of eye pain is characteristic and may hinder physical examination. Topical anaesthesia may facilitate eye examination but can result in further epithelial damage.
- Eye pain is accompanied by conjunctival injection, tearing, photophobia, blepharospasm, and decreased visual acuity.
- Other features include corneal infiltrates, epithelial defects (visualized by fluorescein stain under cobalt blue light), stromal suppuration, corneal oedema, corneal neovascularization, intraocular inflammation (white cells or protein flare in the anterior chamber, hypopyon, synechiae, glaucoma), and loss of corneal tissue (keratolysis).

Diagnosis

- Because of the limited amount of tissue available, extreme care must be taken in the collection, transport, and processing of specimens.
- Corneal scrapings (or biopsies) should be taken using a sterile technique and transferred to glass slides and appropriate culture media. It may also be helpful to culture material from the conjunctivae, eyelids, and contact lenses/solutions/storage cases.
- For viruses, samples should be collected into viral transport media. PCR assays enable rapid diagnosis of HSV and VZV.

Management

Patients may need to be admitted to hospital for management, particularly if there is evidence of corneal thinning.

- Bacterial keratitis—topical fluoroquinolones or topical cephalosporin/aminoglycoside combinations. The use of topical corticosteroids is controversial. Supportive measures: topical cycloplegics, temporary soft contact lens for corneal ulceration.
- Chlamydial keratitis—systemic antimicrobials (e.g. PO doxycycline). Sexual partners should be treated simultaneously.

- Interstitial keratitis—an immune phenomenon associated with syphilis and Lyme disease. Specific therapy may be indicated for the primary disease but has little impact on the cornea. Topical corticosteroids may be helpful.
- HSV keratitis—TOP (aciclovir, valaciclovir). Systemic antiviral therapy may be used in some cases.
- VZV keratitis—acute herpes zoster ophthalmicus requires systemic antiviral therapy (aciclovir, famciclovir, or valaciclovir) and pain management (e.g. amitriptyline). Topical corticosteroids may be helpful.
- Viral keratoconjunctivitis—no specific treatment required; supportive treatment only (e.g. artificial tears ± cycloplegics). If severe symptoms, topical steroids may be helpful.
- Fungal keratitis— may require combined topical (e.g. natamycin, voriconazole, amphotericin) and systemic (e.g. voriconazole) therapy for months.
- Parasitic keratitis—the optimal treatment for *Acanthamoeba* keratitis is unknown, and various agents have been used (e.g. diamidines, biguanides, aminoglycosides, azoles). Onchocerciasis is treated with ivermectin.

Uveitis

Uveitis is an inflammation of the uveal tract (iris, ciliary body, choroid) or adjacent ocular structures such as the retina. Inflammation may occur in different anatomical regions of the eye (e.g. anterior (commonest), intermediate, posterior, or panuveitis). Uveitis may be caused by infections, autoimmune conditions, or rarely trauma; 50% are idiopathic. Some infectious causes may affect particular locations. Aspiration of aqueous or vitreous material may allow identification of the causative organism. Involve an ophthalmologist early in management.

Classification

- **Anterior uveitis**—inflammation affects the iris (iritis), anterior ciliary body (cyclitis), or both (iridocyclitis). It presents with a unilateral red eye, deep ocular pain, a tender eyeball, an irregular/constricted pupil, photophobia, and eye-watering. Most cases are associated with autoimmune conditions (45%) or are idiopathic (40%). Infectious causes include HSV, VZV, syphilis, TB, and Lyme disease.
- **Intermediate uveitis**—inflammation involving the anterior vitreous, ciliary body, and adjacent portion of the retina. The aetiology of most cases is unknown. Infectious causes are rare but include Lyme disease, TB, and leptospirosis (69%). Non-infectious causes include sarcoidosis and multiple sclerosis.
- **Posterior uveitis**—inflammation involving the choroid (choroiditis), retina (retinitis), or both (choroidoretinitis). More likely to be painless and present with floaters. Over 40% of cases are due to infection (e.g. *Toxoplasma* (commonest infectious cause), cytomegalovirus (CMV), acute retinal necrosis (HSV), *Toxocara*, syphilis, and *Candida*).

- **Panuveitis**—inflammation involving all parts of the uvea. Causes: mostly autoimmune, idiopathic (25%), and infections (10%) (e.g. syphilis, TB, and *Candida*).

Aetiology

- **Infectious**—these include bacteria, spirochaetes, viruses, fungi, and parasites (see Table 20.2). These affect different populations and have distinctive clinical presentations.
- **Systemic inflammatory conditions associated with uveitis**—these include spondyloarthritides (e.g. ankylosing spondylitis, reactive arthritis, psoriatic arthritis), inflammatory bowel disease (IBD), sarcoidosis, Behçet's disease, tubulointerstitial nephritis and uveitis (TINU) syndromes, juvenile idiopathic arthritis, Kawasaki disease, relapsing polychondritis, Sjögren's syndrome, systemic lupus erythematosus (SLE), granulomatosis with polyangiitis (GPA).
- **Syndromes confined to the eye**—pars planitis (may be associated with multiple sclerosis or sarcoidosis), sympathetic ophthalmia (inflammation of the contralateral eye that occurs weeks to a year after trauma to one eye), birdshot choroidopathy.
- **Masquerade syndromes**—these include ocular lymphoma, melanoma or retinoblastoma, leukaemia, giant retinal tears, retinal ischaemia, and retinitis pigmentosa.

Table 20.2 Infectious causes of uveitis

Bacteria	Viruses	Fungi	Parasites
TB	CMV	Aspergillosis	Toxocariasis
Syphilis	EBV	Blastomycosis	Toxoplasmosis
Cat-scratch disease	HSV	Candidiasis	*Acanthamoeba*
NTM	VZV	Coccidioidomycosis	Cysticercosis
Leprosy	HIV	Cryptococcosis	Onchocerciasis
Leptospirosis	HTLV-1	Histoplasmosis	
Lyme disease	Mumps	*Pneumocystis jirovecii*	
RMSF	Parechovirus	Sporotrichosis	
Whipple's disease	Rubella		
Brucella	Measles		
	Dengue virus		
	West Nile virus		
	Chikungunya virus		

CMV, cytomegalovirus; EBV, Epstein–Barr virus; HSV, herpes simplex virus; HTLV-1, human T-cell lymphotropic virus 1; NTM, non-tuberculous mycobacteria; VZV, varicella-zoster virus.; RMSF, rocky mountain spotty fever

Diagnosis

- The diagnosis of uveitis is almost always presumptive as the uvea cannot be biopsied without risking sight. The aqueous and vitreous humours may be sampled, but these samples rarely yield a diagnosis.
- Molecular diagnostic techniques may be helpful (e.g. PCR for HSV, VZV, and CMV). Serology is unhelpful, apart from in the diagnosis of syphilis and Lyme disease.
- A CXR may be useful to look for TB or sarcoidosis.

Treatment

Treatment of the infectious causes of uveitis is the same as that for CNS infection caused by the same pathogen. Systemic corticosteroids may be given in some conditions (e.g. ocular syphilis).

Endophthalmitis

Inflammation of the ocular cavity (aqueous and vitreous humours). Usually caused by bacteria or fungi, which may be introduced into the eye from an external (exogenous) source (e.g. trauma, surgery, keratitis, bleb-related) or enter the eye haematogenously from a distant (endogenous) site of infection (e.g. endocarditis). Panophthalmitis refers to inflammation of all ocular tissue.

General features

- Symptoms—eye pain, redness, lid swelling, decreased visual acuity, headache, photophobia, discharge. Fungal endophthalmitis may have a more indolent course, with symptoms developing over days to weeks. Consider in anyone with a history of penetrating injury with a plant substance or soil-contaminated foreign body. Symptoms of the primary source of infection may be seen in endogenous cases (e.g. fever, meningism).
- Signs—lid swelling/erythema, inflamed conjunctiva, hypopyon, chemosis, corneal oedema, discharge, reduced/absent red reflex, papillitis, cotton-wool spots, vitritis, fluffy yellow-white retinal or vitreoretinal lesions of growing fungi, fever, and, late in panophthalmitis, proptosis.

Aetiology

- Bacterial—the commonest infectious cause. Onset is abrupt, and progression rapid. Most cases are seen after intraocular surgery. Slit-lamp examination is necessary to confirm the diagnosis and detect early signs of infection. Two types:
  - exogenous—symptoms develop 24–48h after eye trauma, later in patients undergoing extracapsular cataract extraction (<5 days post-operatively). Ocular surface flora is responsible for the majority of infections, and preoperative conjunctival sterilization may reduce the incidence. Common post-operative causes: CoNS, *S. aureus*, *Streptococcus* spp. Common post-traumatic causes: *Bacillus cereus*, CoNS, *Klebsiella*, *Pseudomonas* spp., moulds. Delayed endophthalmitis

after cataract extraction in patients with an intraocular lens may run a chronic course—the commonest cause is *Cutibacterium acnes*;
* endogenous—rare. Foci of primary infection include meningitis, endocarditis, intra-abdominal abscess, urinary tract infection, and transient bacteriaemia (e.g. endoscopy, IV drug use). Causes: *S. aureus*, *Streptococcus* spp., *Klebsiella pneumoniae*, *Escherichia coli*.
* Fungal—*Candida* endophthalmitis is usually endogenous. Risk factors include indwelling central venous catheters, total parenteral nutrition (TPN), broad-spectrum antibiotics, recent abdominal surgery, and neutropenia. Patients are often sick (e.g. ventilated on the intensive care unit) and may not report early visual symptoms. Have a low threshold for ocular examination of such patients. Mould endophthalmitis is usually exogenous, but endogenous cases may occur in seriously immunosuppressed patients and people who inject drugs (PWID). Common causes: *Aspergillus*, *Fusarium*. Other causes: *Cryptococcus*, *Histoplasma*, *Coccidioides*.

Diagnosis

Early recognition and prompt microbiological investigations are essential if functional vision is to be salvaged in bacterial endophthalmitis. Samples from the vitreous humour (vitreous aspirate, vitrectomy) have the greatest yield. It may also be appropriate to obtain material from the anterior chamber and any wound. Samples should be sent for microscopy (Gram and calcofluor staining), and cultured for both bacteria and fungi. BCs should be taken if the patient is systemically unwell.

Treatment

Successful outcome is dependent upon a low threshold of clinical suspicion for diagnosing infectious endophthalmitis. Urgent specialist referral is indicated.
* Bacterial—broad-spectrum intravitreal antibiotics (e.g. vancomycin and ceftazidime) should be started immediately after urgent diagnostic aspirates and modified in the light of culture results. Those with visual acuity of light perception or worse benefit from immediate vitrectomy; those with better vision than this do no better with vitrectomy and intravitreal antibiotics than with biopsy and intravitreal antibiotics (unless perhaps they are diabetic). Outcome is influenced by the time to diagnosis and appropriate treatment and the virulence of the organism—*P. aeruginosa* and *S. aureus* can destroy the eye within 24h of presentation. There may be a role for early corticosteroids.
* Fungal—*Candida*: intravitreal voriconazole or amphotericin B, systemic antifungals (fluconazole, voriconazole. amphotericin B). Vitrectomy should be considered. *Aspergillus*: intravitreal voriconazole or amphotericin B, systemic voriconazole. Vitrectomy should be considered.

Skin and soft tissue infections

Skin and soft tissue infections: introduction

Impetigo

- Caused by *Staphylococcus aureus* and/or group A *Streptococcus* (GAS). Commonly affects children in tropical/subtropical regions; also prevalent in temperate regions in summer months.
- Clinical features—occurs on the face and extremities. Lesions start as small vesicles that develop into flaccid bullae that rupture, releasing a yellow discharge that forms thick crusts.
- Treatment—mupirocin is the best topical agent. Patients who have numerous lesions or who do not respond to topical treatment should receive oral antibiotics (e.g. flucloxacillin or cefalexin). If meticillin-resistant *S. aureus* (MRSA) is suspected/isolated, then treatment with doxycycline, clindamycin, or co-trimoxazole is appropriate.

Folliculitis

- A superficial infection of the hair follicles and apocrine structures.
- Aetiology—*S. aureus* (commonest), *Pseudomonas aeruginosa* ('hot tub' folliculitis), *Enterobacterales* (complication of acne), *Candida* spp., and *Malassezia furfur* (in patients taking corticosteroids). Eosinophilic pustular folliculitis occurs in patients with uncontrolled HIV.
- Clinical features—lesions consist of small, erythematous, pruritic papules, often with a central pustule.
- Treatment—empirical treatment is with an antistaphylococcal antibiotic (topical or systemic, depending on severity). If the clinical response is slow, consider other pathogens.

Cutaneous abscesses

- Collections of pus within the dermis and deeper skin structures.
- Aetiology—*S. aureus* (commonest), polymicrobial containing skin/mucous membrane flora.
- Clinical features—painful, tender, fluctuant nodules, usually with an overlying pustule and surrounded by a rim of erythematous swelling.
- Treatment—incision and drainage. Antibiotics are rarely necessary, unless there is extensive infection or systemic toxicity, or the patient is immunocompromised.

Furuncles and carbuncles

- A furuncle (boil) is a deep inflammatory nodule that usually develops from preceding folliculitis. Furuncles usually occur in areas containing hair follicles (e.g. face, neck, axillae, buttocks).
- A carbuncle is a larger, deeper lesion made of multiple abscesses extending into the subcutaneous fat. Usually occurs at the nape of the neck, on the back, or on the thighs. Patients may be systemically unwell.
- Outbreaks of furunculosis caused by meticillin-sensitive *S. aureus* (MSSA) and MRSA have been described in groups of individuals with close contact (e.g. families, prisons, sports teams).
- Most furuncles may be treated with application of moist heat, which promotes localization and spontaneous drainage. Large lesions require

surgical drainage. Systemic antibiotics are indicated if fever, cellulitis, or lesions are located near the nose or lip. Control of outbreaks may require washing with chlorhexidine soaps, no sharing of cloths or towels, laundering of clothing, towels and bedclothes, and eradication of staphylococcal carriage in colonized persons.

Ecthyma

- Punched-out ulcers surrounded by raised, violaceous margins.
- Caused by *S. aureus* or GAS. Similar lesions (ecthyma gangrenosum) may occur with *P. aeruginosa* in neutropenic patients.
- Empirical treatment is with flucloxacillin or cefalexin (unless cultures yield streptococci alone, in which case penicillin is appropriate). Antipseudomonal agents (e.g. piperacillin–tazobactam) should be given for *P. aeruginosa* infections.

Erysipelas

- An acute spreading skin infection with prominent lymphatic involvement. Usually affects infants, children, and the elderly. Predisposing factors include skin lesions, venous stasis, paraparesis, diabetes mellitus, and alcohol abuse.
- Causes—GAS (commonest), group C and G streptococci, *S. aureus*, *Streptococcus agalactiae*.
- Clinical features—painful, erythematous, oedematous lesion with an elevated, sharply demarcated border. Usually occurs on the face or legs. Systemic symptoms are common; 5% are bacteraemic.
- Treatment is with flucloxacillin or clindamycin. If cultures yield streptococci, treatment with penicillin is appropriate.

Cellulitis

- An acute spreading infection of the skin that extends into the subcutaneous tissues. *S. aureus* and streptococci are the main causes. Clues to other causes include physical activities, trauma, water contact, animal, insect, or human bites, and immunosuppression. Examples include *Enterobacterales*, *Legionella pneumophila*, *Aeromonas hydrophila*, *Vibrio vulnificus*, *Erysipelothrix rhusiopathiae*, and *Cryptococcus neoformans*.
- Clinical features—spreading erythematous, hot, and tender lesion, usually accompanied by systemic symptoms.
- Diagnosis is usually clinical, as cultures are rarely positive.
- Treatment—empirical treatment is with flucloxacillin, clarithromycin, or doxycycline. For MRSA cellulitis, IV options include vancomycin or teicoplanin; PO options include clindamycin, linezolid, and co-trimoxazole. Gram-negative and anaerobic cover may be required for cellulitis near the eyes/nose and in the context of diabetic ulcers. The affected limb should be immobilized and elevated.

Further reading

National Institute for Health and Care Excellence (2019). *Cellulitis and erysipelas: antimicrobial pre-scribing*. NICE guideline [NG141]. Available at: ℘ https://www.nice.org.uk/guidance/ng141

Bite infections

Animal bites

- Aetiology—these are usually caused by domestic pets (e.g. dogs or cats) but may be caused by exotic pets or wild animals. Most infections are polymicrobial. The predominant pathogens are the oral flora of the biting animal (e.g. *Pasteurella multocida*, *Capnocytophaga canimorsus*, *Bacteroides* spp., *Fusobacterium* spp., *Prevotella* spp., *Porphyromonas* spp., peptostreptococci). Secondary bacterial infection with *S. aureus* or GAS may occur.
- Diagnosis of bite infection is clinical, but samples may be taken to identify the causative organisms. Complications include septic arthritis, osteomyelitis, subcutaneous abscesses, tendonitis, and bacteraemia.
- Management—wounds should be irrigated copiously with sterile saline, and any debris removed; debridement is rarely necessary. Wounds should be Steri-Strips™®, but not sutured (except facial wounds by a plastic surgeon). Empirical antibiotic therapy for bite infection is with PO co-amoxiclav or PO doxycycline and metronidazole. The need for antibiotic prophylaxis for uninfected bites depends on the animal and the depth of the bite. Tetanus vaccination and human normal immunoglobulin (HNIG) need to be considered, depending on the immunization status of the patient and the state of the wound. Rabies vaccination should be considered for animal bites in endemic regions. Prophylactic valaciclovir or aciclovir should be considered for monkey bites (simian herpes B virus).

Human bites

- Aetiology—human bites result from aggressive behaviour and are often more serious than animal bites. The causative organisms are usually the oral flora of the biter (e.g. oral streptococci, staphylococci, *Haemophilus* spp., *Eikenella corrodens*, *Fusobacterium* spp., *Prevotella* spp., *Porphyromonas* spp., and rarely *Bacteroides* spp.). Human bites may also potentially transmit viral infections (e.g. hepatitis B virus (HBV), hepatitis C virus (HCV), HIV).
- Clinical features—bite wounds may be occlusive injuries (where teeth bite the body part) or clenched-fist injuries (where one person's fist hits the other person's teeth). Complications of clenched-fist injuries include tendon or nerve damage, fractures, septic arthritis, and osteomyelitis.
- Management—the principles are the same as those for animal bites (e.g. wound irrigation and consideration of antibiotics for either prophylaxis or treatment) (➔ see Animal bites above). Hand injuries should be evaluated for complications by a hand surgeon. Post-exposure prophylaxis (PEP) against hepatitis B should be considered if the source is potentially infected. HIV PEP following a human bite is only recommended in very specific circumstances.

Further reading

National Institute for Health and Care Excellence (2020). *Human and animal bites: antimicrobial prescribing*. NICE guideline [NG184]. Available at: ℘ https://www.nice.org.uk/guidance/ng184

Surgical site infections

Infections of surgical wounds are common adverse events following surgery. The frequency of surgical site infections (SSIs) is related to the category of operation and is highest with contaminated or high-risk surgical procedures. There are three categories of SSIs:

- superficial incisional SSIs—involve the skin or subcutaneous tissue, occur within 30 days of operation;
- deep incisional SSIs—involve muscle and fascia, occur within 30 days of operation (or 1 year if prosthesis inserted);
- organ/space SSIs—involve any part of the anatomy (organs or spaces) other than the incisional site; occur within 30 days of operation (or 1 year if prosthesis inserted).

Aetiology and pathogenesis

The commonest organisms are *S. aureus* and MRSA. Others include coagulase-negative staphylococci (CoNS), streptococci, enterococci, and aerobic Gram-negative bacilli. SSIs that occur after an operation on the GI tract or ♀ genitalia have a high probability of having mixed flora. The presence of prosthetic material greatly reduces the number of organisms that are required to initiate infection.

Clinical features

- Most SSIs have no clinical manifestations for at least 5 days after the operation, and many may not become apparent for up to 2 weeks.
- Local signs of pain, swelling, erythema, and purulent drainage are usually present. Fever may not be present until a few days later.
- In morbidly obese patients or in patients with deep, multilayer wounds (e.g. thoracotomy), external signs of SSIs may appear late.

Diagnosis

Diagnosis is usually clinical. Swabs from skin surrounding a wound may be polymicrobial, and distinguishing colonization from infection may not be possible. Ideally, samples of fluid or tissue should be taken from a newly opened wound or during surgical debridement, and sent to the laboratory for Gram staining and culture. Negative cultures may indicate atypical infection.

Management

- The primary therapy for SSIs is to open the incision, debride the infected material, and continue dressing changes until the wound heals by secondary intention.
- Although patients commonly receive antibiotics for SSIs, there is little or no evidence supporting this practice.
- A common practice, endorsed by expert opinion, is to open all infected wounds. If there is minimal evidence of invasive infection (<5cm of erythema) and if the patient has minimal systemic signs of infection (temperature <38°C, WCC < × 10⁹/L), antibiotics are unnecessary. For patients with a temperature of >38°C or WCC > × 10⁹/L, a short course of antibiotics may be indicated.
- UK health authorities perform SSI surveillance

Clostridial gas gangrene (myonecrosis)

This is a rapidly progressive, life-threatening skeletal muscle infection caused by *Clostridium* spp. (clostridial myonecrosis).

Aetiology and pathogenesis

- Gas gangrene usually occurs following muscle injury and contamination of the wound by soil or foreign material containing clostridial spores. *Clostridium perfringens* is the predominant cause (80–95%), and its pathological effects are mediated by α and λ toxins.
- Spontaneous or non-traumatic gas gangrene may occur in the absence of an obvious wound. This form is usually caused by *Clostridium septicum* and is associated with intestinal abnormalities (e.g. colon cancer, diverticulitis, bowel infarction, necrotizing enterocolitis).
- Other organisms include *Clostridium novyi*, *Clostridium bifermentans* (now called *Paraclostridium* bifermentans), *Clostridium histolyticum*, and *Clostridium fallax*. Organisms, such as *Escherichia coli*, *Enterobacter* spp., or enterococci, may be isolated, reflecting contamination of the wound.

Clinical features

- The incubation period is usually 2–3 days but may be shorter.
- Patients present with acute onset of excruciating pain and signs of shock (fever, tachycardia, hypotension, jaundice, renal failure).
- Local oedema and tenderness may be the only early signs, or there may be an open wound, herniation of muscle, a serosanguinous and foul-smelling discharge, crepitus, skin discoloration, and necrosis.
- Progression is rapid, and death may occur within hours.

Diagnosis

- Diagnosis is usually clinical but may be confirmed by Gram staining of the wound exudate or debrided tissue.
- Liquid anaerobic cultures may be positive within 6h.
- Plain radiographs may show gas in the affected tissues.

Management

- Emergency surgical exploration and debridement of the affected area should be performed.
- Empirical antibiotic therapy with piperacillin–tazobactam and clindamycin plus vancomycin (if risk of MRSA) is appropriate, pending cultures.
- Definitive treatment for clostridial myonecrosis is with penicillin and clindamycin.
- Hyperbaric oxygen therapy is not recommended, as its benefit is unproven and it may delay resuscitation/surgery.

Necrotizing fasciitis

A severe acute infection involving the superficial and deep fascia.

Aetiology

- Type I (polymicrobial) necrotizing fasciitis involves at least one anaerobic species (e.g. *Bacteroides* or *Peptostreptococcus* spp.), as well as one or more facultative anaerobic species (e.g. non-GAS, *E. coli*, *Enterobacter*, *Klebsiella*, *Proteus* spp.).
- Type II (monomicrobial) necrotizing fasciitis is usually caused by GAS alone or in combination with other species (e.g. *S. aureus*). Infections caused by *A. hydrophila* (associated with freshwater injury) and *V. vulnificus* (associated with seawater injury or oyster ingestion in patients with cirrhosis) have been reported.

Epidemiology

Risk factors include diabetes mellitus, people who inject drugs (PWID), obesity, immunosuppression, surgery, and traumatic wounds.

Clinical features

- Type II: most infections present in the limbs, particularly the legs. Type I: trunk and perineal infections are commoner.
- The affected area is usually red, hot, swollen, and exquisitely tender/painful, with pain disproportionate to clinical findings. There is rapid progression with skin discoloration, crepitus, bulla formation, and cutaneous gangrene. The affected area becomes anaesthetic as a result of small vessel thrombosis and destruction of superficial nerves. Systemic toxicity is common.
- In the newborn, necrotizing fasciitis may complicate omphalitis and spread to involve the abdominal wall, flanks, and chest wall.
- Fournier's gangrene is a form of necrotizing fasciitis that affects the ♂ genitals and is usually polymicrobial.
- Craniofacial necrotizing fasciitis is usually associated with trauma and caused by GAS.
- Cervical necrotizing fasciitis is usually associated with dental or pharyngeal infections, and is polymicrobial.

Diagnosis

- Surgery—the diagnosis of necrotizing fasciitis is a clinical one that is confirmed by surgical exploration and debridement. The tissues appear swollen, with dull, grey fascial appearances, a thin exudate, and easy separation of tissue planes by blunt dissection.
- Microbiology—surgical samples should be sent for urgent Gram staining and culture. Blood cultures (BCs) are positive in about 60% of cases of type II necrotizing fasciitis. Skin swabs are not as reliable as deep tissue samples.
- Histopathology—characteristic features include extensive tissue destruction, blood vessel thrombosis, and abundant bacteria spreading along fascial planes.
- Imaging—plain X-rays and CT or MRI scans may demonstrate subcutaneous and fascial oedema and gas in the tissues, but should never delay surgical exploration.

Management

- Emergency surgical exploration and debridement confirm the diagnosis and are the mainstay of therapy.
- Empirical therapy—this should be broad (e.g. piperacillin–tazobactam plus clindamycin), pending culture results. Add vancomycin if MRSA is a possible cause. Bacterial protein synthesis inhibitors, such as clindamycin, may have anti-toxin effects against toxin-producing strains of streptococci and staphylococci.
- Specific therapy for proven GAS necrotizing fasciitis is with penicillin and clindamycin.
- Adjunctive therapies—more evidence is needed to assess the effectiveness of intravenous immunoglobulin (IVIG). Data support its use in combination with clindamycin in the treatment of those with streptococcal toxic shock.

Outcome

Necrotizing fasciitis is associated with considerable mortality, even with optimal therapy—21% in type I and 14–34% in type II necrotizing fasciitis.

Pyomyositis

Pyomyositis is a purulent infection of skeletal muscle, usually with abscess formation, that arises from haematogenous spread.

Epidemiology

Most cases occur in the tropics where it affects two age groups: children (aged 2–5 years) and adults (aged 20–45 years). In temperate climes, pyomyositis usually affects adults or the elderly. ♂ are more commonly affected than ♀. Patients in temperate regions often have a predisposing condition (e.g. immunodeficient state—HIV infection, diabetes mellitus, malignancy, cirrhosis, renal insufficiency, organ transplantation, immuno-suppressive therapy), trauma, or concurrent infections (e.g. toxocariasis, varicella-zoster virus (VZV)) or are PWID.

Aetiology

S. aureus accounts for 90% of tropical cases and 75% of temperate cases. GAS accounts for 1–5% of cases. *E. coli* ST131 is an emerging cause in patients with haematological malignancy. Uncommon causes include groups B, C, and G streptococci, *Streptococcus pneumoniae*, and *Streptococcus anginosus*. Rare causes include *Enterobacterales*, *Yersinia enterocolitica*, *Neisseria gonorrhoeae*, *Haemophilus influenzae*, *A. hydrophila*, anaerobes, *Burkholderia mallei*, *Burkholderia pseudomallei*, *Aspergillus fumigatus*, *Candida* spp., *Mycobacterium tuberculosis* (MTB), and *Mycobacterium avium* complex (MAC).

Clinical features

Between 20% and 50% of cases have had recent blunt trauma or vigorous exercise of the affected area. The disease usually affects the lower extremity (thigh, calf, gluteal muscles), but any muscle group may be affected.

Multifocal infection occurs in up to 20% of cases. There are three clinical stages:

- stage 1 (invasive stage)—crampy local muscle pain, swelling, and low-grade fever. Induration of the affected muscle and leucocytosis may be present;
- stage 2 (suppurative stage)—this occurs 10–21 days after the onset of symptoms, and most patients present at this stage. Clinical features include fever, exquisite muscle tenderness, and oedema. An abscess may be clinically apparent, aspiration of which yields pus. There is marked leucocytosis;
- stage 3 (systemic stage)—the affected muscle is fluctuant. Patients may present with complications of *S. aureus* bacteraemia (e.g. septic shock, endocarditis, septic emboli, pneumonia, pericarditis, septic arthritis, brain abscess, and acute renal failure). Rhabdomyolysis may occur.

Diagnosis

- Early pyomyositis may be difficult to differentiate from a number of other conditions (e.g. thrombophlebitis, muscle haematoma, muscle rupture, pyrexia of unknown origin (PUO), osteomyelitis). Iliacus pyomyositis may mimic septic arthritis of the hip, and iliopsoas pyomyositis may mimic appendicitis.
- Imaging—MRI is the optimal imaging technique and may show diffuse muscle enhancement and IM abscesses. CT may detect muscle swelling and well-delineated abscesses. Ultrasound may be helpful, both diagnostically and therapeutically.
- Microbiology—diagnostic aspirates prior to antibiotic therapy are helpful to define the microbiology of the infection. BCs are positive in 10% of tropical cases and in 35% of temperate cases.

Management

- Antibiotics—although stage 1 disease can be treated with antibiotics alone, most patients present with stage 2/3 disease and require antibiotics and drainage. Empirical therapy should be directed against *S. aureus* and streptococci (e.g. flucloxacillin or vancomycin (if there is a risk of MRSA)). For immunocompromised patients, broader-spectrum therapy is indicated (e.g. piperacillin–tazobactam ± vancomycin). Antibiotic therapy should be tailored in the light of culture results and continued for 3–4 weeks.
- Drainage—percutaneous drainage can be useful both to secure a microbiological diagnosis and as a therapeutic measure. This may be CT-guided or ultrasound-guided. If there is deep infection or extensive muscle involvement, open surgical intervention, including fasciotomies, may be required.

Further reading

Stevens DL, Bisno AL, Chambers HF, *et al*. Practice guidelines for the diagnosis and management of skin and soft tissue infections: 2014 update by the Infectious Diseases Society of America. *Clin Infect Dis*. 2014;**59**:147–59.

Fungal skin infections

Fungi may cause primary infection of the skin or present with cutaneous manifestations of systemic disease.

Candida

(➜ See *Candida* species, pp. 510–12.)

- Localized skin infections—'erosio interdigitalis blastomycetica' (between fingers and toes), folliculitis, mastitis, intertrigo, nappy rash, paronychia, onychomycosis, balanitis.
- Generalized cutaneous candidiasis—in which lesions spread and become confluent, affecting widespread areas of the trunk, thorax, and extremities (uncommon).
- Chronic mucocutaneous candidiasis—a group of candidal infections that fail to respond to normally adequate therapy, resulting in complications such as oesophageal stenosis, alopecia, and disfigurement of the face, scalp, and hands. These failures seem to be associated with immunological abnormalities such as interleukin (IL)-17 pathway immune deficiencies. Most cases present in infancy or by the age of 20 years. There is a wide spectrum of severity. Up to half of patients subsequently develop certain endocrinopathies (e.g. hypoparathyroidism). Most patients have good life expectancy. The commonest cause of death is bacterial sepsis, rather than disseminated candidiasis. Treatment is with azoles; chronic suppressive therapy is often required. Amphotericin can be used for severe cases.

Malassezia furfur

Causes pityriasis versicolor (a superficial skin infection characterized by hypopigmented or hyperpigmented lesions, usually confined to the trunk and proximal limbs) and folliculitis, as well as IV line infections. *Malassezia* spp. have been implicated in the pathogenesis of seborrhoeic dermatitis (➜ see *Malassezia* infections, p. 519).

Aspergillus

Cutaneous infection is rare, usually occurring in burn wounds or neutropenic patients at the site of intravascular catheter (IVC) insertion. Commoner is otomycosis, caused by *Aspergillus niger*, in those with chronic otitis externa. Cleaning and topical therapy with an agent such as 3% amphotericin or clotrimazole is curative (➜ see *Aspergillus*, pp. 524–30).

Mucormycosis

Infection by fungi belonging to the order *Mucorales*. Risk factors: immuno-suppression, transplantation, diabetes mellitus, trauma. Presents with chronic ulcer or cellulitis—if unrecognized, the organism penetrates deeper into the skin, with vascular invasion, necrosis, and possible dissemination (➜ see Mucormycosis, pp. 530–2).

Eumycetoma

Chronic, slow-growing, destructive fungal infection of the hands or feet. Found worldwide in tropical regions, but rare in temperate areas (➜ see Eumycetoma, pp. 532–3).

Scedosporium apiospermum

May cause eumycetoma, skin and soft tissue infections, and abscesses (➔ see *Scedosporium apiospermum*, p. 811), previously known as *Pseudoallescheria boydii*.

Lomentospora prolificans, formerly known as Scedosporium prolificans

Extremely rare. Focal (e.g. osteoarticular) disease in the immunocompetent, disseminated infection (including skin) in the immunocompromised (e.g. those undergoing bone marrow transplant (BMT)) (➔ see *Scedosporium prolificans*, p. 536).

Fusarium species

Rare in immunocompetent people. Skin lesions start as macules and progress to necrotic papules. Systemic infection is seen in patients with acute leukaemia with prolonged neutropenia and those undergoing BMT (➔ see *Fusarium* species, pp. 536–7).

Sporothrix schenckii

Inoculated into the skin at sites of minor trauma. May cause either a fixed plaque or painless smooth or verrucous erythematous nodular papules, with secondary lesions that follow the routes of lymphatic vessels (➔ see *Sporothrix schenckii*, pp. 537–9).

Chromomycosis

Associated with minor trauma caused during outdoor work. Often starting with a small itchy pink papule, followed by crops of lesions. These may be nodular, tumourous, verrucous, plaque-like, or cicatricial. Satellite lesions may occur. Some people develop annular, papular lesions, with active edges and healing in the centre, which can become scarred or form keloid. Fibrosis of the affected limb and limb distortion, including elephantiasis, may occur in severe cases (➔ see Chromomycosis, pp. 539–40).

Dermatophytes

A group of fungi capable of invading the keratin of skin, hair, and nails. Clinical classification is by the body area involved: tinea capitis (scalp hair and the commonest in children), tinea corporis (trunk and limbs), tinea manuum and pedis (palms and soles, and the commonest overall worldwide), tinea cruris (groin), tinea barbae (beard area and neck), tinea faciale (face), tinea unguium (nail—also known as onychomycosis) (➔ see Dermatophytes, pp. 533–5).

Cutaneous manifestations of systemic fungal infection

Systemic fungal infections that present with cutaneous disease include:
- disseminated candidiasis;
- cryptococcosis (➔ see *Cryptococcus*, pp. 520–2);
- *Talaromyces* (*Penicillium*) *marneffei* (➔ see *Talaromyces* (*Penicillium*) *marneffei*, pp. 551-2);
- *Blastomyces dermatitidis* (➔ see *Blastomyces dermatitidis*, pp. 544–7);
- *Coccidioides immitis* (➔ see *Coccidioides immitis*, pp. 547–50);
- *Paracoccidioides brasiliensis* (➔ see *Paracoccidioides brasiliensis*, pp. 550-1);

- *Fusarium* spp. (➔ see *Fusarium* species, pp. 536–7);
- Lomentospora (*Scedosporium*) *prolificans* (➔ see *Scedosporium prolificans*, p. 536);
- mucormycosis (➔ see Mucormycosis, pp. 530–2).

Viral skin infections

Herpes simplex virus

Cutaneous manifestations of herpes simplex virus (HSV) infection (➔ see Herpes simplex, pp. 438–41) include:

- pharyngitis/gingivostomatitis—the commonest presentation of primary HSV-1, generally seen in children and young adults. General features: fever, malaise, difficulty chewing, cervical lymphadenopathy. Ulcers and exudative lesions are found on the posterior pharynx and sometimes on the tongue, buccal mucosa, and gums. Patients with eczema may develop severe disease (eczema herpeticum), which may disseminate, requiring systemic therapy. HSV has been associated with up to 75% of cases of erythema multiforme;
- recurrent herpes labialis—the most frequent manifestation of HSV-1 reactivation. May be asymptomatic or present with symptoms that are milder and of shorter duration than primary infection. Mild prodromal tingling is followed by the development of lesions within 48h, and they usually resolve within 5 days. Immunosuppressed patients may experience severe mucositis, with spread to skin surrounding the mouth;
- herpetic whitlow—HSV infection of the finger, which may result from auto-inoculation (existing oral or genital infection) or direct inoculation from some other environmental source. Presents with vesicles ± regional lymphadenopathy;
- *Herpes gladiatorum*—mucocutaneous infection that classically occurs on chest, ears, face, and hands in rugby players and wrestlers.

Varicella-zoster virus

(➔ See Varicella-zoster virus, pp. 441-5.)

- Chickenpox—90% of cases occur in children under 13 years of age. Incubation is 10–14 days and may be followed by a 1- to 2-day febrile prodrome before the onset of constitutional symptoms (malaise, itch, anorexia) and rash. Lesions start as maculopapules (<5mm across), progressing to vesicles which quickly pustulate and form scabs, which fall off 1–2 weeks after infection. They appear in successive crops over 2–4 days, starting on the trunk and face and then spreading centripetally. May rarely involve the mucosa of the oropharynx and vagina. Complications include secondary bacterial infection, pneumonitis, and encephalitis. Disease may be severe in pregnancy and the immunocompromised.
- Shingles (herpes zoster—localized recurrence of varicella virus)—causes a unilateral vesicular eruption in a dermatomal distribution (most commonly thoracic and lumbar), often preceded by 2–3 days of pain in the affected area. Maculopapular lesions evolve into vesicles, with new crops forming over 3–5 days. Resolution may take 2–4 weeks.

Complications include keratitis (herpes zoster ophthalmicus), Ramsay Hunt syndrome (ipsilateral facial nerve palsy, ear pain with vesicles in the auditory canal, loss of taste in anterior two-thirds of tongue), encephalitis, and paralysis (anterior horn cell involvement).

Smallpox

(➔ See Poxviruses, pp. 435–7.)

- Smallpox is caused by variola virus, an orthopoxvirus. There are two strains: variola major (mortality 20–50%) and variola minor (mortality <1%).
- The last reported case was in Somalia in 1977, and the virus was declared eradicated by the World Health Organization (WHO) in 1980. Virus stocks exist in two laboratories and there are concerns about its potential use as a bioterrorism agent (➔ see Bioterrorism, pp. 882–3).
- The incubation period is 10–12 days and is followed by a prodromal period of 1–2 days. The centrifugal rash is initially maculopapular and progresses to vesicles, pustules, and scabs over 1–2 weeks. Death may occur with fulminant disease.
- Diagnosis may be confirmed by electron microscopy (EM) or PCR (to differentiate it from other poxviruses).
- There is no specific treatment. Management is by isolation of cases to prevent transmission.

Mpox (previously known as monkeypox)

(➔ See Poxviruses, pp. 435–7.)

- Mpox is an orthopoxvirus.
- It causes a vesicular illness in monkeys and rodents in West and Central Africa. Infection may sporadically be transmitted to humans. A large outbreak in humans in the USA was traced to importation and sale of exotic pets. The disease is similar to, but less severe than, smallpox.
- Prior to 2022, all UK cases either had been imported from countries with endemic infection or had proven links with imported cases. In May 2022, an international outbreak of mpox—not associated with recent travel—was recognized first in the UK and then in other parts of Europe and the USA. It was declared an outbreak of international concern by the WHO in July. Most cases were identified in men who have sex with men—but there were also cases among household contacts. Among the former lesions were mostly anogenital and perioral. Severe cases were unusual and people were admitted to hospital generally for isolation or pain control. Pre-exposure prophylaxis with an orthopoxvirus vaccine (e.g. live non-replicating MVA vaccine) appears effective and may also be used for PEP—ideally within 4 days. Vaccinia immune globulin may be considered as PEP in immunocompromised patients. Severe clinical cases may benefit from the antiviral tecovirimat.
- Diagnosis is by EM or PCR (to differentiate it from other poxviruses).
- Clinical features—incubation is usually 5–13 days (range 4–21 days), averaging 8.5 days in the 2022 outbreak. Systemic symptoms (fever, headache, sore throat, myalgia) last 1–5 days and typically precede rash. Rash lesions crust over and dry up 7–14 days after the first appearance. Lesions are usually painful at first, then itchy.

Other features: conjunctivitis, keratitis, encephalitis, bowel oedema, pneumonia, myocarditis, epiglottitis, severe lymphadenopathy.
• Mortality varies with clade—reported at 10% in Central Africa (clade 1) and at <0.1% in the immunocompetent in West Africa (clade 2). The 2022 outbreak was of a mild phenotype, with an apparent mortality of <0.2% (USA Centers for Disease Control and Prevention data).

Orf

(➔ See Poxviruses, pp. 435–7.)
• Orf is caused by a parapoxvirus and primarily affects sheep, goats, and cattle. Humans are infected following direct exposure to infected animals.
• Lesions develop at sites of contact (e.g. hands and arms). They are initially maculopapular but then progress to target lesions, wet nodules, dry nodules, and finally a regenerative papilloma. Resolution can take 4–6 weeks.
• Diagnosis is clinical but can be confirmed by EM.
• Management is symptomatic, as there is no specific treatment.

Molluscum contagiosum

(➔ See Molluscum contagiosum, p. 437.)
• Molluscum contagiosum is caused by a poxvirus.
• It is spread by close human contact and may cause severe, generalized disease in HIV-infected patients.
• The lesions are small, firm, umbilicated papules, which occur on exposed epithelial surfaces or the genitalia. Lesions may resolve spontaneously or persist for months or years.
• Diagnosis is clinical but can be confirmed by EM.
• Management: treatment is not usually recommended, as infection is benign and usually self-limiting. Treatment may be recommended for those with unsightly lesions or the immunosuppressed. Options include topical treatment, curettage, cryotherapy, and laser treatment. For patients with HIV, starting antiretroviral therapy may be effective.

Miscellaneous skin infections

Cutaneous anthrax

• Cutaneous anthrax is caused by *Bacillus anthracis* (➔ see *Bacillus anthracis*) Advisory Committee on Dangerous Pathogens (ACDP, pp. 291-3). It usually affects humans who are in direct contact with infected animals (e.g. cattle and sheep) or animal products.
• The lesion begins with a pruritic papule that enlarges to form an ulcer surrounded by vesicles and then develops into an eschar surrounded by oedema. There may be regional lymphangitis, lymphadenopathy, and systemic symptoms.
• Diagnosis is confirmed by microscopy and culture of the vesicle fluid. If the patient has received antibiotics or cultures are negative, a punch biopsy may be taken for immunohistochemistry or PCR.
• Antimicrobial therapy does not accelerate healing of the skin lesion but may reduce oedema and systemic symptoms. Empirical therapy

for cases without systemic involvement is with PO ciprofloxacin or PO doxycycline for 7–10 days; the duration of treatment should be increased to 60 days if inhalational anthrax is a possibility or for bioterrorism-associated cases. If there is systemic involvement, empirical therapy would be IV ciprofloxacin plus IV clindamycin or linezolid—anti-toxin treatment may also be indicated.

Erysipeloid

- Erysipeloid is caused by *E. rhusiopathiae* (➜ see *Erysipelothrix rhusiopathiae*, pp. 299). It usually affects people who handle fish, marine mammals, poultry, or swine.
- After exposure, a red maculopapular lesion develops, usually on the fingers or hands. Erythema spreads centrifugally, with central clearing. A blue ring with a peripheral red halo may appear. Regional lymphangitis/lymphadenopathy occurs in approximately one-third of cases. A severe, generalized cutaneous infection may also occur.
- Diagnosis is confirmed by culture of a lesion aspirate and/or biopsy specimen; BCs are rarely positive.
- Untreated erysipeloid resolves during a period of 3–4 weeks, but treatment probably hastens healing and perhaps reduces systemic complications. Treatment is with PO penicillin or amoxicillin for 7–10 days. *E. rhusiopathiae* is intrinsically resistant to vancomycin.

Cat-scratch disease

- Cat-scratch disease is mainly caused by *Bartonella henselae* (➜ see *Bartonella* species, pp. 384–6).
- A papule or pustule develops 3–10 days after a scratch or bite. Regional adenopathy occurs ~3 weeks after inoculation, and ~10% of nodes suppurate. Extranodal disease (e.g. CNS, liver, spleen, bone, and lung) occurs in 2% of cases.
- Diagnosis is by PCR or histology (Warthin–Starry silver staining). Serology is no longer available in the UK.
- Treatment of uncomplicated infection is with PO azithromycin for 5 days. Clinical response is rarely dramatic, but lymphadenopathy usually resolves by 6 months.

Bacillary angiomatosis

Bacillary angiomatosis may be caused by *B. henselae* or *Bartonella quintana*. It usually occurs in immunosuppressed patients, especially those with un-controlled HIV (➜ see *Bartonella* species in chapter 7, pp. 384–6).

Bone and joint infections

Septic arthritis

Joint inflammation caused by an infectious agent, most often bacteria. It can be rapidly destructive and requires prompt diagnosis and treatment to prevent mortality and morbidity.

Aetiology
- *Staphylococcus aureus*, including meticillin-resistant *S. aureus* (MRSA).
- Streptococci (groups A, B, C, and G, *Streptococcus pneumoniae*).
- *Neisseria gonorrhoeae*.
- Gram-negative bacilli, including *Escherichia coli*, *Pseudomonas aeruginosa*.
- *Neisseria meningitidis*.
- *Salmonella* spp.
- *Kingella kingae* (in children aged <5 years).
- Coagulase-negative staphylococci.
- Polymicrobial infections.

Epidemiology
The reported incidence of septic arthritis varies from 3 to 10 cases per 100 000 population, but is 10 times commoner in people with risk factors (immunocompromise, rheumatoid arthritis, diabetes mellitus, people who inject drugs (PWID), and alcoholism). There are two peaks in incidence: young children and older adults.

Pathogenesis
In over 70% of cases, septic arthritis occurs after haematogenous seeding of pathogenic microorganisms. Other cases occur after direct inoculation (injection, surgery, or trauma) and contiguous spread from adjacent infection.

Clinical features
- Monoarticular in 90%, usually accompanied by fever (60–80%).
- Symptoms include pain, swelling, redness, and reduced mobility in the joint.
- Most commonly affects the knee, and also the hip, shoulder, and elbow.
- Polyarticular infections occur in 10–20% of patients, especially those with gonococcal disease, rheumatoid arthritis, and viral causes.

Rarer infectious causes
- *Pasteurella multocida* (cat), *Capnocytophaga canimorsus* (dog), *Streptobacillus moniliformis* (rat), and *Eikenella corrodens* (human) are associated with bites.
- *Brucella* spp. are linked with unpasteurized milk and are commoner in tropical regions.
- *Burkholderia pseudomallei* is endemic in South East Asia and Northern Australia.
- *Clostridium* spp. are related to the GI tract.
- *Borrelia burgdorferi*, *Brucella* spp., *Tropheryma whipplei*, and *Nocardia asteroides* can cause chronic infections.
- Mycobacteria (e.g. *Mycobacterium tuberculosis* (MTB)—commonest), and also non-tuberculous mycobacteria (NTM).

- Fungal arthritis is associated with immunosuppression. Infections with *Candida* spp. are the most frequently seen, but dimorphic fungi, as well as *Sporothrix schenkii*, are uncommon causes.
- Viruses (e.g. parvovirus B19, hepatitis B, mumps, rubella, human T-cell lymphotropic virus 1 (HTLV-1), HIV, lymphocytic choriomeningitis virus, chikungunya virus, Ross River virus).
- Parasites (e.g. filarial infections, schistosomiasis).

Differential diagnosis

- Inflammatory arthritides.
- Gout and crystal-induced arthritis.
- Post-infectious arthritis.
- Haemarthrosis.

Diagnosis

- Laboratory investigations—frequently show a raised WCC and inflammatory markers. Blood cultures (BCs) should be sent and are positive in 75% of cases. Aspiration reveals a purulent synovial fluid, with an elevated WCC (50 000–100 000 cels/mm^3), predominantly neutrophils. Gram staining is positive in 29–50% of cases, and culture is positive in 80–90% of cases. False-positive Gram stains may occur with artefacts from stain, mucin, and cellular debris. Direct inoculation of the synovial fluid into BC bottles may improve recovery of pathogens. Samples should also be sent for microscopy for crystals. 16S PCR may be considered if no causative organism is found and a fastidious organism is suspected.
- Imaging—X-rays of the affected joint may be normal at presentation. Findings may include effusion, soft tissue swelling, fat pad oedema, loss of joint space, and periarticular osteoporosis. CT and MRI are highly sensitive at detecting early septic arthritis. CT is better for imaging bone lesions. MRI can detect cartilaginous damage but may not distinguish septic arthritis from inflammatory arthropathies.

Management

- **Drainage of the joint**—ideally to dryness, should be performed urgently. This can be by either closed aspiration or arthroscopic washout. Open drainage may be required either when repeated drainage has failed to control the infection or for infection of the hip.
- **Antimicrobial therapy**—should be started empirically according to local guidelines and should cover *S. aureus*. Additional cover for Gram-negatives and/or MRSA needs to be considered. Definitive therapy should be tailored to the susceptibility of the organism isolated. Treatment is usually for 2–4 weeks and can be PO when there is clinical improvement.
- Consider the development of adjacent osteomyelitis in those cases that fail to improve as expected or relapse on treatment completion.
- **Adjunctive therapy**—short-course systemic corticosteroid treatment has been shown to be of benefit in children with haematogenous bacterial arthritis.

Septic bursitis

Inflammation of the synovial bursa due to infection.

Pathogenesis

Occurs as a result of bacterial inoculation, which may be direct (e.g. trauma, corticosteroid injection), contiguous from nearby soft tissues (e.g. cellulitis), or haematogenous (e.g. endocarditis).

Aetiology

S. aureus is the commonest cause (>80%), followed by streptococci (usually β-haemolytic streptococci). Other organisms include coagulase-negative staphylococci (CoNS), enterococci, *E. coli*, *P. aeruginosa*, and anaerobes. Polymicrobial infections occur up to a third of cases. Subacute/chronic bursitis may occur with *Brucella abortus*, MTB, NTM, fungi, and algae.

Clinical features

Patients typically present with fever, pain, erythema, and warmth around the affected bursa. The most commonly affected sites are the olecranon and the pre-patellar and infra-patellar bursae. The WCC, ESR, and CRP are usually raised. Bacteraemia is rare in the absence of deep bursitis.

Diagnosis

- Aspiration of the affected bursa is indicated, and the fluid should be examined microscopically for cells, organisms, and crystals, and cultured. A WCC of >2000 cells/mm^3 was reported to have 94% sensitivity and 79% specificity for the diagnosis of septic bursitis. Gram staining is reported to be 15–100% sensitive in septic bursitis.
- Imaging is not usually required, unless there is a history of trauma or concern about foreign body penetration. If septic bursitis of a deep bursa (e.g. ischiogluteal bursa) is suspected, then CT or MRI may be indicated.
- Differential diagnosis includes: cellulitis, crystal-induced bursitis, acute monoarthritis, haemobursa, non-septic bursitis, and patellar osteomyelitis.

Management

- **Aspiration**—is useful both diagnostically and therapeutically.
- **Antibiotics**—should be started empirically to cover *S. aureus* (e.g. flucloxacillin or vancomycin, if there is a risk of MRSA). In immunosuppressed patients, broad-spectrum therapy (e.g. piperacillin–tazobactam ± vancomycin) may be indicated. Antibiotic therapy should be tailored in the light of culture results. The duration of therapy is determined by the clinical response but is typically 2–3 weeks.

Reactive arthritis

Reactive arthritis arises during or soon after an infection elsewhere. The joint itself is sterile. A triad of reactive arthritis, urethritis, and conjunctivitis is described in a subset of patients (previously known as Reiter's syndrome).

- Aetiology—most commonly follows GI (*Shigella* spp., *Salmonella* spp., *Campylobacter*, *Yersinia* spp.) or genitourinary (GU) (*Chlamydia trachomatis*) infection.
- Also described following *E. coli*, *Clostridioides difficile*, or *Chlamydophila pneumoniae*.

Epidemiology

Reactive arthritis is relatively uncommon, with an estimated annual incidence of 0.5–27 per 100 000 adults. It is mostly seen in ♂ aged 20–40 years. Most cases occur sporadically, but clusters may follow point source infection outbreaks.

Pathogenesis

- The pathogenesis of the condition is not fully understood; it probably represents an abnormal host response to infectious agents.
- It is associated with the presence of HLA-B27, which is found in >90% of affected patients.

Clinical features

- Patients may recall previous GI or GU symptoms, and typically present 1–4 weeks after the precipitating infection.
- **Musculoskeletal symptoms**—most often monoarthritis or asymmetric oligoarthritis, affecting the lower limbs. Axial involvement is commoner in HLA-B27-positive patients. Enthesitis (inflammation of ligaments) is common and mostly seen in the Achilles tendon and plantar fascia. Dactylitis (swelling of entire digits) is uncommon.
- **Extra-articular symptoms**:
  - eyes: anterior uveitis, episcleritis, conjunctivitis;
  - GU: urethritis, balanitis, symptoms linked to the original infection;
  - skin: mouth ulcers, keratoderma blennorrhagica, erythema nodosum, nail changes;
  - other: fever, malaise, headache, weight loss. Pericarditis is rare.

Diagnosis

- There is no diagnostic test for reactive arthritis, but investigations are undertaken to look for the causative infection and exclude other pathology.
- Inflammatory markers—ESR and CRP may be elevated.
- Faecal samples are rarely positive for bacterial pathogens, as diarrhoea has usually resolved at the time of clinical presentation.
- Urine and genital swabs may be positive for *Chlamydia* by nucleic acid amplification tests (NAATs), even in the absence of symptoms.
- Serological testing for GI pathogens is not diagnostically helpful but may be epidemiologically useful.
- Patients may be HLA-B27-positive.
- Imaging—X-rays may show evidence of arthritis and enthesitis.
- Joint fluid aspiration shows a raised WCC (2000–64 000 white cells/mm³), with a neutrophil predominance. Histology shows non-specific changes.

Management

- Treatment should aim to treat the triggering infection, manage symptoms, and minimize disability.
- **Antibiotics**—prompt treatment of *C. trachomatis* can reduce the severity of arthritis. Conversely, antibiotics are not indicated in GI disease as they do not alter the disease course. A systematic review and meta-analysis of antibiotics versus placebo for treatment of reactive arthritis found no difference in remission of arthritis.
- **Anti-inflammatory drugs**—use NSAIDs (e.g. naproxen, diclofenac, or indometacin) for symptomatic relief of acute arthritis.
- **Glucocorticoids**—intra-articular or systemic glucocorticoids may be used in patients who do not respond adequately to a prolonged course of NSAIDs (2–4 weeks).
- **Disease-modifying drugs**—can be considered in refractory disease. The best evidence is for sulfasalazine, but methotrexate and azathioprine have been used. Anti-tumour necrosis factor (TNF) drugs (etanercept or infliximab) may also be used.

Prognosis

- The clinical course of reactive arthritis is highly variable, and symptoms can fluctuate.
- In 50% of patients, symptoms will resolve in 6 months.
- Enteroarthritis appears to have a better prognosis than *Chlamydia*-related arthritis. HLA-B27-positive patients are more likely to require ongoing treatment.
- Around 20% can develop chronic arthritis and may require long-term treatment.

Osteomyelitis

An inflammatory process of bone and bone marrow caused by bacterial infection. It results in progressive bone destruction.

Pathogenesis

Infection can occur from either haematogenous seeding (endogenous) or contiguous spread from adjacent infected tissues, or by inoculation from trauma or surgery (exogenous). Bacteria infect the periosteum and spread within the bone; growth and inflammatory reaction result in increased pressure. The periosteum is lifted from the bone, disrupting the blood supply and resulting in necrosis. Pieces of dead bone which become separated are known as sequestra.[1] The new bone which forms is known as the involucrum.

Classification

Two classification systems exist:[2]
- **the Cierny–Mader system**—is a functional classification and is useful in guiding therapy. There are four anatomical stages of osteomyelitis: stage 1 (medullary), 2 (superficial), 3 (localized), and 4 (diffuse). There are three physiological classes: A (normal host), B (host

with local or systemic compromise—B1 and Bs, respectively), and C
(risk of harm from treatment is worse than from disease);
- **the Lee and Waldvogel system**—is based on the duration (acute
  or chronic), mechanism (contiguous or haematogenous), and presence
  of vascular insufficiency. It is less helpful in terms of treatment.

Aetiology

- Haematogenous osteomyelitis is usually monomicrobial, whereas
  contiguous osteomyelitis may be monomicrobial or polymicrobial.
- *S. aureus* is the commonest pathogen, followed by CoNS and other
  Gram-positives. Polymicrobials, Gram-negatives (*Enterobacterales*
  and *Pseudomonas*), and anaerobes are causing an increasing share of
  infection.
- Rare causes (<5%) include MTB, other mycobacteria, dimorphic fungi,
  Candida spp., *Aspergillus* spp., *Mycoplasma* spp., *T. whipplei*, *Brucella* spp.,
  Salmonella spp., and *Actinomyces* spp.

Clinical features

- Acute osteomyelitis usually presents with pain of the affected site.
  Systemic symptoms are common. Local findings (swelling, tenderness,
  warmth, and erythema) may be present in long bone infection but are
  often absent in infection affecting the vertebrae, hip, and pelvis.
- Chronic osteomyelitis also presents with pain; deformity and altered
  function are common. A sinus tract or a deep, poorly healing ulcer
  (especially if bone is felt on probing) may indicate osteomyelitis.

Diagnosis

A high index of suspicion is needed. Diagnosis is by a combination of radiological, microbiological, and histopathological investigations.
- Blood tests—the blood WCC may be normal or raised; inflammatory
  markers (ESR and CRP) are often elevated. BCs are more likely to be
  positive in axial disease and haematogenous osteomyelitis.
- Radiology—although insensitive, a plain radiograph is readily available
  and inexpensive, and may show changes after 10–14 days. Bone scans
  and CT have a low specificity. MRI is the investigation of choice.
- Biopsy—an open or percutaneous bone biopsy should be taken,
  preferably prior to commencing antibiotic therapy. Cessation of
  antibiotics 48–72h prior to biopsy may increase the microbiological
  yield. Samples should be sent for both microbiology and histology. Sinus
  tract swabs are of dubious value, as they may represent colonizing flora,
  rather than the true pathogen.

Management

- **General principles**—owing to the lack of good clinical trial data,
  most recommendations on management come from animal models,
  retrospective cohort studies, and expert opinion. The goal of therapy is
  to eradicate infection and restore/preserve function.
- **Surgery**—the principles of surgical therapy are debridement of
  infected tissue, removal of metalware, management of dead space
  (using a flap), wound closure, and stabilization of infected fractures.

- **Antimicrobial therapy**—choice of therapy depends on the organism isolated and its drug susceptibility results. Rifampicin is often added to β-lactams in staphylococcal infections involving prosthetic material for its biofilm activity. The non-inferiority of oral antibiotics (as demonstrated in the OVIVA trial)[3] has enabled a shift from long courses of intravenous antibiotics towards earlier use of oral antibiotics. Duration is guided by clinical progress but is usually at least 6 weeks.
- **Adjunctive therapy**—hyperbaric oxygen is effective in animal studies, but there are inadequate data to support its use in humans. Negative-pressure wound therapy (vacuum-assisted closure) may accelerate wound healing in complex wounds and in diabetic patients.

Complications

- Haematogenous spread, sepsis.
- Pathological fractures.
- Tumours can develop in patients with long-standing (4–5 years) osteomyelitis; the commonest is squamous cell carcinoma.

References

1 Lew DP, Waldvogel FA. Osteomyelitis. *Lancet*. 2004;**364**:369–79.
2 Mader JT, Shirtliff M, Calhoun JH. Staging and staging application in osteomyelitis. *Clin Infect Dis*. 1997;**25**:1303–9.
3 Li HK, Rombach I, Zambellas R, *et al*. (2019). Oral versus intravenous antibiotics for bone and joint infection. *N Engl J Med*. **31**;**380**:425–36.

Prosthetic joint infections

Epidemiology

- The prevalence of prosthetic joint infections (PJIs) is around 2–4% in 10 years following surgery, highest in the first 2 years, and then reducing.
- Associated with high rates of morbidity, reduced quality of life, and decreased function for the patient, as well as expense to the healthcare system.
- Mortality within 5 years after revision surgery is 26%.
- The biggest risk factor for PJIs is obesity. Other factors include cardiovascular disease, immunocompromise, diabetes mellitus, and previous infection of the joint.
- The risk of relapse depends on the type of surgical procedure, comorbidities, and the organism causing PJI. It can be up to 20%.

Pathogenesis

- The infecting dose of *S. aureus* required to cause an infection is 100 000 times reduced in the presence of a foreign body, due to deactivation of granulocytes.
- Biofilm formation begins within hours and takes 4 weeks to mature. Microorganisms adhere to the prosthesis and proliferate to form a micro-colony. They produce an extracellular polysaccharide matrix, which protects the organism from the action of antimicrobials.

Classification

- **Early-onset PJI** (<3 months after surgery)—result from bacteria acquired during implantation or as a result of post-operative wound infection. Tend to be virulent organisms such as S. aureus, Gram-negative bacilli, anaerobes, and polymicrobial infections.
- **Delayed-onset PJI** (3–12 months after surgery)—also usually acquired during implantation. Often less virulent pathogens such as CoNS, Cutibacterium (formerly known as Propionibacterium), and Enterococci spp.
- **Late-onset PJI** (>12 months after surgery)—usually secondary to haematogenous spread (e.g. sexually transmitted infection (STI), urinary tract infection (UTI), vascular catheter). Commonly S. aureus, β-haemolytic streptococci, and Gram-negative bacilli.
- Rarer causes include corynebacteria, fungi, and mycobacteria.

Clinical features

- **Early-onset PJI**—acute-onset fever, joint pain, swelling and erythema, and wound discharge. Often associated with haematoma formation or superficial necrosis of the skin.
- **Delayed-onset PJI**—presents subacutely with persistent joint pain, with or without implant loosening. Fever occurs in <50%. Sinus tract formation and intermittent discharge may be seen.
- **Late-onset PJI**—acute onset of symptoms in a previously well-functioning joint.

Differential diagnosis

- Aseptic loosening, dislocation, gout, haemarthrosis, and osteolysis.

Diagnosis

There is no single test able to confirm or refute a suspicion of PJI; a combination of clinical features, microbiology, histology, and imaging is required.

- Blood tests—raised ESR and CRP levels are suggestive but can be elevated in inflammatory disease or following surgery. Procalcitonin has low sensitivity for the diagnosis of PJI. Interleukin-6 levels may be helpful. The WCC is often normal.
- BCs—recommended in patients with fever to detect possible haematogenous spread.
- X-rays—should be performed, although will be normal in 50%. Soft tissue swelling, peri-prosthetic lucency, and component loosening are suggestive but cannot differentiate from aseptic disease.
- Imaging—CT (can be limited by artefact from metal) and MRI (some prostheses are not compatible) can be useful, although neither is sensitive enough to be used as a rule-out test. Radioisotope scans are useful in late infection, but in the first 2–5 years after infection, they may give false positives due to normal bone remodelling. None of the above are recommended routinely.
- Arthrocentesis—aspiration of the joint, ideally after antibiotics have been held for 2 weeks, may be diagnostic. Leucocyte count of >1500 and/or polymorphs of >65% make PJI likely. Gram staining is often negative and should not be used to rule out infection. Culture has the

highest specificity but low sensitivity, and needs to be interpreted in combination with other factors.

- Operative samples (arthroscopic or open surgical)—ideally at least five tissue samples (plus fluid) should be taken, using clean instruments. They should be sent for microbiology and histology. Phenotypically indistinguishable organisms cultured from ≥2 samples clearly define infection. 16S PCR can be useful if the culture is negative and there is a clinical suspicion of infection.
- Histological examination showing ≥5 neutrophils in ≥5 high-power fields is the most commonly used criterion, but lower thresholds also have a good specificity at predicting infection.
- Explant sonication—disrupting the biofilm improves the microbiological yield, particularly in patients receiving antibiotics.

Management

Management of PJIs usually involves both surgery and antibiotic therapy. The choice of type of surgery depends on the time frame of the infection, the organism, and the patient's circumstances.

- **Two-stage revision**—recommended in chronic infections where there is an established biofilm or in cases with difficult-to-treat pathogens. Historically the gold standard (success of up to 90%), although recent evidence suggests similar reinfection rates with 1- and 2-stage procedures, and 2-stage procedures can lead to higher morbidity and longer hospital stays. The first stage involves complete resection of the prosthesis, debridement of soft tissue, and insertion of a joint spacer and cement (both often antibiotic-impregnated). Antibiotics are administered for 6 weeks in the interval period before the second stage, when a new prosthesis is implanted.
- **One-stage revision**—used in patients with easily treatable organisms and good bone stock and surrounding soft tissue. Within the same operation, there is prosthesis resection, debridement of soft tissue and bone, and reimplantation of a new prosthesis. Oral antibiotics with good bioavailability, in combination with agents active against biofilm (e.g. rifampicin, daptomycin), are as effective as intravenous treatment. Post-operative duration varies across centres, with many electing to give 3 months for hip PJI and up to 6 months for knee PJI.
- **Debridement and implant retention (DAIR)**—used in early-onset PJI (<30 days' implantation) or in acute-onset haematogenous infection (<3 weeks' symptoms) if the prosthesis is well fixed and there is no sinus tract. Also considered in patients for whom other surgical options are too high-risk. Involves extensive debridement, washout, exchange of polyethylene liner and mobile parts, and retention of the prosthesis. Targeted antibiotic therapy, including anti-biofilm agents, should be given for 3–6 months; differences of opinion on long-term suppressive therapy remain.
- **Permanent resection arthroplasty**—used in patients who are not suitable for any of the previous surgical options. Patients with hip PJI undergo resection arthroplasty (Girdlestone procedure), and those with knee PJI undergo resection arthroplasty and arthrodesis.
- **Long-term suppressive antibiotic therapy**—either alone or following operation (e.g. prosthesis removal impossible, prosthesis not

loose, pathogen relatively avirulent, pathogen highly sensitive to oral antibiotic, patient able to tolerate long-term oral antibiotics).
- **Cure rates**—variable, depending on the host, organism, operative strategy, and antibiotic agent used (e.g. better for Gram-negative infections if ciprofloxacin can be used; DAIR outcomes can be poor with *S. aureus*). Case series range from 30% to 30% infection-free at 5 years.

Prevention

PJIs may be prevented by perioperative antimicrobial prophylaxis, meticulous surgical technique, filtered laminar airflow systems in operating theatres (probably), and early recognition and prompt treatment of wound infections.

Further reading

Osmon DR, Berberi EF, Berendt AR, et al.; Infectious Diseases Society of America. Diagnosis and management of prosthetic joint infection: clinical practice guidelines by the Infectious Diseases Society of America. *Clin Infect Dis*. 2013;**56**:1–25.

Signore A, Sconfienza LM, Borens O, et al. Consensus document for the diagnosis of prosthetic joint infections: a joint paper by the EANM, EBJIS, and ESR (with ESCMID endorsement). *Eur J Nucl Med Mol Imaging*. 2019;**46**:971–88.

Diabetic foot infections

Infected diabetic ulcers are the commonest manifestation. However, the spectrum of disease includes paronychia, cellulitis, myositis, abscesses, tendonitis, septic arthritis, osteomyelitis, and necrotizing fasciitis.

Epidemiology

Foot infections in diabetic patients are common, debilitating, and difficult to manage. All patients with diabetes should have foot checks at least annually to detect early problems. Risk factors for developing disease include neuropathy (sensory, motor, or autonomic), vascular insufficiency, and deformity (e.g. Charcot joint), and are related to poor diabetic control and hyperglycaemia. Other factors include patient disability (vision, mobility), maladaptive behaviours (footwear or foot care), and health system failure (education and management).

Aetiology

A number of organisms may be associated with various syndromes (see Table 22.1).

Clinical features

Diabetic foot infection is defined by the presence of at least two of the following: local swelling or induration, erythema, local tenderness or pain, local warmth, or purulent discharge. Severity is classified as:
- **mild**: skin and subcutaneous tissues, <2cm erythema;
- **moderate**: erythema >2cm or involving deeper structures (abscess, osteomyelitis, septic arthritis, fasciitis);
- **severe**: local infection plus signs of systemic inflammatory response.

Classification systems such as SINBAD or University of Texas are recommended.

Assessment

- **Examination**—should include peripheral pulses and sensation using a monofilament. Doppler ultrasound is used to determine ankle–brachial pressure indices (ABPIs).
- **Imaging**—X-ray can detect osteomyelitis. MRI is the imaging modality of choice in assessing the extent of infection and bony involvement. It is both more sensitive and specific.
- **Microbiology**—deep samples (bone/tissue) ideally before antibiotics and following debridement are most useful. Superficial swabs should be avoided, as they are likely to show colonizing flora only.

Management

(See National Institute for Health and Care Excellence and Infectious Diseases Society of America guidelines.)[1,2]

- Patients with systemic signs of sepsis, limb ischaemia, or deep-seated infection will need to be managed in hospital.
- **Surgery**—necrotizing infection, gas gangrene, and critical limb ischaemia are emergencies, and urgent surgical review is required. Surgical input is also required for debridement, amputation, and revascularization to promote healing.
- **Antibiotics**—do not give antibiotics for uninfected ulcers. Initial empirical therapy should be based on the severity of infection, available microbiological data, and previous antibiotic use. Gram-positive cover may be all that is required in mild infection, but broader therapy, including Gram-negative, pseudomonal, and MRSA cover, should be considered in severe infection. Duration is guided by the clinical picture, but in skin and soft tissue infections, a duration of 2 weeks is likely

Table 22.1 Aetiology of diabetic foot infections

Foot infection syndrome	Pathogens
Cellulitis	β-haemolytic streptococci (groups A, B, C, and G), *Staphylococcus aureus*
Infected ulcer, antibiotic-naïve	Often monomicrobial: *S. aureus* or β-haemolytic streptococci (groups A, B, C, and G)
Infected ulcer, chronic, previous antibiotic therapy	Usually polymicrobial: as above plus *Enterobacterales*, anaerobes
Macerated ulcer	*Pseudomonas aeruginosa* ± other organisms as above
Long-standing, non-healing wound, prolonged antibiotic therapy	Usually polymicrobial with antibiotic-resistant organisms: aerobic Gram-positive cocci (*S. aureus*, CoNS, enterococci), diphtheroids, *Enterobacterales*, *Pseudomonas* spp., non-fermentative GNRs, fungi
'Fetid foot': extensive necrosis or gangrene	Mixed aerobic Gram-positive cocci (*S. aureus*, CoNS, enterococci), *Enterobacterales*, non-fermentative GNRs, obligate anaerobes

CoNS, coagulase-negative staphylococci; GNR, Gram-negative rod.

to be sufficient. Longer treatment is required if there is evidence of
osteomyelitis.
- **Wound care**—combination of debridement of necrotic tissue,
offloading of pressure from the wound, and dressing selection.
Multiple types of dressings are available; the aim is to provide a moist
environment for granulation and to absorb exudate. Promoting good
diabetic control is important. Vacuum-assisted wound closure and larval
therapy can be beneficial. Use of granulocyte colony-stimulating factor
(G-CSF) and hyperbaric oxygen is not recommended.

References

1 National Institute for Health and Care Excellence (2015, updated 2019). *Diabetic foot prob-lems: prevention and management*. NICE guideline [NG19]. Available at: ℛ https://www.nice.org.uk/guidance/ng19/chapter/Recommendations#diabetic-foot-infection

2 Lipsky BA, Berendt AR, Cornia PB, *et al.*; Infectious Diseases Society of America. 2012 Infectious Diseases Society of America clinical practice guideline for the diagnosis and treatment of diabetic foot infections. *Clin Infect Dis*. 2012;**54**:132–73.

Pregnancy and childhood

Congenital infections

Congenital infections may be acquired *in utero* via the placenta or during delivery via exposure to mucous membranes, blood, and birth products.

Background

- The congenital infections included in this chapter have been selected because, although they cause only mild or asymptomatic infection in the mother, they can have significant adverse effects on the neonate. A high clinical suspicion is needed at all times.
- The previously used acronym TORCH (*Toxoplasma*, other, rubella, cytomegalovirus (CMV), herpes simplex virus (HSV)) overlooks other common causes of congenital complications such as syphilis, varicella-zoster virus (VZV), HIV, hepatitis B, and parvovirus B19.
- Some infections are screened for routinely (the advice on this differs from country to country), and some will only be tested for in the presence of specific risk factors or clinical presentations.
- Certain interventions may prevent or reduce neonatal acquisition, or treat infections in exposed neonates.
- Long-term consequences include growth retardation, microcephaly, congenital defects, and progressive disease in childhood.

General management principles

- Pregnancies complicated by congenital infection should be referred to regional fetomaternal medicine centres.
- Infants in whom congenital infection is suspected and those born preterm, where infection may have played a role, need follow-up with paediatric teams (e.g. neurology).
- Congenital infection should be suspected in the following circumstances:
  - maternal symptoms consistent with a target infection;
  - abnormalities on routine fetal scans (including, but not limited to, fetal hydrops, fetal brain lesions, unexplained severe intrauterine growth restriction (IUGR), and *in utero* demise);
  - symptoms including unusual exanthemata, organomegaly, or thrombocytopenia in the neonate.
- Investigation comprises a combination of maternal serology or other blood tests, fetal investigations (USS or invasive sampling), and testing of the neonate.
- Amniocentesis is the method of choice for fetal sampling in possible congenital infection when invasive investigations are warranted.

Infection prevention advice

Strategies aimed at preventing congenital/perinatal infection should start well before conception. Population-wide education and public health measures (e.g. vaccination) are vital. As part of routine antenatal care, disease-specific education should be given to include advice about:

- **measles, rubella, parvovirus, HSV, VZV**—pregnant women should be advised to make urgent contact with health services if they develop a rash or have contact with anyone with a rash;
- **Listeria**—risk can be reduced by avoiding soft cheese, pate, and unpasteurized milk. Caution with reheated ready meals;

- ***Salmonella***—avoid raw or partly cooked food, in particular eggs (and food that may contain them, e.g. mayonnaise) and meat;
- ***Toxoplasma***—promote good hand hygiene and ensure careful washing of food. Avoid contact with cat faeces in litter trays. Suggest use of gloves when gardening.

Routine screening (UK)

Screening for the following infections is offered to, and strongly recommended in, all pregnant women in the UK:
- HIV—starting combination antiretroviral therapy (cART) will greatly reduce the risk of mother-to-child transmission;
- hepatitis B—postnatal interventions, including active and passive immunization, can prevent neonatal infection;
- syphilis—early treatment is beneficial for both mother and baby.

Screening is NOT currently recommended in the UK for the following infections: hepatitis C, CMV, toxoplasmosis, rubella (removed in 2019), group B *Streptococcus* (GBS), asymptomatic bacterial vaginosis, and *Chlamydia trachomatis*.

Cytomegalovirus

(➔ See also Cytomegalovirus, pp. 448–50.)
- **Maternal infection**—primary infection is asymptomatic in 90% of cases but may present with an infectious mononucleosis-like syndrome. Occurs in 1–2% of seronegative women during pregnancy. Viral reactivation can occur in 10% of seropositive mothers; however, the risk of congenital infection is much lower in secondary cases.
- **Transmission**—the rate of transmission rises with increased gestational age, from 30% in the first trimester to 47% in the third trimester. However, infection in early pregnancy (<20 weeks) is associated with a higher risk of severe sequelae.
- **Fetal infection**—infection of the neonate may occur *in utero* or perinatally. Only 15% of infected infants will be symptomatic at birth, but 50% of these will have long-term sequelae such as neurological impairment. The other 85% of infected infants, who are asymptomatic at birth, may not be diagnosed. However, 10% of these will go on to develop long-term disability (e.g. hearing impairment).
- **Investigations**—undertaken in symptomatic mothers or if abnormalities are seen on fetal scanning (to include, but not limited to: microcephaly, periventricular calcifications, and IUGR).
- **Diagnosis**—confirmed by serology showing IgG in a previously seronegative mother, or IgM combined with low IgG avidity. IgM alone is not diagnostic (not specific and persists for many months).
- **Amniocentesis**—PCR for CMV DNA, ideally 6 weeks after infection. Not valid before 20 weeks (relies on fetal urine production).
- **Testing in neonate**—at least 2× urine for CMV PCR before 3 weeks old. If positive, consider blood and/or CSF PCR as well. Examine for symptomatic infection (hepatosplenomegaly, hearing loss, jaundice, thrombocytopenia).

- **Management *in utero***—there are no measures to prevent congenital infection. Antiviral treatment is not recommended in maternal infection. If infection is confirmed on amniocentesis, then regular scans and assessment of the fetal brain are recommended.
- **Treatment of neonates**—valganciclovir is recommended only in symptomatic neonates, and it can reduce hearing loss and neurological sequelae. It must be started within 1 month of birth and is continued for 6 months (FBC and renal function monitoring required).

Enterovirus

(➔ See also Enteroviral infection, pp. 853–5.)
- **Maternal infection**—usually mild or asymptomatic.
- **Transmission**—does not readily cross the placenta or cause fetal disease, miscarriage, or preterm birth. Vertical transmission more likely to occur in the perinatal period than via the placenta.
- **Fetal infection**—there have been rare cases of early-onset neonatal myocarditis, hepatitis, and insulin-dependent diabetes; however, a clear causal relationship with maternal infection is not described.
- **Diagnosis**—enterovirus PCR of clinical specimens or serology (limited utility in acute infection as serotype-specific).
- **Treatment**—no recommendation for investigation of fetus in maternal infection and there are no known preventative measures. Intravenous immunoglobulin (IVIG) has been given to neonates with myocarditis.

Hepatitis B

For more details, ➔ see Hepatitis B, pp. 465–70 (and the UKHSA 2023 guidance at: www.gov.uk/government/publications/hepatitis-b-antenatal-screening-and-selective-neonatal-immunisation-pathway/guidance-on-the-hepatitis-b-antenatal-screening-and-selective-neonatal-immunisation-pathway--2).[1]
- **Background**—in contrast to adult infection, up to 90% of neonates infected with hepatitis B perinatally go on to become chronic carriers. The risk is highest if the mother has high DNA level or is hepatitis B e antigen positive.
- **Diagnosis**—the mother may have pre-existing hepatitis B or symptoms of acute infection in pregnancy. Asymptomatic cases should be picked up on routine screening.
- **Maternal management**—mothers should be referred to specialist care and have frequent monitoring. Decisions around starting antivirals are complex and depend on both the severity of the liver disease and the risk of transmission. As a high viral load (VL) is linked with increased rates of transmission, current guidelines advocate starting antivirals in the third trimester if the DNA level is >200 000IU/mL.
- **Neonatal management**:
  - All babies born to mothers with hepatitis B (hepatitis B surface antigen (HBsAg) +ve) should receive an accelerated vaccine schedule with vaccines at birth (within 24h), 4 weeks, and 1 year. Additional vaccinations will be given as part of routine childhood immunization at 8, 12, and 16 weeks.
  - All infants should be tested for hepatitis B at 12 months to diagnose congenital transmission.

- Unless the mother is anti-HBe positive and HBeAg negative, the infant should be given hepatitis B immunoglobulin (HBIG) within 48h after birth, in addition to vaccination.
- If the baby is premature or weighs <1500g, or the mother has a HepB DNA level of above 1×10^6 IU/mL. HBIG should be given, regardless of the 'e' antigen status.
- Vaccination alone is effective at preventing disease in 90% of cases; with the addition of HBIG, prevention rates are expected to be very high.

Herpes simplex

(➔ See Herpes simplex, pp. 438–41.)

- **Maternal infection**—primary infection presents with a vesicular genital rash. Relapse of previous infection is common (seen in 15% of previously infected women), and ~2% of women with a history of recurrent HSV infection are asymptomatically shedding at the time of delivery.
- **Transmission**—congenital infection *in utero* is extremely rare. Infection later in pregnancy carries a risk of preterm labour or IUGR. The main concern is transmission during delivery—if the primary infection is within 6 weeks of delivery, this risk is 50%. However, the risk of transmission from reactivation is only 2%.
- **Fetal infection**—neonatal herpes can be localized to skin (30%), CNS disease alone (encephalitis), or disseminated disease. Mortality is extremely low in skin disease; however, it is up to 30% (despite treatment) in disseminated disease.
- **Diagnosis**—usually clinical in the mother. May be confirmed by HSV PCR of blister fluid or serology. Attempt to establish if first infection or not—if unsure, test maternal IgG.
- **Maternal treatment**—first and second trimesters: treat with PO aciclovir at time of rash. Restart aciclovir at 36 weeks to prevent recurrence. Vaginal delivery recommended, unless lesions present at the time. Third trimester: start aciclovir (continue until delivery). Caesarean section is recommended.
- **Neonatal management**—if risk of transmission, then screen baby with surface swabs and blood for PCR at 24h. If high risk (vaginal delivery following primary infection within 6 weeks), start treatment of mother and child.

Human immunodeficiency virus

For more details, ➔ see HIV virology and diagnostics—chapter 8, p. 105 (see also British HIV Association, 2020).[2]

- **Background**—congenital acquisition of HIV is entirely preventable with cART but remains a significant problem in countries with a high burden of disease and lower rates of treatment. Untreated, most maternally infected children die by the age of 10.
- **Transmission**—the virus can pass across the placenta. Also risk of transmission during delivery from blood and placental fluids and via breast milk.
- **Mode of delivery**—vaginal delivery can be supported if the mother is taking cART and has an undetectable VL. If the maternal VL is detectable, a caesarean section is recommended.

- **Neonatal post-exposure prophylaxis (PEP)**—in low-risk infants (mother on cART and undetectable VL at delivery), 2–4 weeks of zidovudine monotherapy is recommended. If the VL is detectable, combination therapy should be started in the neonate within 4h of delivery.
- **Breastfeeding**—there is a small, but possible, risk of transmission. In the UK, breastfeeding is not recommended; however, if the woman makes an informed decision to breastfeed, then she should be supported. This would normally be if she has an undetectable VL and agrees to close follow-up and monitoring.

Parvovirus
(➔ See Rash illnesses in pregnancy, pp. 837–41.)

Rubella (German measles)
(➔ See Rash illnesses in pregnancy, pp. 837–41.)

Syphilis
- Caused by *Treponema pallidum* (➔ see *Treponema* species, pp. 369–72).
- **Maternal infection**—should be detected on routine screening. Risk of congenital infection is 50% in primary and secondary syphilis, 40% in latent infection, and 10% in tertiary syphilis.
- **Transmission**—can occur at any stage of pregnancy.
- **Fetal infection**—abnormalities detected on fetal USS include IUGR, hydrocephaly, and hydrops. Also causes miscarriage and stillbirth. Typical features of neonatal infection include jaundice, anaemia, lymphadenopathy, hepatosplenomegaly, pyrexia, failure to move an extremity (pseudoparalysis of Parrot), rhinitis ('snuffles'), rash (classically palmo-plantar), and osteochondritis.
- **Diagnosis**—usually based on maternal serology. Less commonly, dark-field microscopy or staining for treponemes in samples from the placenta or umbilical cord.
- **Maternal treatment**—refer to genitourinary medicine (GUM)/ sexual health services for treatment and follow-up. Treated with IM benzathine benzylpenicillin. Serology following treatment is recommended, to look for falling titres.
- **Neonatal treatment**—ensure birth plan from maternal GUM team is documented before delivery. All children born to mothers treated for syphilis require assessment and investigation (non-treponemal tests and IgM) at least at birth and 3 months. Treponemal antibodies can be passively transferred and are less useful. Treatment depends on timing of maternal infection, maternal antibiotics given, and test of cure. If treatment is required, penicillin is given IV for 10 days.

Toxoplasmosis
- Caused by *Toxoplasma gondii* (➔ see *Toxoplasma gondii*, pp. 562–6)
- **Maternal infection**—may be subclinical (>90%) or present with an infectious mononucleosis-like illness with lymphadenopathy.
- **Transmission**—risk rises from 5% in the first trimester (although associated with more severe abnormalities) to near 80% by the end of the last trimester.

- **Fetal infection**—suspected if risk factors or abnormalities on fetal USS (hydrocephalus, intracranial calcifications, IUGR). Triad of congenital toxoplasmosis is chorioretinitis, hydrocephalus, and intracranial calcifications, but neonates can be asymptomatic or have a combination of fever, seizures, hepatosplenomegaly, petechial rash, and other symptoms. Sequelae include intellectual disability, deafness, and spasticity.
- **Diagnosis**—maternal seroconversion or IgM-positive results can be confirmed with a dye test (performed at a reference laboratory) and IgG avidity. If infection was a few months before conception or in early pregnancy, fetal infection can be confirmed by amniocentesis.
- **Neonatal investigation**—IgM can become positive in the first few days of life. Serology should be monitored throughout the first year, as diagnosis is challenging. IgG is transferred from the mother but wanes over 12 months; high IgG at this point confirms the diagnosis.
- **Antenatal treatment**—spiramycin can be used (if fetal PCR negative) to reduce fetal infection rate, but the efficacy of this is debated. If the fetus is infected, referral to fetal medicine for monitoring is required.
- **Neonatal management**—treat with pyrimethamine, sulfadiazine, and folinic acid for 1 year, under specialist guidance. Will require follow-up from ophthalmology and a developmental specialist.

Varicella-zoster

(⊙ See Rash illnesses in pregnancy, pp. 837–41.)

References

1 Aysha Aslam, *et al*. Management of chronic hepatitis B during pregnancy. *Gastroenterol Rep (Oxf)*. 2018;**6**:257–62. www.gov.uk/government/publications/hepatitis-b-antenatal-screening-and-selective-neonatal-immunisation-pathway/guidance-on-the-hepatitis-b-antenatal-screening-and-selective-neonatal-immunisation-pathway--2
2 British HIV Association (2020). *British HIV Association guidelines for the management of HIV in pregnancy and postpartum 2018 (2020 third interim update)*. Available at: ℘ https://www.bhiva.org/file/5f1aab1ab9aba/BHIVA-Pregnancy-guidelines-2020-3rd-interim-update.pdf

Useful resources

National Institute for Health and Care Excellence (2008, updated 2019). *Antenatal care for uncomplicated pregnancies*. Clinical guideline [CG62]. Available at: ℘ https://www.nice.org.uk/guidance/cg62/resources/antenatal-care-for-uncomplicated-pregnancies-pdf-975564597445
RCOG guidelines
Green book and other PHE documents
https://www.bhiva.org/pregnancy-guidelines
https://www.rcog.org.uk/guidance/browse-all-guidance/green-top-guidelines/chickenpox-in-pregnancy-green-top-guideline-no-13/
https://www.gov.uk/government/collections/immunisation-against-infectious-disease-the-green-book

Rash illnesses in pregnancy

See also the UK Health Security Agency (UKHSA) guidance on rashes in pregnancy and Public Health England's *Green Book*.[3,4]

Background

- There are multiple causes of a rash, both infective and non-infective. Common viral causes of diffuse rash include parvovirus B19, measles, rubella, varicella, human herpesvirus 6 (HHV-6) and 7 (HHV-7), and enterovirus. Infections, such as CMV, Epstein–Barr virus (EBV), and HIV, can include rash as a symptom. Imported infections, such as dengue and zika virus, would be suspected based on the travel history. Bacterial causes include streptococcal or meningococcal disease and syphilis.

- Any febrile illness is associated with an increased risk of fetal loss in the first trimester. Specific risks related to many diseases are not known. Mothers should be managed as normal, and the fetus followed up if there is concern.
- Rubella, parvovirus B19, and VZV are considered here, as there are interventions that will reduce the risk of adverse events in the fetus.
- Although varicella usually impacts the fetus beyond 20 weeks' gestation, investigation is recommended at any age as: (1) age calculation may not be accurate, and (2) diagnosis is helpful in managing contact with other pregnant mothers and neonates.

Patients presenting with a non-vesicular rash

All pregnant women with a non-vesicular rash illness compatible with rubella or parvovirus B19 should be investigated simultaneously for both infections, **regardless** of previous history, immunization, or prior testing.

Rubella

(➲ See Chapter 8.)
- **Background**—maternal infection is extremely rare in the UK. There were 31 cases in pregnancy between 2003 and 2016—in all cases, the country of birth was known, the births were outside the UK, and most infections were acquired outside the UK. However, rates of susceptible pregnant women are rising and are currently about 7%.
- **Maternal infection**—asymptomatic in up to 50%. Symptoms include fever, coryza, maculopapular rash (starting on the face and spreading to the trunk), and conjunctivitis. Subsequent polyarthritis can be seen.
- **Transmission**—risk of transmission to the fetus decreases with gestation: 90% at <11 weeks, reducing to 45% at over 16 weeks. Risk of adverse fetal outcome is highest with early gestation: 90% at <11 weeks, falling to 20% at 16 weeks. There is no increased risk of infection to the fetus past 20 weeks.
- **Fetal infection**—infection can cause major and varied congenital abnormalities (including IUGR, radiolucent bone lesions, microcephaly, microphthalmia, cardiac abnormalities, meningoencephalitis, interstitial pneumonitis, sensorineural deafness, 'blueberry muffin skin', cataracts, hepatosplenomegaly, haemolytic anaemia, and thrombocytopenia). At 16–20 weeks, there is a risk of deafness.
- **Diagnosis**—maternal serology, including IgG and IgM. Can be compared to booking bloods to demonstrate seroconversion. Any IgM-positive result should be referred to the reference laboratory for confirmatory testing, which may include PCR or IgG avidity. Fetal and postnatal diagnosis should be discussed with the reference laboratory, as virological techniques are not widely available.
- **Treatment**—confirmed and suspected cases should be managed in a specialist unit. No specific treatment available. Depending on the gestation when infection occurred, termination may be considered.

- **Neonatal management**—if the mother was infected during pregnancy, or if infection cannot be ruled out, samples of cord blood, placenta, urine, and oral fluid should be sent to the reference laboratory. Neonates should be assessed for complications. Infants with congenital rubella are infectious, and isolation must be considered.

Parvovirus

(⊙ See Chapter 8.)

- **Background**—40–50% of the general population are susceptible, including pregnant mothers. In the UK, seroconversion occurs in up to 13% of susceptible pregnancies, resulting in around 1 in 500 affected pregnancies.
- **Maternal infection**—range of presentations from asymptomatic to rash ('slapped check'/fifth disease/erythema infectiosum or generalized, indistinguishable from rubella), arthropathy, and aplastic crisis. Infection is generally self-limiting.
- **Transmission**—risk increases with gestation: from 15% at 5–16 weeks to 25–70% at over 16 weeks. Risk of adverse effects reduces with gestational age: over 20 weeks, <1% have complications.
- **Fetal infection**—at <20 weeks' gestation, infection is associated with 9% excess fetal loss and 3–11% risk of fetal hydrops (50% mortality if untreated). The virus induces severe anaemia in the fetus, which presents as heart failure and accumulation of fluid in two or more fetal compartments (fetal hydrops).
- **Diagnosis**—testing may be undertaken either following a rash illness in the mother or on detection of fetal hydrops on USS. Parvovirus B19 IgM should be tested as soon as possible after rash onset. If positive, confirmation is recommended via seroconversion (compared to booking blood) or detectable B19V DNA. Fetal blood can also be tested for DNA.
- **Management if no fetal abnormality**—specialist advice should be sought. Serial fetal scanning (e.g. 1- to 2-weekly) and Doppler assessment to detect and treat fetal hydrops are required.
- **Management of fetal hydrops**—intrauterine transfusion has been shown to improve the outcome of infection. It increases resolution of infection from 5% to 55%.

Varicella-zoster virus

(⊙ Varicella Zoster virus (pp. 441–5).)

- **Background**—up to 10% of pregnant women are susceptible to VZV. History of chickenpox should be established at booking visit. If no positive history or vaccination, then pregnant women should be advised to avoid exposure to chickenpox or shingles and seek immediate medical attention if they have a contact with a case.
- **Maternal infection**—primary VZV infection presents with a vesicular rash. Complications of infection are commoner in pregnancy; pneumonitis is seen in 10%, and encephalitis, although rare, has up to 10% mortality. Overall case fatality rate is 1 in 1000.
- **Transmission**—risk increases with gestational age, from 5–10% at <28 weeks to 50% at over 30 weeks. Primary VZV infection before 20

weeks' gestation has been associated with a 1–2% risk of congenital varicella syndrome. There is a risk of neonatal chickenpox with late-term infection.

- **Fetal infection**—risk of spontaneous abortion in the first trimester. Fetal varicella infection is characterized by low birthweight, dermatomal skin scarring, limb hypoplasia, eye defects (chorioretinitis, cataract, micro-ophthalmia), and neurological abnormalities (microcephaly, cortical atrophy, mental retardation, bladder and bowel dysfunction). Primary VZV immediately before or after delivery may cause neonatal chickenpox; lack of maternal IgG is associated with disease severity.
- **Diagnosis**—usually clinical. May be confirmed by VZV PCR of skin lesions in the mother or infant.
- **Maternal treatment**—aciclovir should be given within 24h of onset of rash and continued for 7 days (no evidence of benefit if started after 24h). Caution in <20 weeks' gestation. Can be given PO, but close follow-up with daily review is recommended. Admission for IV therapy is strongly recommended if severe disease (respiratory or neurological symptoms, dense or haemorrhagic rash) or immunosuppression. Also considered if fever persists or new vesicles appear after 6 days. Other risk factors for severe disease include approaching term, poor obstetric history, smoking, chronic lung disease, and lack of social support.
- **Fetal management**—in infection before 20 weeks, perform a specialist USS looking for signs of fetal varicella syndrome. If infection is after 20 weeks, congenital varicella syndrome does not occur, but there are reports of mild fetal damage up to 28 weeks.
- **Neonatal treatment**—90% of neonatal infections are acquired perinatally, 5% congenitally, and 5% postnatally (e.g. from an adult with herpes labialis). Varicella-zoster immunoglobulin (VZIG) should be administered to neonates to prevent infection in specific circumstances:
  - if the mother develops chickenpox from 7 days before to 7 days after delivery (the neonate will not have protective antibody);
  - if born to a susceptible uninfected mother (VZV antibody negative) and exposed to VZV from another source in the first 7 days of life;
  - if born before 28 weeks' gestation or weighing <1kg, then VZV antibody should be tested. VZIG can be given if antibody negative up to 1 year of life for infants who have remained in hospital.

IV aciclovir should also be administered to infants who:
  - develop varicella infection despite VZIG (high dose);
  - are born to mothers who develop chickenpox from 4 days before to 2 days after delivery (prophylactic dose).
- **Other considerations**:
  - If other children in the family have varicella, and the mother has had varicella (or is VZV antibody positive), there is no reason to prevent a new baby from going home. If the mother is susceptible, contact with siblings with varicella should be delayed, until the new baby has reached 7 days of age.
  - Mothers with varicella can breastfeed, but if they have lesions close to the nipple, they should express milk from the affected breast until the lesions have crusted. This milk can be fed to the baby if they are covered by VZIG and/or aciclovir.

References

3 UK Health Security Agency (2022). *Guidance on the investigation, diagnosis and management of viral illness, or exposure to viral rash illness, in pregnancy.* Available at: ⏚ https://assets.publishing.serv ice.gov.uk/government/uploads/system/uploads/attachment_data/file/1116128/viral-rash-in-pregnancy-guidance.pdf

4 UKHSA (2013, updated 2020). *The Green Book: immunisation against infectious disease.* Available at: ⏚ https://www.gov.uk/government/collections/immunisation-against-infectious-disease-the-green-book

Rash contact in pregnancy

See also the UKHSA guidance on rashes in pregnancy and Public Health England's *Green Book*.[5,6]

Contact definition

During pregnancy, all women should be advised to seek urgent medical attention following contact with anyone with a rash. A significant contact is classed as either being in the same room for >15 minutes or having face-to-face contact.

Contact with non-vesicular rash

Rubella, parvovirus B19, and measles have management strategies after contact in pregnancy. This is due to the possibility of asymptomatic infection causing fetal harm, or the need for preventative treatment. Rubella and parvovirus B19 should be assessed for in all cases. Investigation of measles is based on epidemiological and clinical risk factors. If measles or rubella is suspected, then urgent testing of the case and notification to Health Protection Unit are required. In other causes of a rash, no action is required unless the pregnant woman becomes unwell

Rubella

- If the woman has two documented doses of rubella-containing vaccines or a previous IgG-positive rubella antibody, then no further action is needed. She should be reassured and advised to contact her General Practitioner (GP) if she develops a rash.
- If these criteria are not met, then serum should be tested for rubella-specific IgG and IgM. If helpful, serology can also be requested on booking bloods to look for seroconversion:
  - IgG positive/IgM negative—immune and no evidence of recent infection. Reassure as above;
  - IgG negative/IgM negative—susceptible. Advise to seek medical attention if rash develops. Advise immunization with two doses of measles, mumps, and rubella (MMR) vaccine after delivery;
  - IgM positive—confirm with reference laboratory testing. As rubella is so rare in the UK, most IgM-positive results do not reflect rubella. If rubella is confirmed, manage as rubella infections, as detailed in ⏵ Rash illnesses in pregnancy, pp. 837–41.

Parvovirus B19

- All women should be promptly investigated for asymptomatic infection, with serum tested as soon as possible after rash contact. Active management of the fetus reduces the chance of poor outcome.

- Maternal serum should be tested for parvovirus B19-specific IgG and IgM:
  - IgG positive/IgM negative—reassure;
  - IgG negative/IgM negative—repeat in 4 weeks. If remains negative, reassure no active infection;
  - IgM positive—repeat immediately. If still positive, manage as for parvovirus B19 infection as detailed in ➜ Rash illnesses in pregnancy, pp. 837–41.

Measles

- If the woman has two documented doses of measles-containing vaccines or previous documented immunity, then she should be reassured and advised to contact her GP if she develops a rash. No testing is required. Additionally, if the index case is not a 'likely' case of measles, no further action is required.
- If epidemiological and clinical features suggest the source patient has measles and there is a chance the woman could be susceptible (unvaccinated, one dose only, or unknown), then her measles specific-IgG should be tested:
  - IgG positive—immune. Reassure. Contact GP if develop a rash;
  - IgG negative—susceptible.
- If she is susceptible, passive prophylaxis with IM human normal immunoglobulin (HNIG) should be given as soon as possible, but within 6 days. It attenuates maternal illness but does not confer benefit to the fetus. Advise immunization with two doses of MMR vaccine after delivery.

Contact with vesicular rash

Varicella-zoster virus

- A case is deemed infectious from 48h before onset of rash to crusting of all vesicles. In prolonged contact (household), then the day of onset of rash is used to calculate timings.
- If the woman has a history of chickenpox or shingles, or has had two doses of a varicella-containing vaccine, then she can be reassured that she is protected.
- If this cannot be confirmed, her VZV-specific IgG should be measured; if it is >100IU/mL, then she can be considered immune.
- If she is susceptible, VZIG should be given within 10 days of exposure. Without prophylaxis, up to 70% of susceptible individuals will contract the disease. VZIG protects against maternal illness, and therefore also against fetal varicella syndrome (commonest <20 weeks' gestation).
- If there is a shortage of VZIG, and the woman is over 20 weeks' gestation, then prophylactic PO aciclovir can be given instead from day 7 to day 14 following a contact.[7]

References

5 UK Health Security Agency (2019). *Guidance on the investigation, diagnosis and management of viral illness, or exposure to viral rash illness, in pregnancy.* Available at: 🔗 https://assets.publishing.serv ice.gov.uk/media/6565bdac1524e6000da101b2/viral-rash-in-pregnancy-guidance-syphilis.pdf

6 UK Health Security Agency (2019). *Guidelines on post-exposure prophylaxis for measles.* Available at: 🔗 https://www.gov.uk/government/publications/national-measles-guidelines

7 UK Health Security Agency (2019). *Updated guidelines on post-exposure prophylaxis (PEP) for varicella/shingles.* Available at: 🔗 https://assets.publishing.service.gov.uk/media/63e230638fa8f 50e86ff1ae4/UKHSA-guidelines-on-VZ-post-exposure-prophylaxis-january-2023.pdf

Maternal infections associated with neonatal morbidity

Listeria monocytogenes

(➔ See Chapter 7, Listeria, pp. 297–8.)

- **Background**—pregnant women are 20 times more likely to contract listeriosis than other adults; over 33% of all cases of *Listeria* infection occur during pregnancy.
- **Aetiology**—follows ingestion of contaminated foods such as soft cheese, unpasteurized milk, and undercooked ready meals.
- **Presentation**—most commonly asymptomatic. Can cause flu-like illness or febrile gastroenteritis. Rarely septicaemia or meningitis.
- **Congenital infection**—amnionitis, septic abortion, or premature labour. Infected neonates may have sepsis, meningoencephalitis, or disseminated infection with granulomatosis infantiseptica. Mortality is around 50%.
- **Late-onset infection**—(over 7 days) likely due to infection transmitted during delivery. Main presentation is meningitis.
- **Diagnosis**—cultured from blood or CSF.
- **Treatment**—amoxicillin with gentamicin is the treatment of choice for both mother and neonate. Co-trimoxazole in penicillin allergy (not licensed in pregnancy).

Pelvic inflammatory disease

(➔ See Chapter 18, Pelvic inflammatory disease, pp. 750–2.)

Pelvic inflammatory disease (PID) can be associated with chlamydial or gonorrhoeal infection (~50%) or other bacteria comprising vaginal flora (e.g. anaerobes, *Haemophilus influenzae*, enteric Gram-negative rods). Symptoms include lower pelvic pain, fever, cervical discharge, and cervical and uterine or adnexal tenderness. In pregnancy, there is a significant risk of maternal morbidity, preterm delivery, and neonatal complications (e.g. ophthalmia neonatorum). Women should be admitted for IV antibiotics to cover common bacteria, including sexually transmitted infections (STIs).

Group B *Streptococcus* (*Streptococcus cgalactiae*)

(➔ See Chapter 7, Group B Streptococcus pp. 748–750.)

GBS carriage is common and present in up to 40% of adults. Screening is not recommended in the UK due to lack of evidence of clinical benefit. However, GBS is the commonest cause of severe, early-onset neonatal sepsis. If GBS carriage is detected during pregnancy, intrapartum antibiotic prophylaxis with benzylpenicillin is recommended. No treatment is recommended for the neonate in the absence of other risk factors.

Zika virus

(➔ See Chapter 8, Zika, p. 132.)

Zika virus is transmitted via the bite of the *Aedes* mosquito. It is endemic in Asia and the Pacific region, and also in the Americas since the 2015 outbreak. Although illness is generally mild (often asymptomatic), infection during pregnancy has been linked with birth defects, including microcephaly. There is no vaccine or treatment, and pregnant women are advised to avoid countries with a high risk of transmission. Latest travel advice should be checked prior to travel. If travel to a high-risk area has occurred, serology is advised if the woman has symptoms. If not, then additional USS should be done at 18–20 weeks and 28–30 weeks.

Other relevant sections

- Malaria (➜ see *Plasmodium* species (malaria), pp. 556–60).
- Leptospirosis (➜ see *Leptospira* species, pp. 376–8).
- *Ureaplasma urealyticum* (➜ see *Mycoplasma*, pp. 386–8).
- *Mycoplasma hominis* (➜ see *Mycoplasma*, pp. 386–8).

Chorioamnionitis

Inflammation of the chorion (outer) or amnion (inner) membrane, which comprises the amniotic sac. It is usually due to bacterial infection. There are significant maternal and fetal consequences, including long-term morbidity.

Aetiology

In over 96% of cases, the causative organism ascends from the vagina into the (normally sterile) amniotic sac. Rarely, it can be associated with invasive sampling (amniocentesis or chorionic villus sampling) or haematogenous spread (e.g. *Listeria*). Common pathogens include:

- genital mycoplasmas: *U. urealyticum* (47%), *M. hominis* (30%);
- anaerobes: *Gardnerella vaginalis* (25%), *Bacteroides* (30%);
- GBS (15%);
- Gram-negative rods, including *Escherichia coli* (8%);
- Polymicrobial in over 65% of cases.

Clinically apparent infection complicates up to 5% of term deliveries. However, histological inflammation is much commoner.

Risk factors

Both prolonged labour and preterm premature rupture of the membranes (PPROM) are major risk factors for developing chorioamnionitis; the risk rises with duration. However, subclinical chorioamnionitis is also a major cause of PPROM. Other risk factors include: alcohol and tobacco use, GBS colonization, bacterial vaginosis, meconium-stained amniotic fluid, multiple digital examinations after membrane rupture, internal monitoring, and epidural anaesthesia.

Clinical features

Maternal fever (>37.8°C) plus at least two of: maternal tachycardia (>100bpm), fetal tachycardia (>160bpm), uterine tenderness (difficult to establish in labour), and purulent amniotic fluid/vaginal discharge are suggestive of chorioamnionitis, especially in the presence of risk factors.

Asymptomatic mothers presenting with PPROM, premature labour, or rupture of membranes (ROM) at term (prior to contractions) should be investigated for chorioamnionitis.

Diagnosis

- **Blood tests**—WCC and CRP will often be raised, but this is not specific.
- **Microbiology**—blood cultures (BCs), low vaginal swab, and urine for microscopy, culture, and sensitivity (MC&S)
- **Amniotic fluid examination**—risk of obtaining fluid needs to be balanced against benefit. Amniocentesis can be considered and may be used to confirm diagnosis before inducing premature labour. Fluid can be sent for microscopy, culture, pH, glucose, and PCR if appropriate.
- **Histology**—diagnosis may be confirmed or refuted on histological examination of the placenta, fetal membranes and umbilical cord for evidence of inflammation and infection.

Management

- Acute chorioamnionitis—prompt administration of broad-spectrum antibiotics reduces maternal and fetal complications, and neonatal sepsis is decreased by 80%. Delivery should be expedited, but a caesarean section is not recommended unless there is a specific indication (e.g. fetal distress).
- PPROM and no obvious infection—expectant management advised to avoid risks associated with prematurity. However, follow-up (often as an inpatient) is required to diagnose infection or fetal distress promptly. Steroids are offered to promote fetal lung maturation. There is evidence that erythromycin (or penicillin) for 10 days, or until the start of labour, reduces the risk of chorioamnionitis and prolongs the time until delivery.
- Antibiotics should include Gram-positive (e.g. amoxicillin) and Gram-negative (e.g. gentamicin) cover. Although commonly used regimens do not cover genital mycoplasmas, they have good efficacy and there is currently no evidence to suggest a need for additional cover.
- The infant should be assessed and treated for any evidence of infection. BCs are often sent, and a raised CRP level may indicate a need for further investigations.

Complications

Maternal complications

- Rate of caesarean delivery increased by 2- to 3-fold.
- Increase in endometritis, wound infection, pelvic abscess, and post-partum haemorrhage.
- Sepsis, disseminated intravascular coagulopathy (DIC), and death are extremely rare.

Fetal complications

- Associated with 40% of cases of neonatal sepsis.
- Increased rates of pneumonia, sepsis, intraventricular haemorrhage, and death.

- Consequences are more severe when combined with prematurity.
- Associated with a 4-fold risk of cerebral palsy in term infants.

Puerperal infection

Any infection from delivery to up to 6 weeks post-partum is classified as puerperal infection. The spectrum ranges from mild infection to life-threatening sepsis.

Background

Puerperal infection was the leading cause of maternal mortality until the development of antibiotics. In the mid part of the twentieth century, rates were extremely low. However, since 2003, they have been rising, and in 2006, sepsis was the leading cause of direct maternal death. This is largely due to group A *Streptococcus* (GAS) infection.

Aetiology

- The source of infection is most commonly the genital tract, leading to endometritis. Infections are often polymicrobial, and pathogens include GAS, *E. coli*, GBS, *Bacteroides*, and *Clostridium* spp.
- Other sources include: mastitis, urinary tract infection (UTI), pneumonia, and skin and soft tissue infection (including wound infection and perineal cellulitis).
- Risk factors include: diabetes, obesity, immunosuppression, invasive procedures (e.g. amniocentesis, caesarean section), prolonged rupture of membranes, retained products of conception, previous pelvic infection, and carriage of invasive organisms (e.g. GAS).

Clinical features

- Well-described features of sepsis, such as fever, tachycardia, hypotension, hypoxia, and impaired consciousness, may not always be present. Other common features of puerperal sepsis include abdominal pain, diarrhoea and vomiting, abnormal discharge, and rash.
- The onset can be insidious, yet clinical deterioration rapid, and the clinician should have a low threshold for referral to secondary care.
- Other clinical features may indicate the underlying cause.

Diagnosis and management

- **Blood tests**—FBC, U&Es, CRP, lactate, BCs.
- **Microbiology**—BCs, urine cultures, wound swab or discharge for MC&S, other investigations guided by symptoms.
- **Imaging**—if pelvic source suspected, pelvic USS may detect abscesses or infected haematoma. Contrast abdominal CT may be required if non-pregnancy-related abdominal sources of infection are suspected.
- **Management**—fluid resuscitation and other management of sepsis as per national guidelines. Antibiotic therapy should be guided by the likely source of infection; examples and specific features of management are given below:
  - endometritis—PO co-amoxiclav if mild, IV cefuroxime/ metronidazole if severe;

- mastitis—flucloxacillin. Continue to express milk to prevent engorgement. Check for abscess development;
- UTI/pyelonephritis/pneumonia as per local guidelines;
- septic pelvic thrombosis—anticoagulation and broad-spectrum antibiotics;
- infected wounds may need surgical debridement or drainage, in combination with antibiotic therapy.
- Avoid tetracyclines if breastfeeding.
- Considerations if failure to respond:
  - check culture results and exclude resistant organisms;
  - collections or spreading skin infection—may need surgical intervention before clinical improvement occurs (source control).
- GAS, GBS, *Chlamydia*, or *Neisseria gonorrhoeae* may have implications for the neonate. Inform the paediatrician or GP, so treatment can be considered in the child.

Neonatal infection

This is any infection occurring within the first 4 weeks of life. Onset is often rapid, especially in premature infants. Although bacterial infections cause the most concern, certain viral infections can cause an indistinguishable clinical presentation. It accounts for 10% of all neonatal mortality.

Definitions
- Early onset—within 72h of birth (but 85% present within 24h of delivery). Less common (0.9 of every 1000 births) but tends to be more severe.
- Late onset—over 72h from birth. Commoner (7 of every 1000 births).
- Many more infants will be assessed for infection and treated with antibiotics due to non-specific early signs.

Aetiology
- Early onset—associated with microbes from the mother (GBS, *E. coli*, *H. influenzae*, *L. monocytogenes*).
- Late onset—associated with organisms acquired from the environment (coagulase-negative staphylococci (CoNS), *Staphylococcus aureus*, *Enterobacterales, Pseudomonas* spp., *Candida* spp., *Acinetobacter* spp., GBS, anaerobes).

Risk factors
- Early onset—maternal colonization with GBS, maternal fever, maternal chorioamnionitis, prematurity, prolonged ROM.
- Late onset—prematurity, central venous catheter, ventilation, surgery.

Clinical features of sepsis
- Red flag indicators include apnoea, seizures, signs of shock, need for ventilation, and need for cardiopulmonary resuscitation.
- Respiratory features—respiratory distress, hypoxia, grunting.
- Cardiac features—pulmonary hypertension, decreased cardiac output, bradycardia or tachycardia.

- Neurological features—altered behaviour or responsiveness, altered muscle tone (e.g. floppiness), neonatal encephalopathy.
- GI features—feed refusal, intolerance (e.g. vomiting or excessive gastric aspirates), abdominal distension, jaundice within 24h of birth.
- Haematological features—thrombocytopenia, abnormal bleeding, DIC, high or low WCC (50% normal). The immature-to-total neutrophil ratio is a more useful marker of infection ('left shift').
- Other features—temperature abnormality (<36°C or >38°C), hypo- or hyperglycaemia, acidosis (base deficit >10mmol/L).

Clinical syndromes

- Meningitis shows signs in only 30%, so lumbar puncture (LP) must be undertaken if infection is suspected. In early disease, CSF WCC may be normal. Causative pathogens include GBS (36%), *E. coli* (31%), and *Listeria* (5–10%). Complications include obstructing ventriculitis, subdural empyema, and small-vessel thrombi.
- Pneumonia can develop following aspiration of amniotic fluid or aspiration during delivery. CXR can show consolidation. *Klebsiella* spp. and *S. aureus* may cause severe lung damage, with abscesses and empyema. Early-onset GBS pneumonia may be fulminant, with significant mortality.
- Necrotizing enterocolitis (NEC) is much commoner in premature babies. If suspected, then anaerobic cover (e.g. metronidazole) should be added to empirical antibiotic regimens.
- Conjunctivitis, localized umbilical infection, and UTI can cause neonatal infection.

Investigations

- **Blood tests**—FBC, U&Es, and LFTs. Even mild elevations in CRP level (e.g. >10) can be significant.
- **Microbiology**—BCs should be sent prior to antibiotics. They may be negative if the mother received intrapartum antibiotics. Urine culture and skin swabs, as guided by symptoms. LP if there is strong evidence of infection or signs of meningitis.
- **Other tests**—infection markers, such as interleukin (IL)-6, IL-8, and CD64, have been used in the evaluation of sepsis in neonates but are not in general clinical use.
- **Radiology**—CXR may show lobar changes but more usually resembles respiratory distress syndrome, with a diffuse reticulogranular pattern. Cranial USS may show evidence of ventriculitis and chronic changes. CT may be required in complex meningitis with obstruction and abscesses.

Management

- General management for sepsis, with cardiovascular, respiratory, and nutritional support as required.
- Antibiotics should be started as soon as cultures are taken. In early-onset sepsis, IV benzylpenicillin plus IV gentamicin is recommended. In late-onset sepsis, the choice will be guided by local resistance patterns

and depends on whether the baby has been admitted from home or remained in hospital.
- Review antibiotics at 36h. They can be stopped if: BCs are negative, the initial suspicion of infection was not strong, the clinical condition is reassuring, and the CRP level is low.
- If there was a strong suspicion of infection or BCs are positive, then treatment is recommended for 7 days. In some pathogens causing bacteraemia (Gram-negatives, *S. aureus*), treatment will need to be longer.
- **Meningitis**:
  - empirical treatment with cefotaxime (Gram-positive + Gram-negative cover with CNS penetration) plus amoxicillin (*Listeria*);
  - repeat LP at 48–72h to assess for sterility. If not sterile, then consider complication such as ventriculitis or abscess;
  - if Gram-negative pathogen, then continue cefotaxime or base choice on sensitivities. Duration should be at least 3 weeks;
  - in GBS infection, change to IV benzylpenicillin for at least 14 days from sterile CSF culture, with gentamicin for 5 days;
  - in *Listeria* infection, treat with IV amoxicillin for at least 14 days as above with gentamicin until clear improvement (5 days).
- Surgical interventions—the development of hydrocephalus may require placement of a ventriculoperitoneal (VP) shunt. Abscesses may require surgical drainage.

Prognosis and follow-up
- With early diagnosis and treatment, prognosis of non-meningitic disease is good.
- Mortality from meningitis is 8%, and residual neurological disability is seen in 50% of neonates with septic meningitis. Follow-up should be arranged with a paediatric neurologist.
- If aminoglycosides have been given, hearing assessment should be undertaken before discharge and at 3 months.
- If a baby was treated for GBS, the mother needs to be informed of the risk in future pregnancies. Intrapartum prophylaxis is recommended.

Further reading
National Institute for Health and Care Excellence (2021). *Neonatal infection: antibiotics for prevention and treatment*. NICE guideline [NG195]. Available at: ॐ https://www.nice.org.uk/guidance/ng195

Viral causes of childhood illness

(See Table 23.1.)

Table 23.1 Viral causes of childhood illness

Virus*	Typical age	Features
HSV	Neonate	➋ see Congenital infections, pp. 832–7
	Childhood (highest incidence in children aged 6 months to 3 years)	Over 80% of primary HSV infections are asymptomatic. Symptoms of primary infection: fever, anorexia, sore mouth (ulcerative gingivostomatitis), local lymphadenopathy. Contamination of skin by infectious saliva may lead to secondary lesions on the perioral skin, eye, fingers, and vulva. Those with disseminated infection should be isolated. Topical aciclovir is of no benefit in acute primary infection of children. Often self-limiting and no treatment required. Systemic treatment can decrease healing time and is important in the immunocompromised
VZV	90% of cases occur in those under 13 years of age	For prevention and management of neonatal disease, ➋ see Varicella-zoster virus after rash illness in pregnancy, p. 839–41
		Primary infection causes varicella (chickenpox), a maculopapular rash that forms pustulating vesicles. It is spread via the airborne route or by direct contact. Incubation is up to 21 days. Complications: bacterial superinfection, viral pneumonia, encephalitis. Treatment is not required in children, but systemic aciclovir is given in immunocompromised patients

Table 23.1 (Contd.)

Virus*	Typical age	Features
Measles ('first disease')	Uncommon in those populations with vaccination	Acute, highly infectious disease characterized by cough, coryza, fever, and rash (macules start on the face and spread to the trunk and limbs). Airborne spread. Incubation 7–14 days. Infectious from 2 days before to 5 days after symptoms. Severe manifestations and complications include pneumonia, encephalitis, bacterial superinfection, and SSPE. Treatment focuses on supportive care and isolation of cases. Ribavirin can be used in immunocompromise or CNS disease
Rubella ('third disease')	Extremely rare in the UK. Prior to vaccination, the incidence was highest in spring amongst children aged 5–9 years	Acute mild exanthematous viral infection, clinically indistinguishable from measles. Rash starts on the face and spreads to the trunk and extremities. Associated with fever and lymphadenopathy. Incubation 12–23 days. Infectious from 7 days before to 7 days after rash. Spread by airborne transmission. Self-limiting, with few complications, apart from the ability to cause devastating fetal infection
Parvovirus B19 (slapped cheek disease, erythema infectiosum, 'fifth disease')	Infection common in childhood—50% are IgG positive by 15 years	20% asymptomatic. Prodrome (5–7 days) of myalgia, arthralgia, malaise, rhinorrhoea, and fever, then a bright red rash on the cheeks, followed 1–2 days later by a maculopapular rash on the trunk, legs, arms, and buttocks. This clears after a few days, leaving a characteristic lacy pattern, which fades/reappears over the following 3 weeks. Transmission primarily via droplets

(Continued)

Table 23.1   (Contd.)

Virus*	Typical age	Features
HHV-6 (roseola, exanthem subitum, 'sixth disease')	Most children acquire infection between 4 months and 3 years of age	Abrupt onset of fever (± periorbital oedema) is followed 3–5 days later by a rash (rose-pink papules, which are mildly elevated and non-pruritic, and blanch on pressure) on the back and neck, and spreads to the chest and limbs, sparing the feet and face. Lasts ~2 days. Other features: malaise, vomiting, diarrhoea, cough, pharyngitis, lymphadenopathy, febrile convulsions (10% of primary infections). Meningitis and encephalitis are less commonly seen
Mumps	Prior to vaccination, 90% of cases occurred in children aged under 15 years. Now cases occur in older children and those at university	Acute generalized viral infection of children and adolescents, causing swelling and tenderness of the salivary glands, usually bilateral. Other manifestations include epididymo-orchitis (3% ♂) and transient hearing loss. Incubation 12–25 days. Infectious from 1–2 days before to 9 days after symptoms
Enterovirus	All age groups, but commoner in younger children	Includes Coxsackie virus, echovirus, and enterovirus spp. They account for the majority of childhood fever–rash syndromes (➔ See Enteroviral infections, pp. 853–5)
Parechovirus	Infants and young children	Closely related to enterovirus. Can similarly cause rash/fever illness, GI disease, and rarely CNS manifestations
EBV (cause of 90% of cases of infectious mononucleosis)	>50% of UK children are infected by age of 11 years, around 90% by age of 25 years	Primary infection in childhood is asymptomatic. Infection in adolescence may present with an acute infectious mononucleosis syndrome
Adenovirus	Commonest in young children (under 5 years old)	Most commonly respiratory illness, but also gastroenteritis, cystitis, and conjunctivitis. Often mild and self-limiting. Cidofovir can be considered in extremely immunocompromised patients

Table 23.1 *(Contd.)*

Virus*	Typical age	Features
Molluscum (poxvirus)	Children aged 1–10 years	Small, raised, pearly lesions with a central dimple appear anywhere on the body. Usually self-limiting but can take months to resolve. Spread via direct contact or fomites
RSV	Circulates during winter. Most children infected by second birthday	Common cause of respiratory illness in children. Often mild but can cause severe disease in young children (bronchiolitis and pneumonia). Ribavirin can be used in immunocompromised patients
Metapneumovirus	Most children infected by age of 5 years	Common respiratory pathogen causing upper and lower respiratory tract infections
Rhinovirus	Highest rates in children aged under 5 years	Commonest virus to cause common cold
Rotavirus	Peak age 3 months to 3 years	Causes watery diarrhoea and vomiting, often associated with fever and abdominal pain. Incubation ~2 days. Spread via faeco-oral route. PO vaccine included in routine childhood schedule

* ➔ See Chapter 8.

EBV, Epstein–Barr virus; HHV, human herpesvirus; HSV, human simplex virus; RSV, respiratory syncytial virus; SSPE, subacute sclerosing panencephalitis; VZV, varicella-zoster virus.

Enteroviral infections

The enterovirus family contains over 100 distinct strains and these viruses are responsible for a range of clinical syndromes. Poliovirus will not be considered in this chapter. Non-polio enteroviruses (including Coxsackie viruses A and B, enterovirus, and echovirus) are the leading cause of childhood fever–rash syndromes, and can also cause encephalitis, myocarditis, and sepsis. Only hand, foot, and mouth (HFM) disease and herpangina have a clinical presentation distinct enough to allow identification.

Epidemiology

- Enteroviruses are found worldwide. In temperate climates, cases peak in summer months.
- Infections can occur in all age groups, but the highest infection rates are seen in children. Reasons for this include lack of immunity, increased exposure, and poor hygiene.
- Infections are often more severe in neonates and young children. In older children and adults, infections are often mild or asymptomatic.

Clinical features

- Transmission occurs via direct contact with infected bodily fluids (faeces, respiratory secretions, blister fluid). Following infection, the virus can be shed for many weeks.
- Spread can also occur by fomites; the virus can survive at room temperature for several days. Respiratory spread is possible in crowded conditions.
- Incubation period is 3–10 days. Symptoms last for 3–7 days.
- Infections are asymptomatic in over 50% of cases.
- Mild, undifferentiated illness may present as low-grade fever of sudden onset, with malaise, myalgia, and rash.
- Associated syndromes include:
  - respiratory—coryza, pharyngitis, cough, croup, bronchiolitis, bronchospasm, pneumonia;
  - skin—HFM disease, non-specific exanthems (especially echoviruses; can mimic rubella/measles), periodic shedding of nails;
  - neurological—aseptic meningitis, encephalitis, acute flaccid myelitis;
  - GI—nausea, vomiting, diarrhoea, hepatitis, pancreatitis;
  - genitourinary—orchitis, epididymitis;
  - eye—acute haemorrhagic conjunctivitis, uveitis;
  - cardiac—myopericarditis;
  - muscle—pleurodynia (lancinating chest pain attacks), myositis.

Herpangina

- Enteroviral vesicular pharyngitis.
- Organism—Coxsackie viruses A 1–10, 16, and 22 most commonly.
- Typically seen during summer in children aged 3–10 years (may occur in young adults).
- Prodromal symptoms and fever precede rash by 24h. Red spots in the posterior pharynx and tonsils develop into vesicles, and later into small yellow ulcers (<5mm) with a red rim. Usually only 3–6 lesions. Associated lymphadenopathy. They are painful, resulting in reluctance to eat.
- Symptoms last for 3–7 days.

Hand, foot, and mouth disease

- Enteroviral vesicular stomatitis with exanthema.
- Organism—Coxsackie virus A16 and enterovirus A71 are commonest.
- Fever present for 1–2 days. Associated with vesicles of the anterior pharynx/tongue and peripheries, particularly the palms and soles. Vesicles in the mouth may burst and become painful. Cutaneous vesicles do not crust (compared to chickenpox).

- Enterovirus A71 can occur in outbreaks and is more likely to be associated with neurological disease (meningitis, encephalitis, and acute flaccid paralysis).

Diagnosis and management

- Diagnosis of herpangina and HFM disease is clinical (both are mild, self-limiting illnesses that do not warrant laboratory diagnosis), and management supportive (e.g. soft food for those with painful mouth ulcers, antipyretics, TOP analgesics).
- In severe disease, serology can be tested. Diagnosis can be inferred by serology consistent with acute infection.
- PCR is useful and a variety of samples, including blood, CSF, faeces, vesicular fluid, and respiratory secretions, can be tested, with varying sensitivity.
- Even in severe cases of CNS disease, management is supportive and there are no active antivirals.
- Hygiene measures, including handwashing, are important, to prevent continued faeco-oral spread.

Bacterial causes of childhood illness

Scarlet fever (notifiable disease)

One of the common childhood exanthems, previously known as 'second disease'. It is caused by infection with GAS, in particular, a strain producing erythrogenic toxins.

Background

- GAS colonizes the upper respiratory tract of up to 20% of children.
- Disease manifestations of GAS are broad and may include pharyngitis, pyoderma, cellulitis, pneumonia, and bacteraemia.
- Certain subtypes are linked to post-infectious immune-mediated sequelae such as rheumatic fever or glomerulonephritis.
- Usually seen in children aged 5–15 years.
- Subtype emm12 has been associated with severe disease and erythromycin/clindamycin antibiotic resistance.

Clinical features

- Often associated with pharyngitis but can be seen in association with other infections such as skin and soft tissue.
- Rash appears 1–2 days into illness. It is diffuse and red, with points of deeper red, including in the skinfold. It begins on the chest and spreads to the trunk, neck, and extremities sparing the palms and soles. The face tends not to be involved but may be flushed. The skin may have a sandpaper texture. The rash fades over a week, but desquamation follows, which can last several weeks.
- Examination of the oropharynx may reveal exudative pharyngitis, tonsillitis, and small, red haemorrhagic spots on the palate. The tongue may be coated white in early disease but then becomes beefy red ('strawberry tongue').
- Severe forms of the disease (from haematogenous spread and toxaemia) are rare in the antibiotic era.

- Complications—suppurative complications from local spread (e.g. abscess) and non-suppurative (rheumatic fever, post-streptococcal glomerulonephritis, erythema nodosum).

Diagnosis and management
- Throat swab for culture is the gold standard diagnosis.
- Anti-streptococcal O titre (ASOT) detects antibodies against the exotoxin produced by almost all strains of GAS and is a good indicator of recent disease. Higher titres may be associated with the development of acute rheumatic fever.
- Antibiotics are given to prevent rheumatic fever and suppurative complications, and to reduce symptoms and infectivity.
- No strains of GAS resistant to penicillin have been reported. Phenoxymethylpenicillin PO should be given for 10 days. If required, benzylpenicillin can be given IV.
- Differential—measles, infectious mononucleosis, other viral infections with rash, Kawasaki's disease, staphylococcal toxic shock syndrome. Pharyngitis can also be caused by group C and G streptococcal spp. and diphtheria.

Staphylococcal epidermal necrolysis

Also known as (staphylococcal) scalded skin syndrome (SSSS), this condition is caused by an exotoxin produced by *S. aureus*, which leads to exfoliation of the upper layers of the epidermis; 98% of cases occur in children under 6 years of age, due to lack of immunity and immature renal clearance capability. Mortality is low in children (1–5%) but can be higher in adults who are usually immunocompromised or have renal failure.

Clinical features
- An infection commonly occurs at a site such as the oral or nasal cavities, throat, or umbilicus. Epidermolytic toxins are produced locally and act at a remote site, leading to abrupt onset of generalized skin erythema.
- The epidermis beneath the granular cell layer separates due to binding of the toxins to desmoglein-1 in desmosomes. Bullae form, and diffuse sheet-like desquamation may occur 1–2 days later (Nikolsky sign positive). This leaves a raw and tender exposed surface.
- There may be associated conjunctivitis, stomatitis, and urethritis.
- Most patients do not appear very ill, but significant dehydration can develop. Healing occurs over 1–2 weeks.

Diagnosis
- *S. aureus* can usually be cultured from the site of remote infection; WCC is usually normal, but inflammatory markers may be elevated, a PCR test for the toxin is available. BCs are usually negative in children (but may be positive in adults).
- Differential diagnosis—toxic epidermal necrolysis (part of the disease spectrum that contains bullous erythema multiforme and Stevens–Johnson syndrome and associated with a deeper epidermal detachment than that of SSSS), erythema multiforme, burns.

Management
- Antibiotics—flucloxacillin, or erythromycin if penicillin-allergic.
- Fluids—patients can leak a lot of proteinaceous fluid through the skin and may require IV supplementation. Wound care is similar to that given for burns, and very severe cases may require specialist burns unit input. The skin damage can make patients vulnerable to secondary infection.

Pertussis

A highly contagious bacterial infection of the respiratory tract, spread by droplets and characterized by paroxysmal cough ('whooping cough'). Caused by *Bordetella pertussis* (➲ see *Bordetella*, pp. 345–6), a Gram-negative pleomorphic bacillus, of which humans are the sole reservoir, and less commonly *Bordetella parapertussis*.

Epidemiology
- Infection is worldwide, but unusual in the UK and other countries with widespread vaccination. Neither infection nor vaccination provides complete or lifelong immunity. Protection against typical disease lasts for 3–5 years, and immunity is not detectable after 12 years. The UK introduced a preschool pertussis booster in 2001, which has seen morbidity at the lowest levels yet in both vaccinated groups and infants too young to receive the vaccine.
- Most cases occur in infants/children (the majority infected by coughing adults and older children). Adults (10% of cases) experience milder disease. Children aged <1 year are most likely to require hospitalization.
- Worldwide, it remains a major cause of death—around 50 million cases and 600 000 estimated deaths each year.
- Those at risk of severe disease (pneumonia, encephalopathy, death) include premature infants and those patients with underlying cardiac, pulmonary, and neuromuscular/neurological disease.

Clinical features
- Incubation 3–12 days. Patients are infectious from the onset of illness until towards the end of the paroxysmal phase.
- Pertussis is a 6-week illness of three stages, each lasting around 2–4 weeks. Older children and adults may not exhibit these distinct stages:
  - stage 1 (catarrhal phase)—indistinguishable from the common cold: congestion, sneezing, mild fever, and rhinorrhoea. Patients are at their most infectious during this phase;
  - stage 2 (paroxysmal phase)—paroxysms of intense coughing, which can last for several minutes, may be followed by a loud whoop in older infants and toddlers. Infants aged <6 months may have apnoeic episodes but do not whoop. Vomiting is common after coughing. Subconjunctival haemorrhages and facial petechiae may occur. Most deaths occur in infants (coughing leading to choking and apnoea);
  - stage 3 (convalescent phase)—chronic cough, which may last for weeks, triggered by intercurrent viral infections.
- Differential diagnosis—bronchiolitis, *Mycoplasma* pneumonia, chlamydial pneumonia, inhaled foreign body.
- Complications—pneumonia, secondary bacterial infection, pneumothorax, diaphragmatic rupture, surgical emphysema, neurological deficits secondary to hypoxia.

Diagnosis

- Laboratory confirmation is usually delayed. Diagnosis should be made clinically.
- General—leucocytosis is associated with an increased risk of death; CXR may be normal or show peribronchial thickening, consolidation (secondary bacterial infection, rarely pertussis pneumonia), pneumothorax, pneumomediastinum, or air in soft tissues.
- Microbiological culture—requires special media (e.g. Regan–Lowe or Bordet–Gengou agar). Culture specimens are best obtained by flexible swab or deep nasopharyngeal aspirate (NPA) during the catarrhal or early paroxysmal phase. Culture for 7 days. Usually negative in those previously immunized or given antibiotics.
- Serology is useful to confirm the diagnosis retrospectively. PCR-based tests are available.

Management

- General—supportive care is the mainstay. Consider admitting patients at risk of severe disease and complications plus those younger than 3 months or 3–6 months with severe paroxysms; 50% of infants require hospitalization. Infection control measures should be taken for those patients in the contagious phase of the disease.
- Antimicrobial therapy—erythromycin given early in the catarrhal phase shortens the duration of the paroxysmal stage. Once cough is established, antimicrobial agents do not alter the course of the illness but serve to limit the spread of disease. Treatment duration—14 days. Patients should be isolated. Consider treating close contacts of pertussis cases (including children and staff at day centres) who are particularly vulnerable, unvaccinated, partially vaccinated, or under 5 years of age.
- Other agents—there is no evidence for any benefit from corticosteroids or $\beta 2$-adrenergic agents. Pertussis-specific immunoglobulin is an experimental therapy that may be effective in decreasing paroxysms of cough.

Prevention

- There is no transfer of protective maternal antibody, even from mothers with a documented history of infection or vaccination. Nearly all cases of fatal pertussis in developed countries occur in infants too young to be immunized.
- Vaccination is recommended for all babies at 2, 3, and 4 months, as part of the diphtheria, tetanus, polio (DTP) vaccine. It may not prevent the illness entirely but lessens disease severity and duration. In the UK and many other countries, vaccination is offered to pregnant women, with the aim of reducing the risk of exposure for babies until their vaccination. Similarly, children are given boosters at 3–4 (UK) or 11–12 (USA) years of age, with the aim of reducing transmission to pre-vaccination infants.

Other common causes of bacterial infection in childhood

- Bacterial meningitis, including *Neisseria meningitidis* (◐ see Bacterial meningitis, pp. 764–8).

- Bacterial causes of pneumonia (➡ see Community-acquired pneumonia, pp. 649–53).
- Infectious diarrhoea (➡ see Infectious diarrhoea, pp. 691–3).
- UTIs (➡ see Urinary tract infections, Introduction, pp. 724–5).
- Upper respiratory tract infections (➡ See Group A Streptococcus (p. 280), Moraxella (p. 314), Haemophilus (p. 339), Bordetella (p. 345), and Atypical pneumonia (p. 653)).
- Superficial bacterial infections of the skin (e.g. erysipelas) (➡ see Skin and soft tissue infections: introduction, pp. 802–3).

Immunodeficiency

Primary immunodeficiency

Primary immunodeficiencies are a rare and heterogeneous group of disorders. They can arise from either a single-gene mutation (normally X-linked or autosomal recessive) or from a genetic susceptibility combined with environmental factors. New genetic mutations are consistently described. They typically present in childhood, although they can be diagnosed later in life.

Classification

Primary immunodeficiencies can affect either the innate immune system (including phagocyte disorders and complement defects) or the adaptive immune system (B- and/or T-cell deficiencies).

Epidemiology

Primary immunodeficiency is rare, with an estimated 5000 people living with the condition in the UK. However, the effects can be serious, and often life-threatening, requiring expensive medical interventions and lifelong treatments.

Severe antibody deficiency is the commonest serious disease and occurs in fewer than 16 per million births; other primary immunodeficiency syndromes are even less frequent. Partial antibody deficiency syndromes are reported to occur in 1 in 700 Caucasians, although most will remain healthy and often undiagnosed.

Screening

Screening is not currently undertaken in the UK, despite years of campaigning by patient groups. Some other countries, including at least 48 states in the USA, screen for severe combined immunodeficiency disease (SCID).

Infections associated with different immunodeficiencies

(See Table 24.1.)

Antibody deficiency syndromes

X-linked agammaglobulinaemia

Presents from 6 to 9 months (as maternal antibody wanes) but can be diagnosed later. Recurrent respiratory infections and an absence of tonsils are typical. Diagnosis is by low/absent levels of antibody and <2% of CD19 B cells. Mutation in Bruton's tyrosine kinase (BTK) is the commonest cause and can be tested for, but other genetic mutations resulting in failed development of B cells are seen. Treatment is with intravenous immunoglobulin (IVIG) (typically 3- to 4-weekly), and aggressive treatment with antibiotics if infection occurs. Prognosis is good.

Common variable immunodeficiency

Often diagnosed in the second or third decade, presenting with either increased infections or non-infectious sequelae (e.g. autoimmune disease). Lymphadenopathy and splenomegaly are common. Heterozygous disease and a specific mutation are often not identified. Can only be diagnosed >4 years and after exclusion of other causes. Low levels of immunoglobulin G (IgG) with low immunoglobulin A (IgA) or immunoglobulin M (IgM) are seen, and definitive diagnosis is by lack of specific antibody response (e.g.

Table 24.1 Infections associated with different immunodeficiencies

	Antibody deficiency syndromes	Selective T-cell deficiencies	Complement deficiencies	Chronic granulomatous disease
Clinical presentations	Respiratory tract infections, sinusitis, meningitis, osteomyelitis	Intracellular pathogens and opportunistic infections	Respiratory tract infections	Skin infections, liver abscess
Common bacterial pathogens	Encapsulated: *Haemophilus influenzae*, *Streptococcus pneumoniae*		Encapsulated, especially *Neisseria*	*Staphylococcus aureus* *Serratia marcescens* *Burkholderia cepacia*
Atypical bacterial pathogens	*Mycoplasma* *Ureaplasma* *Campylobacter jejuni* *Giardia lamblia*	*Mycobacterium* *Salmonella*		*Nocardia* Mycobacteria
Viral pathogens	Enterovirus Rhinovirus (NOT other viruses)	Herpesviruses Adenovirus Papillomavirus Rotavirus		
Fungi, protozoa, and helminths		*Cryptococcus neoformans* *Candida* *Aspergillus* *Toxoplasma gondii* *Pneumocystis jirovecii* *Cryptosporidium* *Strongyloides*		*Aspergillus*

to vaccination). Treatment is with IVIG, but patients will often still have infections requiring prompt antibiotic treatment and prophylaxis may be required.

Thymoma with hypogammaglobulinaemia (Good syndrome)

Similar to common variable immunodeficiency (CVID), although additional opportunistic infections with *Candida*, herpes simplex virus (HSV), varicella-zoster virus (VZV), PCP, and cytomegalovirus (CMV) are seen. Thymectomy should be performed, although immunity does not return to normal subsequently. Treatment is similar to that for CVID, although prognosis is poorer.

Transient hypogammaglobulinaemia of infancy

Considered a normal variant and is often self-limiting within the first few years of life. Children may have increased infections, although typically invasive infections are not seen. It is a diagnosis of exclusion. Total IgG level may be low, although specific antibodies are present. IVIG can be considered, but often no treatment is required.

Selective IgA deficiency

Commoner (up to 1 in 300), but often asymptomatic or mild. Symptoms are thought to be restricted to individuals who cannot produce mucosal IgA. Can present with respiratory or GI infection and some association with autoimmunity (e.g. rheumatoid arthritis, coeliac disease, malignancy). Many drugs can give a similar picture (e.g. anti-epileptics, gold, sulfasalazine, hydroxychloroquine, NSAIDs). Can progress to CVID, so monitoring should occur. No specific treatment required, although prophylactic antibiotics can be considered.

IgG subclass deficiencies

Diagnosis comprises a history of infections, normal total IgG, IgA, and IgM levels, and one or more subclasses of IgG lower than the fifth percentile on more than one occasion. Associated with atopy, autoimmune disease, and trisomy 21, but not malignancy. IgG1 comprises 60% of total IgG, so deficiency normally results in hypogammaglobulinaemia. IgG4 is present in low levels until the age of 10, so it should not be diagnosed in young children. IVIG can be considered judiciously, and patients may benefit from additional doses of pneumococcal vaccination.

Selective IgM deficiency

Rare deficiency in IgM alone. Increase in infections caused by bacteria, viruses, fungi, and protozoa. Associated with autoimmune diseases, as well as haematological conditions and malignancy. IVIG may be useful.

Specific antibody deficiency

Normal levels of total IgG, IgA, IgM, and IgG subclasses, but abnormal IgG response to polysaccharide vaccines (response to protein antigen and conjugated vaccines is unaffected). If associated with increased respiratory infections, additional pneumococcal vaccination and, rarely, IVIG can be considered.

Selective T-cell deficiencies

Di George syndrome

Triad of cardiac anomalies, hypoplastic thymus, and hypocalcaemia (from parathyroid hypoplasia), associated with facial anomalies. Most commonly associated with deletion on chromosome 22 (22q11.2). Lack of thymic tissue prevents positive or negative selection of T cells for maturation. Immunodeficiency can range from partial (naïve T-cell count >50 cells/microlitre) to complete, which can present similarly to SCID with a high risk of fatal opportunistic infection. FBC shows lymphopenia (which can be confirmed by flow cytometry), and a lack of thymus can be seen on CXR. Treatment for complete di George syndrome is with thymic transplant, but mortality rates remain high. In partial cases, immune function tends to improve with time.

Ataxia telangiectasia

Autosomal recessive, with gradual presentation in childhood. Along with cerebellar ataxia, nystagmus, and telangiectasia, T-cell counts fall and the thymus becomes hypoplastic. Progresses to leukaemia/lymphoma, which is often fatal.

Chronic mucocutaneous candidiasis

Either autosomal recessive or dominant, due to failure of T cells to respond to *Candida* antigens. No increased susceptibility to other infections.

Combined B- and T-cell disorders

Severe combined immunodeficiency (SCID)

Presents in the first weeks of life with failure to thrive, chronic diarrhea, hepatosplenomegaly, and infections, in particular candidiasis, *Pneumocystis* pneumonia (PCP), and aspergillosis. CMV and Epstein–Barr virus (EBV) can be particularly severe, and live vaccines (especially bacille Calmette–Guérin (BCG)) can lead to disseminated disease. Graft-versus-host disease (GVHD) can occur from maternal lymphocytes proliferating in the fetal blood or from blood transfusion with non-irradiated blood, which is often fatal. Lymphopenia is often present (a count of $<2.8 \times 10^9$/L should prompt immunodeficiency screening), although the lymphocyte count may be normal in B-cell variants or in GVHD. T-cell subsets should be requested and immunoglobulin levels will be low.

There are over 50 genetic mutations identified, which result in defective development of T cells ± B cells (see Table 24.2). Rather than preventing cell development, adenosine deaminase (ADA) deficiency results in cell damage due to build-up of toxic metabolites. Purine nucleoside phosphorylase (PNP) deficiency results in gradual loss of mature T cells, as well as in neurological symptoms (developmental delay, spasticity, ataxia, and pyramidal signs).

Protective isolation is vital to preventing infection, either in hospital or at home if suitable. Treatment comprises prophylaxis with trimethoprim–sulfamethoxazole for PCP, fluconazole as an antifungal, and aciclovir against HSV infection. Palivizumab should be considered in respiratory syncytial virus (RSV) season. IVIG can be given when maternal antibodies wane. All live vaccines should be avoided and blood products should be irradiated, leucocyte-depleted, and CMV-negative. Breastfeeding should be stopped, pending CMV testing on the mother. Haematopoietic stem cell

Table 24.2 Genetic mutations in severe combined immunodeficiency affecting development of T and B cells

Mutation/deficiency	Frequency (%)	Inheritance	Cells affected
IL-2R common γ chain	50	X-linked	T and NK
JAK-3	10	AR	T and NK
RAG1 or 2	10	AR	T and B
DCLRE1C (Artemis)	10	AR	T and B
ADA deficiency	10–20	AR	T, B, and NK
PNP deficiency	<1	AR	Progressive loss of T cells

ADA, adenosine deaminase; AR, autosomal recessive; IL-2R, interleukin 2 receptor; NK, natural killer; PNP, purine nucleoside phosphorylase.

transplantation (HSCT) is the definitive treatment, although gene therapies are being developed and may be promising.

X-linked immune deficiency with associated hyper-IgM

Abnormal expression CD40 T-cell ligand prevents antibody class switching from IgM to IgG (also to IgA and IgE). Pyogenic infections, PCP, and *Cryptosporidium* infection are common. IVIG is effective, although HSCT is curative.

Disorders of the innate immune system

Chronic granulomatous disease (CGD)

Phagocytes are unable to produce superoxide due to mutations in nicotinamide adenine dinucleotide phosphate (NADPH) oxidase genes (the commonest being X-linked mutation in the gp91phox subunit). Diagnosis is by the dihydrorhodamine assay. Lifelong prophylaxis with trimethoprim–sulfamethoxazole and itraconazole has dramatically increased survival. γ Interferon gamma-1b and HSCT may have a role.

Leucocyte adhesion deficiency (LAD)

Neutrophils are unable to leave the vasculature to act in infected tissues, resulting in impaired ability to form abscesses. Presents with late umbilical cord separation, periodontal disease, and *Staphylococcus aureus* infection. Leucocyte counts can be elevated (cannot leave the circulation) and it can be fatal without HSCT.

Complement deficiency

Rare conditions causing bacterial infections (due to reduced lysis, opsonization and phagocytosis of bacteria) as well as autoimmune conditions. C2 deficiency is the best described, resulting in recurrent respiratory and sinus infections. Approximately 10% of patients also have systemic lupus erythematous. All pathways converge on C3, so a defect here results in the greatest risk of infection. Terminal pathway (C5 to C9) deficiencies lead to greatly increased risk of *Neisseria* spp. infection.

Further resources

British Society for Immunology (2017). *Immunodeficiency*. Available at: ℘ https://www.immunology. org/policy-and-public-affairs/briefings-and-position-statements/immunodeficiency

Darian T, Freij JB, Seth D, Poowuttiku P, Secord E (2020). *A review of primary immune deficiency disorders*. Available at: ℘ https://www.emjreviews.com/allergy-immunology/article/a-review-of-primary-immune-deficiency-disorders/

Secondary immunodeficiency

Secondary immunodeficiency is impairment of a patient's immune response, resulting from factors or conditions extrinsic to the immune system. It can be either transient or permanent. Different causes can affect either primarily humoral or cell-mediated immunity (CMI).

Important causes and their effects can be seen in Table 24.3.

Assessment

Clinical history should be thorough, especially relating to the pattern, type, and frequency of infections. Concurrent medical issues and any medications are important. Blood tests to consider include: FBC, lymphocyte phenotyping (neutrophils; T, B, and natural killer (NK) cells), serum immunoglobulins, antibody response to previous vaccinations, and albumin and total protein levels.

Table 24.3 Important causes of secondary immunodeficiency

Cause	Examples	Description
Infections	HIV	Depleted CD4 cells
	Measles virus	Depleted T and B cells
	Mycobacteria	Depletion of antigen-presenting cells Increased interferon-γ
	Influenza	Reduced activity of neutrophils
Malignancy	Chronic lymphocytic leukaemia	Hypogammaglobulinaemia Altered phagocyte and NK function
	Myeloma	Reduced T cells Hypogammaglobulinaemia

(Continued)

Table 24.3 (Contd.)

Cause	Examples	Description
Drugs	Glucocorticoids	Reduced cell-mediated immunity (T cells and phagocytes)
	Tacrolimus Ciclosporin	Reduced T-cell function
	Methotrexate Cyclophosphamide Azathioprine Mycophenolate	Inhibited T- and B-cell proliferation
	Bleomycin Vincristine Cisplatin	Neutropenia
	JAK inhibitors	Impaired T- and B-cell proliferation
	Anti-B-cell therapy (anti-CD20, etc.)	B-cell lymphopenia Hypogammaglobulinaemia
	IL-1 inhibitor	Decreased T- and B-cell activity
	IL-6 inhibitor	Decreased innate and adaptive immunity
	TNF-α inhibitors	Downregulate cytokines
Metabolic	Diabetes mellitus	Reduced neutrophil function
	Renal failure	Impaired innate and adaptive immunity
	Nephrotic syndrome Protein-losing enteropathy	Hypogammaglobulinaemia
Malnutrition	Zinc deficiency	Prevents T-cell maturation
	Vitamin A deficiency	Reduced CD4 and CD8 cells
Surgery	Splenectomy	Reduced innate immunity
	Trauma Burns	Persistent rise in inflammatory cytokine levels resulting in immunosuppression
Extremes of age	Prematurity	Reduced migration of neutrophils Immature B-cell response
	Old age	Decreased antigen-specific cellular immunity
Environmental factors	Stress	Non-specific immune activation
	Radiation	Reduced blood cell lineages

IL, interleukin; NK, natural killer; TNF, tumour necrosis factor.

Management principles

The first step is to remove, or improve, the primary condition or environmental factor. General measures include reducing exposure to infections, immunizations, antibiotic prophylaxis, and immunoglobulin replacement.

Infections in asplenic patients

The spleen plays a vital role in protecting the body from infections by activating the adaptive immune response. Asplenia may be congenital but is more often acquired (traumatic or surgical). Hyposplenia or functional asplenia can result from sickle-cell disease, coeliac disease, haemoglobinopathies, allogeneic bone marrow transplant (BMT), untreated HIV infection, and autoimmune disease. Asplenia or hyposplenia results in an increased risk of severe and overwhelming infection, with a high mortality rate.

Pathogens

- Encapsulated organisms: *Streptococcus pneumoniae*, *Haemophilus influenzae*, *Neisseria meningitidis*.
- Other bacteria: *Capnocytophaga canimorsis*, *Bartonella*, *Bordetella*, *Salmonella*.
- Intracellular protozoa: *Plasmodium falciparum*, *Babesia*, *Ehrlichia*.
- CMV.

Clinical features

- The highest risk of post-splenectomy sepsis (PSS) is in the first 3 years, but it may occur many years later.
- PSS has a short prodrome with fever, chills, pharyngitis, muscle aches, vomiting, and diarrhoea.
- In adults, there is usually no obvious site of infection, whereas in children, meningitis is common.
- Deterioration is usually rapid and occurs over hours with septic shock, disseminated intravascular coagulopathy (DIC), seizures, and coma.

Management

- Asplenic patients should be given a supply of antibiotics for self-administration at the first sign of serious illness.
- If the patient presents acutely with PSS, they should receive immediate treatment with IV antibiotics (e.g. ceftriaxone plus vancomycin).[1]

Prevention

- Prophylactic antibiotics—PO phenoxymethylpenicillin should be given to patients with an absent or dysfunctional spleen. It should be given at least for the first 3 years and is often recommended to be lifelong.
- Ensure all vaccinations are up to date, according to the national schedule. Additional vaccinations against *N. meningitidis* (group B and ACWY), *S. pneumoniae* (repeated every 5 years), and influenza (yearly) are advised. See UK Health Security Agency (UKHSA) guidance in the *Green Book* (available at: https://www.gov.uk/government/collecti ons/immunisation-against-infectious-disease-the-green-book).

Neutropenic sepsis

Neutropenia is associated with an increased risk of bacteraemia and severe infection. Although neutropenia is defined as an absolute neutrophil count of $<0.5 \times 10^9$ cells/L, many experts believe that the risk of infection increases when the neutrophil count falls below 1×10^9 cells/L. Febrile neutropenia occurs in around 8 in 1000 patients receiving chemotherapy. It is a medical emergency, and appropriate antimicrobial therapy should be started immediately.

Clinical features

- In immunocompromised patients, localizing signs and symptoms of infection may be absent.
- Fever (>38°C) may be the only clinical feature.
- Even fever may be absent, and patients who are generally unwell should be assessed.
- Typically occurs 5–7 days following cytotoxic chemotherapy.

Aetiology

- Often no microbiological pathogen is found; bacteraemia is documented in only 10–15% of neutropenic fever episodes.
- Gram-positive pathogens predominate, probably related to the use of long-term vascular access devices.
- Gram-negative pathogens, including *Pseudomonas aeruginosa*, are also seen, although rates have dropped since the recommendation for antimicrobial prophylaxis.

Patient evaluation

The following factors should be considered:
- underlying disease and any recent chemotherapy;
- previous history of infections and risk of drug-resistant organisms;
- comorbidities;
- non-infectious causes of fever (e.g. blood transfusion, disease progression);
- symptoms—fever, organ-specific symptoms;
- examination—skin and mucous membranes, inferior vena cava (IVC) sites, lungs, abdomen, ear, nose, and throat (ENT), perianal region, sinuses;
- investigations—FBC, biochemistry, lactate, urinalysis, blood cultures (central and peripheral), other cultures (e.g. urine, faecal samples, swabs, sputum, CSF, as clinically indicated), serum fungal markers such as galactomannan and β-D glucan (in high-risk patients);
- imaging—CXR in low-risk patients and CT chest in high-risk patients;
- risk stratification—scores such as the Multinational Association for Supportive Care in Cancer (MASCC) Risk Index[1] can be used to identify low-risk patients.

Management

- Broad-spectrum antimicrobial therapy with pseudomonal cover (e.g. piperacillin–tazobactam) should be started as soon as possible, and certainly within 60 minutes of presentation.

- Antistaphylococcal cover (e.g. vancomycin) may be added if there is a high-risk of vascular access infection or the patient is critically unwell.
- Combination therapy with aminoglycosides is not recommended, unless there are specific microbiological indications.
- Consult local guidelines for penicillin-allergic patients. Alternative regimens include vancomycin and aztreonam or ciprofloxacin and clindamycin.
- Empirical antifungal agents can be considered in high-risk patients with no response after 4–7 days. Investigations should include fungal biomarkers and CT chest imaging as a minimum. Agents must cover *Aspergillus*.
- Colony-stimulating factors are not recommended routinely but may be used in particular instances.
- Patients should be examined daily, and persistent/recurrent fever should prompt a search for occult infection.
- Therapy should continue until there is a good clinical response (e.g. resolution of fever) or a non-infectious cause of fever is suspected.

Outcomes

The incidence of neutropenic sepsis is rising, due to the increased use of anti-cancer treatments. Although mortality is declining, it remains significant, with an in-hospital mortality of 10%. This rises to 18% in patients with Gram-negative bacteraemia, and to 40% in highest-risk patients, when using the MASCC Risk Index score.

Prevention

Guidelines from the National Institute for Health and Care Excellence (NICE) recommend consideration of fluoroquinolone prophylaxis in patients at high risk of profound, prolonged neutropenia ($<0.1 \times 10^9$ cells/L for >7 days) for the duration of the risk period.[2]

References

1 Klastersky J, Paesmans M, Rubenstein EB, *et al*. The Multinational Association for Supportive Care in Cancer risk index: a multinational scoring system for identifying low-risk febrile neutropenic cancer patients. *J Clin Oncol*. 2000;**18**:3038–51.

2 National Institute for Health and Care Excellence (2012). *Neutropenic sepsis: prevention and management in people with cancer*. Clinical guideline [CG151]. Available at: ℞ https://www.nice.org.uk/guidance/cg151

Infections in transplant recipients

Outcomes from organ transplantation continue to improve due to better surgical techniques and advances in immunosuppressive regimens. However, infections remain a significant cause of mortality, with deaths from infection varying from 13% in patients with kidney transplant to 50% in those with liver transplant.

Risk factors

The risk of infection at any time results from a combination of epidemiological exposures of both the patient and the donor, combined with the

patient's net state of immunosuppression. Factors contributing to a patient's immunosuppressive state include:
- immunosuppressive therapy (type, intensity);
- comorbidities—diabetes, organ dysfunction, malnutrition, extremes of age;
- technical features relating to transplant surgery;
- use of broad-spectrum antimicrobials;
- breaks in mucosal defences;
- GVHD.

Pre-transplantation screening

A detailed history should be taken to assess the risk of infectious diseases (as well as other factors) before a HSCT donation, to include lifestyle factors and medical and travel history, as no screening tests are 100% sensitive or specific.

Specific screening tests will vary by type of transplant and transplant centre but, in general, will include screening for:
- hepatitis B and C;
- HIV, and sometimes human T-cell lymphotropic virus (HTLV);
- EBV and CMV;
- syphilis;
- *Toxoplasma*;
- sometimes VZV and HSV;
- consideration of malaria, *Trypanosoma cruzi*, coccidioidomycosis, schistosomiasis, *Strongyloides*, West Nile virus, and Chagas' disease based on the travel history;
- CXR and interferon-γ release assay (IGRA) for *Mycobacterium tuberculosis* if high risk.

Solid-organ transplantation

The frequency of infection and specific pathogens tend to follow a predictable time frame following transplantation. An outline of typical infections and their time points is given in Table 24.4.

Haemopoietic stem cell transplantation

The risk of infection varies (see Table 24.5) with:
- patient-related factors—age, comorbidities, frailty;
- disease-related factors—underlying disease requiring HSCT and immunosuppressive treatment used prior to transplant;
- transplant-related factors—type of graft (e.g. allogeneic transplant has a higher risk of infection than autologous transplant), type of conditioning chemotherapy, human leucocyte antigen (HLA) match, ongoing immunosuppression.

Post-transplantation management

Detailed assessment for early signs of infection in the post-transplant period is vital, and symptoms, clinical observations, and blood tests should be monitored closely. Fever or suspicion of infection should be thoroughly investigated. Specific considerations in the post-transplant period include:
- **infection control**—high-risk patients (allogeneic HSCT, prolonged neutropenia) should be treated in positive pressure rooms, with >12 air

Table 24.4 Infection timelines after transplantation of solid organs

	Infection type	Examples
First 30 days	Health-care associated bacterial infections (consider drug-resistant organisms)	Hospital-acquired pneumonia, central line infection, *Clostridioides difficile*, surgical site infections, UTI
	Donor-transmitted infections	*Candida* (most commonly) or other fungi Viral (e.g. viral hepatitis, HIV, CMV) Bacterial (e.g. *Mycobacterium tuberculosis* or from donor bacteraemia)
30–180 days	Opportunistic infections*	*Pneumocystis jirovecii* Fungi *Toxoplasma gondii* *Nocardia*
	Viral infections	CMV** Herpesviruses Viral hepatitis BK virus Respiratory viruses
	GI parasites	*Cryptosporidium* *Microsporidium*
Over 6 months	Typical community-acquired infections	
	Herpesvirus infections	Herpes zoster- and EBV-related lymphoproliferative syndrome

* Trimethoprim–sulfamethoxazole prophylaxis has decreased the incidence of both *P. jirovecii* and *T. gondii* infections.

** Due to routine use of anti-CMV prophylaxis, CMV disease now often occurs later, after prophylaxis is ceased.

CMV, cytomegalovirus; EBV, Epstein–Barr virus; UTI, urinary tract infection.

Table 24.5 Risk factors for infections associated with haematopoietic stem cell transplantation

	Immunology/risk factors	Typical pathogens
Pre-engraftment period	Prolonged neutropenia Breaks in mucocutaneous barrier	Gram-negative and positive bacteraemia HSV reactivations Respiratory viruses *Candida* *Aspergillus* Rare fungi (e.g. *Fusarium*)
First 100 days post-engraftment	Impaired cell-mediated immunity	Herpesviruses (especially CMV) Adenovirus *Pneumocystis jirovecii* *Aspergillus*
Late period (over 100 days)	B- and T-cell function continues to recover (takes longer in allogeneic transplant or if GVHD) Phagocytic cell defects may persist	CMV VZV EBV-related lymphoproliferative syndrome Respiratory viruses Encapsulated bacteria Parvovirus BK/JC virus

CMV, cytomegalovirus; EBV, Epstein–Barr virus; GVHD, graft-versus-host disease; HSV, herpes simplex virus; VZV, varicella-zoster virus.

exchanges per hour and point-of-use high-efficiency (>99%) particulate air (HEPA) filters (➲ see Chapter 6);

- **multidrug-resistant pathogens**—common, and cultures should be sent regularly to guide optimal therapy;
- **inflammatory markers**—CRP may be non-specifically raised, and some centres will use alternative tests (e.g. procalcitonin);
- **molecular tests**—preferred for many viral pathogens (e.g. adenovirus, EBV, CMV) due to unreliability of serology;
- **antigen tests**—(beta-D-glucan, galactomannan) can be used to screen for fungal infections (although beware low sensitivity); imaging and tissue diagnostics are critical in fungal disease.

Prevention of infection

- Prophylactic antimicrobials are commonly used (e.g. ganciclovir for CMV, aciclovir for HSV, fluconazole for candidiasis, and trimethoprim–sulfamethoxazole for PCP). Protocols differ across centres.

- Post-HSCT patients should be viewed as 'never vaccinated', and repeat immunizations (including childhood vaccinations) should be considered in line with local protocols.
- In solid-organ transplantation, immunizations can be given prior to transplantation; specific additional vaccinations include influenza, pneumococcal, and hepatitis B.
- In both HSCT and solid-organ transplantation, live vaccinations should be avoided and only be given if benefit outweighs risk.
- Blood products—red blood cells, platelets, and plasma products should be leucocyte-depleted (to reduce the risk of CMV infection) and irradiated (to reduce transfusion-associated GVHD). In allo-HSCT, products must be ABO-matched to both donor and recipient.
- Food hygiene—HSCT patients should avoid undercooked meat, eggs, and shellfish.
- Detailed advice should be given about travel to areas with high-risk endemic diseases, and safe sex practices should be highlighted.
- Chimeric antigen receptor T-cell (CAR-T) therapy. This new therapy involves reprogramming the patient's own immune system cells, which are then used to target their cancer. It is highly complex and may cure some patients with B-cell acute lymphoblastic leukaemia (B-ALL). Side effects include cytokine release syndrome (CRS), neurotoxicities, cytopenia, hypogammaglobulinaemia, and increased risk of infection. Seek expert input.

Further reading

Centers for Disease Control and Prevention (2000). *Guidelines for preventing opportunistic infections among hematopoietic stem cell transplant recipients* Available at ⌖ https://www.cdc.gov/mmwr/preview/mmwrhtml/rr4910a1.htm

Dykewicz CA; Centers for Disease Control and Prevention (US), Infectious Diseases Society of America, American Society of Blood and Marrow Transplantation. Summary of the guidelines for preventing opportunistic infections among hematopoietic stem cell transplant recipients. *Clin Infect Dis.* 2001;**33**:139–44.

Health protection

Immunizations

Routine childhood immunizations

All children in the UK are entitled to free immunizations to protect them from childhood illnesses. The introduction of immunization has resulted in dramatic declines in certain diseases (e.g. meningitis caused by *Haemophilus influenzae* type b and *Neisseria meningitidis* serogroup C). Routine childhood immunization schedules vary from country to country. The UK routine immunization schedule is summarized in Table 25.1.

Table 25.1 Routine immunization schedule

Child's age	Vaccine(s) given	Diseases protected against
2 months	DTaP/IPV/Hib/hep B, PCV*, rotavirus (oral), MenB	Diphtheria, tetanus, pertussis, polio, *Haemophilus influenzae* type b, hepatitis B, rotavirus, meningococcal B
3 months	DTaP/IPV/Hib/hep B, rotavirus (oral), PCV13*	Diphtheria, tetanus, pertussis, polio, *H. influenzae* type b, hepatitis B, rotavirus, pneumococcal infection
4 months	DTaP/IPV/Hib/hep B, MenB	Diphtheria, tetanus, pertussis, polio, *H. influenzae* type b, hepatitis B, meningococcal B
12–13 months	Hib/MenC, PCV13, MMR, MenB	*H. influenzae* type b, meningococcal C, pneumococcal infection, measles, mumps, and rubella, meningococcal B
2, 3, and 4 years	Flu (annually)	Influenza
3 years and 4 months	DTaP/IPV, MMR	Diphtheria, tetanus, pertussis, polio, measles, mumps, and rubella
12–13 years	HPV (two injections)	Cervical, oral, throat, and anal cancers caused by HPV types 16 and 18
14–18 years	Td/IPV / MenACWY	Diphtheria, tetanus, polio / Meningococcal types A, C, W, and Y
50 and over	Flu (annually)	Influenza
65 years	PPV	Pneumococcal infection
70 years	Shingles vaccine	Shingles

* There are three types of pneumococcal vaccines: PPV23 (polysaccharide), PCV13 (conjugate), and PCV10 (conjugate).

Non-routine immunizations

Some children who may be at increased risk of certain diseases (e.g. tuber-culosis) may be given additional vaccines, as may those in other risk groups. The indications shown in Table 25.2 are not exhaustive, and full guidelines can be found in the UK *Green Book*. For up-to-date vaccination schedules against severe acute respiratory syndrome coronavirus 2 (SARS-CoV-2), see UK Health Security Agency (UKHSA) website.

Vaccinations in those infected with HIV

HIV-infected adults who are susceptible on serological screening should be considered for vaccination against hepatitis B, measles/mumps/rubella (if CD4 count >200), and varicella (if CD4 count >200). The pneumococcus vaccine should be given once, and the influenza vaccine annually.

Inactivated vaccines may be used safely in all HIV-infected adults, if re-quired. These include cholera WC/rBS, hepatitis A and B, *H. influenzae*, parenteral influenza, meningitis C and ACWY, pneumococcus PPV23, ra-bies, Td/IPV (tetanus, diphtheria, parenteral polio), and typhoid ViCPS. Certain live vaccines are contraindicated in all HIV patients, regardless of the CD4 count. These include cholera CVD103-HgR, intranasal influ-enza, oral poliovirus vaccine (OPV), typhoid Ty2´a, and bacille Calmette–Guérin (BCG).

Table 25.2 Indications and vaccines for at-risk groups

Recipient	Vaccine	Diseases protected against
At birth, for babies who are more likely to be exposed to TB	BCG	TB
Individuals with an absent or dysfunctional spleen (e.g. sickle cell disease, coeliac disease)	Pneumococcal vaccination*, Men B, Men ACWY	Pneumococcal infection, meningococcal types B, A, C, W, and Y
PWIDs, MSM, anyone receiving regular transfusions of blood products, sex workers, medical staff, etc.	Hep B	Hepatitis B
Those in close contact with the immunocompromised (e.g. children of a patient undergoing chemotherapy)	Varicella	Chickenpox
Pregnancy	Influenza during flu seasons	Influenza
	Pertussis from 16 weeks pregnant	Whooping cough

BCG, bacille Calmette–Guérin; MSM, men who have sex with men; PWID, people who inject drugs; TB, tuberculosis.

Further reading

British HIV Association (2015). *British HIV Association guidelines on the use of vaccines in HIV-positive adults 2015*. Available at: ℘ https://www.bhiva.org/file/NriBJHDVKGwzZ/2015-Vaccination-Guidelines.pdf

NHS (2023). *NHS vaccination and when to have them*. Available at: ℘ https://www.nhs.uk/conditions/vaccinations/nhs-vaccinations-and-when-to-have-them/

UK Health Security Agency (2013). *Immunisation against infectious disease (the Green Book)*. Available at: ℘ https://www.gov.uk/government/collections/immunisation-against-infectious-disease-the-green-book

Notifiable diseases

- The statutory requirement for the notification of certain infectious diseases (e.g. cholera, diphtheria, smallpox, typhoid) started towards the end of the nineteenth century.
- Originally, the head of the family or landlord had the responsibility of reporting the disease to the local authority 'Proper Officer'; the attending medical practitioner now does this.
- The prime purpose of the notification system is to detect possible outbreaks or epidemics. Accuracy of diagnosis is secondary, and a clinical suspicion of a notifiable infection is all that is required. If a diagnosis later proves incorrect, it can always be changed or cancelled.
- Doctors in England and Wales have a duty to notify the Proper Officer of suspected cases of diseases shown in Table 25.3. They should not wait for laboratory confirmation. The notification certificate should be sent within 3 days or verbally within 24h for urgent cases. Requirements differ slightly for Scotland (exclude some of the diseases shown in Table 25.3, but specifically include *Escherichia coli* O157, meningococcal infection, *H. influenzae* type b, necrotizing fasciitis, and tularaemia).

Table 25.3 Notifiable diseases

Acute encephalitis	Malaria
Acute infectious hepatitis	Measles
Acute meningitis	Meningococcal sepsis
	Monkeypox
Acute polio	Mumps
Anthrax	Plague
Botulism	Rabies
Brucellosis	Rubella
Cholera	Severe acute respiratory syndrome (SARS)
Covid-19*	
Diphtheria	Scarlet fever
Enteric fever (typhoid/paratyphoid)	Smallpox
Food poisoning	Tetanus

Table 25.3 *(Contd.)*

Haemolytic uraemic syndrome	Tuberculosis
Infectious bloody diarrhoea	Typhus
Invasive group A *Streptococcus*	Viral haemorrhagic fever
Legionnaire's disease	Whooping cough
Leprosy	Yellow fever

Note that individual notifiable diseases may vary by region; check with the UK Health Security Agency.

See ℘ https://www.gov.uk/guidance/notifiable-diseases-and-causative-organisms-how-to-report

* Since 1.4.22 only cases of COVID-19 due to either deliberately working with the virus (e.g. in a laboratory) or being incidentally exposed to the virus from working in environments where people are known to have COVID-19 (e.g. in health and social care) are reportable.

Bioterrorism

Biological warfare has a long and unpleasant history. Around 400 BC, the Scythians were attempting to poison their arrows with blood and manure, and in the fourteenth century, the Tartar catapulted the corpses of plague victims into the city of Kaffa, with the intention of initiating an outbreak. The years after the Second World War saw a race to develop more effective biological agents, before various treaties later led to the limitation, and even destruction, of biological weapon stockpiles by many nations (UK 1957, USA 1973). Today, around 17 countries are suspected of having biological weapon programmes. The threat of biological warfare is seen as issuing not primarily from states, but from independent organizations and terrorists. The term 'deliberate release' refers to any intentional spread of a biological or chemical agent. Such a release may be **overt** (e.g. a prior warning or the release may be apparent, either due to the use of an explosive device or because a suspicious substance is obviously visible) or **covert** (the release not becoming apparent until the first cases of disease arise). Only two proven deliberate releases have recently affected a large number of people: contamination of restaurant salads with *Salmonella typhimurium* in Oregon in 1984 and dissemination of *Bacillus anthracis* via the US mail in 2001.

Organisms with the potential to be used as weapons agents

The ideal biological weapon agent has low visibility and high potency, is accessible with a long shelf life, is relatively easy to deliver, and shows limited epidemic spread. A small amount of the agent may be capable of killing a large number of people (particularly in a metropolitan environment) and creating a disproportionate level of fear and disruption—a key part of their attractiveness to terrorist organizations.

- Category A agents—those organisms are easily disseminated or transmitted from person to person, with high mortality rates and the potential for major public health impact and requiring special action for public health readiness:
  - anthrax (➜ see *Bacillus anthracis*, pp. 291–3)—pulmonary anthrax presents with severe febrile illness or sepsis with respiratory failure (massive mediastinal lymphadenopathy). The organism may be identified in blood cultures or the sputum;
  - smallpox (➜ see Poxviruses, pp. 435–7)—the previously vaccinated lose protection after 10–20 years. Vaccination provides moderate protection if given within 2–4 days of exposure. Disease may develop 1–3 weeks after exposure;
  - botulism (➜ see *Clostridium botulinum*, pp. 301–3)—toxin may be inhaled or food-borne; anti-toxin is available;
  - plague (➜ see *Yersinia pestis*, pp. 349–50)—inhaled as aerosol, causing pneumonic plague;
  - tularaemia (➜ see *Francisella*, pp. 352–3);
  - Viral haemorrhagic fevers (VHFs) (➜ see Viral haemorrhagic fevers, pp. 485–7).
- Category B agents—moderately easy to disseminate, moderate morbidity rates and low mortality rates, require enhancement of both diagnostic capacity and disease surveillance. They include: glanders (➜

see Treatment, p. 338), melioidosis (⮕ see *Burkholderia pseudomallei*, pp. 337–8), brucellosis (⮕ see *Brucella*, pp. 347–9), psittacosis (⮕ see *Chlamydophila psittaci*, pp. 390–1), and Q fever (⮕ see *Coxiella burnetii* (Q fever), pp. 382–4).

- Category C agents—emerging pathogens that might be engineered for mass dissemination (e.g. SARS, H1N1 flu, hantavirus).

Recognizing an attack

In the absence of issued warnings or a very obvious release (e.g. explosive device), the first indicator of an outbreak may be a cluster of symptomatic cases. Such clusters may present acutely or over a period of days or weeks. Isolated fatalities due to undiagnosed febrile illness are not uncommon. Prompt epidemiological inquiry is essential. Features indicative of deliberate release include:

- an unusually large number of patients over a short time period;
- cases that are linked by epidemiological or geographical features;
- signs/symptoms that are unusual or very severe;
- unknown cause or an identified cause unresponsive to normal therapy or unusual in the UK or where acquired.

Remember that symptoms may also be due to radiological or chemical contamination.

Responding to an attack

Consider the risk of transmission to, or contamination of, staff and other patients—it may be appropriate to isolate affected patients and use personal protective equipment (PPE). Decontamination of potentially exposed individuals is vital for suspected releases of *B. anthracis*. Expert advice must be sought locally, and the health protection unit (HPU) informed. Empirical antibacterial prophylaxis is indicated for possible exposure to certain bacterial agents such as anthrax, plague, and tularaemia (ciprofloxacin) or *Brucella*, *Burkholderia*, and Q fever (e.g. doxycycline). National agencies have stockpiles of suitable antibiotics for such emergencies. Early cases should be managed according to the best available advice, until more detailed epidemiological information and laboratory tests are available. In the UK, management of all incidents is led by the police, with involvement of other emergency and health services, as appropriate. All microbiological testing of suspect material must be done in **specialist** laboratories.

More information

The UKHSA website has extensive information on the management of deliberate release incidents, including clinical and diagnostic algorithms, antibiotic protocols, and guidelines for dealing with 'suspect packages' (available at: ℅ https://www.gov.uk/government/collections/deliberate-and-acc idental-releases-investigation-and-management).

Migrant health

A mix of social, economic, and political factors mean more people are migrating across the world than ever before. The 2011 census of England and Wales demonstrated that 13% (7.5 million) of residents were born outside the UK (up from 4.6 million in 2001). Most are young and healthy adults, but many will have a number of risk factors that put them at increased risk of ill health. These include:

- an early life in regions with a high prevalence of infectious disease. In the UK, >70% of new cases of HIV, TB, and malaria are diagnosed in those who were born overseas;
- frequent travel to the country of origin or contact with those who do;
- many may live in crowded or deprived regions in the UK, mixing with other at-risk groups;
- some people are at increased risk of diabetes and cardiovascular disease, particularly if moving to a 'Western' diet and lifestyle. In the UK, diabetes is three times more prevalent among those of Bangladeshi, Pakistani, or Indian origin, and the highest rates of heart disease are seen amongst the Black Caribbean population;
- risk of preventable infections due to an incomplete vaccine history;
- mental health issues, perhaps related to the circumstances of the departure from their home country, social isolation, or racism in the UK.

For example, the relative risk for developing schizophrenia is three times higher for migrants to European countries, and increases to four times for black migrants to European countries

New arrivals

New arrivals presenting to secondary care should be encouraged to find a general practitioner (GP). It is important to remember that all people living in the UK are entitled to primary care, regardless of the legal immigration status.

Treatment of notifiable diseases (see Table 25.3) and HIV infection is also free for everyone. Those presenting to primary care should have the standard new patient check (e.g. medical history, allergies, social, smoking, alcohol). Attention should also be given to:

- the circumstances of their migration—are they likely to have specific economic or mental health needs (e.g. refugee, persecution, human trafficking)?;
- their social situation in the UK;
- any specific infectious disease risk—those from high-prevalence countries should automatically be offered screening for HIV, TB, and hepatitis, as well as certain parasitic infections if symptoms suggest it;
- if immunizations are not in keeping with the UK schedule, then they should be brought up-to-date, including for Covid-19;
- any specific nutritional concerns (e.g. vitamin D or A deficiency);
- education regarding lifestyle, diet, exercise, and sexual health;
- information about the structure and use of the National Health Service (NHS), including considering the need for language interpretation and translation;
- visits back home—if they are planning to make trips home, they should be advised to seek travel advice, if relevant. For example, those from countries in which malaria is endemic may be unaware of their increased risk of acquiring malaria and the need for prophylaxis.

Further reading

The UKHSA has a comprehensive migrant health resource, which includes country-specific health risks and advice for primary care (available at: ℅ https://www.gov.uk/government/collections/communicable-diseases-migrant-health-guide).

The British Medical Association (BMA) has a resource for doctors treating refugees and asylum seekers which contains helpful legal definitions and clarifies eligibility for NHS services (available at: ℅ https://www.bma.org.uk/advice-and-support/ethics/refugees-overseas-visitors-and-vulnerable-migrants/refugee-and-asylum-seeker-patient-health-toolkit).

Liverpool John Moores University hosts an online hub providing accessible and up-to-date information on the rights and well-being of asylum seekers and refugees (available at: ℅ https://www.ljmu.ac.uk/microsites/resources-for-professionals-who-support-asylum-seekers-and-refugees).

Index

For the benefit of digital users, indexed terms that span two pages (e.g., 52–53) may, on occasion, appear on only one of those pages.
Tables, figures, and boxes are indicated by an italic *t*, *f*, and *b* following the page/paragraph number.

The manufacturer's authorised representative in the EU for product safety is
Oxford University Press España S.A. of el Parque Empresalial San Fernando
da Henares, Avenida da Castilla, 2 - 28830 Madrid (www.oup.es/en)